DISEASES AND DISORDERS IN INFANCY AND EARLY CHILDHOOD

DISEASES AND DISORDERS IN INFANCY AND EARLY CHILDHOOD

EDITORS-IN-CHIEF

JANETTE B. BENSON
and
MARSHALL M. HAITH
Department of Psychology, University of Denver,
Denver, Colorado, USA

ELSEVIER

AMSTERDAM • BOSTON • HEIDELBERG • LONDON • NEW YORK • OXFORD
PARIS • SAN DIEGO • SAN FRANCISCO • SINGAPORE • SYDNEY • TOKYO
Academic Press is an imprint of Elsevier

ACADEMIC
PRESS

Academic Press is an imprint of Elsevier
The Boulevard, Langford Lane, Kidlington, Oxford OX5 1GB, UK
525 B Street, Suite 1900, San Diego, CA 92101-4495, USA

First edition 2009

British Library Cataloguing in Publication Data
A catalogue record for this book is available from the British Library

Library of Congress Catalog Number: 2009927180

ISBN: 978-0-12-375068-6

For information on all Elsevier publications
visit our website at books.elsevier.com

Printed and bound by CPI Group (UK) Ltd, Croydon, CR0 4YY
Transferred to Digital Printing, 2013

CONTENTS

S

T

V

CONTRIBUTORS

B Ackerson
University of Illinois at Urbana–Champaign, Urbana, IL, USA

D Adams
National Institutes of Health, Bethesda, MD, USA

A Ahuja
National Jewish Hospital, Denver, CO, USA

J B Asendorpf
Humboldt-Universität zu Berlin, Berlin, Germany

D H Ashmead
Vanderbilt University Medical Center, Nashville, TN, USA

J Atkinson
University College London, London, UK

L A Baker
University of Southern California, Los Angeles, CA, USA

R Barr
University of British Columbia, Vancouver, BC, Canada

A Belden
Washington University School of Medicine, St. Louis, MO, USA

C A Boeving
Yale University School of Medicine, New Haven, CT, USA

C F Bolling
Children's Hospital Medical Center, Cincinnati, OH, USA

O Braddick
University of Oxford, Oxford, UK

A W Burks
Duke University Medical Center, Durham, NC, USA

M L Campbell
Kennedy Krieger Institute, Baltimore, MD, USA

R L Canfield
Cornell University, Ithaca, NY, USA

I Chatoor
Children's National Medical Center, Washington, DC, USA

A I Chin
University of California, Los Angeles, Los Angeles, CA, USA

S R Daniels
University of Colorado Health Sciences Center, Denver, CO, USA

R B David
St. Mary's Hospital, Richmond, VA, USA

G Dawson
University of Washington, Seattle, WA, USA

R R Espinal
University of Chicago, Chicago, IL, USA

F Farzin
University of California, Davis, Davis, CA, USA

D J Fidler
Colorado State University, Fort Collins, CO, USA

D R Fleisher
University of Missouri School of Medicine, Columbia, MO, USA

B Forsyth
Yale University School of Medicine, New Haven, CT, USA

D R Gemmill
California Sudden Infant Death Syndrome Advisory Council, Escondido, CA, USA

I R Gizer
Emory University, Atlanta, GA, USA

M M Gleason
Tulane University Health Sciences Center, New Orleans, LA, USA

E L Grigorenko
Yale University, New Haven, CT, USA

R J Hagerman
University of California, Davis, Medical Center, Sacramento, CA, USA

J Harel
University of Haifa, Haifa, Israel

K M Harrington
Emory University, Atlanta, GA, USA

R W Hendershot
University of Colorado Health Sciences Center, Denver, CO, USA

A H Hoon
Kennedy Krieger Institute, Baltimore, MD, USA

J Isen
University of Southern California, Los Angeles, CA, USA

J S Jameson
Colorado State University, Fort Collins, CO, USA

T Jirikowic
University of Washington, Seattle, WA, USA

M V Johnston
Kennedy Krieger Institute, Baltimore, MD, USA

T A Jusko
University of Washington, Seattle, WA, USA

T G Keens
Keck School of Medicine of the University of Southern California, Los Angeles, CA, USA

S King
University of Washington, Seattle, WA, USA

S E Lerman
University of California, Los Angeles, Los Angeles, CA, USA

H Liang
King's College London, London, UK

J Luby
Washington University School of Medicine, St. Louis, MO, USA

M Macaoay
Children's National Medical Center, Washington, DC, USA

L J Miller
Sensory Processing Disorder Foundation, Greenwood Village, CO, USA

M C Moulson
Massachusetts Institute of Technology, Cambridge, MA, USA

M E Msall
University of Chicago, Chicago, IL, USA

M Muenke
National Institutes of Health, Bethesda, MD, USA

C A Nelson
Harvard Medical School, Boston, MA, USA

H Carmichael Olson
University of Washington, Seattle, WA, USA

M Y Ono
University of California, Davis, Medical Center, Sacramento, CA, USA

T Ostler
University of Illinois at Urbana–Champaign, Urbana, IL, USA

K P Palmer
University of Arkansas for Medical Sciences, Little Rock, AR, USA

F S Pedroso
Universidade Federal de Santa Maria, Santa Maria, Brazil

S L Pillsbury
Richmond, VA, USA

J A Rudolph
Children's Hospital Medical Center, Cincinnati, OH, USA

P A Rufo
Children's Hospital Boston, Boston, MA, USA

R C Schaaf
Thomas Jefferson University, Philadelphia, PA, USA

A Scher
University of Haifa, Haifa, Israel

R Seifer
Brown University, Providence, RI, USA

E Simonoff
King's College London, London, UK

D P Sladen
Vanderbilt University Medical Center, Nashville, TN, USA

D L Smith
The Children's Hospital, Denver, CO, USA

M M Stalets
Washington University School of Medicine, St. Louis, MO, USA

L Sterling
University of Washington, Seattle, WA, USA

D M Teti
The Pennsylvania State University, University Park, PA, USA

A M Tharpe
Vanderbilt University Medical Center, Nashville, TN, USA

N Towe-Goodman
The Pennsylvania State University, University Park, PA, USA

I D Waldman
Emory University, Atlanta, GA, USA

S E Watamura
University of Denver, Denver, CO, USA

P D Zeanah
Tulane University Health Sciences Center, New Orleans, LA, USA

C H Zeanah
Tulane University Health Sciences Center, New Orleans, LA, USA

PREFACE

In 2008, Elsevier published the three-volume Encyclopedia of Infant and Early Childhood Development, encompassing all aspects of development in the 0–3 age range. Articles were selected on the basis of significant bodies of research and/or significant interest in what constitutes normal development, how it progresses, milestones, and what may adversely or positively affect that development. The original three-volume work was a successful publication for library purchase. It seems a shame, however, to have such succinct, eminently readable research summaries by our most distinguished researchers be limited only to libraries. Hence the birth of this volume, selecting only those articles relating to diseases and disorders of infancy and early childhood, and intended for individual purchase.

Because the articles are only those that were included on this topic in the larger work, we cannot say that the coverage is necessarily soup to nuts on all topics relating to diseases and disorders in infancy and early childhood. We were looking for balance in the larger work across all elements of development, and hence we were selective in topic coverage relative to other aspects of development. What this means is that you have larger, more inclusive articles on those topics with the strongest research base rather than more numerous but narrowly focused topics that could have been largely theoretical.

Contents

Several strands run through this work, and they reflect the current themes inherent in the work of developmental psychologists, including the interaction of genes and environment. Of course, the nature-nurture debate is one strand, but no one seriously stands at one or the other end of this controversy any more. Although advances in genetics and behavior genetics have been breathtaking, even the genetics work has documented the role of environment in development, and researchers acknowledge that experience can change the wiring of the brain as well as how actively the genes are expressed. There is increasing appreciation that the child develops in a transactional context, with the child's effect on the parents and others playing no small role in his or her own development.

There has been increasing interest in brain development, partly fostered by the Decade of the Brain in the 1990s, as we have learned more about the role of early experience in shaping the brain and, consequently, personality, emotion, and intelligence. The "brainy baby" movement has rightly aroused interest in infants' surprising capabilities, but the full picture of how abilities develop is being fleshed out as researchers learn as much about what infants cannot do as well as of what they are able. Parents wait for verifiable information about how advances may promote effective parenting.

The central focus of the articles in this work is on diseases and disorders, with considerable attention paid to psychological and medical pathology in our attempt to provide readers with a broad view of the state of knowledge about diseases and disorders in infancy and early childhood. We asked authors to tell a complete story in their articles, assuming that readers will come to this work with a particular topic in mind, rather than reading the volume whole or many articles at one time. As a result, there is some overlap between articles at the edges; one can think of partly overlapping circles of content, which was a design principle in as much as nature does not neatly carve topics in human development into discrete slices for our convenience. At the end of each article, readers will find suggestions for further readings that will permit them to take off in one neighboring direction or another, as well as web sites where they can garner additional information of interest.

Coverage in this volume includes articles that span a broad array of topics that straddle the psychological – medical continuum, although often that distinction is illusory, at best. For example, there are articles on what are broadly classified as more on the psychological continuum of disorders (e.g., ADHD, autism spectrum disorder, depression, Down syndrome, intellectual disabilities, learning disabilities), others typically classified as more on the medical diseases and disorders end of the continuum (e.g., allergies, asthma, auditory development and hearing disorders, bedwetting, cerebral palsy, colic, obesity, SIDS, vision disorders and visual impairment), along with articles that emphasize the genetic, systems, and environmental influences (e.g., endocrine system, fetal alcohol syndrome disorders, Fragile X Syndrome, genetic disorders, immune system and immunodeficiency, lead poisoning, parental chronic mental illness). We also include articles that are broad in terms of approaches taken to study diseases and disorders in early life (e.g., birth defects, developmental disabilities, infant mental health, teratology, and reflexes).

Interest in and opinion about early human development is woven through human history, from as early as the Greek and Roman eras, and repeated through the ages to the current day. Even earlier, the Bible provided advice about nutrition during pregnancy and rearing practices. But the science of human development can be traced back little more than 100 years, and one cannot help but be impressed by the advances in methodologies that are documented in this volume for learning about infants and toddlers. Scientific advances lean heavily on methods, and few areas have matched the growth of knowledge about human development over the last few decades. The reader will be introduced not only to current knowledge in this field but also to how that knowledge is acquired and the promise of these methods for future discoveries.

Audience

Articles have been prepared for a broad readership, including advanced undergraduates, graduate students, working professionals in allied fields, parents, and even researchers in their own disciplines. We plan to use several of these articles as readings for our own seminars.

A project of this scale involves many actors. We are very appreciative of the advice and review efforts of our original editorial advisory board, as well as the efforts of our authors, to abide by the guidelines that we set out for them. Nikki Levy, the editor at Elsevier for this work, has been a constant source of wise advice, consolation, and balance. Her vision and encouragement made this project possible. Barbara Makinster, also from Elsevier, provided many valuable suggestions for us, and we thank her, along with the Production team in England. It is difficult to communicate all the complexities of a project this vast; let us just say that we are thankful for the resource base that Elsevier provided. Finally, we thank our families and colleagues for their patience over the past few years.

Janette B. Benson
and
Marshall M. Haith

A

ADHD: Genetic Influences

I R Gizer, K M Harrington, and I D Waldman, Emory University, Atlanta, GA, USA

Glossary

Allele – One of the alternate forms of a DNA marker.

Association – A nonrandom difference in the frequency of alternate forms of a DNA marker between individuals with and without some diagnosis or across levels of a trait.

Candidate gene study – A study that conducts a targeted test of the association of one or more DNA markers in a specific gene with a disorder or trait.

Endophenotype – Constructs posited to underlie psychiatric disorders or psychopathological traits, and to be more directly influenced by the genes relevant to disorder than are manifest symptoms.

Exon – The nucleotide sequences of a gene responsible for the coding of proteins that comprise the gene product.

Genome scan – An exploratory search across the whole genome for genes related to a disorder or trait.

Haplotype – A particular configuration of alleles at multiple DNA markers in close contiguity within a chromosomal region.

Insertion/deletion – An insertion (deletion) occurs when one or more nucleotides are added to (removed from) the genetic sequence. It can be difficult to discern whether a given polymorphism is the result of an insertion or a deletion, and thus, such polymorphisms are often referred to as insertion/deletions.

Intron – The nucleotide sequences of a gene that lie between the exons and are not involved in the coding of proteins that comprise the gene product.

'Knockout' gene studies – Studies in model organisms, such as mice, in which one or both copies of a gene are deactivated and the effects on behavior and/or cognition are examined.

Linkage – The correlation of a disorder and DNA markers within families, typically tested by examining the co-segregation of the presence or absence of the disorder with sharing particular allele(s) of a DNA marker.

Polymorphism – A DNA marker that varies among individuals in the population.

Population stratification – An association between a DNA marker and a disorder or trait that is not due to the causal effects of the gene, but is instead due to the mixture of subsamples (e.g., ethnic groups) that differ in both allele frequencies and symptom levels or diagnostic rates.

Promoter – A DNA sequence involved in the initiation of transcription of the associated gene.

Repeat sequences (STR and VNTR) – DNA markers that consist of a number of base pairs that are repeated a varying number of times across individuals in the population. The length of the repeat can vary, with repeats of just 2 or 3 base pairs (bp) (i.e., dinucleotide repeats or short-tandem repeats (STRs)) to repeats of between 10 and 60 bp (i.e., variable number of tandem repeats (VNTRs)).

SNP – Single-nucleotide polymorphism: a single nucleotide base that varies among individuals in the population.

Transmission disequilibrium test (TDT) – A within-family test of association and linkage that is robust to the potentially biasing effects of population stratification, the TDT contrasts the transmitted and nontransmitted alleles from heterozygous parents only (i.e., parents with two different alleles) to their children diagnosed with the target disorder.

UTR – An untranslated region of the gene, meaning a part of the gene that is not involved directly in the coding of proteins, but which may contain regulatory elements that are involved in gene expression.

3′ and 5′ – The nucleic acid sequences of genes are written from left to right with the 5′ end lying to the left of the genetic sequence and the 3′ end lying to the right.

Introduction

Since the mid-1980s, considerable progress has been made in understanding the etiology of childhood 'attention deficit hyperactivity disorder' (ADHD), largely due to the publication of numerous twin studies of ADHD symptoms conducted in both clinically referred and large, nonreferred, population-based samples. Findings from these studies are consistent in suggesting substantial genetic influences (i.e., heritabilities ranging from 60% to 90%), nonshared environmental influences that are small to moderate in magnitude (i.e., ranging from 10% to 40%), and little-to-no shared environmental influences. Following from the findings of these quantitative genetic studies, numerous molecular genetic studies of association and linkage between ADHD and a variety of candidate genes have been conducted since the mid-1990s. While the majority of the candidate genes studied underlie various facets of the dopamine neurotransmitter system, researchers also have examined the etiological role of candidate genes in other neurotransmitter systems (e.g., norepinephrine, serotonin), as well as those with functions outside of neurotransmitter systems (e.g., involved in various aspects of brain and nervous system development).

The current review describes recent findings from the behavior genetic and candidate gene literatures of childhood ADHD. It begins with an introduction to the key features of ADHD. This is followed by a brief review of quantitative behavior genetic studies that have attempted to estimate the genetic and environmental influences underlying ADHD. This leads to a review of the extant molecular genetic literature on ADHD, first summarizing genome scan studies and then summarizing candidate gene studies of childhood ADHD. Finally, the review concludes with a consideration of some of the emergent themes that will be important in future studies of the genetics of ADHD.

Background of ADHD

ADHD is a childhood disorder characterized by inattention, hyperactivity, and impulsivity. The prevalence of ADHD has been estimated as 3–7% in school-age children, with male-to-female ratios ranging from 2:1 to 9:1. The definition of ADHD has evolved over time and has been known previously as hyperkinetic reaction of childhood, hyperkinetic syndrome, hyperactive child syndrome, minimal brain damage, minimal brain dysfunction, minimal cerebral dysfunction, minor cerebral dysfunction, and attention deficit disorder with or without hyperactivity.

Currently, ADHD is defined by two distinct, but correlated symptom dimensions, namely an inattentive and a hyperactive–impulsive symptom dimension, each consisting of nine symptoms. The inattentive symptoms consist of behaviors such as 'often has difficulty sustaining attention in tasks' and 'often has difficulty organizing tasks and activities'. The hyperactive–impulsive symptoms consist of behaviors such as 'often fidgets with hands or feet' and 'often has difficulty waiting turn' (see **Table 1** for a complete list of symptoms). Because an individual can present with just inattentive symptoms, with just hyperactive–impulsive symptoms, or with both inattentive and hyperactive–impulsive symptoms, three subtypes of ADHD corresponding to these patterns of presentation have been defined: the predominantly inattentive type, the predominantly hyperactive–impulsive type, and the combined type, respectively.

Theoretical accounts of ADHD have long focused on deficits in sustained attention, and more recently, executive functions deficits have been hypothesized as another possible core feature of the disorder. The term 'executive functions' refers to a list of 'higher-order' cognitive processes required for goal-directed behavior, which includes inhibitory control, working memory, strategy generation and implementation, shifting between subordinate tasks, and monitoring. Common assessment measures hypothesized to assess executive functioning include the 'Wisconsin card sorting task', 'go/no-go tasks', and the 'Stroop color/word task'. The presence of

Table 1   The symptoms of ADHD

Inattentive symptoms
1. Often does not give close attention to details or makes careless mistakes in schoolwork, work, or other activities.
2. Often has trouble keeping attention on tasks or play activities.
3. Often does not seem to listen when spoken to directly.
4. Often does not follow instructions and fails to finish schoolwork, chores, or duties in the workplace (not due to oppositional behavior or failure to understand instructions).
5. Often has trouble organizing activities.
6. Often avoids, dislikes, or does not want to do things that take a lot of mental effort for a long period of time (such as schoolwork or homework).
7. Often loses things needed for tasks and activities (e.g., toys, school assignments, pencils, books, or tools).
8. Is often easily distracted.
9. Is often forgetful in daily activities.

Hyperactive symptoms
1. Often fidgets with hands or feet or squirms in seat.
2. Often gets up from seat when remaining in seat is expected.
3. Often runs about or climbs when and where it is not appropriate (adolescents or adults may feel very restless).
4. Often has trouble playing or enjoying leisure activities quietly.
5. Is often 'on the go' or often acts as if 'driven by a motor'.
6. Often talks excessively.

Impulsive symptoms
1. Often blurts out answers before questions have been finished.
2. Often has trouble waiting one's turn.
3. Often interrupts or intrudes on others (e.g., butts into conversations or games).

executive functions deficits in ADHD has been well documented in recent reviews, which provide strong support suggesting that both children and adults diagnosed with ADHD show impaired performance on these tasks relative to control subjects. Though the term 'executive functions' has long been synonymous with the frontal lobes, more recent accounts of the neurobiology of executive functions have begun to take seriously the reciprocal connections between the prefrontal cortex and subcortical brain areas such as the basal ganglia, and as a result, these brain regions have been implicated in the pathophysiology of ADHD.

The most common treatments for ADHD consist of psychostimulant medications such as methylphenidate and psychosocial treatments focusing on behavior management. Treatment outcome studies have tended to suggest that the gains achieved with medication are greater than those achieved by psychosocial treatments, though there are beneficial aspects to both approaches. Nonetheless, psychostimulant medications have proven extremely effective with studies demonstrating that between 75% and 92% of children diagnosed with ADHD will show improvement in symptoms following treatment. These medications have been shown to act on the dopamine, norepinephrine, ans serotonin neurotransmitter systems, which allow for communication between neurons throughout the brain including the frontal lobes and basal ganglia. Importantly, studies focusing on the specific mechanisms by which psychostimulant medications influence these neurotransmitter systems have been highly informative for molecular genetic studies of ADHD, as will be reviewed.

Behavioral Genetic Studies of ADHD

Research designs for investigating genetic and environmental influences include family studies, adoption studies, and twin studies all of which have suggested that ADHD is transmitted within families from parents to their offspring. Twin study designs have certain advantages over both family and adoption studies, however, in that they are more generalizable, more powerful, and better able to provide accurate estimates of the magnitude of genetic and environmental influences. Twin studies examine the etiology of a trait by taking advantage of the fact that MZ twin pairs share 100% of their genes identical by descent, whereas DZ twin pairs share 50% of their genes on average. By using this information and comparing the correlations of the trait or disorder in MZ and DZ twin pairs, the magnitude of genetic and environmental influences acting on a trait or disorder can be estimated.

More than 20 twin studies have now been published that have attempted to disentangle the genetic and environmental influences underlying ADHD, and though

these studies have differed in many ways including how attention/hyperactivity problems are operationalized, the source of participants, the age range of the subjects, and the statistical methods used, several general conclusions about the etiology of ADHD can be drawn. Most importantly, both ADHD symptoms in the general population and extreme levels of ADHD in selected populations appear to be highly heritable (with most h^2 estimates ranging from 0.6 to 0.9), and demonstrate little evidence of shared environmental influences. Further, researchers who have conducted behavior genetic studies examining the etiology of inattention and hyperactivity–impulsivity as two separate dimensions rather than as a single disorder have reported similarly high heritability estimates for each symptom dimension.

Molecular Genetic Studies of ADHD

Before proceeding with the review, a brief introduction to some key concepts commonly used in molecular genetic studies is necessary. With the discovery of the double-helix structure of DNA, it was determined how paired nucleotide bases form the basic building blocks of life. These bases, defined by the letters A, C, G, and T, for adenine, cytosine, guanine, and thymine, respectively, make up the basic language of DNA. Each base on one strand of DNA forms a pair with its complement on the second strand to form the double helix structure with adenine and thymine always pairing together and cytosine and guanine always pairing together. The human genome has been shown to be made up of approximately three billion such base pairs (bp). Importantly, these three billion bp do not occur on a single length of DNA, but are divided into 23 pairs of chromosomes, with one set of chromosomes inherited from the mother and one set inherited from the father. The structure of a chromosome consists of a centromere at the center and two arms, a short arm and a long arm, that project from the centromere.

Population geneticists have estimated that 99.9% of the human genome is identical across individuals, which means that 1 in every 1000 bp represents a point of variation across individuals. These points of variation or polymorphisms are the source of genetic variation that contribute to differences between individuals, and thus, are the focus of attention for molecular genetic studies. There are several types of polymorphisms, though two commonly studied types are repeat sequences and single-nucleotide polymorphisms (SNPs). Repeat sequences consist of a set of bp that can be short in length (i.e., 2–4 bp) or quite long (i.e., 10–60 bp), and the different variants of the polymorphism, or alleles, are defined as how many times the sequence is repeated (e.g., two-repeat vs. four-repeat vs. seven-repeat). A SNP consists of a

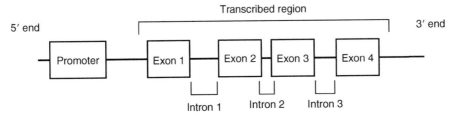

Figure 1 Diagram of a gene.

change in a single bp, however; thus, the alleles at a SNP are defined by the observed bp (e.g., A vs. C).

Polymorphisms throughout the genome are of interest to molecular geneticists, but those that lie within or near actual genes are of particular interest. The human genome is estimated to contain around 20 000 genes, each of which is responsible for the production of a specific protein(s). The structure of a gene consists of a promoter region that is involved in the initiation of transcription of the gene, a process that ultimately leads to the production of the gene product, and the gene sequence itself. The gene sequence consists of exons, which are elements of the gene sequence responsible for the coding of proteins, and introns, which are elements of the gene sequence not involved in the coding of proteins (see **Figure 1** for an illustration). As a result, polymorphisms that lie within the exons are the most likely to result in functional changes in the gene product, though recent research suggests that polymorphisms in the promoter region and introns may also result in functional changes in the gene product and differences in levels of gene expression. Ultimately, the aim of molecular genetic research is to identify polymorphisms that result in these types of functional changes that are related to disorders of interest.

Genome Scans for ADHD

Given the strong evidence suggesting that genetic influences are substantively involved in the etiology of ADHD, researchers have begun conducting molecular genetic studies that attempt to identify the specific genes or genomic regions related to ADHD. Broadly speaking, such studies use one of two general strategies to accomplish this. The first is a genome scan, in which linkage or association is examined between a disorder and evenly spaced DNA markers (approximately 10 000 bp apart, though this spacing continues to decrease as genotyping technologies continue to advance) distributed across the entire genome. Evidence for linkage or association between any of these DNA markers and the trait or disorder of interest implicates a broad segment of the genome that may contain hundreds of genes. Thus, genome scans may be thought of as exploratory searches for putative genes that contribute to the etiology of a disorder.

Four independent genome scans for ADHD have been published to date. Across these studies, 22 different genetic loci have provided evidence that was either significant or at least suggestive of linkage, and although many of these linkage regions were unique to a particular study, several loci demonstrated replicable evidence of linkage with ADHD in multiple studies. The most robust finding is a linkage region on the short arm of chromosome 5 with each of the published genome scans reporting evidence that was suggestive of linkage for this region. Interestingly, the dopamine transporter gene (*DAT1*), which will be discussed in detail, is found near this region, though further studies are needed to determine whether the linkage peak can be attributed to this gene. Nonetheless, the consistent evidence of linkage across the four genome scans provides strong support for a gene or genes in this region to be involved in the pathophysiology of ADHD.

In addition to the short arm of chromosome 5, three loci have been independently identified in three of the four genome scans, which include the long arms of chromosomes 9 and 11 and the short arm of chromosome 17. Further, two loci have been independently identified in two of the four genome scans, which include the short arm of chromosome 8 and the long arm of chromosome 20. Thus, there are now six promising regions of the genome that have been identified for future studies attempting to identify the actual genes in these regions involved in the etiology of ADHD.

Although the initial findings from these genome scans are encouraging, the 16 novel loci identified that are unique to each study also highlight some of the difficulties inherent in drawing inferences regarding linkage from a few studies with relatively small samples, in which it is likely that the genomic regions suggestive of linkage will differ appreciably across studies for statistical reasons alone; that is, although there may be other reasons for the discrepant findings across these samples, such as differences in the populations sampled or in the assessment or diagnostic methods used, the stochastic fluctuations associated with few studies of small sample size are sufficient to cause such discrepancies. Thus, while these findings provide promising directions for future research, they also highlight the necessity for future studies conducted with larger samples and for meta-analytic reviews of the results of genome scans, as have appeared for schizophrenia and bipolar disorder.

Candidate Genes for ADHD

The second strategy for finding genes that contribute to the etiology of a disorder is the candidate gene approach. In many ways, candidate gene studies are polar opposites of genome scans. In contrast to the exploratory nature of genome scans, well-conducted candidate gene studies represent a targeted test of the role of specific genes in the etiology of a disorder as the location, function, and etiological relevance of candidate genes is most often known or strongly hypothesized *a priori*. With respect to ADHD, genes underlying the various aspects of the dopaminergic, and to a lesser extent the noradrenergic and serotonergic, neurotransmitter pathways have been widely studied based on several lines of converging evidence suggesting a role for these neurotransmitter systems in the etiology and pathophysiology of ADHD. For example, stimulant medications, the most common and effective treatment for ADHD, appear to act primarily by regulating dopamine levels in the brain, and also affect noradrenergic and serotonergic function. In addition, 'knockout' gene studies in mice have further demonstrated the potential relevance of genes within these neurotransmitter systems. Such studies breed genetically engineered mice lacking one or more specifically targeted genes. These mice are then studied, and if they display behaviors similar to those that characterize the disorder of interest, it can be inferred that the gene that has been 'knocked out' may be causally related to the disorder. Results of such studies have markedly strengthened the consideration of genes within the dopaminergic system, such as the dopamine transporter gene and the dopamine D1 and D4 receptor genes, as well as genes within the serotonergic system, such as the serotonin 1β receptor gene, as candidate genes for ADHD.

In the following section, studies of association and linkage between ADHD and candidate genes within the dopaminergic and other prominent neurotransmitter pathways, including the noradrenergic and serotonergic pathways, are reviewed. These studies are being published at a rapid rate, and the number of candidate genes that have been explored in relation to ADHD is continually increasing. Further, many genes that have been examined have led to largely negative results (e.g., the dopamine D2 receptor gene (*DRD2*), the dopamine D3 receptor gene (*DRD3*), and the tyrosine hydroxylase gene (*TH*)) that will not be discussed in the current review. Thus, the following is meant to be a representative though not exhaustive review and should provide the reader with a sense of current findings from studies of association and linkage between ADHD and several prominent candidate genes.

Dopamine Transporter

The dopamine transporter is involved in regulating dopamine neurotransmitter levels in the brain. Neurons transmit impulses from one neuron to the next across small junctions called synapses. This is accomplished when a nerve impulse causes the first, or presynaptic neuron, to release a neurotransmitter into the synapse, which then triggers the postsynaptic neuron. Once this is accomplished, any excess neurotransmitter is cleared from the synapse to allow for effective transmission of future nerve impulses. Transporter proteins help to accomplish this by binding to the neurotransmitter and transporting it back to the presynaptic neuron. The dopamine transporter is an example of such a protein. It is densely distributed in the striatum and nucleus accumbens, which are areas in the brain involved in motor control and reward pathways, respectively, and represents the primary mechanism of dopamine regulation in these brain regions.

The gene that codes for the dopamine transporter, *DAT1*, has generated interest as a candidate gene for ADHD based on several lines of converging evidence. For example, stimulant medications (e.g., methylphenidate), which are among the most effective treatments available for ADHD symptoms, act by inhibiting the function of the dopamine transporter and thereby increasing the levels of available dopamine in the synapse. Further, a study of *DAT1* 'knockout' mice demonstrated that mice lacking both copies of the gene, and thus lacking any dopamine transporter, exhibit behaviors analogous to ADHD, such as greater motor activity, compared to mice with intact copies of the gene. This suggests these nice experience a downregulation of the dopamine system as a compensatory mechanism for the lack of dopamine transporter, and this downregulation results in a hypoactive dopamine system. In addition, studies using single photon emission computed tomography (SPECT), which can measure levels of targeted proteins in the brain, have suggested that adult participants with ADHD show differences in dopamine transporter availability that is related to a specific polymorphism in *DAT1*.

Each of the lines of research described above suggests involvement of the dopamine transporter in the etiology and pathophysiology of ADHD. Thus, *DAT1* has been one of the most widely researched genes in relation to ADHD. These studies have focused almost exclusively on a repeat polymorphism at the 3′ end of the gene in an untranslated region (UTR) of *DAT1* that consists of a variable number of tandem repeats (VNTR) in the genetic sequence. This repeat sequence is 40 bp in length and the most common alleles are the 10 (480 bp) (71.9%) and 9 (440 bp) (23.4%) repeats. By the end of 2005, approximately 20 published studies had evaluated this relation in clinic-referred samples, and of these studies, approximately half reported positive evidence suggesting that the 10-repeat allele was associated with increased risk for developing ADHD. Given that a large number of studies failed to detect a significant relation between *DAT1* and ADHD, it is not surprising that recently published meta-analyses of these studies suggest that there is not a significant relation between *DAT1* and ADHD across studies. Nonetheless, these meta-analyses have also reported that there is greater heterogeneity in the effect sizes across studies than would be expected by chance with odds ratios ranging from 0.81 to 2.90. An odds ratio represents the ratio of having a risk factor to not having the risk factor, and thus, values of 1 indicate no increased risk, values less than one indicate reduced risk, and values greater than indicate 1 increased risk. As stated, the odds ratios for studies testing for association between *DAT1* and ADHD ranged from 0.81 to 2.9, which suggests there may be important moderating variables related to the sample characteristics of each study that influence the strength of the relation. Thus, meta-analyses evaluating specific variables that quantify specific sample characteristics (e.g., use of a clinic-referred sample vs. community-based sample, ethnicity of the sample, proportion of ADHD subtypes in each sample, etc.) as moderators of the relation between *DAT1* and ADHD are needed to elucidate what role, if any, *DAT1* plays in the pathophysiology of ADHD.

Further, as stated, the studies described thus far that have tested for association and linkage between *DAT1* and ADHD have focused almost exclusively on a single polymorphism, the VNTR in the 3' UTR of the gene. Although the 10-repeat allele of the VNTR has been shown to be associated with increased *DAT1* transcription, it is not currently known whether the VNTR itself is a functional polymorphism that contributes directly to susceptibility for ADHD, or whether the VNTR simply is in close linkage disequilibrium with a functional polymorphism that represents the actual susceptibility allele. Linkage disequilibrium (LD) refers to the nonrandom association of alleles at multiple DNA markers that results from their close proximity to one another within a chromosome and co-inheritance. Researchers have begun to examine multiple markers in candidate genes, including *DAT1*, and to create haplotypes, which summarize the genetic information across a set of identified markers in close proximity to one another into a single descriptor. In doing so, these haplotypes capture a greater degree of the genetic variation in that region than a single marker and, thus, provide a more powerful method to test for association and linkage. These studies have suggested a relation between *DAT1* and ADHD, and importantly, the results from these studies have tended to yield stronger and more consistent results than studies that include only tests of individual markers. Thus, studies that test for association and linkage between ADHD and multiple markers that lie within or near *DAT1* have the potential to further our understanding of the potential involvement of *DAT1* in the pathophysiology of ADHD.

Dopamine D4 Receptor

As described, neurotransmitters convey nerve impulses from one neuron to the next across small junctions called synapses. When these neurotransmitters successfully cross the synapse, they bind to specific receptor on the postsynaptic neuron which then trigger that postsynaptic neuron to give. Abnormalities in the dopamine neurotransmitter system have been hypothesized to underlie ADHD, and thus, the five genes that code for the five different types of dopamine receptors have been identified as candidate loci for ADHD. The dopamine D4 receptor gene (*DRD4*) has been the most widely studied of the dopamine receptor genes in relation to ADHD primarily due to association studies that initially linked the gene to the personality trait of novelty seeking, which has been compared to the high levels of impulsivity and excitability often seen in ADHD. It is also highly expressed in the frontal lobes, which are significantly involved in executive functioning. As a result, the deficits in executive functioning associated with ADHD also suggest a possible relation between *DRD4* and ADHD. Further interest has been generated from studies of *DRD4* knockout mice. For example, one study compared the behavior of *DRD4* knockout mice and 'wild-type' controls following administration of cocaine and methamphetamine, which belong to the same family of drugs as methylphenidate that is commonly used to treat ADHD. The investigators noted that the knockout mice showed a heightened response to cocaine and methamphetamine injection relative to controls, as measured by increases in locomotor behavior. In addition, it has been suggested that the seven-repeat of a 48-bp VNTR in exon 3 of the gene differs, albeit slightly, from the two- and four-repeats in secondary messenger (i.e., cAMP) activity and also possibly in response to the antipsychotic medication, clozapine.

Following from this suggested involvement of *DRD4* in the pathophysiology of ADHD, several studies have investigated the relation between the exon 3 VNTR of *DRD4* and ADHD, the findings and methods of which have been described in a number of previous reviews. The findings of association between ADHD and *DRD4* were replicated in some studies but not in others, similar to the pattern of findings reported for *DAT1*. Thus, it is noteworthy that meta-analytic reviews of these studies have repeatedly suggested a significant *DRD4*–ADHD association with odds ratios of approximately 1.4. Further, some studies have also examined whether the strength of the association between *DRD4* and ADHD might differ by subtype, and though these studies are few in number, they tend to suggest that *DRD4* is more strongly associated with the inattentive than with the combined subtype of ADHD.

More recently, studies testing for association and linkage between *DRD4* and ADHD have examined other polymorphisms in addition to the exon 3 VNTR. The most frequently studied marker after the exon 3 VNTR has been a 120-bp VNTR in the 5′ UTR of the gene. These studies have typically created haplotypes using multiple markers within *DRD4* to test for association and linkage with ADHD. Overall, this has tended to strengthen the relation between *DRD4* and ADHD, but such studies still yielded both significant and nonsignificant results, again demonstrating the necessity for meta-analytic reviews before drawing substantive conclusions from the existing literature regarding the relation between *DRD4* and ADHD.

Catechol-*O*-Methyl-Transferase

Catechol-*O*-methyl-transferase (COMT) is an enzyme responsible for the degradation of catecholamines, such as dopamine and norepinephrine. COMT is highly expressed in the frontal lobes and plays an important role in regulating synaptic dopamine levels in this region because the dopamine transporter is not significantly expressed in the frontal lobes. Thus, because frontal lobe dysfunction has been hypothesized as a possible causal factor in ADHD several studies have recently tested for association and linkage between this gene and ADHD. These studies have focused on a functional SNP in exon 4 that leads to an amino acid substitution (valine → methionine), and has been shown to substantially affect COMT enzyme activity such that homozygosity for valine shows 3–4 times greater activity than homozygosity for methionine. Given that the higher activity of the valine allele leads to less synaptic availability of dopamine than does the methionine allele, it is reasonable to consider the valine allele as the high-risk allele for ADHD.

Despite such evidence suggesting that the *COMT* gene would represent a strong candidate gene for ADHD, the results from studies testing for association and linkage between *COMT* and ADHD have been largely negative. The initial study to test this relation yielded positive evidence for association, suggesting that the valine allele was associated with increased risk for ADHD. Nonetheless eight studies that have attempted to replicate this association have failed to support this relation with one exception. A single study examined the relation between *COMT* and ADHD and examined subtype and gender differences as moderators of genetic association. They found that the evidence for association and linkage was strengthened when analyses were restricted to male subjects with the inattentive ADHD subtype, showing significant preferential transmission of the methionine allele (rather than the valine allele) to boys with ADHD. Furthermore, there was significant evidence for association between *COMT* and ADHD among girls with the valine allele being over-represented, consistent with the original association reported. Thus, these findings suggest an important sex difference in the relation of *COMT* to ADHD. Importantly, these results are consistent with the findings from a study of *COMT* knockout mice, which found similar gender differences.

As a result, additional studies of association and linkage between *COMT* and ADHD are needed that focus on identifying moderating variables such as children's sex and ADHD subtypes or symptom dimensions.

Dopamine D5 Receptor

The dopamine D5 receptor belongs to a class of dopamine receptors distinct from the dopamine D4 receptors and is expressed in different areas of the brain, most predominantly in the hippocampus which is involved in spatial mapping and memory. Studies that have tested for association and linkage between ADHD and the dopamine D5 receptor gene (*DRD5*) have almost exclusively focused on a highly polymorphic dinucleotide repeat 18.5 kb 5′ of the gene. Initial studies reported at least suggestive evidence for association and linkage between ADHD and *DRD5*, but an interpretation of their results was not straightforward with respect to allelic association, given that some of the studies' findings differed as to which allele was being preferentially transmitted.

In an attempt to clarify the nature of the relation between *DRD5* and ADHD, a combined analysis of the data from 18 independent samples was performed that examined the evidence for association and linkage between ADHD and the 148-bp allele of the *DRD5* dinucleotide repeat. Importantly, the authors of this combined analysis did not detect significant heterogeneity among samples, and thus were able to conduct their analyses on the combined samples. The combined samples showed clear evidence for the preferential transmission of the 148-bp allele ($p = 0.00005$, odds ratio $= 1.24$) providing strong support for association and linkage between *DRD5* and ADHD.

Dopamine D1 Receptor

The dopamine D1 receptor gene (*DRD1*) gained attention as a candidate gene for ADHD due to several converging lines of evidence suggesting its involvement in the development of ADHD symptoms. First, dopamine D1 receptors are present in the prefrontal cortex and striatum, two brain regions widely believed to be involved in ADHD. Second, dopamine D1 receptors have been shown to influence working memory processes localized in the prefrontal cortex, which appear to be impaired in ADHD. Third, *DRD1* knockout mice have displayed hyperactive locomotive behavior, and thus provide a promising animal model of ADHD.

Based on these converging lines of evidence, two studies of association and linkage between ADHD and *DRD1* have been conducted. The first used four previously identified nonfunctional, biallelic polymorphisms including one marker in the 3′ UTR, two in the 5′ UTR, and one that lies upstream of the promoter region. Tests of association at each marker yielded statistical trends toward association for the two markers in the 5′ UTR and the marker in the 3′ UTR. There was less evidence for association and linkage between ADHD and the marker upstream of the promoter region. The authors then constructed haplotypes from the four markers, and found three that were common in their sample, one of which was preferentially transmitted to ADHD children. Further, it was demonstrated that this haplotype appeared to be more strongly associated and linked with inattentive than hyperactive–impulsive symptoms. These findings were partially replicated in an independent sample that tested for association and linkage between ADHD and *DRD1* using the two identified SNPs in the 5′ UTR. Thus, the studies conducted to 2007 provide promising evidence suggesting a relation between *DRD1* and ADHD.

Dopamine Beta Hydroxylase

Norepinephrine is a widely distributed neurotransmitter in the brain hypothesized to be involved in processes of behavioral arousal and learning and memory. Dopamine beta hydroxylase converts dopamine to norepinephrine and thus represents an interesting candidate gene for ADHD given the suggestion that the underlying pathophysiology of ADHD involves norepinephrine as well as dopamine. Further, a functional polymorphism within the *DβH* gene has been shown to strongly influence dopamine beta hydroxylase levels in plasma and cerebrospinal fluid, providing strong evidence for *DβH* involvement in noradrenergic regulation in the brain. Of direct relevance to ADHD, *DβH* knockout mice display hypersensitive responses to amphetamine treatment, such that they exhibit increased locomotive behavior relative to wild-type, control mice.

Five research groups have published studies of association and linkage between ADHD and *DβH*, with most of these studies focusing on a *Taq*I polymorphism in intron 5 of the gene. Of the studies that have focused on this marker, each one reported evidence that was significant or suggestive of association with ADHD, but importantly the studies differed with regard to which allele was associated with increased risk for developing the disorder. More specifically, four studies suggested that the A2 allele was related to ADHD, whereas one study reported that the A1 allele was associated with increased risk. Nonetheless, it is noteworthy that those studies that examined additional markers found no evidence for association between any polymorphisms other than the *Taq*I polymorphism and ADHD. Further, of those studies that conducted haplotype analyses, the authors reported that the evidence for association with these haplotypes were no stronger than those for the *Taq*I polymorphism by itself. Thus, given the potential role of both norepinephrine and dopamine in ADHD, as well as the positive association reported in several studies, *DβH* represents an interesting candidate gene for ADHD that warrants further study.

Norepinephrine Transporter

Like the dopamine transporter, the norepinephrine transporter is a protein responsible for the reuptake of neurotransmitters, in this case norepinephrine, from the synaptic cleft back to the presynaptic neuron. Unlike the dopamine transporter, however, it is highly expressed in the frontal lobes, and thus represents an important mechanism for the regulation of norephinephrine activity in the prefrontal cortex. Given the hypothesis that noradrenergic dysregulation might be an underlying cause of ADHD, researchers have begun to examine the potential role of the norepinephrine transporter in ADHD. Much of this attention has come from pharmacological studies demonstrating that stimulant medications lead to reductions in ADHD symptoms through increases in dopamine and norephinephrine activity, as well as from studies showing that tricyclic antidepressant medications also lead to reductions in ADHD symptoms, via blocking activity of the norepinephrine transporter. Most recently, treatment outcome research has shown that a drug that specifically blocks the reuptake of norephinephrine (i.e., atomoxetine) leads to significant improvements in ADHD-related symptoms. Thus, the gene that codes for the norepinephrine transporter (*NET1*) has recently received attention as a candidate gene for ADHD.

Four studies have been published examining the relation between *NET1* and ADHD, which have yielded largely negative results. An initial study examined three polymorphisms within the gene, located in exon 9, intron 9, and intron 13, and a second study examined a SNP in intron 7 and the same intron 9 SNP genotyped in the first study. Although both studies failed to detect evidence of association between *NET1* and ADHD, it is important to note that the markers selected in both studies were located at the 3′ end of the gene and were in strong LD with each other. As a result, these studies might have failed to detect an association between *NET1* and ADHD if the susceptibility locus was found to be at the opposite end of the gene (i.e., the 5′ end). To evaluate this possibility, a more recent study examined the relation between *NET1* and ADHD using 21 SNPs that were spaced across the length of the gene to provide a more comprehensive test of association. Nonetheless, this study also failed to detect a significant relation between *NET1* and ADHD. Despite these negative findings, another study that examined just two SNPs within *NET1* did report significant evidence of association and linkage between these SNPs and ADHD. Nonetheless, this study tested for association and linkage between ADHD and 11 other genes, in addition to *NET1*, without correcting for multiple testing. Thus, it is possible that this result represents a false positive. As a result, there is little current evidence to support a relation between *NET1* and ADHD, though this gene is likely to receive further interest as a candidate for

ADHD given the research literature suggesting that noradrenergic dysregulation may represent an underlying cause of ADHD.

Adrenergic 2A Receptor Gene

The noradrenergic and adrenergic neurotransmitter systems are hypothesized to influence attentional processes and certain aspects of executive control. More specifically, it has been suggested that adrenergic neurons influence attention and executive processes through the inhibition of noradrenergic neurons and that abnormalities in this regulatory system might contribute to a specific subtype of ADHD. Thus, genes involved in the adrenergic neurotransmitter system represent interesting candidate genes for ADHD. As specific genes in the noradrenergic system have already been discussed (i.e., *DβH* and *NET1*) the following section focuses on published studies that have examined evidence for association and linkage between the adrenergic 2A receptor gene (*ADRA2A*) and ADHD.

The *ADRA2A* gene has been widely studied and there are now seven published studies that have examined the relation of this gene with ADHD. Each of these studies has focused on a *Msp*I restriction site polymorphism in the promoter region of the gene, though some studies have also genotyped additional polymorphisms. The first association that was reported between *ADRA2A* and ADHD was detected in a sample that was initially selected for the presence of Tourette's syndrome and was subsequently diagnosed with ADHD. The authors reported that the G allele of the *Msp*I polymorphism, which indicates the presence of the restriction site, was positively associated with ADHD. Given that the sample was originally selected for Tourette's syndrome, several additional research groups tested this relation in samples of children selected for ADHD, without the presence of comorbid Tourette's syndrome, to determine if the original reported association would generalize to the wider ADHD population. Of the six studies that followed up this initial report, four have yielded significant evidence for association between the G allele of the *Msp*I polymorphism and ADHD, one yielded evidence suggesting a trend for such an association, and one study failed to detect any evidence of such an association. It is also noteworthy that two of these studies yielded evidence suggesting that *ADRA2A* is strongly associated with both the hyperactive–impulsive and inattentive ADHD symptom dimensions. Thus, the results are fairly consistent across studies providing support for the involvement of *ADRA2A* in the pathophysiology of ADHD.

Serotonin Transporter

Like the dopamine and norepinephrine transporters, the serotonin transporter is a solute carrier protein responsible for the reuptake of neurotransmitters, in this case serotonin, from the synaptic cleft back to the presynaptic neuron. Serotonin dysregulation has been related to impulsive and aggressive behavior in children and thus has been hypothesized as a causal factor in ADHD. Involvement of the 5-HT transporter gene (*5-HTT*) in ADHD is suggested by studies that have demonstrated that the binding affinity of the platelet serotonin transporter shows a positive relation with impulsive behavior, such that increases in binding affinity, which corresponds to lower levels of available serotonin, are associated with increases in impulsive behavior in children with ADHD. In addition, pharmacological studies have demonstrated that the serotonin-selective reuptake inhibitors used to treat depression by blocking activity of the serotonin transporter, thereby increasing levels of available serotonin, also lead to reductions in ADHD symptoms. In light of this evidence, *5-HTT* has been widely studied as a candidate gene for ADHD.

Seven studies have been published examining the relation between *5-HTT* and ADHD, and all of these have focused on a 44-bp insertion/deletion in the promoter region leading to long and short alleles that are believed to have functional consequences. More specifically, the long variant appears to be associated with more rapid serotonin reuptake, and thus, lower levels of active serotonin, whereas the short variant appears to be associated with reduced serotonin reuptake. Of the seven studies, five have reported evidence suggesting that the long allele is associated with ADHD providing fairly strong evidence for a relation between *5-HTT* and ADHD. In addition, one of these studies also found that the evidence for association was stronger among the ADHD combined subtype than the inattentive subtype, and, while this finding clearly requires replication, such studies have the potential to further our understanding of the relation between *5-HTT* and ADHD.

Serotonin 1B Receptor Gene

As described, serotonin dysregulation has been hypothesized to underlie the impulsive symptoms of ADHD. In addition to the serotonin transporter, the serotonin 1B receptor gene (*HTR1B*) has received attention as a candidate gene for ADHD. Specific evidence supporting *HTR1B* involvement comes from a study of knockout mice lacking this gene suggesting that these mice show increased aggression and impulsive behavior and fail to show the normal hyperlocomotion associated with amphetamine administration.

Five studies have been conducted examining *HTR1B* as a candidate gene for ADHD, with all of the studies focusing on the G861C polymorphism. Four of these studies utilized clinic-referred samples and the fifth study utilized a community-based sample. Importantly, each of the studies utilizing a clinic-referred sample reported evidence that the 861G allele was associated with increased risk for ADHD, whereas the single study utilizing a community-based sample failed to detect a relation between the G861C polymorphism and ADHD. This difference in findings might suggest that the association between *HTR1B* and ADHD may not generalize beyond clinic-referred samples, but additional studies utilizing community-based samples are needed before such a conclusion can be made. Nonetheless, several of the studies utilizing clinic-referred samples conducted important follow-up analyses in an attempt to explain the relation between *HTR1B* and ADHD further. For example, two studies found that the evidence for association and linkage between *HTR1B* and ADHD was stronger for the inattentive subtype than the combined subtype. Taken together, the evidence suggesting a relation between *HTR1B* and ADHD is fairly consistent, providing strong support for the involvement of this gene in the pathophysiology of ADHD.

Tryptophan Hydroxylase and Tryptophan Hydroxylase 2

Tryptophan hydroxylase (TPH) is an enzyme crucial to the synthesis of the neurotransmitter serotonin. The *TPH* gene was originally thought to be solely responsible for TPH production, but more recently, a second gene, *TPH2*, was identified that is highly involved in TPH production. Researchers have since focused on both genes as candidates for behavioral disorders characterized by impulsivity and aggressiveness, which have been related to serotonin dysregulation. Nonetheless, results from studies testing for an association between *TPH* and ADHD have been largely negative, and thus, are not reviewed.

The two studies that have tested for association between *TPH2* and ADHD, however, have yielded positive evidence suggesting that this gene may be involved in the etiology of ADHD. The authors of the first study genotyped eight SNPs located in introns 4, 5, 7, 8, and 9 of *TPH2*, and they reported significant evidence for association between a SNP in intron 5 and ADHD that was strengthened when a haplotype was created using this SNP as well as a second SNP in intron 5. The second study genotyped three different SNPs, two of which were located in the regulatory region of the gene at the 5′ end of the gene and a third that was located in intron 2. The authors reported significant evidence for association between the two SNPs in the regulatory region of *TPH2* and ADHD. In addition, the evidence for association was strengthened when a haplotype constructed from the two regulatory region SNPs was tested in relation to ADHD. Thus, despite including SNPs from different regions of *TPH2*, both studies were suggestive of an association between *TPH2* and ADHD.

Monoamine Oxidase Genes

The monoamine oxidase genes (*MAOA* and *MAOB*) are located in close proximity to one another on the X chromosome and encode enzymes involved in the metabolism of dopamine, serotonin, and norepinephrine. Treatment studies have suggested that monoamine oxidase inhibitors (MAOIs) can reduce ADHD symptom levels. Given that each of these neurotransmitters are thought to be involved in the etiology of ADHD, the two monoamine oxidase genes, *MAOA* and *MAOB*, represent interesting candidate genes for ADHD. More specific support for *MAOA* comes from a linkage study conducted in a large Dutch family, demonstrating a relation between *MAOA* and impulsive, aggressive behavior. In addition, *MAOA* knockout mice have been shown to display increased levels of aggressive behavior associated with increased levels of monoaminergic neurotransmitter levels.

Five published studies have examined a possible relation between *MAOA* and ADHD, largely focusing on a dinucleotide repeat in intron 2 of the gene, a 30-bp VNTR in the promoter region of the gene, and a SNP in exon 8. The VNTR has received particular interest due to studies suggesting an association between this polymorphism and impulsive, aggressive behavior. The VNTR consists of alleles containing 2, 3, 3.5, 4, and 5 copies of the repeat sequence. The two- and three-repeat alleles have been shown to be less efficiently transcribed and have been associated with impulsivity and aggression in previous studies. Thus, the two- and three-repeat alleles have been designated 'low-activity' alleles, while the remaining alleles have been designated as 'high-activity' alleles.

Studies testing for association and linkage between *MAOA* and ADHD have all reported significant evidence suggesting such a relation. Nonetheless, the reported findings differed across studies, both with regard to which polymorphism yielded significant evidence of association and which allele within a polymorphism was the risk-inducing allele. As a result, there is consistent evidence implicating *MAOA* in the pathophysiology of the disorder, but the differences across reports make it difficult to offer substantive conclusions regarding the nature of this association. In contrast, findings from two published studies that have tested for association between *MAOB* and ADHD have been more consistent. These studies focused on a dinucleotide repeat in intron 2 of the gene and both studies failed to detect evidence for association, suggesting that *MAOB* is not involved in the pathophysiology of ADHD.

Synaptosomal-Associated Protein 25 Gene

Researchers have also examined association and linkage of ADHD with candidate genes outside of the major neurotransmitter systems. Synaptosomal-associated protein

25 gene (*SNAP-25*) is an example of such a gene, as it codes for a protein involved in the docking and fusion of synaptic vesicles in presynaptic neurons necessary for the regulation of neurotransmitter release. The *coloboma* mouse strain, which has been bred lacking one copy of the *SNAP-25* gene following a radiation-induced deletion of a segment of DNA on one chromosome, displays hyperactive behavior and provides a potential animal model of ADHD. Thus, several studies have tested for linkage and association between *SNAP-25* and ADHD.

The two most commonly studied markers in the *SNAP-25* gene are SNPs at positions 1065 and 1069. Three initial studies tested for association between *SNAP-25* and ADHD using these two markers, and each study reported evidence suggestive of such a relation. The first published study also reported that a haplotype constructed from these markers showed significant evidence of association and linkage with ADHD. The second study reported a significant association between the polymorphism at position 1069 and ADHD, but the result conflicted with the association reported in the initial study as to which allele within the polymorphism was the risk-inducing allele. Nonetheless, the third study reported results that were consistent with the initial published report. The authors of this study reported a trend for biased transmission of the same haplotype implicated in the first study, and importantly, follow-up analyses revealed a parent-of-origin effect for the transmission of this haplotype. They found that the evidence for association became significant when paternal transmission of the haplotype was examined but not when maternal transmission was examined suggesting that genomic imprinting may be involved. Imprinting refers to specific regions of the genome where only the maternal or paternal copy of a gene is expressed. Thus, the expressed copy of an imprinted gene is either paternally or maternally inherited, and as result, if a disorder is associated with an imprinted gene it will follow the same inheritance pattern.

Evidence suggesting association and linkage between *SNAP-25* and ADHD has also been detected in studies that have examined polymorphisms other than the two SNPs described. For example, association between *SNAP-25* and ADHD has been reported in one study that identified a tetranucleotide repeat polymorphism that lies in the first intron of *SNAP-25*. Further, the authors of this study expanded their analyses to include seven additional polymorphisms, including the SNPs at positions 1065 and 1069. They reported significant evidence for association between three individual polymorphisms and ADHD, namely a SNP in the promoter region of the gene, the tetranucleotide repeat, and a SNP in exon 7. In addition, they reported that several haplotypes showed significant evidence for association that was stronger than the evidence obtained from the individual markers. Finally, follow-up analyses suggested that the findings for the individual markers were

stronger when only paternal transmissions of the putative 'high-risk' alleles were included in the analyses. Thus, this study not only provides additional evidence supporting the involvement of *SNAP-25* in the etiology of ADHD, but it also provides additional evidence suggesting that genomic imprinting may be involved in the transmission of genetic risk for ADHD at the *SNAP-25* gene.

Future Directions

This review concludes with a consideration of some of the more important themes emerging from molecular genetic studies of ADHD and related psychopathology that will inform future research in this area. These include the replicability and consistency of findings of association and linkage between a candidate gene and a disorder, the transition from testing single to multiple markers in candidate genes, the specificity of association and/or linkage findings to particular diagnostic subtypes or symptom dimensions, the heterogeneity of association and/or linkage with a particular disorder due to characteristics of individuals such as age, sex, or age of onset, or due to aspects of the environment (i.e., gene–environment interactions). The last theme involves the use of endophenotypes in molecular genetic studies of psychopathology, namely examining association and/or linkage with some underlying biological or psychological mechanism that is thought to reflect the gene's action more directly than does the disorder of interest.

It should be clear from the preceding section that for each candidate gene studied, there is a mixed picture of positive and negative findings. This is true not only for candidate gene studies of ADHD, but also for those of all other psychiatric and complex medical disorders. Such mixed findings tend to appear as studies of a particular candidate gene accumulate and the effect size typically diminishes from that in the original published study. This phenomenon is well illustrated by the studies of *DAT1*, *DRD4*, and *DRD5* reviewed above. Fortunately, meta-analytic procedures are becoming more common as a framework for systematically evaluating the consistency and replicability of findings of association and linkage of candidate genes with disorders across multiple studies. Such analyses can also test whether there is significant heterogeneity of the effect sizes across studies and are capable of mapping such heterogeneity on to substantively meaningful or methodologically important differences across studies. Meta-analytic methods have recently been used to good effect in reviewing the findings of association and linkage between ADHD and *DRD4* and *DRD5*, as they demonstrated consistent, significant association across studies, even in the presence of mixed findings.

A second theme in the research literature on association of candidate genes with ADHD is the transition from studying a single marker to studying multiple markers in candidate genes. In the literature reviewed above, most of the studies examined a single polymorphism in a particular candidate gene for its association with ADHD. This is problematic for at least two reasons. First, negative findings for the association between a single polymorphism in a candidate gene and a disorder are ambiguous because they would appear to indicate that the gene is not involved in the disorder's etiology. It may be the case, however, that a studied marker in an etiologically relevant candidate gene may not be associated with a disorder simply because it is not in strong enough LD with (e.g., not close enough to) the functional, etiologically relevant polymorphism(s) in the gene. Second, and somewhat paradoxically, positive findings for the association between a single polymorphism in a candidate gene and a disorder also are ambiguous because one may not know whether the studied polymorphism is functional, and thus the risk-inducing polymorphism. Further, it is possible that certain genes contain multiple functional, etiologically relevant polymorphisms. Thus, even if the studied marker is known to be functional, it may not be the only functional marker in the gene. The difficulty this poses is that even if one finds a significant association between a disorder and a single marker in a candidate gene, one cannot estimate accurately the magnitude of the gene's role in the etiology of the disorder because one is limited to inferring this from only one of the possible functional, etiologically relevant markers in the gene.

A third theme for future studies of candidate genes and ADHD involves the specificity of association and/or linkage findings to particular diagnostic subtypes or symptom dimensions. It is highly unlikely that whatever genes confer risk for ADHD work at the level of the overall diagnosis, and that nature so closely resembles the current version of the Diagnostic and Statistical Manual (DSM). Thus, it is possible that whatever genes contribute to risk for ADHD do so by conferring risk for specific diagnostic subtypes or symptom dimensions. Although this area of molecular genetic research is only in its infancy, there have been a few examples of such findings in this research domain. For example, some studies have suggested that *DRD4* is more strongly associated and linked with the inattentive than the combined ADHD subtype, and appears to be related more strongly to inattentive than to hyperactive–impulsive symptoms. Although other researchers have focused on examining genetic influences on higher-order diagnostic constructs, such as an externalizing symptom dimension, and have advocated the utility of studying the genetics of broad diagnostic constructs that span several DSM-IV diagnoses, the results cited above suggest that examining association and linkage with more specific diagnostic subtypes or symptom dimensions also will be a fruitful approach. Pursuing both of these possibilities simultaneously in a two-pronged approach is ideal,

given the primitive stage of our knowledge of the association between specific genes and disorders, and the likelihood that some genes will be risk factors for several related disorders whereas others will only confer risk on narrower disorder phenotypes.

A fourth theme that is important for future studies of candidate genes and ADHD involves the heterogeneity of association and/or linkage with a particular disorder due to characteristics of individuals such as age, sex, or age of onset, or due to aspects of the environment (i.e., gene–environment interactions). Few molecular genetic studies of ADHD have examined such sources of heterogeneity, and, given that additional analyses such as these will increase the rate of false-positive results due to multiple statistical tests, some caution is warranted when conducting such analyses. Nonetheless, prudently selected characteristics, particularly those shown to be biologically relevant to the disorder of interest and/or the candidate gene being studied, have the potential to inform future candidate gene studies. For example, age and sex represent potential sources of heterogeneity given research showing that several candidate genes show important sex or age differences in expression. Within the dopamine system, for instance, levels of the dopamine transporter have been shown to be higher in males than females and to decline appreciably with age. Despite these findings, none of the published studies of *DAT1* and ADHD have examined sex or age differences in association. As reviewed above, studies of association and linkage between *COMT* and ADHD have yielded mixed findings. In the most recent of these studies, however, analyses were conducted separately by sex and suggested sexually dimorphic findings, with the low-activity methionine allele being associated with ADHD in boys but the high-activity valine allele being associated with ADHD in girls. Although these results are preliminary, confined to one study, and need to be replicated, they embody the type of heterogeneity analyses that may be useful for elaborating the nature of the relations between candidate genes and ADHD.

Although developmental psychopathology researchers have long been excited by the prospect of gene–environment interaction, and many have contended that one cannot understand the development of psychopathology without the consideration of such processes, initial studies identifying specific gene–environment interactions for psychopathology have only recently been published. For example, one such study found that risk for adolescent antisocial behavior and violence was in part determined by an interaction between the presence of abuse during early childhood and alleles at a functional polymorphism in the *MAOA* gene. Importantly, it remains an empirical question whether such gene–environment interactions are present in the etiology of ADHD. As described above, twin studies suggest substantial genetic influences, small-to-moderate nonshared environmental influences, and little-to-no shared environmental influences in the etiology of ADHD. Thus, such gene–environment interactions may not be as relevant to molecular genetic studies of ADHD as for other conditions. Nonetheless, twin studies typically assume that genetic and environmental influences combine in an additive rather than multiplicative fashion and cannot be used either to support or refute the presence of gene–environment interactions. Thus, studies of gene–environment interactions in ADHD should be pursued, but few such interactions have been posited and/or studied in the ADHD literature.

Gene–environment interactions that have been studied in relation to ADHD include interactions between *DAT1* genotype and maternal smoking and maternal alcohol consumption during pregnancy, two environmental risk factors that have been related to ADHD. Unfortunately, the results from these studies have been mixed in their support of such interactions, and thus are not described in detail here. Nonetheless, the relation of such environmental risk factors, as well as other factors such as pre- or perinatal complications and early child abuse, to genetic influences underlying ADHD represents an important line of research that is likely to gain further consideration.

The final theme of this review involves the use of endophenotypes in molecular genetic studies of ADHD. Clearly there is a large gap between candidate genes and the manifest symptoms of disorders such as ADHD as typically assessed by interviews or rating scales. It is desirable from both a conceptual and empirical perspective to find valid and meaningful mediational or intervening constructs that may help to bridge this gap. The term 'endophenotype' is often used to describe such constructs and the variables that are used to measure them. More generally, endophenotypes refer to constructs that are thought to underlie psychiatric disorders. Thus, they are hypothesized to lie closer to the immediate products of such genes (i.e., the proteins they code for) and are thought to be more strongly influenced by the genes that underlie them than the manifest symptoms that they in turn undergird. Endophenotypes also are thought to be 'genetically simpler' than the manifest disorders or their symptom dimensions such that there are fewer individual genes (or sets thereof) that contribute to their etiology suggesting that they may be more straightforward to study.

The use and evaluation of putative endophenotypes in molecular genetic studies of ADHD is in its infancy, such that only a few studies have examined association and linkage between candidate genes and plausible measures of endophenotypes for ADHD. These studies have focused almost exclusively on measures of sustained attention and executive functions as endophenotypes for ADHD, given their posited relation to ADHD. Researchers proposing that sustained attention and executive functions might serve as useful endophenotypes for ADHD cite empirical studies demonstrating that children with

ADHD perform poorly on these tasks relative to control children. Importantly, such studies provide the basis for recent theoretical accounts of ADHD that focus on deficits in executive functioning as the core mechanisms underlying the disorder.

Results from early studies that have included measures of sustained attention and executive functions as endophenotypes for ADHD, however, have yielded a mixture of positive and negative findings that have proven to be as complex as those reported for the ADHD diagnosis itself. As such, these studies have yet to provide results that are more informative or more consistent in explaining the relation between specific candidate genes and ADHD than studies that have focused solely on ADHD as the phenotype. Nonetheless, there are several possible explanations as to why sustained attention and executive function measures have thus far proved of limited utility in molecular genetic studies of ADHD. For example, a prerequisite for the validity and utility of putative endophenotype measures is that they represent heritable traits and demonstrate shared genetic influences with the disorder of interest. Nonetheless, large-scale, quantitative genetic studies with sufficient statistical power to estimate the heritability of such measures and the etiology of their overlap with ADHD symptoms have yet to be conducted. Thus, some measures may prove to be inappropriate as endophenotypes. Therefore, while putative endophenotypic measures hold much promise for identifying susceptibility genes and explaining their relation to psychiatric disorders, such issues must be addressed before any findings of association between candidate genes and endophenotypes can be fully interpreted.

Summary

This review has attempted to summarize current studies and some of the most exciting recent developments in molecular genetic research on ADHD. In addition to reviewing extant findings for the association and linkage of ADHD with candidate genes, the review also focused on several emerging themes in this literature that should guide future research. These themes include the 'replicability and consistency' of findings of association and linkage between candidate genes and ADHD, the transition from the use of single to multiple polymorphisms to characterize variation in candidate genes, the 'specificity' of association and/or linkage findings to particular ADHD diagnostic subtypes or symptom dimensions, the 'heterogeneity' of association and/or linkage between candidate genes and ADHD due to characteristics of individuals or to aspects of their environments (i.e., gene–environment interactions), and the use of 'endophenotypes' (i.e., underlying biological or psychological mechanisms thought to reflect more directly the gene's action) in molecular genetic studies of ADHD. It is hoped that these themes not only provide a glimpse of extant molecular genetic research on ADHD and its development, but will help to set the research agendas for future studies.

Acknowledgments

Preparation of this article was supported in part by NIMH grants F31-MH072083 to I R Gizer and K01-MH01818 to I D Waldman.

See also: Developmental Disabilities: Cognitive; Fetal Alcohol Spectrum Disorders; Fragile X Syndrome; Genetic Disorders: Sex Linked; Genetic Disorders: Single Gene; Learning Disabilities; Mental Health, Infant; Sensory Processing Disorder.

Suggested Readings

Doyle AE, Faraone SV, Seidman LJ, *et al.* (2005) Are endophenotypes based on measures of executive functions useful for molecular genetic studies of ADHD? *Journal of Child Psychology and Psychiatry and Allied Disciplines* 46: 774–803.

Faraone SV, Perlis RH, Doyle AE, *et al.* (2005) Molecular genetics of attention-deficit/hyperactivity disorder. *Biological Psychiatry* 57: 1313–1323.

Heiser P, Friedel S, Dempfle A, *et al.* (2004) Molecular genetic aspects of attention-deficit/hyperactivity disorder. *Neuroscience and Biobehavioral Reviews* 28: 625–641.

Thapar A, O'Donovan M, and Owen MJ (2005) The genetics of attention deficit hyperactivity disorder. *Human Molecular Genetics* 14: R275–R282.

Waldman ID (2005) Statistical approaches to complex phenotypes: Evaluating neuropsychological endophenotypes for attention-deficit/hyperactivity disorder. *Biological Psychiatry* 57: 1347–1356.

Waldman ID and Gizer I (2006) The genetics of attention deficit hyperactivity disorder. *Clinical Psychology Review* 26: 396–432.

AIDS and HIV

C A Boeving and B Forsyth, Yale University School of Medicine, New Haven, CT, USA

Glossary

Adherence – Routine maintenance of illness management regimen, typically referring to successful compliance with the medication schedule.

Health-related quality of life (HRQOL) – Inclusion of the impact of a disease and its treatment in the assessment of a person's functioning and life satisfaction; domains include physiological, social, educational, emotional, and cognitive functioning.

Highly active antiretroviral therapy (HAART) – Approved in 1998 for use with children, this medication regimen includes a combination of at least three medicines from different classes of medications. The aim of treatment is to suppress viral replication and reduce the emergence of resistant viral variants.

Mother-to-child transmission (MTCT) – Route of HIV infection by which the infant acquires HIV either prenatally, during the birth process, or postnatally (typically through breast milk).

Opportunistic infection – Illnesses incurred as a result of suppression of the immune system. HIV diminishes the ability of the individual's immune system to respond to infections that would be innocuous in immunocompetent individuals. Opportunistic infections are considered AIDS-defining illnesses.

Introduction

Since the first description of AIDS in the 1980s, the epidemic has exploded to impact millions of adults and children throughout the world. As the epidemic has expanded, children have become increasingly affected, both by infection with the virus as well as by parental illness and death. With more recent advances in prevention and treatment science, the current impact of the epidemic is glaringly disproportionate between the western world and resource-poor settings. In developed countries, the infection rates of children living with the virus have dropped dramatically, as have rates of orphaning since those individuals who are infected are remaining healthier longer due to availability of life-saving medications. A very different picture has emerged in the developing world where the epidemic continues to expand. The implementation of prevention programs and availability of treatment in these parts of the globe have grown slowly, and healthcare systems in these settings need substantial revision and bolstering to handle the care of millions of people living with the virus.

For those children who have access to treatment, pediatric HIV infection is now considered a chronic, although life-threatening, illness. This is in contrast to earlier in the epidemic when it was almost certainly viewed as a terminal illness. The advent of life-prolonging treatment facilitates infected children's development into adolescents and young adults living with HIV, only recently creating the opportunity to research the impact of HIV/AIDS throughout the developmental trajectory. This article presents a synthesis of the current state of knowledge regarding infant and young child development in the context of pediatric HIV/AIDS. Great strides have been made in prevention and treatment, and there is now a considerable body of work examining the neurodevelopmental sequelae of HIV in children. However, in many respects, developmental research in the context of HIV is in its nascency. The majority of pediatric HIV research has been conducted in developed nations, which, for certain aspects of child development, may have limited translatability to low-resource settings. Child development is inextricably linked with the environment, thus a child's physiological, psychological, and social development is closely tied to the child's community and familial resources. Further research on the impact of the epidemic upon the development of children in low-resource settings (e.g., in sub-Saharan Africa) is essential to combat the effects of the epidemic and to increase our understanding of the developmental impact of pediatric HIV/AIDS upon the world's children.

Epidemiology of Pediatric HIV/AIDS: Global Epidemic

The epidemiology of HIV/AIDS is an ever changing landscape. Not only does the absolute number of infected people continue to grow, but the demographic of people living with HIV has broadened. Whereas AIDS was first identified in homosexual men and intravenous drug users in the 1980s, currently, heterosexual transmission drives the epidemic in most parts of the world. Likewise, the reach of HIV/AIDS now extends beyond adults to children across the globe. HIV/AIDS exerts a harrowing impact on the world's children, reflected in the World Health Organization (WHO) estimates that a child is newly infected with HIV every minute. Global estimates indicate that approximately 2.3 million children were living with the virus in 2006, which is quite likely to be an underestimate (higher estimates reach 3.5 million).

The epidemic has followed a very different course in the developed world as compared to low-resource settings. In the West, findings from a landmark study were released in 1994 that identified a protocol to successfully prevent transmission of the virus from a mother to her child, and now, in the US, fewer than 200 babies are born infected with the virus each year. The advent of highly active antiretroviral therapy (HAART) followed just a few years later, prolonging life and greatly improving the functioning of infected individuals.

These improvements in prevention and treatment have not been widely implemented in other parts of the world, resulting in a differential impact of the HIV/AIDS epidemic upon the children living in developing nations. According to the United Nations Children's Fund (UNICEF), approximately 1% of women worldwide are infected with HIV; however, the vast majority (95%) of these infected women live in developing countries. The impact of the epidemic upon children is not only due to infection with the virus; parental loss due to AIDS has created 15 million AIDS orphans, the vast majority of whom live in the developing world (**Figure 1**).

Specifically, children living in sub-Saharan Africa have born the brunt of the pediatric epidemic. According to the UNAIDS 2006 Epidemic Update, a preponderance (87%) of children living with HIV/AIDS live in sub-Saharan Africa. Further, estimates released from WHO

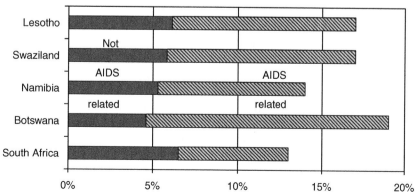

Figure 1 Percentage of children in sub-Saharan Africa who were orphans in 2005. Source UNAIDS/UNICEF, 2006.

and UNAIDS indicate that 1400 children die every day from causes attributable to AIDS and about 90% of these deaths occur in sub-Saharan Africa.

The context of HIV disease is also important when considering how children are affected by the epidemic. It is a disease that is commonly associated with poverty and, in the developed world, may also be associated with intravenous drug use. In developing countries, poverty is aligned with nutritional concerns and an increased prevalence of other illnesses such as tuberculosis. Advances in decreasing high child mortality have been reversed. In all societies, AIDS is a stigmatizing disease which contributes to the isolation of those affected by the disease, both those who are infected and also their family members. Millions of children have been orphaned by AIDS. Others are experiencing the illness of parents, sometimes taking on roles of caregiver for their ill parents or assuming the parenting role for younger siblings. Aging grandparents take an expanding number of children into their homes and, with fewer adults generating incomes, food is dispersed more thinly among members of the household.

Transmission of HIV/AIDS to Infants

The growth of the global pediatric HIV epidemic is primarily due to transmission of the virus from HIV-positive mothers to their children. Before the routine use of preventive medications in Europe and the US, approximately 15–25% of children born to HIV-infected mothers were infected with the virus. Rates of transmission vary, however, between developing and developed nations. The virus can also be transmitted through breastfeeding, so in parts of the world where breastfeeding is prevalent, or even essential, rates of transmission may reach as high as 45%. Aside from availability of preventive measures, transmission rates may be influenced by rates of Cesarian section (a protective factor), breastfeeding patterns, prematurity (influenced by availability of obstetric care and the woman's access to proper nutrition), and the extent to which the mother's disease has advanced.

There are three primary mechanisms through which a woman's HIV infection may be transmitted to her infant: (1) *in utero* (prenatally), (2) during the birth process (intrapartum), and (3) via breast milk (postnatally). Although less common than other modes of transmission, the fetus can become infected with HIV *in utero* during pregnancy, particularly if exposed to the mother's blood through bleeding in the placental lining. Invasive procedures, high maternal viral load, vaginal delivery, and prolonged rupture of the amniotic sac during the birth process are all factors associated with increased rates of intrapartum transmission. Postnatally, breastfeeding can pass the virus to the child through colostrum and breast milk. Again, higher maternal viral loads

increase the risk of transmission to the infant. Furthermore, likelihood of transmission is enhanced if the infant has sores in his or her mouth or if the mother's nipples are cracked and bleeding. Infants who become infected via breastfeeding typically acquire the virus in the first 6 months although transmission can occur anytime during the period of breastfeeding.

Researchers have striven to identify the transmission mechanisms as well as effective prevention methods. In 1994, results were released from a landmark study conducted by the US and France indicating that mother-to-child transmission (MTCT) can be reduced by two-thirds with the targeted use of antiretroviral medication. Within 2 months of analysis of initial data, the randomized controlled trial was ceased and the protocol (referred to as the AIDS Clinical Trial Group Study, ACTG 076) was deemed the standard of care for HIV-positive pregnant women in countries where it can be afforded. The protocol involves administering the drug to a woman while she is pregnant, giving it intravenously during labor, and then to her newborn for the first 6 weeks of life. Because this regimen is considered too expensive for most resource-poor countries, there has been extensive research to identify less expensive interventions to reduce perinatal transmission. Now, in a number of developing countries, the accepted regimen is the use of two doses of one of the antiretroviral medications, nevirapine. One dose of the drug is given to the mother when she is in labor and one dose to the child shortly after delivery. In total, this regimen costs only about $4.

Along with this protocol, breastfeeding guidelines have been developed to reduce transmission rates. In countries where it is considered affordable, safe, and sustainable, it is suggested that HIV-infected women feed formula to their infants rather than breastfeed. In developing countries (e.g., in sub-Saharan Africa), however, women often do not have consistent access to canned formulas or to clean water to mix with powder formulas; thus, the use of infant formulas can lead to an increase in child mortality due to increased rates of infectious illnesses, malnutrition, and dehydration. In these circumstances, the medical community advises that women exclusively breastfeed, meaning that nothing else, not even water, should be given to the baby. There is now evidence that mixed feeding (i.e., the combination of other liquids, such as water and formula, with breastmilk) results in higher rates of HIV transmission than exclusive breastfeeding, although the mechanism for this is poorly understood.

It is important to note that dissemination of prevention of mother-to-child transmission (PMTCT) programs has been slow in the developing world. Barriers to widespread implementation of these protocols have included low rates of HIV testing of pregnant women, lack of availability of medications, and systems of care that cannot handle the influx of women and newborns in need of care. As a first step, it is of paramount importance that women have access to and utilize HIV testing to determine whether they need to be placed on a PMTCT protocol. Equally essential, there must be a concomitant scale-up of the systems of medical care in these resource-poor settings. More health professionals need to be trained and retained (as many leave to work in developed countries) to provide care for the HIV-affected population.

Social–Ecological Model of Child Adaptation: Application to Pediatric HIV

The information presented in this article is conceptually organized according to a social–ecological framework of child adaptation and development, which has been widely applied in research with chronically ill children. The 'transactional stress and coping model' described by Robert Thompson, Jr. and Kathryn Gustafson in 1997 is an application of social–ecological theory to childhood chronic illness that further explicates the role of environment in the child's development. The transactional model incorporates developmental processes with attention to the family and social environments as influences upon the illness–outcome (medical and psychological) relationship. Chronic illness is conceptualized as a stressor to which the child and his or her family must adapt. Thompson indicates that adaptation to pediatric illness is impacted by family functioning, methods of coping, and cognitive processes. Specifically, cognitive processes include expectations, self-esteem, and a sense of ability to control one's own health (health locus of control). Family environment is conceptualized as one of three types: supportive, conflictive, and controlling. Descriptors of the child's illness, such as severity and treatment demands, as well as demographic indices (e.g., socioeconomic status) are included in the model. All of these elements interact to influence child development and adaptation.

Pediatric HIV particularly fits with a social–ecological model because of the many influential environmental and familial factors relating to this disease. The model also lends well to cross-cultural adaptation. In keeping with the transactional perspective, this article highlights the medical, psychological, and social (including familial) aspects of child development in the context of pediatric HIV/AIDS.

Medical Aspects of Pediatric HIV/AIDS

When considering the impact of HIV/AIDS upon infant and early child development, it is important to understand key aspects of the progression and treatment of the disease.

Medical Impact of Pediatric HIV/AIDS

HIV manifests and progresses differently in children than in adults. The clinical course of the disease in children is much faster than in infected adults. Even without treatment, adults often live for many years with HIV before becoming symptomatic, but this is generally not true for children. The disease tends to follow a bimodal presentation in children, with some children having very rapid progression to AIDS and others experiencing a more indolent course. In western countries before treatment was available, approximately 25% of children progressed to AIDS within 1 year. These 'rapid progressors' usually became seriously ill during their infancy, whereas the majority of children progress more slowly, developing AIDS later in childhood (typically between the ages of 6 and 10 years). In developing countries children fare even more poorly – in an analysis using data from seven prospective studies in Africa, 35% of untreated children died by 1 year of age and over half (52%) of infected children did not reach their second birthday.

Comorbid physical conditions

By definition, AIDS is a condition in which the damage to the immune system by HIV leads to the development of opportunistic infections and other disorders such as cancers. The most common of these infections is *Pneumocystis carinii* pneumonia (PcP). Without appropriate HIV management, this pneumonia often occurs in perinatally infected children from 3 to 6 months of age and has a very high mortality. *Mycobacterium avium* complex disease is another prevalent opportunistic infection, typically presenting with fever, diarrhea, and night sweats. Other opportunistic infections include tuberculosis, chronic herpes viruses, and infections of the central nervous system (CNS) with organisms such as *Cryptococcus* and *Toxoplasma*. Children living with HIV have increased risk of malignancies (most commonly lymphoma). The disease can also directly affect different organ systems such as the heart, kidneys, liver, gastrointestinal tract, and bone marrow, the latter causing hematologic abnormalities such as anemia.

Growth and physical development

Pediatric HIV disease is associated with growth deficiencies in over half of untreated children. These children not only experience difficulties maintaining their weight, but also may have problems with linear growth and depletion of lean muscle. Chronically poor growth, or progressive stunting, is associated with a higher risk of mortality. The causes of growth abnormalities are multiple and include neuroendocrine abnormalities, gastrointestinal dysfunction and malabsorption, vitamin and mineral deficiencies, and low levels of growth hormone; however, study results have been varied and therefore these linkages are not conclusive and sometimes are not considered to be causal.

Impact upon CNS

Unlike adult HIV, which begins in a fully mature and myelinated nervous system, pediatric HIV infects infants and children with developing and vulnerable central nervous and immune systems. Hence, children tend to become symptomatic faster than adults with a higher incidence of CNS disease.

Manifestations of the virus's impact upon a child's developing CNS include encephalopathy, neoplasms, opportunistic infections, disruption of the blood–brain barrier, and vascular changes associated with strokes. HIV-associated progressive encephalopathy presents with three primary clinical symptoms: impaired head growth, loss of developmental milestones or stagnation of developmental progression, and progressive motor dysfunction. The clinical course follows one of three patterns: (1) early presentation with a rapid course, (2) subacute course with periods of stability, and (3) static, slower progression. The early, rapid encephalopathy occurs over 1–2 months and is accompanied by a loss of developmental milestones. The typical postdiagnosis survival rate without treatment is less than 2 years. The children presenting with static encephalopathy do not lose milestones, but rather fail to achieve new milestones at an age-appropriate rate, evidencing increasing developmental delay over time.

Medical Treatment of Pediatric HIV/AIDS

In the 1980s and early 1990s, treatment for pediatric HIV/AIDS consisted of single medication regimens that were far less effective than the cocktail, or combination, approach used today. This includes the use of at least three antiretroviral medications with at least one of the three being from a different class of medication. This approach to treatment, referred to as HAART, was first tested and approved for use with adults and approximately 2 years later became approved for use with children (1998). The present approach is to initiate HAART when there is evidence of progression of disease such as a decrease in CD4 T lymphocyte count, which are part of the immune system and suppressed by the activity of the virus.

HAART is a complex medication regimen that can place significant adherence demands upon a child and family. It is extremely important that infected individuals do not forget to take the medicines; lack of adherence can lead to drug resistance, which can be very problematic, particularly in settings in which the different types of available medications are limited.

There are a number of adverse effects of long-term antiretroviral use that can have both physiological and psychiatric consequences. Lipodystrophy syndrome is a condition that is associated with changes to the body shape, including thinning of the face, arms, and legs accompanied by fattening of the abdomen. This can obviously be very distressing for a child or adolescent. Other potential side effects include metabolic abnormalities such as increasing cholesterol and glucose levels (**Figure 2**).

Psychological Aspects of Pediatric HIV/AIDS

Neurodevelopment and Cognitive Functioning

Neurological functioning is very closely tied to a child's cognitive development and brain abnormalities resulting

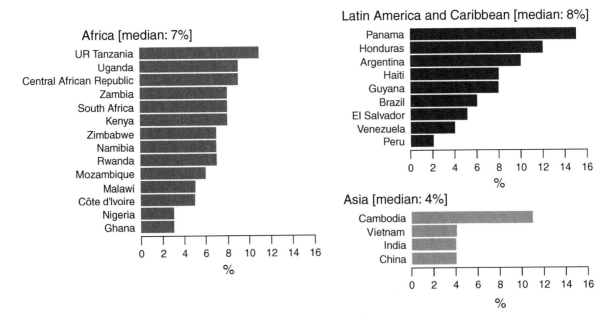

Figure 2   Percentage of people on treatment who are children by country, 2005.

from CNS disease can broadly influence a child's functioning. Deficits that have been associated with pediatric HIV infection include impaired cognitive functioning, attentional difficulties, behavioral and emotional disruption, and problems in academic performance. Children may experience difficulty with expressive language as well as visual–spatial skills and memory tasks. Research has demonstrated that environmental elements (e.g., poverty, correlates of maternal illness) that often accompany pediatric HIV infection can also impact a child's performance on these tasks. At times it can be very difficult for researchers to tease apart the specific contribution of the medical illness and environmental factors to a child's developmental outcomes. In addition, small sample sizes and variability in findings have increased the complexity of interpreting research for clinical application.

In light of these challenges, researchers have striven to identify mechanisms and pathways via which HIV affects a child's cognitive development. Studies have linked structural abnormalities in the brain to cognitive dysfunction. In 1995, Pim Brouwers and colleagues examined brain scans of 87 children with symptomatic HIV who were previously untreated. The scans indicated a higher rate of brain abnormalities in perinatally infected children than in children who acquired the virus from blood transfusions. The severity of abnormalities (including cortical atrophy, white matter changes, and ventricular enlargement) was found to be predictive of cognitive deficits. However, other studies have reported neuropsychological deficits without the accompanying structural abnormalities, indicating that deficits may also be influenced by other factors.

In an effort to examine the role of CNS disease in the neurodevelopment of HIV-infected children further, Wanda Knight and colleagues undertook a prospective study of children's mental and psychomotor development. At two time points, 20 HIV-infected and 25 noninfected infants who had been born to infected mothers (aged 3–30 months) participated in neurological examinations that included the Bayley Scales of Infant Development (BSID). Specific information regarding the children's antiretroviral treatment was not available to the researchers, but all the children were receiving care at an HIV primary care clinic and consistent treatment guidelines were applied. The results of the study demonstrated that HIV-infected infants scored significantly lower at baseline than noninfected infants on the mental development component of the BSID. At follow-up, the infants no longer differed significantly on mental development, but HIV-infected children scored lower than noninfected children on the motor scale. Interestingly, at both time points, the HIV-infected infants with CNS disease scored significantly lower on both mental and psychomotor indices than all other children. These findings suggest that HIV affects children's mental and psychomotor development via the CNS as a primary mechanism.

There is now evidence that treatment with HAART results in clinical improvement of certain cognitive deficits and adaptive behavior, including communication and daily living skills. Although asymptomatic children living with HIV still tend to fall below the average (or norm) on neuropsychological tests, the results are certainly improved since the advent of HAART. Unfortunately, however, children living with HIV in many parts of the world continue to have limited access to these life-saving treatments.

Psychological Distress

A great deal of research has been conducted on the psychological adjustment of HIV-positive adults and a number of interventions have been described for adults living with the virus. Adolescents have also received attention in investigations of mental health and prevention, and, not surprisingly, results suggest that adolescents living with HIV suffer greater psychological distress than their healthy peers. There is, however, a relative paucity of research on the mental health of infants and young children infected with HIV.

Psychiatric disorders including major depression, anxiety, attentional disorders, and behavioral disruption (conduct and oppositional defiant disorders) have all been associated with pediatric HIV infection. In 2006, Claude Mellins and colleagues published findings based upon clinical interviews with 47 perinatally infected youths (aged 9–16 years) and their primary caregivers and reported that 55% of these youths met criteria for a psychiatric disorder, a rate that is substantially higher than that found in the general population (although, these children were not directly compared to a control group with similar environmental stressors). In a second investigation, Mellins examined rates of behavioral problems among very young perinatally infected children (aged 3 years) and compared these to perinatally exposed, but uninfected, children. Very interestingly, the results of this study failed to demonstrate a relationship between HIV status and behavioral problems; instead, the findings showed that sociodemographic characteristics were the strongest predictors of behavioral symptoms.

In other studies, perinatally infected children have been reported to have higher rates of psychiatric symptoms than children infected via blood transfusion. Again, it is important to consider the social–ecological framework in interpreting these findings; it may be that children who acquired the virus earlier in development are physiologically more prone to psychiatric distress than those who became infected later. Alternatively, perinatally infected children are more likely to experience additional stressors, including maternal illness and correlates of maternal HIV (poverty, poor nutritional status, higher rates of intravenous drug use). Likely, the impact of

HIV/AIDS upon children's psychological development is exerted environmentally as well as physiologically. Family stress related to childhood chronic illness can be conceptualized in terms of the overall illness burden in the family (including medication demands, hospital visits, emotional strain); if the child and mother are both infected, the family will experience a very high illness burden. As demonstrated in the model, family stress directly impacts the child's psychological and emotional adjustment, so this constellation of stressors presents significant challenges.

Quality of Life

The quality of a child's life has become an increasingly important consideration as many children with chronic illnesses (including HIV/AIDS) are living longer, but not necessarily more comfortable, lives. The concept of quality of life generally refers to an individual's health, culture, beliefs, values, and life conditions that support the person's wellbeing. In considering an HIV-positive child's health-related quality of life (HRQOL), it is very important to assess the impact of the HIV disease and its treatment upon the child's functioning and life satisfaction.

Quality of life has emerged as a significant marker of how well any particular medical regimen works, as a primary goal of treatment is to not only increase the child's longevity, but also to improve the child's adaptive functioning and ability to enjoy life. In evaluating the impact of pediatric HIV disease and the effectiveness of treatment, it is important to consider child-oriented aspects of quality of life. These include access to education, positive social structure with peers and family, emotional health, physical health, and age-appropriate cognitive and attentional ability. HIV/AIDS can exert a negative influence upon each of these elements. Although HAART has been extremely instrumental in reducing CNS disease and facilitating children's healthy physical functioning, as discussed, this treatment approach involves some trade-offs in adverse effects. Thus, the field still has a great challenge to improve the quality of life of these children.

Coping

Young children living with HIV face a sobering set of challenges. Many of these children must cope with environmental stressors, educational problems, and missing school due to their own or even their parents' illnesses, as well as the physical symptoms and treatment demands associated with their illness.

Children's coping strategies for stressful experiences can render the child either vulnerable or resilient to subsequent stressors. According to the original conceptualization by Richard Lazarus and Susan Folkman in 1988, coping can be broadly delineated into two categories of behavior: problem-focused and emotion-focused coping. Problem-focused coping efforts directly target the stressor in an attempt to resolve the stressful situation. Emotion-focused coping efforts are the individual's attempts to regulate the negative emotional state that is aroused by the stressor, without directly targeting the stressor itself. Pediatric HIV poses complex challenges to the child and family, requiring an array of coping strategies. Controllable aspects of the illness (such as the taking of medications) call for an approach to coping that is problem focused. However, many aspects of the illness cannot be directly ameliorated, requiring coping strategies that facilitate the child's healthy emotional and social adjustment in the midst of illness-related stress. Coping interventions developed for children must be targeted and developmentally flexible.

Social Context of the HIV Epidemic: Impact upon Child Development

Public health and social consequences of the epidemic, including the escalating numbers of children being orphaned, widespread poverty, unpredictable availability of food and safe shelter, and lack of medical and requisite psychosocial care all contribute to poorer outcomes for children. HIV/AIDS has been referred to as a social disease, as it often affects the marginalized, underserved, or socioeconomically disadvantaged segments of a population. The challenges already present in individuals' lives are compounded by the illness and treatment demands of HIV. The stigma associated with the disease can also have a detrimental impact. Families often suffer an emotional exile because of fears of others knowing about the infection, not disclosing their diagnosis to others who might ordinarily provide support. This may also affect an individual's use of healthcare and taking of medications.

The social context for children's development with HIV/AIDS is significantly impacted by parental illness and loss due to the illness. UNICEF released sobering estimates in 2006 indicating that 15.2 million children worldwide had lost one or both parents to AIDS; 12 million of these children live in sub-Saharan Africa. The impact of parental loss on a child's developmental trajectory can be obviously detrimental in the absence of protective factors, particularly if the child has his or her own illness demands and functional limitations. Additionally, lack of schooling, either due to their own illness or due to the necessity of providing for ill parents or younger siblings, can disadvantage these children even further.

Caregiver and Family Functioning in the Context of Pediatric HIV/AIDS

Globally, families have become increasingly stressed and resources fewer due to the consequences of HIV/AIDS. Many children who are perinatally infected will lose their mothers to AIDS, and grandmothers will assume the caregiving role. Particularly in the developing world, HIV-related trauma is intergenerational; grandmothers who have lost children to AIDS are now caring for a grandchild infected with HIV. Grandmothers are often the primary caregiver for more than one grandchild and the majority of families with an infected child has at least one additional HIV-infected person living in the household. Children may also be cared for by multiple caregivers, usually in an extended family network. This may pose a distinct challenge for the management of the child's HIV, particularly if there is secrecy and lack of disclosure regarding the child's HIV diagnosis.

The research investigating the influence of family functioning upon the child's adjustment to chronic illness has been primarily conducted in the western world. However, given the cultural import regarding familial relationships, it is likely that family functioning is similarly, if not more, influential in children's adaptation to illness in African cultures. Family functioning is consistently a strong predictor of the child's adjustment to chronic illness, and many studies have linked maternal coping and adjustment to child psychosocial functioning and illness adaptation. Family functioning has also been linked to specific disease correlates, such as adherence and disease management over time. Findings across studies suggest that family cohesion and emotional expressiveness, as well as open communication and hopeful attitudes about the child's illness, are characteristics of system functioning that reliably predict desirable child adjustment outcomes. Given these demonstrated relationships, harnessing the strength of families for pediatric HIV intervention is considered critical.

Illness Management of Pediatric HIV

As conceptualized in the social–ecological framework, child and family psychosocial functioning directly impact the management of pediatric illness and adaptation. In the following discussion of disclosure and adherence, the role of the family is illustrated as central to the child's successful adaptation to illness demands.

Disclosure: Beginning the Process of Illness Management

Disclosure of the child's HIV status to the child and within the family system is an important aspect of illness

management of pediatric HIV. The American Academy of Pediatrics strongly urges caregivers to discuss the diagnosis with their HIV-infected child, and it is the policy in many pediatric infectious disease clinics to promote disclosure to school-aged children.

Family functioning is closely tied to successful negotiation of the disclosure process. Open communication within the family about the child's HIV status is linked to improved psychological and behavioral adjustment outcomes of the child and greater family expressiveness has been linked to earlier diagnostic disclosure to HIV-infected children. Children who know their HIV status also display fewer symptoms of depression than those children who do not know their diagnosis. In addition, anxiety has been shown to increase when children are not allowed to discuss their fears regarding illness. In research conducted by Des Michaels and colleagues in 2006, 126 caregivers of children on antiretroviral therapy in South Africa were interviewed regarding HIV infection in the family and disclosure to the child. The majority of caregivers indicated a belief that children should learn their HIV status between the ages of 6 and 10 years. However, only a small minority of caregivers interviewed had disclosed to their children. This discrepancy reflects the barriers to disclosure, including fear of familial stigmatization, the caregiver's own difficulty in coping with the child's diagnosis, fear of the child's emotional reaction, and lack of psychosocial support in disclosing to the child.

Clearly, disclosure to the child is crucially important in preparing him or her to cope with and manage the HIV infection, and to develop skills and patterns early for adherence and health-promoting behaviors. However, the timing and method of disclosure is critical with regard to the child's emotional reaction to diagnosis. The child will invariably learn his or her HIV status, and it is clearly best for this process to occur in a controlled, supportive environment. Disclosure of HIV status to the child is best conceptualized as a process, not a one-time conversation with the child, and should be developmentally appropriate. There is significant need for support of the family during the disclosure process. Although research has indicated the benefits of disclosure, empirical investigations of interventions to facilitate disclosure are limited and there is little information and understanding of the importance of the cultural context in issues of disclosure.

Treatment Adherence – Critical to Illness Management

Pediatric HIV is an illness that demands lifelong adherence to a challenging medical regimen. Research on children's medical adherence indicates that adherence is most poor for regimens that are complex, interfere with the child's activities, produce negative side effects, and are long-term and future oriented. By these criteria, pediatric HIV poses clear challenges for children's lifetime adherence. Complicating the demands upon adherence, many children (particularly in the developing world) are diagnosed with comorbid conditions (such as tuberculosis) that require additional medications. Although medication adherence is a challenge in the developed world, when drug resistance does develop because of nonadherence, there are other medications that can sometimes be used. As previously discussed, however, nonadherence in the developing world can have dire consequences given the few pediatric HIV medications available to children. Near-perfect adherence is required for medications to be successful; thus, children's adherence to HAART requires substantial attention and is a crucial target of pediatric intervention.

Children's adherence is positively influenced by disclosure. The child's adaptive functioning and coping also impact adherence, as do the social–ecological processes of family functioning and parenting. Similarly to facilitating disclosure, family environments that are low in conflict and high in support facilitate children's adherence. Communication and consistency among caregivers as well as parent–child communication are critical in promoting adherence to pediatric HIV-treatment regimens.

Future Directions for Intervention Efforts in Pediatric HIV/AIDS

Intervention goals for children living with HIV/AIDS must be targeted and developmentally applicable to the child's particular mental health and illness management needs. As discussed throughout this article, intervention with HIV-affected families requires attention to the social–ecological framework. It is important for interventions to promote coping skills and bolster resiliency within the family for adapting to illness-related stress (**Figure 3**).

Additionally, there is significant need for structured interventions that directly target children's acquisition of illness management skills and engage the caregiver in supporting the child's adaptation to HIV. Given the significance of family functioning, coping, and resiliency to successful illness management, it is of the utmost importance to integrate psychosocial intervention with adherence intervention for children. Further, it is critical to intervene early to bolster the child's skills for illness management and prevent nonadherence and engagement in risky health behaviors, which is often the typical trajectory in adolescence.

Along with providing appropriate medical treatment and family-based support, the child's cognitive development should be monitored with routine neuropsychological testing. Consistent evaluation provides a baseline of cognitive functioning and alerts the child's caregivers and medical providers if there is a drop-off in skills. Based upon a child's functioning, she or he may require treatment from a child psychologist to mitigate loss of functioning. Intervention may include cognitive remediation tasks such as memory work and focus on expressive language. Unfortunately, very few of the millions of children living with HIV have access to monitoring or remediation therapy.

Finally, intervention with children and families should be grounded in the cultural context. Little is currently known about the psychosocial impact of pediatric HIV in African children, and there is sobering potential for unfolding psychological effects of HIV-related trauma. As advances in the availability of antiretroviral therapy improve children's survival rates, health researchers have a responsibility to address these children's needs through specific and targeted efforts to alleviate distress and supply resources with which to face their challenges. Pediatric HIV/AIDS is a complex medical illness that is accompanied by an array of familial and societal stressors. It is of paramount importance to the world's children

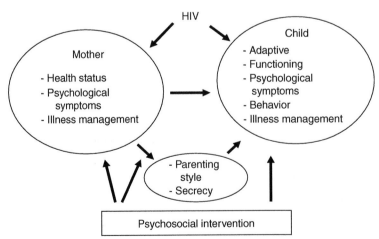

Figure 3 Model of psychosocial intervention with HIV-affected families, attending to the social–ecological processes of the mother and the child.

that researchers continue to attend to the amelioration and mitigation of children's suffering attributable to this disease.

See also: Birth Complications and Outcomes; Endocrine System; Immune System and Immunodeficiency; Mental Health, Infant; Teratology.

Suggested Readings

Brouwers P, DeCarli C, Civitello L, Moss H, Wltrs P, and Pizzo P (1995) Correlation between computed tomographic brain scan abnormalities and neuropsychological function in children with symptomatic human immuno-deficiency virus disease. *Archives of Neurology* 52: 39–44.

Brown LK, Lourie KJ, and Pao M (2000) Children and adolescents living with HIV: A review. *Journal of Child Psychology and Psychiatry* 41(1): 81–96.

Chakraborty R (2005) HIV-1 infection in children: A clinical and immunologic overview. *Current HIV Research* 3: 31–41.

Forsyth BWC (2003) Psychological aspects of HIV infection in children. *Child and Adolescent Psychiatric Clinics* 12: 423–437.

Knight WG, Mellins CA, Levenson RL, Arpadi SM, and Kairam R (2000) Brief report: Effects of pediatric HIV infection on mental and psychomotor development. *Journal of Pediatric Psychology* 25(8): 583–587.

Lazarus R and Folkman S (1988) The relationship between coping and emotion: Implications for theory and research. *Social Science and Medicine* 26: 309–317.

Mellins CA, Brackis-Cott E, Dolezal C, and Abrams EJ (2006) Psychiatric disorders in youth with perinatally acquired human immunodeficiency virus infection. *The Pediatric Infectious Disease Journal* 25(5): 432–437.

Mellins CA, Smith R, and O'Driscoll P (2003) High rates of behavioral problems in perinatally HIV-infected children are not linked to HIV disease. *Pediatrics* 111(2): 384–393.

Michaels D, Eley B, Ndhlovu L, and Rutenberg N (2006) *Horizons Final Report: Exploring Current Practices in Pediatric ARV Rollout and Integration with Early Childhood Programs in South Africa: A Rapid Situation Analysis.* Washington, DC: Population Council.

Thompson RJ and Gustafson KE (1997) *Adaptation to Childhood Chronic Illness.* Washington, DC: American Psychological Association.

Relevant Websites

http://www.nih.gov – National Institutes of Health (NIH), Department of Health and Human Services.
http://www.unaids.org – The Joint United Nations Programme on HIV/AIDS.
http://www.unicef.org – UNICEF, Unite for Children.

Allergies

A W Burks, Duke University Medical Center, Durham, NC, USA
K P Palmer, University of Arkansas for Medical Sciences, Little Rock, AR, USA

Glossary

Allergens – Normally harmless proteins or glycoproteins encountered in the environment which stimulate the production of IgE and result in allergic responses when bound by IgE on the surface of mast cells and basophils.

Atopy – The genetic predisposition to develop IgE-mediated responses to allergens encountered in the environment.

CAP FEIA – CAP Fluorescent Enzyme Immunoassay; newer, more sensitive *in vitro* assay used to detect allergen-specific IgE.

Cross-linkage of IgE – The process of allergen binding to multiple IgE molecules on the surface of mast cells and basophils which leads to signaling through the IgE molecule and the resultant allergic response.

Hypersensitivity – Immune-mediated response directed toward normally harmless substances; may be IgE-mediated but also includes various other immune mechanisms.

IgE – One of the immunoglobulin isotypes secreted by immune plasma cells which binds to IgE receptors on the surface of mast cells and basophils; cross-linking of surface-bound IgE by allergen leads to the signs and symptoms of immediate hypersensitivity.

Immunoglobulin – Protein produced by plasma cells of the immune system that acts to neutralize invading microorganisms and toxins.

Immunotherapy – The repeated administration of specific allergens to an individual that changes the IgE-mediated response so as to reduce symptoms when naturally exposed.

RAST – Radioallergosorbent test; commonly used *in vitro* assay used to detect allergen-specific IgE.

Spirometry – Technique for measuring lung function that is used for the diagnosis and management of asthma.

Introduction

Allergic diseases affect over 20% of the US population, and the prevalence of these conditions is rising. They are the sixth leading cause of chronic disease; an estimated 14.1 million physician office visits occur each year for allergic rhinitis alone. These disorders significantly impact quality of life of affected individuals and account for billions of dollars in direct and indirect costs every year.

The Allergic Response

Immunologically mediated events directed at common, harmless substances characterize the allergic response. Although many parts of the immune system are involved, the principal mediator is immunoglobulin E (IgE). IgE was first discovered in 1967 and, along with IgG, IgA, and IgM, is one of the immunoglobulin isotypes produced and secreted by plasma cells. Production of allergen-specific IgE depends on both the genetic predisposition of an individual to form IgE and the pattern and timing of environmental allergen exposure. Individuals not affected by allergy do not produce allergen-specific IgE and therefore do not respond immunologically to allergens.

The IgE-mediated allergic response, or immediate hypersensitivity reaction, is shown in **Figure 1**. Sensitization occurs during the initial exposure to a specific allergen and is the process whereby an individual initially forms allergen-specific IgE. In order for sensitization to occur, the allergen must first be recognized by specialized cells called antigen-presenting cells that process the allergen into antigenic peptides and present these peptides to T cells. This process triggers the production of cytokines by T cells which directly interact with B cells to stimulate the production of allergen-specific IgE. Secreted IgE then binds to high-affinity IgE receptors on the surface of mast cells and basophils that are located in the skin, mucosal surfaces, and circulation.

Upon re-exposure, allergen binds to and links multiple surface-bound IgE molecules on mast cells and basophils, and thus initiates the early-phase response. Mast cells and basophils contain granules with numerous preformed chemical mediators such as histamine, tryptase, and heparin, which are released upon binding of the allergen to IgE on these cells. Newly synthesized mediators,

such as leukotrienes and prostaglandins, are also released. These mediators, of which histamine is paramount, cause increased vascular permeability, mucus secretion, smooth muscle constriction, vasodilatation, and sensory nerve stimulation. When these changes occur in various organs, they result in the clinical symptoms observed in an immediate allergic reaction (**Table 1**). The late-phase response, which usually occurs 2–4 h after allergen exposure, is due to infiltrating inflammatory cells, such as eosinophils and mononuclear cells. These cells release various cytokines, protein mediators that have various inflammatory effects on other types of cells, and this process results in clinical chronic allergic inflammation.

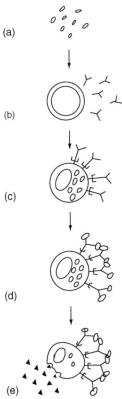

Figure 1 Mechanism of IgE-mediated allergy. (a) Allergen enters the body via inhalation, ingestion, injection, or direct contact. (b) B cells secrete allergen-specific IgE. (c) IgE binds to high-affinity IgE receptors on the surface of mast cells. (d) Upon re-exposure, allergen cross-links allergen-specific IgE on the surface of mast cells. (e) Mast cells degranulate, releasing chemical mediators such as histamine.

Table 1   The allergic response in target organs

Eye	Nose	Lung	Gastrointestinal tract	Skin	Heart and blood vessels
Ocular itching, redness, watery eyes	Nasal itching, runny nose, sneezing, congestion	Cough, shortness of breath, wheezing	Abdominal pain, vomiting, diarrhea	Hives, itching, angioedema, flushing	Decreased blood pressure

Characteristics of Common Allergens

Allergens are common proteins or glycoproteins found in the environment. They may function as enzymes, structural or regulatory proteins, or ligand-binding proteins, thus representing a variety of biologic activities. Their solubility allows them to penetrate the respiratory mucosa when inhaled, but they can gain entry by other means including ingestion, injection, and direct contact. House-dust mite, animal dander, and cockroach are important indoor allergens, whereas the primary source of outdoor allergens are plants and fungi, although the latter may be present in both settings. Other important allergens are found in foods, latex, drugs or drug metabolites, and insect venom.

Pollens

Allergenic pollen grains typically originate from wind-pollinated trees, grasses, and weeds. They are usually 10–100 μm in diameter, allowing them to reach the upper and lower respiratory tract. Exposure and sensitization to pollens is largely dependent on the geographic distribution of these plants and individual characteristics of the pollen grain such as size, dispersibility, and buoyant density. In the US, trees pollinate in early- to mid-spring, whereas grasses pollinate in late spring to early summer and weeds in late summer to early fall. Although there are numerous species of trees, grasses, and weeds in the US, only a limited number of these are responsible for allergic disease.

Fungi

Fungi are organisms with rigid cell walls that are classified according to their sexual reproductive structures. Allergenic fungi are usually microscopic (mold spores); however, macroscopic fungi like mushrooms may also be allergenic. Fungi are common throughout the US, and outdoor mold spore counts are usually highest in the summer and early fall. Common indoor mold sources include damp indoor spaces, baths, showers, crawlspaces, and basements.

Animal Dander

Animal allergens are proteins found in saliva, urine, and secretions from sebaceous oil glands in the skin. Allergenic proteins from cats and dogs comprise the most common, clinically relevant animal allergens; however, birds, rabbits, and multiple other animals can also produce allergenic proteins. The major allergens of cat and dog are extremely lightweight and can be carried through the air easily so that they accumulate on furniture, clothing, and carpets. Therefore, their distribution is virtually ubiquitous with measurable amounts of allergen located in homes with and without pets, schools, offices, and public buildings.

House-Dust Mite

The allergenic proteins of house-dust mite are enzymes excreted in mite feces. Two species of dust mite, *Dermatophagoides pteronyssinus* and *D. farinae*, account for over 90% of allergen found in house-dust samples in the US. Dust mites tend to thrive in warm environments with high humidity, and primary reservoirs include mattresses, carpets, upholstered furniture, draperies, and stuffed toys.

Food Allergens

Food allergens are 10–70 kDa proteins or glycoproteins that are relatively resistant to heat, acidity, and digestion. Although any food can cause an IgE-mediated allergic reaction, reactions to milk, soy, egg, wheat, peanuts, tree nuts, fish, and shellfish account for 90% of food allergies. Proteins identified as major allergens include whey and casein in milk, tropomycin in shellfish, ovomucoid in egg white, and the seed storage proteins vicilin and conglutin in peanuts.

Allergic Diseases in Childhood

Allergic Rhinitis

The term rhinitis refers to inflammation of the nasal mucous membranes which may be due to underlying allergic disease, nonallergic disease, or both. Allergic rhinitis is one of most common allergic diseases in the US affecting approximately 40 million individuals. It has a significant impact on health-related quality of life and results in millions of school and work days missed each year. Children with allergic rhinitis may have sleep disturbances, school problems, anxiety, difficulty concentrating, and familial dysfunction. Furthermore, allergic rhinitis and the use of first-generation antihistamines, such as diphenhydramine, have been found to adversely impact learning in children. Characteristic symptoms of allergic rhinitis include repetitive sneezing, nasal itching, congestion, and clear nasal drainage. These symptoms often develop in young children and may persist into adulthood. Furthermore, allergic rhinitis is commonly associated with other conditions such as asthma, allergic conjunctivitis, and atopic dermatitis.

Allergic rhinitis accounts for approximately 50% of all rhinitis and the symptoms are frequently similar to various forms of nonallergic rhinitis, so it is important to differentiate the two. Infectious rhinitis, often confused with allergic rhinitis, is commonly caused by respiratory viruses and may be accompanied by low-grade fever and purulent nasal secretions predominantly containing neutrophils. Nonallergic eosiniphilic rhinitis is characterized by sneezing, nasal itching, congestion, and nasal discharge, but differs from allergic rhinitis in that there is no evidence of allergen-specific IgE. As the name implies, significant nasal eosinophilia is present on nasal scrapings obtained from these patients. Other forms of nonallergic rhinitis include vasomotor rhinitis, the result of mucosal hyperresponsiveness to various changes in environmental stimuli such as humidity, temperature, strong odors, and chemicals, and hormonally induced rhinitis which may occur during pregnancy, puberty, menses, or in endocrine disorders such as hypothyroidism. Various anatomic abnormalities, such as nasal septal deviation, nasal foreign body, choanal narrowing, and adenoidal hypertrophy can cause rhinitis because normal respiratory mucosal physiology may be altered in these conditions. Finally, medications such as antipsychotic and antihypertensive drugs can induce rhinitis. Topical decongestants, in particular, can lead to significant rebound rhinitis if used for a prolonged time period.

Allergic rhinitis can be classified as either seasonal, caused by allergens such as trees, grasses, and weeds, or perennial, usually caused by allergens such as house-dust mite and animal dander, which do not have seasonal variation. Perennial allergic rhinitis and mixed patterns of perennial rhinitis with seasonal exacerbations account for the majority of cases. In pure seasonal allergic rhinitis, symptoms are episodic and correlate with the implicated seasonal allergen. The profuse watery nasal drainage, repetitive sneezing, and nasal and ocular itching characterize what is commonly referred to as hay fever. Perennial symptoms are similar but are more prominently characterized by postnasal drainage and chronic nasal congestion.

Important risk factors for the development of allergic rhinitis include an immediate family history of allergic disease and a personal history of other allergic diseases such as asthma or atopic dermatitis. The relationship between allergic rhinitis and asthma is particularly important, and the same allergens can be responsible for exacerbations of both diseases. Both the nose and the lungs share a common respiratory mucosa and poorly controlled IgE-mediated responses in the nose can potentially lead to or worsen allergic inflammation of the lower airway.

When evaluating a patient with suspected allergic rhinitis, one must identify the onset and duration of symptoms, severity, relationship of symptoms to seasons, and other identifiable triggers such as dust, animals, or pollen. Examination of the eyes, ears, nose, and throat may reveal characteristic findings that are helpful. Allergic shiners are darkened areas of skin underneath the eyes which result from chronic venous congestion and nasal obstruction (**Figure 2**). Persistent nasal obstruction may also lead to mouth breathing, and nasal pruritis can lead to the formation of a horizontal crease of the mid-to-lower nose due to repetitive rubbing and wiping. The nasal turbinates may appear pale and boggy, at times almost completely obstructing the nasal airway.

The first step in the management of allergic rhinitis is allergen avoidance, and recommendations should be based on tests for allergen-specific IgE (discussed later),

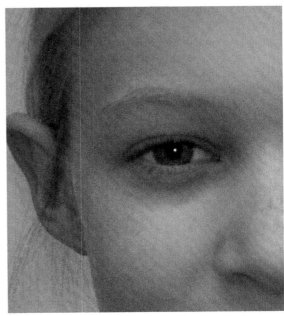

Figure 2 Allergic shiners in a child with perennial allergic rhinitis. Reproduced with permission from the parent.

in combination with the clinical history. Occasionally, allergen avoidance alone is all that is required for symptom control; however, in most cases pharmacologic therapy is needed. Medications used to treat allergic rhinitis include antihistamines, decongestants, intranasal steroids, leukotriene modifiers, mast cell stabilizers, and anticholinergics. In many comparison studies with antihistamines and leukotriene modifiers, intranasal steroids have proved to be most effective in the treatment of all symptoms of allergic rhinitis. In severe or refractory cases, immunotherapy should be considered as it is effective in alleviating symptoms. Ongoing education and follow-up regarding allergen avoidance and compliance with medication and/or immunotherapy is imperative.

Asthma

Asthma is the most common chronic disease of childhood affecting approximately 4.8 million children in the US. Morbidity rates have increased since the mid-1970s despite significant advances in the understanding of pathophysiology and treatment. Asthma can develop at any time, but approximately 80% of individuals who have asthma develop symptoms before 5 years of age. The most important risk factor is atopy, but, a personal or immediate family history of allergy, passive tobacco smoke exposure in childhood, and sensitization to certain inhalant allergens are also important.

Individuals with asthma have recurrent episodes of coughing, shortness of breath, chest tightness, and wheezing. Infants may also demonstrate difficulty feeding, rapid breathing, and grunting. These symptoms are a result of chronic airway hyperresponsiveness, inflammation, and partially reversible airway obstruction. The inflammation of airways in asthma is characterized by mast cell activation, infiltration of inflammatory cells, edema, mucus hypersecretion, and damage to the bronchial epithelium. Over time, these changes lead to airway wall remodeling with collagen deposition underneath the basement membrane, mucus gland hyperplasia, smooth muscle hypertrophy, and vascular proliferation. Once airway remodeling has occurred, it is irreversible. Asthma that is predominantly triggered by allergens may be referred to as extrinsic asthma. In contrast, some asthmatic patients have no identifiable allergies and so are referred to as having nonallergic, or intrinsic, asthma. Triggers such as upper respiratory infections, exercise, cigarette smoke, and cold air can contribute to disease in both types of asthmatic patients.

Objective measurements of airway hyperresponsiveness and pulmonary function are useful for diagnosis and management. Spirometry, measurement of the volume and speed of inhaled and exhaled air, is the most commonly performed method of measurement and is used both for diagnosis and for determining asthma control and response to therapy. Spirometry is used to produce a flow–volume curve which depicts changes seen with inspiration and expiration. The expiratory portion of the flow–volume curve in an asthmatic patient characteristically appears concave. The forced expiratory volume at 1 s (FEV1), measured before and after the administration of a short-acting bronchodilator, can be used to confirm the diagnosis. Reversibility, or response to bronchodilator, is defined as an FEV1 increase of 12% or more. In children who are too young or unable to complete spirometry, a diagnostic trial of inhaled bronchodilators or anti-inflammatory medication can be useful.

Asthmatic patients demonstrate airway hyperresponsiveness to nonspecific parasympathomimetic stimuli such as methacholine, and measurement of this response is commonly known as a methacholine challenge. Histamine can also be used because both these agents act directly on bronchial smooth muscle to cause constriction. Inhaling these pharmacologic agents induces a decrease in lung function – usually a minimum 20% decrease in FEV1. These challenges are particularly useful in clinical trials and in the presence of normal spirometry when the diagnosis of asthma is questionable.

Another useful tool is the peak expiratory flow rate (PEFR), which is a measure of the maximum ability to expel air from the lungs and primarily reflects large airway function. Because it is highly effort-dependent, it is not as sensitive as FEV1 for diagnosing obstruction and should not be used as a diagnostic tool for asthma. Serial measurements are helpful, however, as a monitoring tool that can be performed at home using a peak flow meter. While diurnal variation (difference between measurements obtained in the morning and evening) of PEFR in nonasthmatic individuals is about 5%, variation of more than 20% commonly occurs in individuals with asthma.

The treatment of asthma is aimed at preventing symptoms, maintaining normal pulmonary function, and minimizing exacerbations and need for hospitalization and emergency care. The National Asthma Education and Prevention Program (NAEPP), a multidisciplinary coalition coordinated by the National Heart, Lung, and Blood Institute (NHLBI) of the National Institutes of Health have published guidelines regarding the evaluation and management of asthma. These guidelines use specific criteria to classify asthma severity, and pharmacologic therapy is escalated or decreased in a stepwise fashion according to severity classification (**Table 2**).

There are multiple medications available for the treatment of asthma. Quick relief medications are used for the rescue of acute symptoms, and long-term controller medications treat underlying airway inflammation and prevent the long-term remodeling changes of chronic asthma. Rescue medications, called β-agonists, can be either short acting or long acting. These medications act on airway smooth muscle and cause relaxation resulting in bronchodilation. While all individuals with asthma require short-acting bronchodilators for rescue, those with persistent asthma, in particular those with night-time symptoms, may benefit from the addition of a long-acting bronchodilator. Asthmatic patients with persistent symptoms require a long-term controller medication, of which the most effective are inhaled corticosteroids. Well-designed studies have shown that treatment with inhaled corticosteroids leads to decreased airway hyperresponsiveness as well as decreased frequency of asthma symptoms, exacerbations, hospitalizations, death from asthma, and improved quality of life. Systemic corticosteroids may be needed for individuals with acute exacerbations or in those with severe, refractory asthma. Leukotriene modifiers such as

Table 2 Approach to asthma management

Measurements of asthma control
Frequency of daytime symptoms
Frequency of night-time symptoms
FEV1
Peak flow variability
↓
Classification of asthma severity
Mild intermittent
Mild persistent
Moderate persistent
Severe persistent
↓
Pharmacotherapy based on severity classification
Short-acting-β-agonist
Low-, medium-, or high-dose inhaled corticosteroids
Long-acting β-agonist
Leukotriene modifiers
Oral corticosteroids

montelukast can also be used for long-term control in those with mild, persistent asthma and as adjuncts in those with more severe asthma. Finally, allergen immunotherapy is effective in the treatment of allergic asthma, and can be particularly useful in those patients with co-morbid, poorly controlled allergic rhinitis. However, the risk of systemic reactions from allergen vaccines may be increased in those with poorly controlled symptoms and decreased pulmonary function.

Atopic Dermatitis

Atopic dermatitis is a chronic remitting and relapsing inflammatory disease of the skin affecting 10–20% of children. While skin of normal individuals is usually well hydrated and free from redness or irritation, the skin of those affected with atopic dermatitis is chronically dry, extremely itchy, red, and inflamed. It is usually present in infancy and early childhood, with half of all affected individuals developing symptoms during the first year of life. Atopic dermatitis can cause significant morbidity and adversely affects quality of life leading to missing days at school and emotional stress. It may precede the development of allergic rhinitis and asthma, and so is usually the first manifestation of what is commonly referred to as the atopic march.

The pathophysiology of atopic dermatitis is complex and a result of both genetic and environmental factors. Sensitization to aeroallergens and food allergens, atopy, colonization with *Staphylococcus aureus*, and an altered skin barrier all play significant roles in the inflammatory process. Most individuals with atopic dermatitis have positive skin prick tests or *in vitro* assays for allergen-specific IgE. Multiple controlled studies have demonstrated that these specific allergens especially food allergens, house-dust mite, and animal danders, contribute to the severity and course of skin disease. Food allergy plays a significant role in approximately one-third of those with moderate-to-severe atopic dermatitis. The most commonly implicated foods are milk, soy, egg, wheat, peanuts, and fish. Relevant food allergens are identified by dietary history, skin prick testing, *in vitro* assays for food-specific IgE, and double-blind, placebo controlled food challenges. This is discussed in more detail in further sections.

Recent studies have elucidated an important role of *S. aureus* in the pathophysiology of atopic dermatitis. This organism is found on approximately 90% of skin lesions. *S. aureus* secretes exotoxins, such as enterotoxins A and B and toxic shock syndrome toxin, which act as super-antigens that polyclonally stimulate immune cells and contribute to persistent and worsening inflammation. Furthermore, IgE to these toxins has been found in affected individuals.

Significant itching is a hallmark feature of atopic dermatitis and is usually worse at night. Itching leads to repetitive

scratching that increases inflammation and leads to additional itching, a pattern commonly called the itch–scratch cycle. The mechanical trauma from repetitive scratching and the immunologic changes in the skin result in an altered skin barrier. This altered barrier allows increased evaporative losses and an increased portal of entry for allergens and chemical irritants that can lead to exacerbations of the disease.

The diagnosis of atopic dermatitis is based on the presence of major and minor clinical criteria. Central to the diagnosis of atopic dermatitis is the presence of intense itching and scratching. Other major criteria include a chronically relapsing course, lichenification of the skin, and a personal or family history of atopy. Skin lesions have variable appearance, but acute lesions are typically red patches of intensely itchy, excoriated, dry skin (**Figure 3**). Vesiculations with thin, clear, or discolored oozing may also be present. Chronic lesions generally are thickened or lichenified. The classic distribution of skin lesions in children is on the face and extensor surfaces of the extremities. In adults, involvement of the flexor surfaces is more common. Affected skin contains infiltration of activated lymphocytes, eosinophils, mast cells, and macrophages.

Treatment of atopic dermatitis is aimed at maintaining hydration and restoring the skin barrier, treating and controlling ongoing inflammation, controlling the itch–scratch cycle, and using anti-infective therapy when appropriate. Daily soaking or baths in lukewarm water followed by the application of an emollient act to hydrate the skin and seal in moisture. Moisturizers in the form of creams or ointments should be applied several times daily. Antihistamines act by blocking histamine receptors in the skin and are used in an effort to suppress the itch–scratch cycle. There are numerous anti-inflammatory medications available to treat atopic dermatitis, and the most commonly used are topical corticosteroids of varying potencies. Potency of the topical agents is based on severity of inflammation and

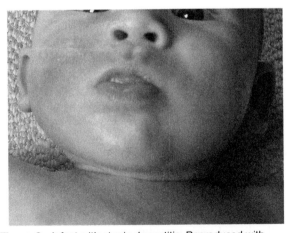

Figure 3 Infant with atopic dermatitis. Reproduced with permission from the parent.

location of affected areas. Also available are topical immunomodulators such as tacrolimus and pimecrolimus that can be used in place of, or in addition to, topical steroids. Systemic and/or topical antibiotics are useful in the treatment of individuals colonized with *S. aureus*. In cases of severe atopic dermatitis refractory to these therapies, the addition of systemic immunosuppressants, phototherapy, or wet dressings may be of added benefit.

Food Allergy

Adverse food reactions can result from both immune and nonimmune mechanisms, and such reactions are common in children. One study of 480 children under 3 years of age revealed that 28% reported an adverse food reaction, but only 8% of these were actually proven to be food related and even fewer were IgE mediated. Examples of nonimmune adverse food reactions include food toxin-mediated effects, such as in scromboid fish poisoning, and host metabolic or enzymatic alterations, as in lactose intolerance. Adverse food reactions due to immune mechanisms can be further classified into IgE-mediated and non-IgE-mediated reactions. IgE-mediated food allergy occurs in approximately 6–8% of young children and 3–4% of adults. These reactions may be severe and are the leading cause of anaphylaxis in children.

The prevalence of IgE-mediated food allergy is greatest during the first few years of life, and children with atopic disease, particularly atopic dermatitis, are more likely to have coexisting food allergy. Ninety percent of food allergies in children are caused by six foods: milk, egg, peanuts, wheat, soy, and tree nuts. In older children and adults, the majority are due to peanuts, tree nuts, fish, and shellfish. Allergies to milk, eggs, wheat, and soy are more likely to be outgrown than those to peanuts, tree nuts, fish, or shellfish.

Food allergens are heat and acid stable proteins that are absorbed via the gastrointestinal tract, crosslink food-specific IgE on the surface of mast cells, and lead to the signs and symptoms of immediate hypersensitivity. When an allergic food reaction occurs, symptoms occur within minutes to a few hours after ingestion. Symptoms may include hives, swelling of the lips or tongue, flushing, itching, wheezing, shortness of breath, abdominal cramping, vomiting, decreased blood pressure, or loss of consciousness. A history of a temporal relationship between the ingestion of a particular food and onset of symptoms is important in establishing a diagnosis of food allergy. When skin-prick testing to the suspected allergen is performed properly and quality extracts are used, a negative test essentially excludes food allergy. Conversely, a positive skin-prick test has a positive predictive value of approximately 50%, so it is important that testing be correlated with clinical history. *In-vitro* measurements for food-specific IgE, preferably the CAP fluorescent immunoassay (CAP FEIA), are particularly useful in food allergy diagnosis because predictive values have been established for the major food allergens based on CAP FEIA levels and results of double-blind, placebo-controlled food challenges in children. These challenges are the gold standard for the diagnosis of food allergy, and decisions regarding food challenges are often based on a combination of clinical history, skin-prick testing, and CAP FEIA results.

Current treatment of IgE-mediated food allergy involves strict elimination of the offending allergen, and ongoing patient and family education regarding how to respond to accidental ingestions and reactions. Food allergic individuals with a history of a severe allergic reactions or anaphylaxis should carry and be able to use injectable epinephrine. (epinephrine is a medication with adrenergic activity that reverses the pathophysiologic changes observed in anaphylaxis.)

Non-IgE-mediated food reactions are usually present in the first few months of life and include food protein-induced gastrointestinal disorders. A comparison of these processes with IgE-mediated reactions is shown in **Table 3**. The most common foods implicated are milk and soy, although foods such as rice, wheat, and poultry have also been implicated. Food-induced enterocolitis can cause protracted vomiting and diarrhea leading to failure to thrive or episodic vomiting and diarrhea 2 h or more following ingestion. The latter may lead to severe dehydration and decreased blood pressure and may be confused

Table 3   Comparison of immune-mediated food reactions

	IgE-mediated food allergy	*Non-IgE-mediated food allergy*
Time course of symptoms	Immediate symptoms – usually within minutes to 2 h following ingestion	Delayed symptoms – usually >2 h following ingestion
Commonly implicated foods	Milk, soy, egg, wheat, peanut, tree nuts, fish, shellfish	Milk and soy
Signs and symptoms	Hives, angioedema, itching, wheezing, cough, vomiting, abdominal pain, throat tightness, shortness of breath	Vomiting, diarrhea, failure to thrive, bloody stools
Examples	Anaphylaxis to peanut	Food protein-induced • enterocolitis • enteropathy • proctocolitis

with fulminant infection, especially in young infants. Food-induced enteropathy is a malabsorption syndrome characterized by vomiting, failure to thrive, and greasy, foul-smelling stools. In contrast, protocolitis, inflammation of the lower part of the gastrointestinal tract or rectum, is not associated with vomiting or diarrhea but rather is characterized by gross or occult blood in the stools. Although the exact pathophysiologic mechanisms of these processes are not well understood, studies have demonstrated that T cells and cytokines such as tumor necrosis factor (TNF)-α and transforming growth factor (TGF)-β1 play important roles in food protein-induced enterocolitis. Treatment of all of these entities involves strict elimination of the suspected food, and they are usually outgrown within the first several years of life.

Anaphylaxis

Anaphylaxis is a severe, IgE-mediated allergic reaction to a specific allergen to which an individual has been sensitized and results from the systemic, rather than local, release of inflammatory mediators from mast cells and basophils. These reactions are potentially life threatening and are considered medical emergencies. In children, foods are the most common cause of anaphylaxis outside of the hospital setting, but other common causes include medications, latex, and insect stings. Anaphylaxis may also occur with exercise or in rare cases, the cause may be unknown. Risk factors include a prior history of reaction, asthma, food allergy, atopy, sensitivity to multiple antibiotics, and use of certain cardiovascular medications.

Symptoms of anaphylaxis may include hives (urticaria), swelling of the face or other body parts (angioedema), itching, repetitive vomiting, anxiety, shortness of breath, wheezing, throat fullness, decreased blood pressure, and collapse. Tryptase is one of the mediators released upon degranulation of mast cells and may be elevated following an anaphylactic reaction for up to 24 h. Measuring serum tryptase levels can be useful particularly if the diagnosis of anaphylaxis is in question.

The primary treatment of anaphylaxis involves initiating basic cardiopulmonary support measures and administering epinephrine.

Additional medications such as antihistamines, steroids, bronchodilators, and intravenous fluids are often required as well. Close monitoring of vital signs, airway patency and breathing, and perfusion is extremely important. Approximately 20% of anaphylactic episodes have a late phase component 2–4 h later during which symptoms may recur.

Latex Allergy

Latex allergy is an IgE-mediated response to the proteins of natural rubber latex which is the fluid obtained from the cultivated rubber tree, *Hevea brasiliensis*. Healthcare workers, individuals who have had multiple surgeries, patients with *spina bifida*, and those who work in the rubber industry are most at risk because sensitization to latex proteins is more likely to occur with repeated exposure. Accordingly, the prevalence of latex allergy has increased since the application of universal precautions in the healthcare industry and the resultant routine use of latex gloves. Atopy is also an important risk factor for the development of latex allergy. Sensitization to latex can occur by wearing latex gloves, inhaling powder from latex gloves, or using medical devices, such as barium enema applicators or urinary catheters, which contain latex.

Allergic reactions to latex present with signs and symptoms similar to other allergic reactions, and some individuals may have anaphylactic reactions. Diagnosis of latex allergy involves a consistent history and positive laboratory testing for latex-specific IgE. Skin-prick testing in latex is not usually performed due to lack of a standardized latex reagent and reports of life-threatening anaphylaxis associated with latex skin testing. *In-vitro* measurements are available and should be correlated with the patient's history. Treatment involves strict avoidance of all latex products and the prescription of injectable epinephrine to be used in case of accidental exposure and reaction.

Insect Hypersensitivity

IgE-mediated systemic reactions can occur to the venoms of several stinging insects. These insects are members of the order *Hymenoptera* and include honeybees, bumblebees, yellow jackets, hornets, and fire ants. While reactions to fire ants are particularly common in the Gulf Coast region, most insect sting reactions in the United States are due to yellow jackets.

Most individuals develop localized swelling, redness, and pain at the site of an insect sting which resolves within several hours. However, some individuals may experience more extensive swelling and redness over a larger but still localized area that may last for several days. Both these types of local reactions can be treated symptomatically and are not indicative of future, more severe reactions. In contrast to local reactions, signs and symptoms of a systemic sting reaction occur at sites distant to the site of sting and may include, generalized urticaria, itching, flushing, angioedema, wheezing, shortness of breath, nausea, vomiting, hypotension, and collapse. These symptoms generally occur within minutes of the sting. Studies have shown that children under 16 years of age with isolated skin symptoms (i.e. hives and angioedema), even if generalized, are not at increased risk for a more severe reaction with subsequent stings.

Individuals with a history consistent with a systemic reaction to an insect sting should undergo skin testing. Venoms of the order *Hymenoptera* are available for immunotherapy and this is the preferred treatment for individuals with a history of systemic reaction to an insect sting confirmed by skin testing or radioallergosorbent assay test (RAST). Affected individuals should continue to carry self-injectable epinephrine in case of accidental sting.

Urticaria and Angioedema

Both urticaria and angioedema can occur as part of an acute, IgE-mediated allergic reaction but may be due to other disease processes as well. Urticaria are red, itchy, blanchable, elevated areas of the skin that are due to mast cell degranulation, venule dilatation, and dermal edema. Lesions can coalesce or be discreet, with individual lesions usually resolving within 24 h. Angioedema is similar but also involves the deep dermis and subcutaneous tissue causing swelling of the face, tongue, genitalia, or extremities.

Urticaria which consistently appear shortly following exposure to a particular allergen are likely IgE-mediated while those that occur on a regular basis with no clear, identifiable triggers may be idiopathic or a sign of other processes such as autoimmune disease, chronic infection, or neoplasm. Viral infections are an important common cause of acute urticaria in children. Likewise, angioedema may be IgE-mediated; idiopathic; or induced by certain physical conditions such as cold, heat, or pressure. Hereditary angioedema is an autosomal dominant condition that results from deficiency of C1 esterase inhibitor and results in recurrent angioedema of the face and extremities as well as repetitive attacks of severe abdominal pain due to bowel wall edema.

Drug Allergy

Adverse reactions to medications include any unintended response elicited by the drug. Those that are immune-mediated are called allergic, or hypersensitivity reactions, and approximately 5–10% of all adverse drug reactions are in this category. Drug reactions can be classified based on underlying immune mechanisms. Immediate hypersensitivity reactions are IgE-mediated and have been extensively described above. In another type of reaction, certain components of the immune system, such as antibodies, interact with drug allergens that associate with cell membranes. This interaction leads to destruction of cells such as platelets, and red and white blood cells. Drug reactions can also be mediated by immune complexes in which the drug acts as antigen and is bound by antibody. These antigen–antibody complexes aggregate in blood vessels and basement membranes and cause significant inflammation. Serum sickness is an example of this type of reaction, occurring when immune complexes enter the circulation, leading to joint pain, enlarged lymph nodes, rash, fever, and hepatitis. Finally, some drug reactions are mediated primarily by T cells. Following drug exposure, these cells become activated and mediate a robust inflammatory response as is seen in allergic contact dermatitis.

The most common medications causing IgE-mediated drug reactions are antibiotics although, theoretically, any drug can be implicated. Many drugs act as haptens which bind to carrier proteins which go on to elicit the immune reponse. In many of these reactions, IgE is specific for metabolites of the drug rather than for the parent drug.

The evaluation for drug allergy is complicated by the lack of standardized skin-testing reagents for drugs other than penicillin. Diagnosis is based on clinical history and the appropriate tests for drug-specific IgE when available. When these are consistent with an IgE-mediated event, the drug should be avoided, and if alternative unrelated medications cannot be used, desensitization can be performed in a controlled medical setting.

Diagnostic Testing for Allergies

Specific testing for allergies is necessary to confirm that certain symptoms are allergic in nature and to guide treatment for allergic diseases. This is especially true when symptoms persist or worsen despite therapy or when immunotherapy is being considered. Currently available tests for allergen-specific IgE include skin testing and in-vitro assays for allergen-specific IgE.

Skin-prick tests are performed by introducing a small amount of allergen extract just underneath the top layer of skin and measuring the size of wheal and flare response. These tests are commonly placed on the back but can be performed on the inner surface of the forearm as well. Extracts of a wide variety of allergens can be used and results are obtained within a short time period. The results of skin-prick tests alone are not diagnostic and should always be correlated with the individual's history. Furthermore, the size of a reaction to a skin test is not related to clinical significance and does not predict severity of reaction. There are certain circumstances in which skin tests administered intradermally are indicated. Intradermal tests are generally more sensitive than prick tests and can be useful in the evaluation of medication allergy, venom hypersensitivity, or when the prick test is negative to an allergen that is strongly suspected by history (but not in food allergy).

The second method for detecting allergen-specific IgE is by in-vitro assays such as the RAST and CAP FEIA. These tests detect the presence of allergen-specific IgE antibody in the serum. As with skin testing, these results must be correlated with the individual's clinical history and environmental exposures.

Allergy skin-prick testing is generally the preferred method of testing and is more sensitive than in-vitro assays. Furthermore, these tests are less expensive, and the results are available immediately. Under certain circumstances, however, in-vitro assays are particularly useful, such as in individuals with severe eczematous rashes or in those who cannot discontinue the use of antihistamines (which suppress skin-prick test results).

Management of Allergic Diseases

Although each of the allergic diseases affecting children must be approached differently, there are several general principles of management that are common to all. These include environmental control of allergen exposure, pharmacologic therapy, allergen immunotherapy, and ongoing education.

Environmental Control of Allergen Exposure (Allergen Avoidance)

The development and pathology of allergy depends on initial and ongoing exposure to allergen. Therefore, the first line in management of allergic disease is identification of clinically relevant sensitivities and education about how to minimize exposure to these allergens effectively. In doing so, it is important to take into consideration the individual's lifestyle, occupation, and hobbies. Because it is not always practical or feasible to remove the individual from the allergen source completely, advice must be tailored to the individual family.

Reservoirs for house-dust mite include bedding, carpet, upholstered furniture, and draperies. Effective techniques for minimizing dust-mite exposure include covering the bed with dust-mite impermeable encasings, laundering bed linens in hot water at least once weekly, and vacuuming frequently or removing carpet. Other suggestions may include minimizing the amount of upholstered furniture pieces and draperies, and reducing the indoor humidity to less than 50%.

Sources of indoor mold include bathrooms without vents or windows, crawl spaces, sites of water damage, and moldy air conditioners, and humidifiers. To minimize mold growth and exposure, indoor humidity should be kept low, water leaks promptly repaired, and crawlspaces ventilated. Complete avoidance of outdoor mold exposure is virtually impossible, but exposure may be minimized by refraining from walking through wet forests and raking leaves.

When animal dander is identified as a clinically relevant allergen, the animal should be removed from the home. If this is not acceptable for the family, the pet can be washed weekly, kept off upholstered furniture, and out of the child's bedroom. In order to minimize cockroach allergen exposure, food and garbage should be kept in closed containers and disposed of regularly.

Pharmacologic Therapy

In some cases, controlling exposure to the offending allergen is sufficient, particularly when an individual has only a limited number of sensitivities. However, because complete avoidance is often not feasible, additional treatment is needed. Multiple medications are available to treat allergic diseases, and the pharmacologic treatment of each allergic process has been outlined in the preceding sections. The general characteristics of the most commonly used medications will be discussed in more detail here. These medications include antihistamines, decongestants, corticosteroids (oral, inhaled, and intranasal), and leukotriene modifiers.

Antihistamines are generally used for allergic rhinitis, atopic dermatitis, allergic conjunctivitis, urticaria, and in the treatment of acute allergic reactions or anaphylaxis to foods, medications, insect stings, and latex. These medications target the histamine receptor and are classified according to their chemical structure and sedative properties. They affect histamine release, the production of adhesion molecules, and recruitment of inflammatory cells. First generation antihistamines have been available for over 50 years and are effective in treating allergic disease; however, they penetrate the central nervous system and have a variety of side effects such as sedation, changes in appetite, dry mouth, and urinary retention. They also may cause psychomotor impairment, and studies have shown evidence of this effect while driving. However, second-generation antihistamines are now available that are not associated with these side effects.

When nasal congestion is the predominant symptom of allergic rhinitis, patients may benefit from decongestants that decrease respiratory mucosal edema. These are available in oral and topical formulations and are often used in conjunction with antihistamines. It is important to emphasize that prolonged use of topical nasal decongestants can lead to rebound effects with a paradoxical increased nasal congestion.

Corticosteroids are anti-inflammatory agents used to treat a variety of allergic diseases and are available in oral, intranasal, and inhaled formulations. They act by binding to special receptors inside the cell and altering the transcription of genes encoding inflammatory proteins. They are usually used in combination with other agents and are the mainstay of therapy for persistent asthma as described above. Intranasal and inhaled corticosteroids are the preferred method of delivery; however, systemic corticosteroids may be required in patients with severe, persistent symptoms.

Leukotrienes are newly synthesized mediators produced by mast cells during the allergic response. Medications, called leukotriene modifiers, are available that interfere with the interaction of leukotrienes with their receptor. These medications are administered orally and are used in the treatment of asthma and allergic rhinitis.

Allergen Immunotherapy

Immunotherapy, or allergy vaccines, is the repeated administration of specific allergens to an individual that changes the IgE-mediated response so as to reduce symptoms when naturally exposed to these allergens. Circumstances in which immunotherapy must be considered include: (1) when symptoms are severe or persistent despite maximal pharmacologic and avoidance management and (2) when allergen exposure is unavoidable. Immunotherapy is effective in the treatment of allergic rhinitis, allergic conjunctivitis, allergic asthma, and stinging-insect hypersensitivity. There are no well-controlled studies that support the use of conventional immunotherapy for food allergy or atopic dermatitis. Allergy vaccines are usually administered over a period of 3–5 years, and studies have shown that improvement in symptoms persists for at least 3 years following vaccine discontinuation. Immunotherapy should only be given under the supervision of a specialist in allergy and immunology and in a setting where trained personnel are available to respond to allergic emergencies.

Education

Individuals with allergic diseases should have ongoing education regarding their diagnosis, allergen avoidance, and medication regimen. This is most helpful when tailored to the child and family and reinforced at regular intervals. Furthermore, written emergency action plans containing guidelines for managing exacerbations and/or severe allergic reactions are useful for individuals with food allergy, stinging-insect hypersensitivity, and asthma.

Summary

Allergic disease is one of the most common chronic conditions in childhood. At a cellular level, it results from the interaction of allergen with allergen-specific IgE on the surface of mast cells and basophils, resulting in the release in chemical mediators and the influx of inflammatory cells. The effect of this process in various target organs results in the clinical signs and symptoms of allergy. Asthma, atopic dermatitis, allergic rhinitis, and food allergy are the most common allergic diseases affecting children, and the prevalence of these conditions has risen in recent years. Recent advances in the understanding of allergic pathophysiologic mechanisms are leading to advancement in the prevention and treatment of these diseases.

See also: Asthma; Immune System and Immunodeficiency.

Suggested Readings

Adkinson NF, Yunginger JW, Busse WW, *et al.* (eds.) (2003) *Middleton's Allergy Principles and Practice,* 6th edn., 2 vols. Philadelphia, PA: Mosby.

Bielory L, Bock SA, Busse WW, *et al.* (eds.) (2000) *The Allergy Report,* 3 vols. The American Academy of Allergy, Asthma and Immunology.

Bock SA (1987) Prospective appraisal of complaints of adverse reactions to foods in children during the first 3 years of life. *Pediatrics* 79: 683–688.

Leung DYM, Sampson HA, Geha RS, and Szefler SJ (eds.) (2003) *Pediatric Allergy Principles and Practice.* St. Louis, MO: Mosby.

Meltzer EO (2006) Allergic rhinitis: Managing the pediatric spectrum. *Allergy and Asthma Proceedings* 27(1): 2–8.

National Asthma Education and Prevention Program (1997) Expert Panel Report 2: Guidelines for the diagnosis and management of asthma. NIH publication 4051. Bethesda, MD.

Sicherer SH and Leung DYM (2005) Advances in allergic skin disease, anaphylaxis, and hypersensitivity reactions to foods, drugs and insects. *The Journal of Allergy and Clinical Immunology* 116: 153–163.

Sicherer SH and Sampson HA (2006) Food allergy. *The Journal of Allergy and Clinical Immunology* 117: S470–S475.

Relevant Websites

http://www.aaaai.org – American Academy of Allergy, Asthma & Immunology.

http://www.theallergyreport.com – The Allergy Report.

http://www.foodallergy.org – The Food Allergy & Anaphylaxis Network.

Asthma

R W Hendershot, University of Colorado Health Sciences Center, Denver, CO, USA

Glossary

Airway – The part of the respiratory system through which air is carried, from the mouth, through the trachea, bronchi, and throughout the alveoli of the lung.

Airway or bronchial hyperreactivity – A term used to describe one of the three main features of asthma. It describes how the airways of the lungs in an asthmatic patient are easily triggered to constrict causing an acute asthma attack and airflow obstruction.

Albuterol – A generally inhaled medication, known as a bronchodilator, that relieves narrowing of the airways caused by bronchospasm.

Allergen/antigen – A substance, usually a protein, that can cause an allergic reaction.

Allergy – A clinical condition in which the body has an exaggerated response to an allergen, usually hypersensitivity; the expression of atopy.

Asthma action plan – A written summary of what actions a patient and their family are to take when their child's asthma worsens. In young children, the asthma action plan is based on symptoms.

Atopic march – The progression of allergic disease an individual may undergo as they mature; generally begins with eczema (atopic dermatitis) and food allergies as an infant and progresses through to asthma and eventually allergic rhinitis (hay fever).

Atopy – A genetically determined state of IgE-mediated hypersensitivity to allergens, the likelihood of being clinically allergic.

Basophil – A type of circulating immune cell that plays a role in the allergic response by releasing chemicals such as histamine when exposed to allergens.

β-blocker – A medicine used to treat high blood pressure and heart disease by blocking β-adrenergic receptors. Its use can make asthma worse.

Bronchoscopy – A procedure performed to examine the airways of the lungs (bronchi) visually with a flexible lighted tube.

Bronchospasm – A tightening of the muscles around the airways of the lungs (bronchi) causing the diameter of the airways to constrict.

Endotoxin – A molecule found in the outer membrane of Gram-negative bacteria, exposure to which is hypothesized to protect against the expression of atopy–allergy and asthma.

Eosinophil – A type of immune cell generally used by mammals to fight parasitic infections but primarily responsible for the damaging effects of atopic disease.

FEV1 – The volume of air an individual can exhale in the first second of a forced exhalation.

Gastroesophageal reflux disease (GERD)/acid reflux – A disease in which acid 'refluxes' into the esophagus from the stomach.

IgE – Allergic antibody that triggers allergic reactions when it comes in contact with allergen.

Inflammation – The body's response to injury typically manifested by redness and swelling.

Lymphocyte – A type of circulating immune white blood cell responsible for coordinating the immune response to infection or injury.

Mast cell – A type of tissue immune cell that, like the basophil, is part of the allergic response.

Mendelian genetics – The set of primary tenets that govern the transmission of an organism's physical characteristics to its offspring. Based upon principles originally put forth by Gregor Mendel. Mendel was a nineteenth-century Austrian monk who discovered and published his results based upon plant hybrid experiments. Mendel explained that an organism inherits two copies of each gene, one from each parent. Each gene is either dominant or recessive in its physical expression. A dominant gene expresses itself as a physical characteristic no matter what gene is inherited from the other parent. A recessive gene is only expressed when both inherited genes are the same.

Nebulizer – A machine that aerosolizes medicine for inhalation into the lung.

Obstructive lung disease – A category of lung disease classified as such because it makes getting air out of the lungs more difficult. In its most severe form it traps air in the lungs making air exchange impossible, which can lead to death.

Peak flow meter – A tool used to measure the severity of a patient's asthma by measuring the maximal velocity with which air exits the lungs.

Reactive airway disease (RAD) – A disease that commonly causes wheezing in infants and young children. It differs from asthma in that RAD is common and transient, usually resolving by the time the child is 5 years old. If the child has persistent wheezing the diagnosis is more likely asthma.

Spirometry – A lung test that evaluates how well air moves in and out of a patient's lungs. It requires patient coordination and cooperation to perform the test.

Therapeutic index – A way of comparing the benefits and risks of medical interventions such as a medication or surgery.

Upper respiratory infection (URI) – Most commonly called a 'cold', the technical term for a viral infection of the nose and sinus.

Wheeze – The sound created as air is breathed through constricted airways.

Introduction

The word asthma is derived from the Greek *aazein*, which means to exhale with an open mouth or to pant. It was first used in the Iliad to describe a short-drawn breath. From a clinical standpoint, Hippocrates was the first Western physician to write about it in *Corpus Hippocraticum*. By AD 1, when asthma was described by the clinician

Aretaeus of Cappadocia, its place as a clinical entity became well known. Sir William Osler was among the first to describe asthma as inflammation of the bronchi, and by 1909 allergenic sensitization of smooth muscle in animals was demonstrated. Today asthma is defined as a chronic disease of the lung manifest clinically as episodic obstruction of pulmonary airflow. Airflow obstruction is caused by inflammation, mucous plugging, and bronchial hyperreactivity that leads to wheezing, chest tightness, excessive mucous production, shortness of breath, and sensitivity to irritants.

The American Lung Association marks asthma as the seventh-ranked chronic health condition in the US and the leading cause of chronic illness among children. While many patients perceive their disease to be only episodic in nature, 80% of asthmatics have persistent symptoms. There are estimated to be over 20 million Americans who suffer from asthma. Of these, approximately 9 million are under 18 years of age, with 3–5% of adults and 7–10% of children affected. The Centers for Disease Control and Prevention (CDC) estimated that for 2004, asthmatic children missed 12.8 million schooldays, made 7 million outpatient visits, had 750 000 emergency room visits, and 198 000 hospitalizations for asthma. Asthma hospitalizations alone represented 3% of all hospitalizations among children. There were 186 deaths from childhood asthma in 2004 in the US. Asthma continues to be the leading cause of school absenteeism due to a chronic illness, and asthma-related direct and indirect healthcare costs are estimated to exceed $14 billion a year. Even though the prevalence of asthma increases with age, healthcare use is highest among the very young.

The prevalence of asthma has steadily increased since at least 1980. However, since 1997 the frequency of asthma-related hospitalizations and deaths have declined. We assume this is due to the progress made in both, treatment and education, of those affected with the disease. Despite great progress in therapy, there remains a major disparity in both morbidity and mortality among racial and ethnic populations. Specifically African–American inner-city asthmatics have a threefold higher risk of both death and hospital admission than asthmatics in other segments of the population.

It is estimated by the Asthma and Allergy Foundation of America that everyday in the US:

- 40 000 people miss school or work due to asthma,
- 30 000 people have an asthma attack,
- 5000 people visit the emergency room due to asthma,
- 1000 people are admitted to hospital, and
- 14 people die due to asthma.

Asthma is defined as a triad of inflammation, airway hyperreactivity, and mucous plugging. However, patients identify most with episodes of acute episodic airflow obstruction causing wheezing and chest tightness. These episodes are extremely anxiety-inducing and very memorable. While 20% of asthmatics have what is referred to as mild intermittent disease, 80% have persistent disease that requires a daily medication. Many asthmatics, with good control, feel completely well between acute episodes and have no symptoms. Most asthmatics achieve that control through strict adherence to their daily medications. In general, asthma does not mean limiting an individual's activity. It is rarely grounds for labeling a child as 'brittle' or the reason why an individual cannot compete on the athletic field. John Weiler, reporting about the 1996 Summer Olympics, commented that more than 20% of the athletes who participated might be considered asthmatic, and that 10.4% of the athletes stated that they took asthma medications either during the games or on a regular basis. While asthma has no cure and there is no treatment that will end the disease, there are some asthmatics that experience a spontaneous remission or outgrow their childhood disease. For most, asthma is a significant but manageable disease, and appropriate care and attention to detail allows the asthmatic to live a normal life.

Effects of Asthma on the Airways

Asthma targets the airways of the lungs. It interferes with our ability to breathe by impeding the process with which our lungs move air in or out. For this reason asthma is referred to as an obstructive disease. In an acute exacerbation, as an asthmatic inhales, air moves into the lungs because expansion of the chest wall creates a negative pressure, allowing air to flow into the lung. However, during exhalation, outflow is obstructed. As the chest wall collapses and pushes air out, the resultant force compresses the airways of an asthmatic, and air is trapped in the lungs. This process can continue until the lungs are hyperexpanded to the point that no more air can get in and a catastrophic failure occurs.

In the 1950s asthma was thought to be a disease characterized by reversible airway obstruction that either resolved spontaneously or resolved following therapy. In the 1960s asthma was viewed as an episodic disease with airway obstruction caused by airway hyperreactivity. The goal of therapy then became relief of bronchoconstriction. This was and still is accomplished by bronchodilator medications known as relievers. In 1969, Dunhill and co-workers detailed the first histopathological evidence of inflammation in asthma when postmortem examinations were performed on asthmatics who died from the disease. It became obvious that tissue damage from airway edema, infiltration by immune cells (especially eosinophils) and excessive mucus secretion were complications of fatal asthma. However, the extent to which inflammation played a role in patients with more mild disease was still unclear. In the 1980s and 1990s, laboratory research and the use of flexible bronchoscopy as a diagnostic tool, led to the understanding that inflammation plays a part in all asthmatics. The beneficial effect of inhaled corticosteroids (ICSs), introduced in the 1970s and coming into wide acceptance in the 1980s for even mild asthmatics, emphasizes the central role of inflammation in asthma. ICSs are now referred to as controllers because of the long-term effect they have in controlling inflammation.

The asthma inflammatory process begins with an acute insult such as an allergen causing both an early (5–15 min) and late (2–6 h) response. The early response, characterized by immediate bronchial constriction and relieved by bronchodilators, begins as antibodies in the immunoglobulin E (IgE) class bind allergen, causing mast cell activation. IgE is the class of antibody responsible for allergies. Activated mast cells then release inflammatory mediators such as histamine and tryptase. These mediators lead to airway hyperreactivity and bronchoconstriction. The late response occurs because mast cell tryptase induces an influx of neutrophils and eosinophils into the airways. The contents of these immune cells are also released causing further inflammation and airway hyperreactivity. These two phases of asthma, early bronchoconstriction and late inflammation, are what reliever and controller medications, respectively, treat.

The director of the asthma orchestra is the T cell, particularly a subgroup known as T-helper cells (Th cells). T cells are so-called because they mature in the thymus, an organ found in the chests of young children which, if not functioning properly *in utero*, leads to immunodeficiency in the newborn. Two distinct Th-cell populations are described, based on which cytokines they release. Th1 cells preferentially secrete interleukin (IL)-2, interferon-γ (IFN-γ), and tumor necrosis factor (TNF)-β. IFN-γ directly inhibits B cells from producing IgE antibodies. Asthmatics are skewed toward responding to allergen exposure with a Th2 response. Th2 cells preferentially secrete IL 4, IL 5, and IL 13. IL 4 and IL 13 induce B cells to produce IgE antibodies. IL-5 is important for eosinophil survival, maturation, and migration from blood into tissues. Th1 cells and their cytokines are important for fighting viral and bacterial infections. Th2 cells, eosinophils, and IgE are important for fighting parasitic infections. Immunotherapy (allergy shots) works in part by shifting the immune system from a Th2 to a Th1 response.

Eosinophils are the primary immune cells believed to cause most of the damage in the lung that leads to asthma. This damage causes increased mucus production, a thickening of the basement membrane that surrounds the airways of the lung, and bronchial hyperreactivity. These processes reduce the caliber of the airway causing

wheezing and the disease we refer to as asthma. If this process goes unchecked, it can lead to airway remodeling and an irreversible loss of lung function.

The amount of inflammation in the lungs of an asthmatic can be quantified several ways. It was first measured by bronchoscopy. Bronchoscopy is a procedure performed that allows a visual examination of the bronchi via a flexible lighted tube and permits the bronchoscopist to obtain microscopic samples of the airways and bronchoalveolar lavage (BAL) fluid washed from the alveoli of the lung. With the tissue, BAL fluid, and a microscope the pathologist can directly measure the amount of inflammation. However, because the risks involved with sedating a child and introducing a foreign object into the lungs is significant, this is only done when essential to help the patient. More commonly, a specialist may measure the inflammation indirectly. This can be accomplished by measuring the percentage of eosinophils in a patient's sputum or the amount of exhaled nitric oxide (NO, a byproduct of eosinophilic inflammation). The long-term treatment of asthma focuses on interruption of the inflammatory cascade via ICSs. The success of that treatment can be evaluated by measuring the response of an asthmatic's inflammation to therapy, as described earlier. This makes these tools very valuable.

In addition to inflammation, asthma is characterized by airway hyperreactivity. 'Reactivity' here refers to the contraction of smooth muscles around the airways resulting in a clinically significant reduction in the internal diameter of the airway, which leads to wheezing. Hyperreactivity denotes an airway that constricts with a minimal amount of stimulus. Stimuli are varied but most commonly include cold air, exercise, allergen, infection, or toxic stimuli such as tobacco smoke and pollution. Of the primary physiological responses in asthma, hyperreactivity is the most widely appreciated because of its immediate clinical effect. Patients understand that if they are exposed to one of their exacerbating stimuli, asthma worsens.

Hyperreactivity is quantifiable. Done by performing an evaluation known as a methacholine, or bronchoprovocational, challenge, it is useful because the more reactive a patient's airways, the more severe their disease. A bronchoprovocational challenge is performed by delivering an agent such as methacholine or histamine in increasing doses until the patient experiences a 20% decrease in their forced expiratory volume in 1 second (FEV1). FEV1 is the volume of air an individual can exhale in the first second of a forced exhalation as measured with a spirometer. A spirometer is a machine used to measure lung function by measuring the volume and flow rate of air during both inhalation and expiration. The PC20 in a bronchoprovocational challenge is the dose of methacholine or histamine at which the patient's FEV1 drops by 20%. There is an inverse relationship between the dose of the agent needed to drop an individual's FEV1 by 20% and the severity of their disease.

Asthma in Young Children

Generally children under 5 years old are incapable of performing the spirometry studies necessary to calculate a PC20. However, some specialists are successful in getting children as young as 4 years old to do it. There is a fair amount of cooperation needed to perform the test. When a child is unable to cooperate to the degree needed, a physician may evaluate a child by performing the provocational challenge and measuring tissue oxygenation and auscultating the chest as the agent is given. Auscultation is the act in which a physician listens to a patient's chest with a stethoscope as they breathe. This allows the physician to assess if a child wheezes or develops other symptoms of concern. While this test is generally unnecessary, it can be helpful if the diagnosis is questionable after the history and physical examination are completed.

Infants are born with small airways compared with adults. Because of their smaller airways and frequent exposure to viral upper respiratory infections (URI), infants and young children are prone to wheezing. If a small child experiences an insult to the airways, they need constrict only minimally before wheezing and increased work of breathing occur. Asthma is the most common cause of wheezing in children 5–18 years old. This is not so in infants and toddlers, whose wheezing is classified as 'reactive airway disease' (RAD). This response is most commonly associated with a viral URI, which causes inflammation and constriction of the infant's airways, leading to wheezing. Most children who experience URI-induced wheezing, however, will not go on to develop asthma. According to the Tucson Respiratory Children's Study:

- 60% of all children will wheeze transiently in early life ('transient wheezers'),
- 85% of children who transiently wheeze will not have asthma,
- 15% of transient wheezers will go on to develop asthma, and
- the most common cause of transient wheezing is a viral URI like the respiratory syncytial virus (RSV), rhinovirus, or the parainfluenzae virus.

In most asthmatics, allergy (or atopy) plays a major role. Atopy is the hereditary predisposition to develop IgE-mediated hypersensitivity to foods, pollen, and animal dander. Allergy is the clinical manifestation of atopy. The immune processes that are in disarray in asthma are stimulated by the interaction of allergens with IgE.

For most patients: good control of allergies, strict adherence to asthma medications, and avoidance of asthma triggers allows them to live normal lives.

Natural History of Allergic Diseases

Allergic diseases are closely related. These include atopic dermatitis (commonly called eczema), food allergy, allergic rhinitis (hay fever), and asthma. Most people who are allergic have more than one of the allergic diseases and having one increases the chances of a child having a combination of them. For example, if a child has severe atopic dermatitis there is a more than 80% chance that the child will eventually have asthma as well. More than 80% of adult asthmatics become so before 6 years of age. Most start down the path toward asthma going along what is referred to as the 'atopic march'. Atopy is a genetically determined state of IgE-mediated hypersensitivity to allergens, the likelihood of being clinically allergic. The atopic march often begins in infancy when the child may have food allergy and atopic dermatitis. Many children grow out of these conditions but others progress toward having asthma and allergic rhinitis. The peak prevalence of atopic dermatitis and food allergy is at 1 year of age. Asthma peaks between 7 and 9 years old, while the peak prevalence of allergic rhinitis occurs in adolescence.

Most infants and young children will wheeze at some time in their life as mentioned earlier. Of course predicting which wheezing children will advance to asthma and which will not is of great interest. A clinical study from the Tucson Children's Respiratory Group in 2000 sought to define an asthma-predictive index for children. In this study it was shown that risk factors for the development of asthma were: a parent with asthma, physician-diagnosed atopic dermatitis, evidence of allergy shown by a positive allergic skin test, wheezing apart from colds, and eosinophilia. (Eosinophilia occurs with increased numbers of circulating eosinophils.) Risk factors for adult-onset asthma include: respiratory infections, tobacco smoke, obesity, occupational exposures, medications, and allergies. A triad of asthmatic disease more common in adults than children is chronic sinusitis associated with nasal polyposis (a condition in which small sac-like growths of inflamed nasal tissue occur in the nose), and a hypersensitivity to nonsteroidal anti-inflammatory medications such as aspirin or ibuprofen.

What Causes Asthma

The etiology of asthma is not straightforward. Asthma is not inherited based on the principles of simple Mendelian genetics. This means that there is no single asthma gene that works in either an autosomal recessive or autosomal dominant manner. Instead, asthma is linked to multiple genes, and the likelihood that an individual will have the disease is multifactorial. Not only are the genetics difficult but asthma, as a disease, is a complex interaction between the environment and the genetic make-up of the individual. It appears that both contribute equally. Research studying the influence genes have on asthma is ongoing and should increase our understanding of, and ability to treat, the disease. Studies attempting to understand the impact the environment has on asthma are ongoing. This research includes everything from allergens to viral and atypical bacterial infections to endotoxin, a component of Gram-negative bacteria. There are several theories about how the interaction between a human's genes and environment leads to asthma. Some studies lend credence to the theories (**Figure 1**).

Originally it was assumed that air pollution was the primary driver behind the increase in asthma worldwide. However, in 1992 and again in 1994, Erika Von Mutius compared the rates of allergy and asthma in East and West Germany. She hypothesized that in these two genetically identical populations, individuals growing up in the more polluted East would suffer from increased allergies, especially asthma. To her surprise, her studies found the opposite to be true. East Germany had less allergic disease than West Germany.

Extending Von Mutius's findings, D. J. Keeley noted that asthma was more prevalent in children from wealthier,

urban environments than in those from poor rural areas. Further studies proposed various causes for the increased prevalence of asthma, including increased tobacco exposure, vaccinations, antibiotic use, obesity, acetaminophen (Tylenol) use during pregnancy, decreased parasite exposure, breastfeeding, or endotoxins. Altered patterns of microflora in the gastrointestinal tract, daycare attendance, and birth order have all been scrutinized. Presently the most popular theory as to the cause of the increasing prevalence of asthma is the 'hygiene hypothesis'.

The 'hygiene hypothesis' states that, from the uterus, the immune system is primed to fight infection. Once the baby is born, if minimal infectious exposures occur, the immune system will expend energy responding to proteins such as animal dander and pollen, and the individual will be allergic. Thus, the good hygiene of contemporary society allows the developing infant to avoid infection, and, as a result, allergies occur and the prevalence of asthma increases.

Diagnosing Asthma

Asthma can be difficult to diagnose. A child who presents with complaints of a persistent cough, wheezing, shortness of breath, or chest tightness likely has asthma. With these complaints, an alternative diagnosis might include acute viral or bacterial infections, postnasal drip secondary to chronic sinusitis or rhinitis, gastroesophageal reflux disease (GERD), chronic lung disease, cystic fibrosis,

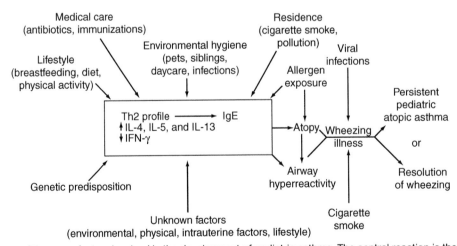

Figure 1 Diagram of the many factors involved in the development of pediatric asthma. The central reaction is the interaction of an individual's genetic composition and their environment that leads to a Th-2 immune response, as indicated by increased release of the mediators of allergy (interleukins 4, 5, and 13) and decreased release of the central mediator of the Th1 response (IFN-γ). The end result is an increase in the key mediator of atopy, IgE, which leads to the symptoms of atopy and bronchial hyperreactivity. This can result in wheezing and potentially persistent atopic asthma. Th, T-helper cell; Ig, immunoglobulin; IL, interleukin; IFN-γ, interferon gamma. Adapted from Johnson CC, Ownby DR, Zoratti EM, et al. (2002) Environmental epidemiology of pediatric asthma and allergy. *Epidemiologic Reviews* 24: 154–175.

Table 1 Differential diagnosis for asthma in infants and young children

Infectious
Bronchiolitis
Pneumonia
Croup
Bronchiectasis (consider cystic fibrosis, aspiration, and ciliary dyskinesia)
Bronchiolitis obliterans
Chronic sinusitis and rhinitis

Anatomic
Gastroesophageal reflux
Cystic fibrosis
Tracheomalacia or bronchomalacia
Congenital heart disease with failure
Tracheoesophageal fistula
Fixed upper airway obstruction (vascular rings or laryngeal webs)
Tumor or enlarged lymph nodes
Aspiration from swallowing disorder

Other
Foreign object in the lung
Bronchopulmonary dysplasia
Allergic bonchopulmonary aspergillosis
Churg–Strauss syndrome

aspiration, or a congenital anatomic abnormality. By evaluating a patient's history, doing a physical examination, and performing appropriate testing, a physician is usually able to differentiate between asthma and the alternatives (**Table 1**).

An asthma evaluation begins with the history and physical examination. Historical elements important in the diagnosis of asthma include when and how the symptoms began, what were the symptoms and their frequency and severity, what triggers symptoms, and how do they respond to therapy like albuterol or prednisone. A history consistent with a diagnosis of asthma includes: onset at an early age with symptoms of cough and wheeze triggered by URIs, tobacco smoke, or allergen exposure such as dogs and cats. Patients may complain of coughing and wheezing that awakens them from sleep or occurs shortly after waking. More severely affected patients will experience symptoms all the time. Infants and young children may even be hypoxic. A positive response to albuterol or prednisone, while helpful, is not definitive.

Once the diagnosis is made, a physician will focus on potential comorbidities. For example, GERD is known to make asthma worse, as will a dog or cat in the home, chronic sinusitis or rhinitis, and tobacco-smoke exposure.

Classification System for Asthma

The National Institutes of Health (NIH) established the National Asthma Education and Prevention Program (NAEPP) in March of 1989 as a task force to reduce asthma-related illness and death, and to improve the quality of life of asthmatics. Today there are 40 major medical associations and health organizations in addition to numerous Federal agencies that comprise the NAEPP Coordinating Committee. The NAEPP published its first set of guidelines for dealing with asthma in 1991. The guidelines were updated in 1997 to include:

- A stepwise approach to asthma putting an emphasis on the early use of inhaled corticosteroids.
- A classification system for asthma severity used to guide therapy.
- A discussion about asthma prevention.
- A discussion about reducing environmental exposures, including tobacco smoke, as a part of asthma therapy.
- Information about identifying an individual's specific triggers.
- Emphasis on education and self-management.
- Recommendations for aggressive detection and treatment of children.
- Tools to help physicians incorporate the guidelines into their practices.

The guidelines were again updated in 2002 with the incorporation of a new class of medication, the leukotriene receptor antagonists (LTRA) as an alternative controller medication in mild persistent asthma. Another update of the guidelines is expected in 2007. Today, once asthma is diagnosed it is classified according to a patient's clinical severity, pulmonary function, and the amount of medicine required to maintain control of symptoms. In infants and young children, where pulmonary function is difficult to obtain, a physician focuses on the clinical symptoms. The goal of therapy is to reduce a patient's symptoms to what would be consistent with mild intermittent asthma.

A mild intermittent asthmatic is defined as an individual with symptoms requiring use of their albuterol medication no more than twice a week, and with nocturnal symptoms no more than twice a month. Patients who have more persistent symptoms need more intensive therapy. The NAEPP guidelines for a stepwise approach to the treatment of asthma are illustrated ahead. The classifications of asthma are: mild intermittent, mild persistent, moderate persistent, and severe persistent (**Table 2**).

Specifically, the goals of the NAEPP guidelines are: minimal or no chronic symptoms day or night, minimal or no exacerbations, no limitations on activities, no missed work days for parents, maintenance of normal or near-normal pulmonary function, minimal use of albuterol, and minimal or no adverse effects from medications.

Table 2　Classification of asthma severity in infants and young children

Severity	Frequency of symptoms day/night	Most commonly used medications used to establish control in infants and young children
Mild intermittent	≤2 days/week ≤2 nights/month	No daily medication needed
Mild persistent	>2 days/week, <1 time/day <2 nights/month	Recommend: low-dose ICSs, alternatives available
Moderate persistent	Daily symptoms >1 night/week	Medium-dose inhaled corticosteroids, addition of a leukotriene antagonist
Severe persistent	Continous daytime symptoms Frequent nocturnal symptoms	High-dose ICSs, LTRA, and if needed, systemic corticosteroids

Adapted from the National Asthma Education and Prevention Program (NAEPP) guidelines. ICSs, inhaled corticosteroids; LTRA, leukotriene receptor antagonists.

Asthma Therapy

Therapy revolves around the triad of asthma and is the reason all persistent asthmatics need two categories of therapy. Controller therapy is prescribed to treat inflammation and reliever therapy is given to treat bronchoconstriction. Controller therapies are anti-inflammatory in nature and include medications such as ICSs, cromolyn, and LTRAs. Reliever medications are primarily the β-agonists but may also include anticholinergics or theophylline to dilate the airways. Next comes good compliance. No matter how effective a treatment may be, if a medication is not taken as it should be, it will not work. Additionally, triggers that make asthma worse must be avoided. The simplest interventions are often the most effective. Sometimes smoking cessation or removing a cat from the home will work well; and while this seems obvious, this is frequently the most difficult choice for parents or asthmatics to make. Finally, the acute exacerbation must be treated.

The NAEPP guidelines for therapy are based upon expert opinion derived from clinical experience and multicenter, double-blind, placebo-controlled studies. The studies and expert clinicians support the model that the basis of asthma is inflammation of the airway. Consequently, ICSs are the safest and single most effective therapy for asthma reducing both morbidity and mortality. It is because of ICSs that the majority of asthmatics can live relatively normal lives.

There are side effects with all medications. With ICSs the most common side effect is a growth delay of 1 cm in height in the child's first year of use. In long-term studies this delay does not accumulate over the years or affect the ultimate height of the child. Another less common adverse affect is thrush or oral candidiasis (a yeast infection of the mouth), which is usually mitigated by rinsing the mouth or brushing teeth after the ICSs are administered. Less commonly, high-dose ICSs can cause suppression of the adrenal–hypothalamic axis, which is the means with which our bodies make and regulate endogenous cortisol (a corticosteroid). So, while there can be adverse effects from using

ICSs, by placing the medicine where it is needed most, the total amount of corticosteroids are reduced. This decreases the likelihood of side effects from the medication and makes the risk–benefit ratio of ICSs favorable.

In mild persistent asthmatics, LTRA are another treatment option, which may limit the amount of ICSs needed. In young children, ICSs and LTRA are the most frequently used and best-studied medications available. Most other medications such as long-acting β-agonists (salmeterol) are unavailable for use in young children because of the difficulty in administering them. There are orally administered medications such as theophylline and albuterol that have a less favorable risk–benefit ratio.

The medications for treating asthma are generally effective. The limiting factor in achieving control is rarely the medicine. Most frequently it is poor compliance, poor technique in administering ICSs, or both. Often it is a combination of poor compliance and a trigger of some sort that leads to an exacerbation. While the appropriate diagnosis and therapeutic plan is essential to a patient's health, ultimately the most important factor is that medication is taken regularly and appropriately. The final piece of controller therapy is avoidance of triggers. Some would rather live with an annoying cough than not have a cigarette or the family cat, however.

Therapy for an acute severe asthma exacerbation has not changed much in recent years. Inhaled short-acting β2-agonists in combination with systemic corticosteroids are the mainstay. Generally, this is effective. However, on occasion an exacerbation is severe enough to require supplemental oxygen or epinephrine (adrenaline). Either way, ambulance transport to the nearest hospital with the resources to care for such a patient is necessary.

Self-Care and Monitoring: Asthma Action Plans

The asthma action plan is a written summary of what actions a patient and his or her family are to take and is considered the standard of care. In young children, the asthma action plan is based on symptoms. An asthma action plan has three zones. The green zone means all is well and to continue routine medications. The yellow zone indicates caution; a patient should begin using their reliever medications, continue routine medications, and if there is no improvement, contact their physician. Sometimes a physician may recommend that a patient double the dose of ICS if in the yellow zone. The red zone means immediate therapy with a reliever medication is needed, followed by contact with a physician. Asthma is a disease that causes a lot of anxiety; the asthma action plan allows patients to take control of their disease.

Taking control is what makes the asthma action plan work. Asthma that is difficult to treat results most often from a lack of 'buy-in' from patients and their families. As with all chronic diseases, if an asthmatic understands that regular use of their medication will improve their life, they will probably take it. A recent study showed that almost 70% of patients with moderate-to-severe disease would be classified as mild if they took their medications appropriately.

Asthma in Special Populations

Infants and young children are a unique challenge to diagnose and treat. There is no blood test to diagnose asthma, and because infants are unable to perform spirometry, evaluating breathing problems is difficult. For similar reasons the treatment of their asthma is difficult. ICSs depend on patient-coordination to work and are much more difficult to administer than a pill or a liquid. In infants and young children, ICSs take time and effort from the parent. When one combines the difficulty of administering the medication with parental concerns about delayed growth, many parents give up, leaving their child at risk for a severe exacerbation.

The inner city is a difficult environment for an asthmatic. The living conditions may include cockroaches, dust mites, pollution, tobacco smoke, and animal dander, all potential triggers of asthma. Additionally, the inner city is often overcrowded. Asthmatics may have challenging social situations as well. There is often a lack of access to healthcare and limited education or family support. Young inner city asthmatics require close monitoring to avoid a catastrophic outcome.

The asthmatic athlete deserves special attention. Most importantly, with appropriate care almost all of them should be able to compete at their highest level. For example, Jerome Bettis, an all-pro National Football League running back, often speaks about how asthma nearly sidelined his career, and that following his physician's advice on how to control his asthma allowed him to perform. Too many athletes try to power their way through

an asthma exacerbation as they do many of the challenges faced in athletics. If an athlete is hindered by asthma, good care of his asthma will generally fix the problem.

Conclusion

Asthma is one of the most common ailments in society today, and its effect is far-reaching in both human and financial terms. The good news is that for most asthmatics, therapy can result in an active normal life.

Some of the key points can be stated as below:

- Asthma is a chronic disease characterized by airway inflammation, bronchial hyperreactivity, and mucous plugging causing airflow obstruction and wheezing.
- While 85% of children with early wheezing do so transiently, the prevalence of asthma has risen for decades and only now seems to be leveling.
- The mainstay of asthma therapy is control, with ICSs as the first-line agents. If a patient is using a short-acting bronchodilator medication more than twice a week for their asthma symptoms, their disease is out of control and their management plan needs revision.
- In general, asthma should pose no limitation to normal activity with appropriate monitoring, therapy, and symptom awareness.
- Compliance with taking medications is the key to asthma control.
- If asthma is limiting a person's lifestyle they need to see their doctor.

See also: Allergies; Immune System and Immunodeficiency.

Suggested Readings

Hannaway PJ (2002) *Asthma – An Emerging Epidemic.* Marblehead, MA: Lighthouse Press.
Johnson CC, Ownby DR, Zoratti EM, *et al.* (2002) Environmental Epidemiology of Pediatric Asthma and Allergy. *Epidemiologic Reviews* 24: 154–175.
Leung DYM, Sampson HA, Geha RS, and Szefler SJ (2003) *Pediatric Allergy Principles and Practice* 2–3, 32–43: 10–38, 337–472.
Plaut TF and Jones TB (1999) *Asthma Guide for People of All Ages.* Amherst, MA: Pedipress.

Relevant Websites

http://www.aaaai.org – American Academy of Asthma, Allergy and Immunology.
http://www.aap.org – American Academy of Pediatrics.
http://www.aafa.org – Asthma and Allergy Foundation of America.
www.nhlbi.nih.gov – National Heart Lung and Blood Institute.
http://health.nih.gov – National Institutes of Health (NIH).

Auditory Development and Hearing Disorders

D H Ashmead, A M Tharpe, and D P Sladen, Vanderbilt University Medical Center, Nashville, TN, USA

Glossary

Auditory brainstem response (ABR) – Electrical activity in the auditory nerve and brainstem in response to sound.

Cochlear implants – A hearing technology in which environmental sounds are picked up by a microphone and converted to electrical signals that are delivered to the inner ear.

Decibel – A measure of the relative intensities of two sounds, expressed in logarithmic units.

Evoked otoacoustic emissions (OAE) – Faint sounds produced in the inner ear in response to external sounds, used to screen for auditory function in infants.

Hearing aids – A hearing technology in which environmental sounds are picked up by a microphone, amplified, and delivered as sounds to the ear canal.

Hearing level (HL) – Measure of the intensity of a sound relative to the intensity at which young adults with good hearing can hear a sound of that frequency.

Sound pressure level (SPL) – Measure of the intensity of a sound relative to a single reference value of 20 Pa.

Introduction

The auditory system responds to sounds, which are fluctuations in the pressure of a medium such as air or water. Sounds are created by physical events, many of which are important to listeners, such as approaching footsteps, spoken words, or falling water. **Figure 1** shows the overall structure of the outer, middle, and inner parts of the ear.

Overview of Auditory System

Sound is gathered by the pinna and directed along the ear canal to the eardrum, or tympanic membrane, which is the boundary between the outer and middle ear. The shape of the pinna funnels sound toward the ear canal, and also filters sound differently depending on the direction of the sound source, which provides a cue for localizing sounds. The pressure changes in the arriving sound make the eardrum vibrate. The middle ear is a cavity normally filled with air. The Eustachian tube connects the middle ear to the throat, allowing the air pressure in the middle ear to equalize to the outside air pressure. Movement of the eardrum is picked up by the three bones, also called the ossicles, in the middle ear (malleus, incus, and stapes). The stapes connects to the cochlea of the inner ear at a flexible membrane called the oval window, so that movement of the stapes creates pressure waves in the fluid inside the cochlea. The overall path from the outer ear to the oval window works to amplify sound by a substantial amount. Some of this amplification comes from the funneling effect of the outer ear and the mechanical structure of the middle ear bones, but most comes from the fact that the area of the eardrum is about 17 times larger than that of the oval window, just as the head of a nail is much larger than its tip. The amplification is greater at middle sound frequencies than at low or high frequencies.

The cochlea in mammals is a snail-shaped coil, making about two-and-a-half turns in humans. The cochlea has three fluid-filled spaces running along its length, with a surface called the basilar membrane also running lengthwise. A complex sensory structure called the Organ of Corti rests on the basilar membrane. Among other details, the Organ of Corti has a single row of inner hair cells and three rows of outer hair cells running along its length. The inner hair cells, about 3500 to 4000 per ear, are activated when pressure changes in the cochlear fluids cause motion of the basilar membrane, to which the bases of the hair cells are attached. These hair cells are the sensory transducers of the auditory system, converting sound energy into neural signals going to the brain. When an inner hair cell moves, the stereocilia (hairs) at its tip are deflected. This deflection allows potassium ions to enter the cell, which in turn sends neurotransmitter chemicals to the nearby auditory nerve fibers. Action potentials (spikes of electrical energy) arise in those fibers and are carried along the auditory nerve toward the brain. About 40 000 auditory nerve fibers connect to each ear, so each inner hair cell is linked to a number of nerve fibers.

The mechanical properties of the inner ear are elegantly structured so that sounds of high frequency mostly activate inner hair cells closer to the oval window or base of the cochlea, while sounds of lower frequency activate inner hair cells further along toward the apex. This 'place principle' is an important part of how the auditory system

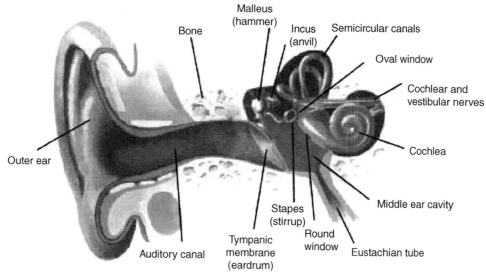

Figure 1 Structure of the auditory system. Reproduced from Widex South Africa, Understanding your Ear.

distinguishes between sounds of different frequencies. A Nobel Prize was awarded to Georg von Békésy for research begun in the 1920s on cochlear mechanics. The other way that the auditory system keeps track of sound frequency is that the action potentials in the auditory nerve fibers can be timelocked to the sound frequency. This process works for low-to-middle frequency sounds.

The outer hair cells, about 11 500 per ear, are also activated by sounds, but their activity is, for the most part, not relayed to the brain. Instead, the outer hair cells change their length slightly in response to sounds, which has the effect of making that section of the basilar membrane vibrate more strongly, providing a stronger signal to the inner ear cells. This process is especially important when the incoming sound intensity is low to medium. For this reason, the activity of the outer hair cells is referred to as the cochlear amplifier. An important practical point is that this outer hair cell activity generates faint noises that can be recorded by a microphone placed in the ear canal. These 'otoacoustic emissions' provide the basis for testing if young infants can hear. Another key point about both the inner and outer hair cells is that, in mammals, they cannot regenerate after being damaged. The term 'sensorineural hearing impairment' is used to refer to such damage.

Proceeding from the inner ear toward the brain, the auditory nerve of each ear connects to brainstem structures called the cochlear nuclei, one on each side. The ventral part of each cochlear nucleus projects to the superior olivary complex structures in the brainstem, on both the same and opposite sides. The superior olives in turn project to the inferior colliculi. The dorsal part of each cochlear nucleus projects to the same and opposite side inferior colliculi. An important functional point is that all structures in the ascending auditory pathways

beyond the cochlear nuclei receive input from both ears. In many listening situations, such as noisy settings, the differences between sounds arriving at the two ears provide a basis for enhanced perception.

The absolute auditory sensitivity of adults varies with sound frequency. Sensitivity is best for the middle range of frequencies from about 500 to 4000 Hz. At frequencies below and above this range, sensitivity worsens substantially. Comparing measures of auditory sensitivity across studies is complicated by the fact that subtle details of the methodology can have a big effect on the results. For this reason, audiologists conduct clinical measures of sensitivity using standardized procedures and instruments.

Another complication is that there are several measurement systems for reporting sensitivity. Each system uses units called decibels (dB). In hearing science the decibel expresses the ratio between the pressures of two sounds, p_1 and p_2:

$$dB = 20 \log_{10}\left(\frac{p_1}{p_2}\right)$$

The term p_1 is the pressure of a sound of interest, such as the softest sound someone can detect in a hearing test, and the term p_2 is a reference value. There are two widely used reference systems, known as the SPL system and the HL system. SPL stands for 'decibels, relative to a sound pressure level of 20 μPa. That reference pressure was selected a century ago as the level at which young adults with excellent hearing could just barely detect a 1000 Hz tone. Any observed sound pressure (p_1, measured in micropascals, μPa) can be related to this reference pressure by the formula

$$dB \ SPL = 20 \log_{10}\left(\frac{p_1}{20}\right)$$

For example, normal conversational speech measures about 65 dB SPL at the listener's position, in which case p_1 is approximately 36 000 µPa. This illustrates the wide dynamic range of the auditory system, allowing us to hear both faint and more intense sounds. We can tolerate brief exposure to very intense sounds, such as machinery sounds above 100 dB SPL. To make matters even more complicated, sound measurements can be made with different filters. A commonly used filter is the 'A-weighted' one, designed to mimic the natural frequency filtering of human hearing. Such a measure might be described in units of dB SPL A-scale. As a semantic note, the terms pressure, intensity, and level are all used to refer to the amount of energy in a sound. Although these terms have distinct physical meanings, there is a tendency to use them interchangeably.

The HL or 'hearing level' sound measurement system is used by audiologists when measuring hearing sensitivity to specific sounds. Instead of using a single reference value, this system uses a different reference value for each sound. For example, an audiologist might measure someone's sensitivity to each of a set of tones ranging from 250 to 8000 Hz. For each tone frequency there is a reference level at which typical young adults can just hear the tone. If someone hears the tone at that reference level, then their sensitivity is 0 dB HL. If the person needs the tone to have a pressure four times the reference level in order to hear it, then their sensitivity is about 12 dB HL. In the HL system, then, 0 dB HL corresponds to typical hearing of young adults, while positive values indicate worse hearing sensitivity.

Development of Auditory Structures

The auditory system begins to develop at a gestational age of 25 days, becomes well differentiated by 9 weeks, and is probably functional by 22 weeks or so. The external, middle, and inner ear parts have distinct embryonic histories and can be associated with different kinds of hearing loss if their development is interrupted. There is currently a strong research focus on molecular and genetic influences on ear development, especially using mouse models in which specific genes are altered.

External Ear

At 6 weeks the outer ears start developing from folds on the front neck area of the embryo. A set of six auricular hillocks or bumps arises for each ear. These hillocks are visible as early features of the adult ear. The ear canal forms at 5 weeks, and at about 12 weeks a plate forms at the inner end of the canal. This plate remains until about 7 months, when it dissolves and the remaining tissue forms the tympanic membrane or eardrum. The outer ear and ear canal continue to grow longer after birth, reaching adult size at about 9 years. Failure of the outer ear to develop at all is called anotia, limited growth is called microtia, while partial or complete closure of the ear canal is called atresia.

Middle Ear

At 5 weeks the middle ear cavity begins as an indentation. Meanwhile the three middle ear bones take shape, and are enveloped by the cavity structure. Part of the cavity also forms the Eustachian tube. Disorders of the middle ear can involve the mechanical connections (either loose connections between the bones or total fusion of the bones) for which surgical adjustment is often possible. There are also hearing aids that bypass the middle ear by transmitting sounds to bones of the skull.

Inner Ear

The inner ear development begins around 3.5 weeks of gestational age as the otic placode, which forms into a pit and over the next 12 days closes to become the otic vesicle. The otic vesicle consists of three parts, each leading to different components of the vestibular (balance) and auditory functions of the inner ear. The cochlea develops as an offshoot of one part of this early structure. The turns of the spiral-shaped cochlea are complete by about 9 weeks' gestational age, and the size of the bone structure of the inner ear is adult-like by 17–19 weeks. The structures of the inner ear, including the hair cells and connected auditory nerve fibers, develop on a timetable so that from a neuroanatomical perspective, it is likely that functional hearing begins around 22 weeks' gestational age. Tests of behavioral or electrophysiological responses to sound by fetuses are complicated by methodological problems, but prematurely born infants show brain activity related to sounds by 25 weeks. Also, full-term infants have been shown to respond preferentially to sounds to which they were exposed *in utero*. Considering that full-term gestation is about 40 weeks, it is clear that during the last 3–4 prenatal months the auditory system is actively processing sounds. Nevertheless, the inner ear continues to develop during this period and for many months following full-term birth.

Approximately half of the cases of hearing loss in infants are from known causes. Of these, about 40% are from confirmed genetic causes and 60% from others. Genetic factors are thought to underlie many of the currently unknown cases of infant hearing loss. One example of a genetically based hearing loss involves a protein called connexin 26, which is critical for the formation of junctions between cells. Development of the inner ear can also be affected by prenatal exposure to viruses, bacteria, and drugs. For example, maternal infection by the rubella virus during pregnancy can cause hearing loss, as documented in numerous epidemics across different countries.

Auditory Pathway

A consistent finding in neuroscience studies of the development of vision and hearing is that sensory brain organization depends on neural activity. This can be understood as an efficient way for the brain to adjust to the fine-grained details of the individual's sensory structures. For example, the cochlea maps sounds from high to low frequency, but the specific relationships between individual inner hair cells and sound frequency must be 'learned' by each developing nervous system. Similarly, language development requires exposure to the specific sound system of one's linguistic environment. For many aspects of auditory development, from basic sensitivity to complex activities such as speech perception, it is agreed that refinement of the auditory pathways above the level of the inner ear has a time course extending for months and even years after birth. One important question in this regard is the age at which to provide hearing aids or cochlear implants for infants with hearing loss, an issue taken up later in this article.

Sensitive Periods and Teratogens

As noted earlier, although many cases of hearing loss evident during infancy are the result of genetic causes, the developing auditory system is susceptible to a variety of teratogenic influences from viruses, bacteria, chemicals, and drugs. There appear to be different sensitive periods, that is, times of greatest risk for these influences. For example, rubella infection during pregnancy can cause damage to a number of organs including the ear, but the prospects are worse during the first 16 weeks of gestation than later on. Effects of cytomegalovirus follow a different and more complex time course. Although most infants exposed to this virus do not experience hearing loss, among those who do, the impairment may exist at birth or may become apparent later. Clearly, the timing of sensitive periods differs for different teratogenic agents. Also, some genetically based hearing losses are progressive in nature or have late onset, so that hearing worsens following birth. An important practical implication is that not all hearing losses are apparent in the newborn period, so that regular ongoing assessment of infant hearing is important.

Age Trends in Hearing Sensitivity

Measurement Considerations

The goal in measuring hearing sensitivity is to find the lowest sound level at which a person can just barely detect

a sound, a value known as auditory threshold. In clinical settings this is usually done separately for each ear, and for sounds of different frequencies. A distinction is made between behavioral and electrophysiological measures of infant hearing sensitivity. Several behavioral testing procedures have been devised, somewhat independently, by pediatric audiologists and developmental psychologists. All of these procedures involve presenting infants with sounds and noting whether they make an observable response. Unfortunately, infants do not tend to make reliable, robust responses to soft sounds, especially during the first half year or so after birth. One procedure used with these younger infants is behavioral observation audiometry (BOA), in which the tester looks for any sign of a response to sound, such as eye widening, head turning, or cessation of movement. However, this method is difficult to interpret because of their low responsiveness, so audiologists do not consider it a valid measure of infants' level of hearing sensitivity. Developmental psychologists doing research studies tend to use procedures like BOA, sometimes called observer-based psychoacoustics (OBP). Generally, in research studies by either audiologists or psychologists, measures are taken to keep the observer 'honest' by not knowing whether a weak or strong sound was presented. In clinical settings the observer typically knows the sound level, in order to enhance assessment in a limited time period. Audiologists use a method called visual reinforced audiometry (VRA) for infants older than about 6 months. Infants are taught to turn their heads when a sound occurs in order to see an attractive toy display or a video event. With this method, the question is whether a head turn was made following a given sound.

For most clinical and some research purposes it is customary to present sounds to one ear at a time using small insert earphones. Otherwise, sounds may be played through loudspeakers, an arrangement known as free field. By presenting sounds with different intensities, the examiner finds a threshold intensity at which the infant can just hear the sound. In clinical settings, it is often necessary to obtain thresholds at several different sound frequencies in order to characterize an infant's hearing. One problem with behavioral tests of infant hearing, noted above, is that they are relatively ineffective at ages below about 6 months. This is because young infants do not reliably make overt responses to sounds, even when we know they can hear the sounds well. Therefore, electrophysiological measures of hearing sensitivity also have an important role.

Several electrophysiological measures are used to estimate infant hearing, but the real workhorse is the auditory brainstem response (ABR). The ABR consists of electrical potentials measured by surface electrodes placed on the head, primarily reflecting neural activity of the auditory nerve and along the brainstem. Usually this response is recorded from sounds presented to one ear at a time through insert earphones, although binaural stimulation is possible. It is not only possible but desirable to do this testing while infants are sleeping or sedated, otherwise body movements interfere with the electrical signal. A threshold is found by noting the sound intensity below which the characteristic waveform of the electrical response is absent. A consistent finding, especially during the first year or so after birth, is that hearing sensitivity estimated by the ABR is more acute than by behavioral measures. One reason is that during behavioral testing infants are easily distracted by nonauditory events. However, it is also likely that the ABR reflects auditory processing at a very peripheral level, whereas behavioral testing reflects not only the entire auditory pathway, but also motor responses linked to hearing. Thus, behavioral testing of infants may reveal immaturities in higher-level auditory processing which are not reflected in the ABR. In fact, audiologists regard the ABR and the otoacoustic emissions test (discussed next) not as measures of 'hearing' but rather as measures of functioning in particular parts of the peripheral auditory system.

Another important means of estimating infant hearing is by measuring the presence or absence of otoacoustic emissions (OAE), a technique widely used in screening programs. As noted earlier, these emissions reflect activity of the outer hair cells. This test is not generally used for measuring hearing thresholds, but rather for determining whether a young infant can hear moderately intense sounds. A probe tip is placed in one ear and a sound is delivered through the probe. A very short time later, a microphone in the probe picks up faint sounds produced in the inner ear as part of the auditory system's response to an incoming sound. Most screening programs for newborn-hearing ability use OAE as the initial test. If these emissions are absent or very weak, then follow-up testing with the ABR is carried out.

Age Trends

Newborn infants are much less sensitive to sounds than adults, but typical newborns can hear sounds in the intensity range of normal conversational speech. It is a cause for concern if a newborn infant does not seem to hear sounds of moderate intensity, and the goal of newborn-hearing screening programs is to identify those infants. We turn now to measures of the absolute sensitivity of newborns to sounds of different frequencies. **Figure 2** shows newborn- and adult-hearing sensitivity measured by ABR at frequencies ranging from 500 to 8000 Hz.

Whereas adults have a bow-shaped curve with better sensitivity at middle frequencies, newborn sensitivity is modest across the entire audible frequency range. In fact, an older child or adult with the hearing sensitivity of a newborn would be considered to have a mild-to-moderate hearing loss. The newborn–adult difference is

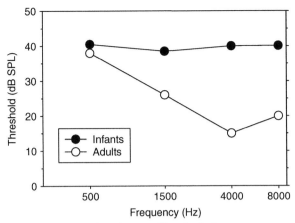

Figure 2 Adult and newborn auditory brainstem response thresholds as a function of sound frequency. SPL, sound pressure level. Adapted from Sininger YS, Abdala C, and Cone-Wesson B (1997) Auditory threshold sensitivity of the human neonate as measured by the auditory brainstem response. *Hearing Research* 104(1–2): 27–38.

least at low frequencies, but this is because adults do not hear low-frequency sounds very well. Thus, auditory sensitivity improves during development at all frequencies, but there is more room for improvement with respect to middle- and high-frequency sounds compared to lower frequencies. The modest hearing sensitivity of newborns is partly attributable to peripheral factors, including the acoustic resonance properties of the ear canal, the mechanical efficiency of the middle ear bones, cochlear function, and coordination of activity across auditory nerve fibers. However, neural organization of the auditory pathways from brainstem to cerebral cortex is also responsible for age changes in auditory sensitivity.

Postnatal development of auditory sensitivity can be characterized by two general trends. First, the pace of development is quite rapid during the first 6–9 months after birth, by which time adult-like sensitivity is approached for middle-to-high frequencies. Second, the rate of development is greater for high-frequency sounds than for low frequencies. In fact, adult sensitivity levels for low-frequency sounds are not achieved until about 4–6 years of age. **Figure 3** shows behaviorally tested sensitivity thresholds across a range of frequencies in 3- and 6-month-olds and adults (9-month-olds were also tested, with results virtually identical to the 6-month-olds).

The general pattern of age-related improvement in auditory sensitivity is paradoxical in that infant–adult differences are initially smallest at low frequencies, yet low-frequency sensitivity reaches adult levels latest during development. This can be understood as a high-to-low-frequency gradient of development, superimposed on the overall human audibility function that has rather poor low-frequency sensitivity.

Most studies of infant hearing sensitivity have been conducted with single age groups, or cross-sectionally with different infants across ages. Longitudinal studies are required to reveal patterns of change within individuals.

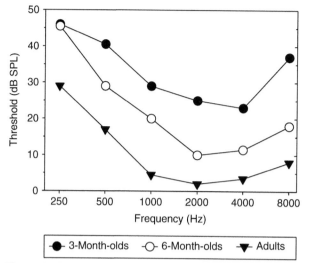

Figure 3 Behavioral thresholds for absolute auditory sensitivity in 3-month-olds, 6-month-olds, and adults. The study also included 12-month-olds, for whom the thresholds were nearly identical to those of the 6-month-olds shown here. SPL, sound pressure level. Adapted from Olsho LW, Koch EG, Carter EA, Halpin CF, and Spetner NB (1988) Pure-tone sensitivity of human infants. *Journal of the Acoustical Society of America* 84(4): 1316–1324.

Figure 4 shows findings from a study of infants followed during the first year, tested for sensitivity to a noise stimulus filtered to match the frequency composition of speech.

These findings confirm, for individual infants, the pattern of rapid development during the first 6–9 months after birth, followed by continued but very gradual improvement in sensitivity. This developmental profile is an important factor when parents and clinicians make intervention decisions about infants with hearing loss.

The factors underlying both the overall rate and the frequency dependency of the development of auditory sensitivity are not well understood. Some of the changes are the result of physical factors in the external and middle ear. The size and shape of the outer ear and ear canal act as frequency filters, and young infants' ears are tuned to favor somewhat higher frequencies than children or adults. Part of the ear canal itself undergoes a cartilage-to-bone transition during infancy. Another physical factor is the transmission of acoustic energy from the ear canal to the middle ear. Again there is a filter property, with an age-related increase in the amount of energy passed to the middle ear, especially at frequencies above about 1500 Hz. In young infants this may be offset to some extent by higher sound levels in the ear canal at some frequencies. Another likely developmental factor is the transmission of energy through the middle ear to the cochlea. As we know from shouting to underwater swimmers from above the surface, sound does not travel well from air to water. The fluid-filled cochlea is essentially an 'underwater'

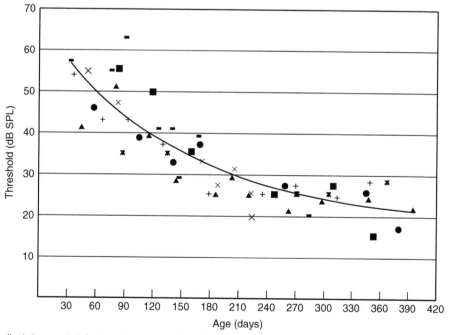

Figure 4 Longitudinal changes in infant auditory sensitivity during the first year after birth. Each symbol style represents a different infant. The curve showing the overall group function was closely matched by individual curves (which are not shown here). SPL, sound pressure level. From Tharpe AM and Ashmead DH (2001) A longitudinal investigation of infant auditory sensitivity. *American Journal of Audiology* 10(2): 104–112.

device which would strongly limit direct transmission of airborne sound (technically, there is an impedance mismatch). The middle ear overcomes this problem by transforming sound energy into mechanical energy, which drives the cochlear fluid via the oval window. Most of the mechanical advantage of the middle ear is because the tympanic membrane is much larger than the oval window, while some additional power comes from the lever action of the middle ear bones. Although it seems likely that middle ear function changes during development, little systematic research has been reported. However, we do know that there is a change in the angle of the tympanic membrane and that the middle ear bones become sleeker over time, thus contributing to some of the changes in sensitivity noted. Although the overall size of middle ear does not change much after birth, its shape and mechanical properties do change in subtle ways.

Cochlear function is an obvious candidate for explaining age changes in hearing sensitivity, but it is difficult to assess cochlear processes independently. Studies of transient otoacoustic emissions (TEOAE) evoked by click stimuli (which carry a wide frequency spectrum) show that even in newborns the response can be elicited by clicks only slightly stronger than needed in adults. This provides some indication that cochlear function is intact by early infancy, but the method is not well suited for assessing thresholds or frequency effects. Another variation on this kind of testing is distortion product otoacoustic emissions (DPOAE), in which several tones differing in frequency serve as the stimuli. Good hearing requires frequency selectivity, but there is a tendency for lower frequency components of sounds to mask or suppress higher frequencies. Studies using this method indicate that cochlear frequency selectivity is immature across the age range of newborn to 3 months, and perhaps older. This could reflect both the passive mechanical properties of inner ear structures and the process of active mechanical adjustments via activity of the outer hair cells. Although these findings on frequency selectivity cannot be applied directly to absolute auditory sensitivity, there is a strong implication that cochlear processes change during the months following birth.

Even when factors involving the external, middle, and inner ear are taken into account, the magnitude of infant–adult threshold differences makes it likely that more central processes are also involved in the development of auditory sensitivity. Studies of postnatal development of the auditory cortex in various species indicate, for example, that although there is a basic plan for frequency-specific zones of cortical neurons, the response properties of these cells depend strongly on an animal's auditory experience. Another idea that has been proposed is that there may be more 'internal noise' (e.g., variability in auditory nerve signal transmission) in infants than in adults.

Hearing Disorders

Classification and Incidence of Hearing Disorders

It is estimated that approximately 278 million people worldwide have some form of disabling hearing loss and that two-thirds of those reside in developing countries. Hearing loss is commonly described in terms of severity and type. Severity of hearing loss is broken into the following five categories based on the individual's auditory thresholds: normal range = 0–20 dB HL; mild loss = 20–40 dB HL; moderate loss = 40–60 dB HL; severe loss = 60–80 dB HL; and profound loss = 80 dB HL or more.

Hearing loss is also classified by type. Specifically, hearing loss is described as conductive, sensorineural, or mixed. Conductive hearing loss refers to a decrease in auditory thresholds resulting from an interruption in the conduction of sound along the ear canal, ear drum, middle ear space, or the middle ear bones (i.e., an impaction of the ear canal, middle ear fluid, or otosclerosis). A purely conductive hearing loss does not involve the cochlea or remaining auditory system and can often be treated with medical intervention (i.e., surgery or antibiotics). The severity of conductive hearing loss may range from mild to moderate, depending on the cause and severity of the pathology. For example, disarticulation of the ossicles completely interrupts the transmission of energy to the cochlea and can result in hearing thresholds up to 60 dB HL.

A sensorineural hearing loss originates from either the cochlea (sensory) or auditory nerve (neural). This type of hearing loss may occur when there is damage or congenital malformation to the cochlea or the auditory nerve, and is most often permanent. The causes of sensorineural hearing loss in children typically include disease (e.g., meningitis), ototoxic medications (e.g., gentamicin, vancomycin), maternal teratogens (e.g., ethanol ingestion), and genetic factors (e.g., connexin 26). A sensorineural hearing loss in adult years may occur because of excessive noise exposure, the aging process, head trauma, or tumors along the auditory nerve.

It is possible for hearing loss to have both a conductive and sensorineural component. For example, an individual may have an ear infection in addition to an already diagnosed sensorineural hearing loss. In this case, the conductive component is expected to resolve. In other cases, an individual may have a permanent conductive hearing loss in addition to a permanent sensorineural hearing loss.

The prevalence of permanent hearing loss with onset in gestation or infancy in European and North American countries is about 1–6 per 1000, with the lower number referring to more severe degrees of bilateral impairment. Many infants and young children experience transient hearing loss as a result of otitis media, a condition in which there is inflammation and possibly fluid buildup in the middle ear, usually associated with bacterial or viral infection. Young children are at greater risk of this condition because the angle of their Eustachian tube does not favor drainage of infectious organisms. Otitis media is among the leading conditions for pediatric office visits. The degree of hearing loss secondary to otitis media is variable. About half of infants and young children with otitis media experience mild hearing loss and 10% have moderate loss. However, evidence for long-term consequences for hearing and language development does not suggest a strong linkage. Practice guidelines have shifted away from aggressive treatment with antibiotics and surgical intervention toward an emphasis on 'watchful waiting'.

Congenital hearing loss can be syndromic or nonsyndromic. A syndromic hearing loss presents itself with other symptoms. For example, Usher syndrome results in visual impairments as well as auditory deficits. However, most children with genetic hearing loss are nonsyndromic and are born to parents who have no family history of hearing loss.

Screening for Hearing Loss

Efforts to identify infants with hearing loss are based on the reasonable assumption that communication skills are a critical component of infant development, with a goal of providing intervention by 6 months of age. Some known risk factors such as premature birth or family history of genetically based hearing loss can be used to target infants for audiological assessment. However, the application of risk-based screening programs is generally thought to miss substantial numbers of infants with hearing problems. Therefore, the goal of universal screening has become popular as a public health approach. These programs have been directed at screening of full-term newborns or prematurely born infants when they are approaching full-term gestational age. A drawback of the focus on newborns is that these programs miss some infants and children with progressive or late-onset hearing loss, as well as some infants with mild degrees of hearing loss.

Newborn hearing screening
Most newborn screening programs use a two-stage procedure. In the first stage, each ear is evaluated separately using an automated OAE test. These tests are usually administered by nursing staff with little training in audiology. As noted earlier, OAE reflect activity of the outer hair cells, which provides an indirect measure of whether the peripheral auditory system is functioning. If either ear fails the OAE test, then an ABR screen is typically performed on each ear. Infants who fail this second screening are referred for a complete audiological evaluation.

Infants born prematurely who have extended hospitalization should be tested as close as possible to their discharge date or their full-term date (whichever comes first), in order to reduce the possibility of failing the screening because of various changes in the ear canal, middle ear, or brainstem.

In general, these screening programs have rather modest epidemiological specificity, meaning that quite a few infants fail the test even though their hearing is normal. This not only has financial costs but also a psychological impact on parents, who are in the position of wondering whether their child really has a hearing loss. The screening programs also have a problem with sensitivity, or failing to identify some infants with hearing problems. By some estimates, about 20% of infants with hearing loss at 1 year of age were missed by newborn screening programs. This may reflect a combination of examiner error, equipment error, failure to screen, and occurrence of progressive or late-onset hearing loss that would not have been evident in the newborn period. However, the lesson is that ongoing assessments of infants after the newborn period are essential.

Screening in older infants and children
Mild, progressive, and late-onset hearing loss may not be detected by newborn hearing screening. Therefore, infants and older children should be screened for hearing loss during regular visits to the pediatrician's office or at least once during the preschool period. Overall communication development can effectively be screened using structured parent-interview scales. It is also possible to screen older infants using OAE, as described earlier for newborn screening. Children over about 2 years of age can be screened using behavioral techniques such as play audiometry. Play audiometry involves instructing a child to respond to sound by performing a motor act such as putting a block in a box. Typically, screening is recommended at 1000, 2000, and 4000 Hz in both ears at 20 dB HL. If a child does not respond at least two out of three times at any frequency in either ear, or if the child cannot be conditioned to the task, a referral to an audiologist with pediatric experience is recommended.

Audiological Management of Children with Hearing Loss

Pediatric audiological assessment
When an infant or young child does not pass a hearing screening or is suspected of having a hearing loss for any reason, an audiological evaluation should be performed by an audiologist who has expertise with infants and young children. The evaluation of infants and young children incorporates a test battery approach that should include tests of middle ear function, hearing sensitivity,

and functional use of hearing. The specific procedures used to measure hearing sensitivity depend on the age and developmental abilities of the infant or child, but typically include a combination of the ABR, OAE, immittance audiometry, and one of several available behavioral procedures discussed previously. Sensitivity should be assessed for both ears across a range of sound frequencies including those that predominate in speech (i.e., 0.5, 1.0, 2.0, and 4.0 kHz). Through the use of a test battery, the audiologist can determine the level of hearing sensitivity and, if hearing sensitivity is not normal, the degree, type, and configuration of the hearing loss.

An important component of the evaluation process is engagement of parents, both in assessing the infant's or child's communication needs and abilities, and in planning for rehabilitation services. This can involve a number of caregiver questionnaires used to gain information about the infant's or child's functional use of hearing and language in real-world settings.

Modes of communication

A primary consequence of severe-to-profound hearing loss is the inability to hear spoken language. This problem is compounded by the finding that approximately 90% of all children with congenital hearing loss are born into hearing (speaking) families. Therefore, families of children with severe hearing loss are faced early on with making a decision about which communication modality to use for teaching language to their child. The modalities are distinguished as an oral approach with spoken language, a manual approach with sign language, or a total communication approach using a combination of speech and signs. With current technology, such as hearing aids and cochlear implants, and under ideal rehabilitative circumstances, it is possible for many young children with hearing loss to have access to auditory information and develop spoken language skills that are comparable to normal hearing peers. However, several factors need to be considered when deciding which communication modality to use with a child who has hearing loss. For example, consideration should be given to the child's capacity to develop spoken language, the severity of the child's hearing loss, access to various forms of intervention, and how the family feels about deaf culture'. Ultimately, a family is not tied to any modality and may change among them as the needs of the child and family shift. Regardless of which communication modality a family chooses to use with their child, the goal is to facilitate the development of a fluent communication system by school age.

Hearing technology

Many infants with permanent hearing loss can benefit from hearing aids or cochlear implants. Hearing aids can be effective for mild-to-profound degrees of conductive or sensorineural hearing loss. Most hearing aids work by presenting amplified acoustic signals to the ear canal, with the understanding that inner ear function in that individual is adequate to take advantage of the input. The primary goal of amplification for infants and young children is to make speech input comfortable and audible. Thus, it is crucial, for purposes of spoken language development, that infants be fitted with hearing aids as soon as their hearing loss is identified and that they wear their hearing aids all of their waking hours. Unless there is a contraindication, children are fitted with bilateral hearing aids because two ears are optimal for sound localization and for hearing in the presence of background noise.

Hearing aids can take many different styles including body, behind-the-ear (BTE), in-the-ear (ITE), and in-the-canal (ITC) aids. Style will be dictated by a child's degree of hearing loss, potential for growth of the outer ear, and individual needs. The outer ear may continue to grow until around 9 years of age, thus dictating the BTE style. Otherwise the hearing aid would need to be re-cased on a regular basis. If using a BTE hearing aid, when growth occurs, only the earmold (the piece that couples the hearing aid to the ear) has to be replaced. Other reasons for fitting young children with BTE aids are that it is more durable (with no circuitry directly exposed to ear wax) than ITE styles, is less likely to produce feedback (the whistling noise produced by amplified sound re-entering the hearing aid microphone), and allows for a variety of features that may be desirable for children (i.e., circuitry for using the aid with a telephone, connections for coupling to television, stereo, or computer inputs).

As described previously, some infants have conductive hearing loss, meaning that sound is not transmitted well by the ear canal or middle ear, with intact inner ear function. In many cases, these problems can be addressed through surgery. If not, and if a traditional air-conduction hearing aid cannot be fitted properly because of a malformation, a bone-conducted hearing aid may be used. Acoustic input is converted into vibrations that are transmitted by the bones of the skull to the cochlea. Two varieties of bone-conducted hearing aids are available, with the stimulator either worn externally on the skull surface, or surgically implanted near the ear ('bone-anchored'). At the time of this writing, the bone-anchored aids are not used with infants and young children in the US.

Another type of hearing technology commonly used with children is a frequency-modulation (FM) system. Because the microphone on a hearing aid will amplify everything in the surrounding area, it is often desirable (especially when there is background noise) to have just an individual's voice amplified. An FM system includes a microphone worn by the speaker, which is typically pinned to the clothes or hung around the neck, to pick up his or her voice, a transmitter to send the signal to the listener, and a receiver worn by the listener. The FM system can be coupled to a child's hearing aid or can be worn alone depending on the style. Regardless of the style used, FM systems are noted for providing a clear acoustic signal to the listener and are often used in educational settings.

Many infants with sensorineural hearing loss that cannot be compensated by hearing aids can benefit from cochlear implants. A cochlear implant is a small ribbon-like array of electrodes that is surgically implanted in the cochlea. The electrodes are wired to a receiver/stimulator, which is implanted in the skull near the ear. An external microphone and acoustic processor transmit signals to the receiver through the skin, causing the stimulator to activate the electrodes in the cochlea. Contemporary cochlear implants have between 12 and 20 electrodes or frequency channels, which are distributed approximately along the natural sound frequency gradient of the cochlea. The match to the natural frequency gradient is not exact, mainly because the implant does not fit all the way to the end of the cochlea. The frequency mismatch requires some adaptation on the part of the cochlear implant user. Thus, when the incoming sound to the microphone has energy at a certain frequency, the stimulator activates a corresponding electrode. Cochlear implants have been widely used with adults since the mid-1980s, and are now approved for use with infants and young children. Regulations about the youngest age at which implants may be used vary by country but implanting children as young as one year of age has become common practice. The question naturally arises as to the optimal age for initiating cochlear implant usage with respect to language development. Research on this topic is complicated by ethical constraints on study designs and by the rapid pace of technical improvement. However, there is general consensus that spoken language development is optimized by use of cochlear implants before the age of 3 years.

It is now common for adults to receive cochlear implants in both ears. Several studies have shown a binaural advantage for adult bilateral cochlear implant users and there is also a growing trend for children to receive bilateral implants as well. There is evidence that implanting bilaterally at a young age will facilitate the development of binaural neurons and allow young children to enjoy the benefits of binaural hearing, although some argue the logic of saving one ear for future technology.

Family support services

It is generally accepted that it is not the lack of hearing but rather the lack of language that can result in psychoeducational and psychosocial difficulties for deaf children. Therefore, regardless of the communication approach decided upon by the family, the early introduction of services that enhance the development of language is crucial. These services should start as soon as an infant is identified with hearing loss, often in the newborn period. Families have repeatedly indicated that they want factual information about the hearing loss and its effects on their child's development. They express interest in learning about causes of hearing loss, communication and educational options, and medical and technological interventions. There are many different models for the provision of services to these families. Services such as these should optimally be delivered via a team approach including audiologists, speech-language pathologists, otologists, deaf educators, and early interventionists. Some service delivery models include home-based services and others include center-based services. There are also numerous online information sources available to families worldwide.

Infant–parent services typically consist mostly of educating the family on the impact of hearing loss and the importance of creating a rich language-learning environment for the child. This includes learning about hearing technology (use and care of hearing aids or cochlear implants), good communication strategies (selecting an effective mode of communication), and creating a good listening environment (reduction of background noise in the home). As the child gets older, more direct intervention with the child occurs. This intervention is likely to include speech-language therapy, preliteracy skill development, and auditory training. The family, including the child when appropriate, should receive information on the services available to them through government and other agencies.

See also: Developmental Disabilities: Cognitive; Developmental Disabilities: Physical; Genetic Disorders: Single Gene; Neurological Development.

Suggested Readings

Abdala C (2004) Distortion product otoacoustic emission (2f1–f2) suppression in 3-month-old infants: Evidence for postnatal maturation of human cochlear function? *Journal of the Acoustical Society of America* 116(6): 3572–3580.

McConkey Robbins A, Koch DB, Osberger MJ, Zimmerman-Phillips S, and Kishon-Rabin L (2004) Effect of age at cochlear implantation on auditory skill development in infants and toddlers. *Archives of Otolaryngology Head and Neck Surgery* 130(5): 570–574.

Olsho LW, Koch EG, Carter EA, Halpin CF, and Spetner NB (1988) Pure-tone sensitivity of human infants. *Journal of the Acoustical Society of America* 84(4): 1316–1324.

Sininger YS, Abdala C, and Cone-Wesson B (1997) Auditory threshold sensitivity of the human neonate as measured by the auditory brainstem response. *Hearing Research* 104(1–2): 27–38.

Tharpe AM and Ashmead DH (2001) A longitudinal investigation of infant auditory sensitivity. *American Journal of Audiology* 10(2): 104–112.

Trehub SE, Schneider BA, and Endman M (1980) Developmental changes in infants' sensitivity to octave-band noises. *Journal of Experimental Child Psychology* 29(2): 282–293.

Werner LA and Marean GC (1996) *Human Auditory Development.* Boulder, CO: Westview Press.

Widex South Africa, Understanding your Ear. http://www.widex.co.za/guide-book/your-ear.htm.

Relevant Websites

http://www.agbell.org – Alexander Graham Bell Association for the Deaf.
http://www.asha.org – American Speech–Language–Hearing Association (ASHA).
http://www.shhh.org – Self-Help for Hard of Hearing.
http://www.nidcd.nih.gov – US National Institutes of Health.
http://www.med.unc.edu – UNC School of Medicine.

Autism Spectrum Disorders

G Dawson and L Sterling, University of Washington, Seattle, WA, USA

Glossary

Autistic regression – A period of typical development for at least 18–24 months followed by a significant decline or loss of language and/or social skills, and the development of autism symptoms.

Broader autism phenotype – The presence of one or more impairments in social functioning, communication, and/or a restricted range of interests/behaviors, but without sufficient severity to meet criteria for a diagnosis of an autism spectrum disorder.

Concordance – The presence of a given diagnosis or impairment in both members of a pair of twins.

Dizygotic twins – Fraternal twins (derived from separately fertilized eggs), sharing approximately 50% of genetic material.

Functional play – The conventional and appropriate use of an object or toy as it is intended, or the association of two or more objects according to their common functions.

Joint attention – The coordination of attention between interactive social partners with respect to objects or events in the environment in order to share awareness of the objects or events.

Monozygotic twins – Identical twins (derived from a single fertilized egg), sharing 100% of genetic material.

Parallel play – Play that occurs independently but alongside another child or group of children.

Social orienting – Volitional visual orienting to naturally occurring social stimuli in one's environment.

Symbolic or pretend play – The engagement in imaginative activities with toys involving substituting one object (the symbol) for another or reference to objects that are not actually present.

Introduction

Autism spectrum disorder (ASD) is the term used to describe the broad range of pervasive developmental disorders, including autistic disorder, asperger syndrome, and pervasive developmental disorder-not otherwise specified (PDD-NOS). As described in the fourth edition of *Diagnostic and Statistical Manual of Mental Disorders* (DSM-IV), individuals with ASD have qualitative impairments in reciprocal social interaction and language and communication, in addition to stereotyped, repetitive, or restrictive behaviors and interests. Of these impairments, deficits in social interaction are considered to be a core aspect of the disorder. The prevalence of ASD is currently estimated to be 1 in 166, which is 3–4 times higher than in the 1970s. Males are affected about 3–4 times more often than females. On average, females diagnosed with ASD are more severely affected (in terms of cognitive functioning and symptomatology) than males.

Impairments in social interaction can include a general lack of interest in others, a lack of affective sharing, and poor peer relationships, among others. Some children with ASD may appear disinterested or disconnected from their peers or their caregivers, whereas others may seek others out for interaction but do so in an odd or awkward manner. Specific signs of social impairment include lack of eye contact with others, restricted range of facial expressions or facial expressions that are not appropriate to the particular situation, lack of seeking to share enjoyment with others, lack of showing and directing attention to things that are of interest (also referred to as 'joint attention'), and difficulty initiating social interactions and establishing peer relationships. In infants, particular social difficulties may also include poor eye contact, failure to orient to their name being called, delayed or absent joint attention, and lack of reciprocal social smiling. Even high-functioning individuals with

ASD tend to have difficulty interpreting social cues from others. This can be especially apparent when interacting or conversing, during which the person with ASD may not read subtle changes in someone else's tone of voice, facial expression, or eye gaze.

Communication impairments include delay in language without use of gestures or other nonverbal forms of communication to compensate. Unlike children with autism and those with PDD-NOS, children with Asperger syndrome do not show significant delays in spoken language, although significant impairments in social use of language are present. Although many children with ASD (about 70%) do develop at least some spoken language, the quality of their speech is often atypical. For example, some children with ASD demonstrate stereotyped use of language, such as repeating lines from videos, repeating phrases they have heard others say, or using odd phrases. The rate, rhythm, or volume can also be atypical. For example, a child with an ASD may consistently talk very loudly, too fast, or speak in monotone. Individuals with ASD also typically have difficulties with the pragmatic use of speech, or language used to start, maintain, or end a conversation, making it difficult to establish a reciprocal conversation.

The third category of impairments includes restrictive, repetitive, and stereotyped behaviors and interests. These can be motor stereotypies, such as hand and finger mannerisms and complicated whole-body movements, such as rocking back and forth and spinning in circles. Symptoms in this domain also include preoccupations, a restricted range of interests, and sensory interests. For example, some children with ASD may engage in prolonged visual examination (e.g., of themselves in the mirror or of objects near them), peering at things out of the corner of their eyes, repetitive feeling of textures, touching, sniffing, biting, and sensitivity to sounds or lights. Other children may use objects in a repetitive manner (e.g., lining toys up, spinning the wheels of a toy car), rather than using the objects or toys flexibly or as they are intended to be used. Some individuals with ASD also engage in specific rituals in routines, which can include exact placement of objects or arrangement of items, as well as following a certain sequence of actions that must be performed in a particular order or will result in anxiety (e.g., touching the doorknob every time he or she leaves a room). Finally, many individuals with ASD have intense interests that can take up the majority of their time. For example, a child with ASD may have a particular interest in trains or cameras, and spend a large proportion of time playing with these items, talking about them, and possess a high degree of factual knowledge about them. Such interests can interfere with engaging in other more functional or prosocial behaviors.

Although there is not currently a 'cure' for autism, behavioral intervention can improve a child's level of functioning, quality of life, and prognosis. The early intervention for infants and toddlers has been a recent focus of research. Current studies suggest that children with ASD are benefiting from approaches such as applied behavioral analysis, especially when delivered in a naturalistic context with a focus on social relationships. Researchers anticipate that as children's behavior improves as a result of early intervention, the neural pathways involved in the development of language and social processing will also change. These implications are promising and underscore the benefits of early diagnosis and intervention at a young age.

Diagnosis and Early Recognition

ASD is a developmental disorder, with symptoms present before the age of 3 years. Speech delay, or the loss of previously acquired speech, is often the first developmental milestone alerting parents and professionals to possible difficulties related to ASD. Deviances from typical development can sometimes be apparent by 8–12 months of age; however, a diagnosis of ASD cannot be reliably made until the age of 2 years. Because there is currently no known biological test for ASD (e.g., blood test), a diagnosis is based on developmental history and observed behaviors. Structured diagnostic measures, such as the Autism Diagnostic Interview and the Autism Diagnostic Observation Schedule, are administered by highly trained clinicians, and are considered gold standards for diagnosing ASD. Clinicians use information from these measures as well as information collected through any other observation to help determine whether an individual meets criteria for ASD based on symptoms outlined in the DSM-IV. Because a significant proportion of children presenting with ASD have an identifiable genetic disorder, such as Fragile X syndrome, karyotyping and other biomedical tests are often conducted to define the cause of the symptoms for a given child better.

Much of current research in the field of autism focuses on methods to detect ASD at even earlier ages, with the goal of providing behavioral and psychosocial interventions to children as early as possible. Clinicians and researchers specializing in early development have begun to make diagnoses of ASD at or before the age of 2 years, and screening measures are currently being tested for infants as young as 6–12 months of age. Given the variability in developmental trajectories and the variability of symptom expression in individuals with ASD, diagnoses before the age of 2 years are considered provisional and the stability of the diagnosis should always be reinvestigated at a later age.

There is great heterogeneity among individuals on the autism spectrum. Many individuals with ASD score in the mentally retarded range on IQ tests, often with significant variability in functioning across subtests. The rate of mental retardation also tends to vary depending on the child's specific ASD diagnosis. For example, recent estimates suggest that the rate of mental retardation in children with autistic disorder is about 67%, compared to approximately 12% of children with PDD-NOS and 0% of children with Asperger syndrome. Virtually all have significant challenges in adaptive functioning and self-care. Up to 25% of individuals with ASD are high functioning, have average-to-above-average cognitive skills, and are able to live independently in society and establish successful relationships. Symptom severity also varies. A portion of children never acquire spoken language, while others achieve a level of communicative competence that is near normal, with subtle impairments in the pragmatic aspects of language. In terms of social interaction, some individuals show high motivation to interact with others, although they may execute this in an awkward or inappropriate manner. Play skills and repetitive behavior also vary across individuals. This variability and range in functioning contributes to the uniqueness of each individual with ASD. It also makes diagnosis and treatment of the disorder complicated. Diagnosing children at earlier ages, and growing recognition of individuals with more subtle impairments who have ASD have broadened the definition of autism.

Genetic Influences in ASD

For approximately 5–10% of autism cases, there is an identifiable disorder with a known inheritance pattern, such as Fragile X syndrome, untreated phenylketonuria, (PKU), tuberous sclerosis, and neurofibromatosis. For the remaining cases of autism, there is no known specific inheritance pattern or genetic test for the disorder. Researchers are currently investigating the role of genetics in the development of ASD.

In order to determine whether a disorder has a genetic basis, it is first necessary to evaluate whether it is familial, that is, whether it runs in families. Evidence suggests that there is a higher rate of ASD and related conditions among family members of individuals with ASD than would be expected in the general population. Much of this evidence comes from studies investigating the concordance of ASD among twins. When one twin has ASD, and the other twin also meets criteria for the disorder, the twins are said to be concordant for ASD.

Studies of monozygotic, or identical twins, are especially helpful in investigating the genetic basis of autism. Monozygotic twins share 100% of their genes, whereas dizygotic or fraternal twins share approximately 50% of their genes. Therefore, for the development of a disorder to be completely determined by genes, in theory monozygotic twins should be nearly 100% concordant for the disorder. Studies have reported concordance rates of

approximately 70%, with rates of concordance reaching 90% if one considered autism-related symptoms, such as social and language impairment. Thus, some monozygotic pairs are discordant for ASD (i.e., when one twin has ASD, the other does not). This suggests that environmental factors (e.g., infectious agents, toxins, trauma, and pre-, peri-, and postnatal factors) must also play a role in the etiology of autism. Nevertheless, the concordance rates for monozygotic twins are substantially greater than those for dizygotic twins, providing evidence for a strong genetic component in the development of the disorder. The concordance rates for dizygotic twins are similar to those reported for siblings. The reported sibling risk rates for ASD range from about 2.8% to 7.0%, which is still much higher than rates found in the general population, though less than rates reported for identical twins. This would suggest that having more genes in common (monozygotic vs. dizygotic twins) is associated with greater risk for ASD concordance. The increased concordance rate for siblings in general, as well as the discrepancy in concordance rates between monozygotic and dizygotic twins, indicates that genes play a significant role in the development of ASD.

Even when siblings do not meet full criteria for the disorder, it has been found that about 10–20% show symptoms related to ASD, including language, learning, and communication impairments, as well as social difficulties. Studies of infant and toddler siblings of children with ASD have shown that young non-ASD siblings can show delays in receptive and expressive language, use of gestures, social smiling, adaptive behavior skills, and social communication and social–emotional functioning. Studies have also shown that parents from families that contain at least two children with ASD have elevated risk of particular personality traits (e.g., aloof, rigid, socially anxious), establish fewer closer relationships than typical adults, have communication impairments (including a history of language delay and pragmatic language deficits), and certain cognitive impairments.

The tendency for some siblings and parents to exhibit one or more difficulties in social functioning, communication, and interests/behaviors, without actually meeting criteria for ASD, has been termed the broader autism phenotype, and is often conceptualized as a 'lesser variant' of autism. Because of the variation and spectrum of autism symptoms and severity, researchers often describe autism as a dimensional disorder, with many different components of varying degrees depending on the individual. Rather than one single gene accounting for the entire autism syndrome, it is possible that multiple genes (perhaps 10 or more) act as risk factors for the development of the components making up the autism disorder. A combination of these susceptibility genes may increase risk for the development of autism, with a greater number of genes leading to a greater risk of development of symptoms. This makes identifying the genes responsible for autism very challenging, given that each of these multiple genes, by itself, could have a very small effect size and the fact that symptoms vary significantly across individuals with ASD. Nevertheless, there is great hope that detection of autism susceptibility genes could ultimately lead to better diagnosis and clues to underlying cause and treatment.

Early Brain Development in ASD

Brain imaging and autopsy studies of individuals with ASD suggest that the disorder affects a wide range of brain regions, including the prefrontal cortex, the medial temporal lobe (especially the amygdala), and the cerebellum. The earliest apparent finding is an abnormal head circumference growth trajectory, characterized by unusually rapid head growth during their first year of life. Although children with ASD do not necessarily have larger head circumferences at birth, by 1 year of age, head circumference, on average, is one standard deviation larger than that reported by the national Centers for Disease Control (CDC) norms. Some evidence suggests that, after 12 months of age, the rate of head circumference growth in children with ASD may decelerate such that the rate of head growth does not differ from the normative CDC sample. It has also been reported that first-degree relatives (e.g., siblings) of children with ASD tend to have larger than normal head circumferences. This is especially relevant given the findings from genetic studies of autism, suggesting that behavioral symptoms associated with ASD occur at a higher prevalence in first-degree relatives than would be expected in the normal population. The possible association between head circumference trajectories and behavioral manifestations of autism is of particular relevance. If it can be established that head circumference trajectories are associated with specific autism-related behaviors, this may become a useful screening marker in alerting professionals to the possibility of the development of autism symptoms.

By 2–3 years of age, brain imaging studies using magnetic resonance imaging have documented larger than normal total cerebral volume and an unusually large amygdala, which is a structure in the medial temporal lobe that is associated with emotional functioning. Autopsy studies have revealed abnormal neuron development in the amygdala, as well. Similar studies of the cerebellum have consistently shown cellular abnormalities. The cerebellum is involved in complex motor activities, attention, and language. These recent findings show promise in implicating brain regions that might play a role in the development of autism-related symptoms. However, it is important to interpret the findings with caution, given that brain imaging studies often contain small sample sizes and results may vary depending on the age of the children in the sample and other individual characteristics.

Recent functional brain imaging studies have also shown that ASD is associated with poor functional connectivity between different brain regions. During resting and complex tasks, whereas typically various regions of the brain operate in synchrony with each other, studies have shown reduced long-range connectivity, especially between the frontal cortex and other regions of the brain. This may help explain why individuals with autism often have difficulty on tasks requiring high-order complex reasoning.

Early Behavioral Development in ASD

Joint Attention

Children with ASD have general impairments in the ability to attend to social stimuli in their environment. Social stimuli can include the sound of a mother's voice, and the movements and features of a human face, particularly eye gaze. Typically developing infants show sensitivity to social stimuli from the first weeks of life. The failure of young children with ASD to attend to these naturally occurring social stimuli in their environment spontaneously has been termed a 'social-orienting impairment'. This impairment is one of the earliest and most basic social deficits in autism and may contribute to social and communicative impairments that emerge later in life.

Young children with ASD also show impairment in joint attention, which refers to the ability to coordinate attention between interactive social partners with respect to objects or events in the environment in order to share awareness of the objects or events. It is a means by which a child can monitor and regulate the attention of another person in relation to objects or events taking place in the outside world. Joint attention behaviors include use of alternating eye gaze, following the attention of someone else by following their eye gaze or point, and directing the attention of someone else through eye gaze or gesture. For example, if a child makes eye contact with an adult, then looks at a toy in the room, and then back to the adult, the child has initiated joint attention by attempting to direct the adult's attention to the toy. Similarly, if a child follows another person's gaze, point, or head turn toward a toy across the room, the child has responded to joint attention.

Typically developing infants tend to demonstrate joint attention abilities by around their first birthday. In children with ASD, this fundamental social-communication impairment is evident by 12–18 months of age and is actually incorporated into the diagnostic criteria for autism. Because joint attention is a discrete observable behavior, it provides a direct measure of social impairment in ASD. Research has shown that joint attention impairments distinguish preschool-age children with ASD from typically developing children and from children who have developmental delay without autism. Degree of joint attention impairment has also been found to be correlated with present and future language ability in children with ASD, and is considered a skill necessary for the acquisition of communicative language.

Play

Typically developing children generally develop symbolic pretend play between 14 and 22 months of age. Pretend play is the engagement in an imaginative activity, and includes using an object to represent another object (e.g., using a block to represent a cup), using absent objects as if they were present (e.g., pretending to feed nonexistent food to a doll), or animating objects and using them as independent agents of action (e.g., making an action figure walk, talk, or interact with other figures). Pretend play is an expression of a child's imagination. Studies have shown that toddlers with ASD produce significantly less pretend play compared with typically developing and developmentally delayed same-aged peers. In addition to the reduced amount of symbolic or pretend play, children with ASD also tend to produce fewer novel play acts, and engage in play that is less elaborate, spontaneous, flexible, and diverse than would be expected given their age. Their pretend play activities tend to be more simplified and rehearsed, as if carried out as part of a ritual, with little variation.

Because pretend play is not typically present until the second year of life, impairment in pretend play is not a distinguishing feature of very young children with ASD; children with other developmental disabilities would also be expected to show deficits in these skills. For example, a child with delayed language development would not be expected to demonstrate elaborate make-believe play skills. However, improving pretend play skills is often a focus of behavioral intervention for children with ASD, as it has been shown to be related to the development of other important skills (e.g., language).

Functional play is defined as the conventional and appropriate use of an object or toy as it is intended to be used, or the use of two or more objects according to their common functions. Examples of functional play include using a spoon to stir in a bowl or playing appropriately with miniatures. In typically developing children, functional play skills tend to emerge during the first year of life. In general, children with ASD engage in less functional play and produce fewer functional play acts. Their functional play also tends to be less diverse and elaborate.

When provided with opportunities to play freely with toys, children with ASD tend to explore toys less, and often play in isolation, without making attempts to involve others in their play. Their play may also be repetitive, often repeating certain activities over and over (e.g., pressing the same button on a pop-up toy). In addition,

a child with ASD is more likely to engage in sensory exploration of a toy or play materials. This can include mouthing a toy or banging toys together, as well as more repetitive activities such as spinning the wheels of a toy car or lining up objects.

Both independent and peer play are considered to be social activities, because children's themes and scripts incorporate aspects of their surrounding environment, in addition to serving as a means of reciprocal social interaction. In terms of peer play, children with ASD often play independently and alongside a group of children, rather than joining them in their play. This is referred to as 'parallel play'. This lack of interactive play with peers can exacerbate the social impairments characteristic of children with ASD, making it difficult to develop the foundations necessary to form friendships or nurture social relations with others. It can also contribute to the isolation often experienced by children with ASD, resulting in fewer opportunities to interact with others and greater social impairment.

Motor Imitation

Impairments in motor imitation – both immediate and deferred – are common in ASD. Typically developing infants demonstrate the ability to imitate actions, such as facial expressions, from birth, and by 9 months of age, can actually imitate actions on objects. An infant's ability to imitate is a manifestation of their social connectedness with others, in that it involves attending, listening, and learning from others. Imitation also serves as a means of communicating and sharing experiences with social partners. Children with ASD show significant impairments in object imitation, imitation of facial and body movements, and imitation of actions on objects.

Studies have shown that the ability to imitate body movements (e.g., waving a hand) is more difficult for children with ASD than the imitation of actions with objects. This pattern of imitation skills is also found among typically developing children and children with developmental delay. In fact, research has indicated that children with ASD acquire simple motor imitation skills in a typical sequence, suggesting that the impairments in imitation in young children reflect a delayed, rather than disordered pattern of acquisition.

Infants and toddlers with ASD also show impairments and delays in the development of social imitative play. This includes engaging in social imitative games with others, such as peek-a-boo and pat-a-cake, that involve the tracking and imitation of another person's movements. Additionally, although infants and toddlers with ASD may participate in such activities with a parent, a child with ASD will rarely initiate such a game or take on both roles, reflecting a lack of social initiation and perspective taking. In fact, it has been suggested that failure to engage in such social imitative activities is associated with deficits in social reciprocity, joint attention, play, and language skills in children with ASD. Imitation skills in general have been shown to correlate with early language ability in children with ASD.

Language

Although social impairments are core diagnostic symptoms in children with ASD, parents of children with ASD often first become concerned about their child's development when speech is delayed or when previously acquired speech is lost. There is extreme variability in the developmental outcome of language ability in children with ASD. While some children (about 30%) never learn to talk, others develop speech but continue to show qualitative communication challenges, such as impairments in nonverbal and pragmatic language skills, atypical speech patterns, and repetitive and stereotyped use of language.

In terms of nonverbal communication, children with ASD tend to use less frequent eye contact, pointing, and other gestures. In very young children, there is a delay in the use of gestures that are used for the purpose of sharing interest and directing social interaction. Examples of these gestures include extending one's arms to show a toy or object that he or she is holding, extending arms to be picked up, requesting something by extending one's arm and opening and closing a hand, and waving goodbye when someone leaves. Children with ASD are more likely to use pointing or other gestures for the purpose of requesting something in particular (e.g., a toy or snack) than for indicating and sharing interest in an object or activity. Even when using language to communicate, children with ASD are less likely to coordinate gestures and eye contact with their vocalizations.

Some children with ASD engage in the direct manipulation of an adult's hand in order to request help. For example, a child with ASD may take the finger or hand of a nearby adult and use their finger or hand as a tool, to press a button, turn a knob, or open a door. In the majority of cases, this act is not accompanied by eye contact or vocalization; it is not a social act, but rather a means of acquiring help without actually involving the adult in the child's play or behavior.

The pragmatic use of speech refers to language used to start, maintain, or end a conversation. Although deficits in these skills are often more apparent and applicable as individuals become older, emerging difficulties with reciprocal conversation are also evident in young children. Deficits in pragmatic language can include a failure to respond to questions and comments made by another person. For example, a young child with ASD may not use eye contact, facial expression, or vocalization to acknowledge that another person has directed a statement or question toward them. This failure to respond to others

marks a lack of reciprocity on the part of the child. Additional examples of pragmatic language impairments include providing excessive details in conversation or a tendency to monopolize a conversation, often when a child is focused on a particular topic of interest. Although the child is participating in conversation, this also makes it difficult to establish reciprocity, as the conversation is one-sided. Children with ASD may also have difficulty understanding how to interact appropriately with someone else during a conversation, such as knowing how close to stand to someone else or how to participate without interrupting.

Atypical speech patterns in children with ASD include immediate or delayed echolalia, (i.e., a child's immediate or delayed repetition of a word or statement), unusual prosody (e.g., atypical intonation, volume, rhythm, or rate), and semantic difficulties such as pronoun reversal (e.g., "you want a drink" or "he wants a drink" instead of "I want a drink"). These atypical speech patterns can persist into adulthood. Repetitive and stereotyped use of language refers to the repetition of phrases that may or may not be used in combination with functional speech. Often, children have heard these phrases in movies, as part of a game, song, or routine. A child with ASD may repeat the phrase while playing on their own, when attempting to converse with someone else, or even when agitated. In some cases, repetition of these phrases becomes compulsive, such that the child feels compelled to repeat the phrase over and over or even insists on someone else repeating the phrase or responding in a particular way. Another example of stereotyped speech includes the use of words or phrases that are more formal than would be expected given the child's developmental level.

Delays in language development affect both receptive and expressive language. Studies have shown that while typically developing children show early signs of language understanding before the end of the first year of life, such signs may not occur in children with ASD until much later in development. The production of words tends to be significantly delayed in children with ASD; word and phrase comprehension have been shown to be even more delayed. Moreover, even once a child has developed the ability to use speech and demonstrates the ability to respond to the speech of others, he or she may continue to have difficulty actually deciphering the meaning of a sentence. For example, children with ASD may interpret phrases in concrete or literal terms, making metaphors or jokes challenging to understand. Studies have also shown that children with ASD not only show a delayed course of language development; in many cases, the course of development is actually atypical. For example, compared to the normative pattern of development, the production of words may be relatively advanced in comparison to the understanding of words and phrases for children with ASD. It is also important to note that among children with ASD, there is great variability in the development of language, with some children achieving language competence in the typical timeframe. Nonetheless, as a whole, children with ASD tend to have significant delay in the development of language compared to typically developing children.

In addition to a frank delay in language development, children with ASD tend to show a lack of communicative intent, or the motivation to communicate with others. In other words, the language impairment evident in young children with ASD is a result of fewer attempts to comment, engage in conversation, or direct someone else's attention through the use of words, gestures, and eye contact, in addition to the lack of specific language skills.

It has been reported that in approximately 20–47% of cases, children with ASD develop typically for about 18–24 months, at which point they experience a decline or loss of language skills. This decline or loss of skill has been termed a 'regression' in development. The period of regression in ASD can be acute or gradual, during which parents report that their child stops using words or word-like sounds that he or she consistently used in the past. Although additional impairments become evident during regression, such as less frequent use of eye gaze and pointing and failure to respond to their name being called, the decline in previously acquired language skills often first alerts parents of a potential developmental problem.

Conclusion

Children with ASD experience deficits in communication and social skills, and have repetitive and restricted interests and behaviors. Individuals diagnosed with ASD are characterized by heterogeneity in terms of their symptom profiles and severity of impairments. High concordance rates are found among identical twins with ASD, and siblings and family members are also at increased risk for the development of autism-related symptoms and the disorder itself. Evidence for a strong genetic component in the development of autism has led to an increase in current research efforts focusing on the genetic etiology of the disorder. It has also been shown that on average, children with ASD exhibit atypical head circumference trajectories, a reflection of abnormal brain growth patterns. One study found that these trajectories correlate with the development of autism symptoms in the second year of life, and may be a useful marker to alert professionals to autism symptom vulnerability. Infants and toddlers with ASD show specific impairments in early development and cognition, specifically in the areas of play, joint attention, language, and imitation. As the age of diagnosis becomes increasingly younger, children with ASD will have the opportunity to receive effective behavioral and psychosocial intervention in the first years of life, hopefully leading to improvement in functioning and preventative methods for the development of the disorder. Recent studies have shown that early intervention can have a significant impact on outcome in individuals with ASD.

See also: Developmental Disabilities: Cognitive; Fragile X Syndrome; Genetic Disorders: Sex Linked; Intellectual Disabilities; Sensory Processing Disorder.

Suggested Readings

Charman T, Baron-Cohen S, Swettenham J, *et al.* (2003) Predicting language outcome in infants with autism and pervasive developmental disorder. *International Journal of Language and Communication Disorders* 38: 265–285.

Charman T, Swettenham J, Baron-Cohen S, *et al.* (1997) Infants with autism: An investigation of empathy, pretend play, joint attention, and imitation. *Developmental Psychology* 33: 781–789.

Dawson G and Toth K (2006) Autism spectrum disorders. In: Cicchetti D and Cohen D (eds.) *Developmental Psychopathology*, 2nd edn., vol. 3, pp 311–357. *Risk, Disorder, and Adaptation*. New York: Wiley.

Dawson G, Toth K, Abott R, *et al.* (2004) Early social attention impairments in autism: Social orienting, joint attention, and attention to distress. *Developmental Psychology* 40: 271–283.

Dawson G, Webb S, Schellenberg GD, *et al.* (2002) Defining the broader phenotype in autism: Genetic, brain, and behavioral perspectives. *Development and Psychopathology* 14: 581–611.

Mundy P and Crowson M (1997) Joint attention and early social communication: Implications for research on intervention with autism. *Journal of Autism and Developmental Disorders* 27: 653–676.

Stone W, Ousley OY, and Littleford CD (1997) Motor imitation in young children with autism: What's the object? *Journal of Abnormal Child Psychology* 25: 475–485.

Stone W, Ousley OY, Yoder PJ, Hogan KL, and Hepburn SL (1997) Nonverbal communication in two- and three-year-old children with autism. *Journal of Autism and Developmental Disorders* 27: 677–696.

Zwaigenbaum L (2001) Autism spectrum disorders in preschool children. *Canadian Family Physician* 47: 2037–2042.

Relevant Websites

http://www.autism-society.org – Autism Society of America.
http://www.autismspeaks.org – Autism Speaks.
http://www.washington.edu – University of Washington, UW Autism Center.

Bedwetting

A I Chin and S E Lerman, University of California, Los Angeles, Los Angeles, CA, USA

Glossary

Atrial natriuretic factor – Hormone produced by the heart involved in homeostatic control of body water and sodium.

Cystometrogram – Test of bladder and urethral sphincter function during the storage and passage of urine, performed by placing a catheter with a sensor into the bladder (catheter cystometry). This procedure is incorporated in urodynamic (see below) testing.

Dysfunctional voiding – Abnormal storage or emptying voiding pattern without neurological or anatomical disease.

Dysuria – Painful or difficult urination, a common voiding symptom.

Encopresis – Repeated involuntary loss of feces in a child of chronologic and mental age of at least 4 years.

Enuresis – Involuntary discharge of urine from the urethra, derived from the Greek word *enourein*, meaning 'to void urine'.

Glomerular filtration rate – Volume of fluid filtered from the kidney often used as a measure of kidney function and typically measured in milliliters per minute.

Hyponatremia – Electrolyte imbalance when the plasma sodium level falls below 135 mmol l^{-1}; severe hyponatremia can cause an osmotic shift of water from the plasma into the brain cells with symptoms including nausea, vomiting, headache, and malaise.

Micturition – Discharge of urine.

Osmolality – Measure of concentration of particles; in humans normal values of serum osmolality is 285–295 mmol kg^{-1}.

Polydipsia – Abnormally large intake of fluids by mouth usually associated with excessive thirst.

Polyuria – Excessive volume of urination; a symptom with multiple etiologies including excessive fluid intake, diabetes, diabetes insipidus, or use of diuretic medications.

Urodynamics – Series of diagnostic tests used to evaluate voiding disorders. These tests may include the measurement of urinary flow, detrusor pressure, sphincter muscle electrical activity, and radiographic imaging.

Voiding cystourethrography – Radiographic study to evaluate anatomic features of bladder and urethra, the ability to empty the bladder, and to diagnose whether urine backs up into the kidneys.

Introduction

The classification of enuresis can be divided into primary enuresis, defined as wetting in patients who have never been dry for extended periods of time, and secondary enuresis, the onset of wetting after a continuous dry period of at least 6 months (**Figure 1**). The degree of incontinence can range from urinary incontinence a few times per week to multiple episodes daily. Enuresis can be further categorized into nocturnal or diurnal enuresis. Nocturnal enuresis is the involuntary wetting that occurs at night or during sleep beyond the age of anticipated bladder control, usually placed at 5 years of age. This condition contrasts to diurnal enuresis, defined as involuntary loss of urine occurring while awake, a problem that is more likely to have an underlying neurologic or physiologic diagnosis. Nocturnal enuresis can be distinguished as monosymptomatic or uncomplicated, defined as nocturnal enuresis associated with normal daytime urination, or polysymptomatic or complicated, defined as nocturnal enuresis associated with other lower tract urinary symptoms. These symptoms include urinary urgency, frequency, poor urinary stream, urinary tract infections, neurological deficit, chronic constipation, or elimination dysfunction.

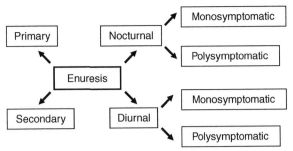

Figure 1 Classification of enuresis. Types of enuresis from primary or secondary to nocturnal or diurnal. Both nocturnal and diurnal enuresis can further by classified into monosymptomatic or polysymptomatic.

Epidemiology

Enuresis beholds no prejudice, seen worldwide in all cultures and races, and has been problematic from antiquity to present. The true incidence of enuresis may not be known because of under-reporting and the lack of uniform definitions of what constitutes a wet child. For instance, a family whose siblings were not dry until later years may not seek medical care concerning a child with enuresis at 5 years of age, while conversely a child still wetting at 4 years may be brought to the pediatrician if his or her siblings were dry at that age. Providing this caveat, 15% of 5-year-old children have primary nocturnal enuresis, having never achieved a period of continent nights. Although the incidence is high in young children, the majority spontaneously resolve, an important consideration when discussing treatment options with parents. In a seminal study of over 1000 enuretics, resolution of symptoms occurred at a rate of approximately 15% each year, such that only 5% of 10-year-olds and 1% of adolescents remain wet. However, historical data suggest that up to 1–2% of adults experience enuresis, based on military recruits during World War II rejected for bedwetting. Monosymptomatic nocturnal enuretics comprise 80–85% of children with enuresis.

The epidemiologic data pose a dilemma on when and if enuretics should be evaluated and treated. Nocturnal enuresis is generally defined as starting at age 5 years, which translates to 15% (or 1 in 6 or 7) 5-year-olds that would require evaluation and treatment for enuresis, which seems impractical. In our experience, most children in this young age group do not consider the bedwetting to be a problem, nor are they sufficiently interested in achieving dry nights through a rigorous treatment program. The economic impact of treating 15% of 5-year-olds is also overwhelming and should not be borne by society. Fortunately, most enuretic children at 5 years of age spontaneously resolve their bedwetting, as anxious parents can be assured that approximately half of children at this stage will improve if treatment is delayed until 8 years of age.

One can then argue that with such a high spontaneous rate of resolution whether or not treatment is necessary at all. Indeed, the 15% per year spontaneous resolution rate of enuresis is the gold standard against which all treatment regimens must be compared. For several reasons, we do not feel these data support a nontreatment approach. First, a lonely, isolated, and painful childhood may evolve while spontaneous cure is awaited. Second, spontaneous resolution does not come to all who wait. The probability that a child at any given age will continue into adulthood with enuresis rises with increasing age. Children who remain enuretic past the age of 8 years have an increasing risk for not resolving their symptoms. Combined with studies concluding that enuresis does not interfere with socialization until 7 years of age, we define enuresis as a clinical condition beginning at age 7–8 years. At this age, most patients are interested in achieving dry nights and their socialization begins to be adversely affected by nocturnal enuresis.

Physiology

Understanding the development of continence provides insight in the etiology and management of enuresis. Bladder storage and emptying requires the activity of sympathetic, parasympathetic, and somatic voluntary nerves coordinated by the spinal cord, brainstem, midbrain, and higher cortical centers (**Figure 2**). The infant bladder relies on the sacral spinal cord micturition center to empty involuntarily and to completion. Bladder distention stimulates the afferent limb to the sacral micturition center, which generates signals through the efferent limb leading to detrusor contraction with coordinated relaxation of the striated muscle of the voluntary external sphincter. Infants empty their bladders approximately 20 times per day, of which roughly 40% occurs during sleep. At 6 months of age, infants decrease the frequency of micturition with a concomitant increase in voided volumes. These changes have been attributed to the development of a cortical inhibition of the voiding reflex and to the proportionately greater increase in bladder capacity relative to increased urine production that occurs with growth. Between 1 and 2 years of age, children begin to achieve conscious sensation of bladder fullness, and the voluntarily ability to void or inhibit voiding until a socially acceptable time is achieved in the second or third year of life, mediated by the frontal lobe and pontine micturition center. Normally inhibited by signals from the frontal lobe, the pontine micturition center coordinates urethral sphincter relaxation and detrusor contraction. When urination is desired, the frontal lobe sends excitatory signals to the pons allowing voiding to occur. By 4 years of age, most children have achieved an adult pattern of micturition. However, like other developmental milestones, bladder control does not

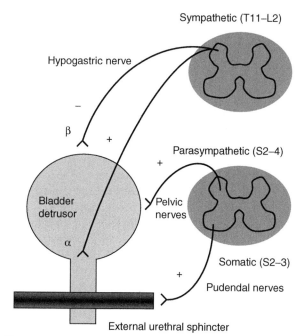

Figure 2 Innervation of the bladder. Sympathetic hypogastric nerves originating from the lateral gray columns of the lumbar spinal cord from T11 to L2 synapse with α-receptors responsible for tonic contraction of the internal sphincter and β-receptors for relaxation of the detrusor muscle to allow bladder filling and storage. Parasympathetic pelvic nerves travel from the ventral gray matter from S2 to S4 to the cholinergic receptors in the detrusor muscle to mediate bladder contraction. Somatic pudendal nerves from the pudendal motor nucleus of S2 to S4 supply the voluntary external urethral sphincter.

appear at a set time in a child's maturation. The typical sequence of developing bladder and bowel control is first nocturnal bowel control, then daytime bowel control, next daytime bladder control, and finally nocturnal bladder control.

Etiology

The persistence of nocturnal enuresis in children has likely multifactorial contributions. Multiple theories have been proposed, including genetic predisposition, physiologic problems including low functional bladder capacity and bladder instability, increased night-time urine production from behavioral or endocrine factors, and maturation delay. These factors ultimately lead to common mechanisms including increased night-time urine production relative to bladder capacity. The following section reviews the current understandings.

Genetic Inheritance

It has been observed that enuresis runs in families. Statistically, at 5 years of age, approximately 15% of children from nonenuretic parents are bedwetters, while 44% of

children with one parent who had enuresis are wet, and 77% of children where both parents had enuresis are afflicted. Other support for genetic predisposition arises from twin studies, with monozygotic twins concordant for enuresis twice as often as dizygotic twins. In one family study, linkage to a region on chromosome 13 has been identified, while other studies have described linkage to regions on chromosome 12 and 22. The practical aspect of this genetic predisposition lies in predicting when a child will likely become dry based on family history, but plays little role in treatment. Currently, no gene for enuresis has been identified and there is no role in gene therapy for treatment of enuresis.

Changes in Bladder Physiology

Two alterations in bladder physiology, detectable by urodynamics, are associated with enuresis, a reduced functional bladder capacity and bladder instability. Prior reports have demonstrated a reduced functional bladder capacity in bedwetters compared with healthy children, with reduction in enuretic children up to 50%. Normal bladder capacity in children can be estimated by the formula age in years plus two equaling bladder capacity in ounces. Enuretic children do not appear to have differences in true or anatomic bladder capacity, which has been shown to be similar to functional bladder capacity when measured in children under general anesthesia. Decreased functional bladder capacity limits night-time urine storage whereby the child either is aroused to void or wets the bed. However, not all studies confirm a generalized decrease in functional bladder capacity among enuretics.

Bladder instability has been widely investigated as an etiology of enuresis, but its contribution is not clear. Initial studies of children with monosymptomatic nocturnal enuresis undergoing awake catheter cystometry showed significant variation in bladder instability, ranging from 16% to 84%. However, subsequent studies found that approximately 16% of children with monosymptomatic nocturnal enuresis experience bladder instability during cystometrograms while awake, a number no different from healthy children. This finding predicts the high failure rate of anticholinergic drugs in the treatment of most enuretics. While performing urodynamic studies it is important not to create false positives by infusing at supraphysiologic flow rates given age and size, as increasing the infusion flow rate can provoke instability. A maximum flow rate at 10% of the patient's normal glomerular filtration rate is recommended.

Endocrine Factors

It has long been observed that less urine is secreted at night than during the day. In 1952, relative nocturnal polyuria was proposed as an etiologic factor for enuresis.

Antidiuretic hormone (ADH) or arginine vasopressin (AVP) is secreted in the hypothalamus, stored in the posterior pituitary, and released by factors such as elevated serum osmotic pressure and low fluid volume. It naturally follows a circadian variation with increased secretion at night. Studies demonstrated lack of the normal circadian variation and increased night-time AVP excretion in enuretic children, suggesting that increased urine production resulting from decreased plasma vasopressin led to urine production exceeding diurnal output. Another study confirmed that 25% of children with enuresis had low nocturnal serum AVP levels compared with controls. Sleep-pattern changes are also known to affect AVP expression.

However, not all studies identify differences in day and night urine production or urine osmolality between enuretics and healthy children when diet and fluid intake are controlled, suggesting that only a subset of children have altered AVP levels as a causative factor for enuresis. Other opponents argue the cause and effect relationship between enuresis and AVP levels. Bladder distention has been shown to stimulate AVP secretion. Thus, lower nocturnal AVP levels may be a response to the smaller functional bladder capacity of enuretics and the empty bladder following an enuretic event.

Developmental Delay and Psychological Factors

Achieving nocturnal urinary control is a normal transitional phase of a child's development between the infant and adult control of urinary function. Another theory of enuresis is that it represents a delay in development by both internal and external factors. Accordingly, children with enuresis may have increased fine and gross motor clumsiness, delayed speech, and perceptual dysfunction compared with healthy children. This theory of developmental delay is supported by the high rate of spontaneous cure and improvement in other aspects of motor skills as well. Furthermore, environmental factors can contribute to this delay. The 2–4-year-old age range is a particularly sensitive time for the development of nocturnal bladder control. Stressors and social pressures during this time have been associated with enuresis, with children in families subject to stressful circumstances such as a divorce experiencing a threefold higher risk. These events are more commonly associated with the development of secondary enuresis. Bedwetting is also more common in lower socioeconomic groups. The theory that enuresis is a psychopathologic disorder has been largely refuted. Several studies have confirmed that enuretics do not have significant differences in psychological disorders compared with healthy children.

Behavioral Factors

Behavioral factors leading to night-time polyuria may also influence enuresis. This may occur with fluid intake

and patterns between daytime and night-time as well as the role of diuretics. In 1886, a pharmacist named Pemberton changed the US and the rest of the world when he created a carbonated beverage to treat hangovers and headaches by mixing an extract of coca with an extract of the African Kola nut. The diuretic activity of caffeine is well documented. Today, consumption of caffeinated soft drinks grows at a dizzying pace, up more than 500% since 1950. A typical 12 oz of soft drink contains anywhere between 30 and 60 mg of caffeine. With a pharmacological dose of caffeine at approximately $2 \, mg \, kg^{-1}$ of body weight, a 30 kg child receives a pharmacologic dose in each 12 oz can. Surveys have shown that people aged 12–24 years consume the most caffeine, followed by people in the 6–11-year age group. A 1986 survey revealed that 25% of 1–3-year-old children consume an average of 7 oz of soft drink per day. Chocolate and cocoa also contain caffeine.

Sleep Factors

The role of sleep disorders in enuresis has long been controversial. A hypothesis suggests that enuresis is a disorder in sleep arousal, with anecdotal evidence reporting that enuretic children are more difficult to arouse. However, controlled studies have found that children with enuresis do not sleep more soundly than do healthy children, with enuretic episodes occurring in random stages of sleep. An association between nocturnal enuresis and obstructive sleep apnea, however, suggested that apneic episodes increased secretion of atrial natriuretic factor. Elevated levels of atrial natriuretic factor lead to inhibition of renin secretion which leads to decreased aldosterone levels and subsequent increased diuresis and night-time polyuria. Treatments of obstructive sleep apnea have been shown to decrease nocturnal enuresis.

Organic Disease

The majority of monosymptomatic nocturnal enuretics are unlikely to have an organic cause for their bedwetting. However, conditions such as urinary tract infections, spinal cord pathology, posterior urethral valves, ectopic ureter, constipation, diabetes insipidus, and diabetes mellitus all need to be considered and understood in the evaluation of enuretic patients. In a study of over 9000 school-aged girls, the prevalence of significant bacteriuria was 1.5% in healthy girls and 5.6% in bedwetters with treatment of infection alone curing a significant number of enuretics. Urinary infection is also commonly associated with diurnal enuresis. In relapsing enuretics, particularly in girls, irritated bladders with chronically inflamed mucosa termed cystitis cystica can cause enuresis with negative urine cultures, but may respond to long-term antibiotic therapy. Although not a common cause of enuresis in the US, pinworm infection is an important cause of sudden onset of enuresis in young girls. Diagnosis is made by recovering eggs in feces, the perineal skin, and under fingernails, and the infection responds well to antihelmintic therapy.

Evaluation

Timing of Presentation

The timing of parents presenting with a child to the pediatrician is individualized depending on that family's concept of 'normal'. It is important to initially present to parents the natural progression of bladder control and to work with them in choosing when to begin treatment. In the initial discussion, it is crucial that the parents understand that the child is not wetting the bed on purpose and that enuresis is not a volitional event. The child also needs to learn to take responsibility for staying dry. Enuresis may disrupt sleep and be a source of turmoil for the entire family and parents may become frustrated with the child. In fact, up to 20–36% of parents punish their children for bedwetting. Although we do not advocate watchful waiting in children older than 8 years, if a child does not view the bedwetting as a problem and is not interested in treatment, then we do not insist.

History

The evaluation of children with nocturnal enuresis begins with a thorough history and physical examination (**Table 1**). Specifically, the timing and onset of enuresis needs to be established. Is it primary, or has the child had previous dry intervals? How many wet episodes occur each night, and how frequently is the child wet? Specific questions need to be asked to characterize the child's voiding. Does the child or parent complain of urgency, diurnal incontinence, frequency, or slow or intermittent stream? Is there a history of constant wetness suggestive of an ectopic ureter? Have the parents noticed posturing such as leg crossing, squatting, or Vincent's curtsey which may be signs of urgency?

Table 1 Common voiding symptoms

Symptoms of voiding dysfunction

- Frequency
- Urgency
   Leg crossing
   Squatting
- Urinary incontinence
   Daytime
   Night-time
- Dysuria
- Urinary tract infections
- Incomplete emptying
- Slow stream
- Constipation
- Stool incontinence

Vincent's curtsey refers to adopting a low crouch position and pressing the heel against the perineum in an attempt to prevent urinary leakage from an uncontrolled bladder contraction by increasing sphincter pressure. What about a history of polyuria or polydipsia? Are there any prior urinary tract infections or dysuria? Does the child have a normal bowel habit, associated constipation, or alternatively encopresis, defined as fecal soiling or the involuntary passage of feces? Indeed, dysfunctional voiding is often associated with bowel changes as 15% of children with enuresis have encopresis, and 25% of children with encopresis have enuresis. A complete voiding and stooling diary for several days to record the timing and volume of voids and stools per day can be extremely helpful (**Figure 3**). In addition, a careful diary of the amounts, timing, and types of fluids consumed is vital with particular notation of caffeinated beverages. Milestones to assess for developmental delay should be evaluated as well as neurological problems such as changes in gait. Other medical problems that may contribute to enuresis such as sleep apnea, diabetes, or epilepsy need to be inquired. It is important to consider that shame and abuse are important elements in the lives of enuretic children who may be subject to abuse and wrongful punishment. This anxiety and embarrassment may make them reluctant to discuss the wetting.

Given the genetic predisposition, a family history of enuresis is required. A history of enuresis in either parent or in any siblings should be ascertained, as well as the age in which nocturnal continence was achieved. A review of socioeconomic conditions and stresses at home may help yield information on precipitating causes of the bedwetting, such as an acrimonious divorce coinciding with the onset of secondary enuresis. The parents and child need to be interviewed regarding their attitudes toward bedwetting and how it has affected their familial relationships. Finally, the physician should question the parents and child carefully for a history of punishment and abuse.

Physical Examination

The physical examination should carefully review several specific systems for signs of underlying abnormalities to suggest organic disease and thus complex enuresis, including a thorough neurologic, genitourinary, and abdominal examination. For the neurological examination, first the child's back should be examined carefully for signs of occult sacral dysraphism such as sacral dimpling, hairy patches, or sacral agenesis. Examination of the L5 to S3 motor and sensory nerves should be made with assessment of muscle tone, strength, and sensation. Peripheral reflexes, anal sphincter tone, and the bulbocavernosus reflex should be tested. An abdominal exam should focus on bladder distention following voiding to identify a large postvoid residual and signs of constipation or fecal impaction. The genitalia should be inspected to evaluate for

Intake and voiding record

Name _____

Start date _____

	Day 1		Day 2	
	Fluid intake	Void/stool	Fluid intake	Void/stool
12 am	_____	_____	_____	_____
1 am	_____	_____	_____	_____
2 am	_____	_____	_____	_____
3 am	_____	_____	_____	_____
4 am	_____	_____	_____	_____
5 am	_____	_____	_____	_____
6 am	_____	_____	_____	_____
7 am	_____	_____	_____	_____
8 am	_____	_____	_____	_____
9 am	_____	_____	_____	_____
10 am	_____	_____	_____	_____
11 am	_____	_____	_____	_____
12 pm	_____	_____	_____	_____
1 pm	_____	_____	_____	_____
2 pm	_____	_____	_____	_____
3 pm	_____	_____	_____	_____
4 pm	_____	_____	_____	_____
5 pm	_____	_____	_____	_____
6 pm	_____	_____	_____	_____
7 pm	_____	_____	_____	_____
8 pm	_____	_____	_____	_____
9 pm	_____	_____	_____	_____
10 pm	_____	_____	_____	_____
11 pm	_____	_____	_____	_____
12 am	_____	_____	_____	_____

Fluid intake: record intake in ounces, c, caffeinated beverage
Void/stool: v, void; a, accident; b, bowel movement; s, bowel accident

Figure 3   Sample intake and voiding record. An example of a 48-h voiding diary.

aberrant anatomy that may result in incontinence such as meatal stenosis, epispadias, bifid clitoris or labial adhesions, or evidence of meatal pits which correlate with the incidence of ectopic ureters. The physician should also be aware of signs of sexual abuse including tearing, scars, or trauma. Hypospadias itself is not an etiology for incontinence. Observed voiding is essential for evidence of slow stream or intermittency. Furthermore, we always inspect the child's underwear for evidence of wetness, suggesting diurnal and therefore complex enuresis. Physical examinations in monosymptomatic nocturnal enuresis are almost always completely normal.

Laboratory and Radiographic Examination

Part of the goal for the history and physical examination is to identify the small number of children who need further investigation and treatment. A routine urinalysis and culture identifies children who may have a urinary tract infection and rules out inadequate urine concentration by the kidneys if a specific gravity of 1.022 or greater can be achieved. If dilute urine is identified, it can be confirmed by a morning void. Glucose in the urine may identify children with diabetes and resulting polyuria.

Approximate functional bladder capacity can be ascertained by two described methods: physiological voluntary end fill whereby the child keeps a 48-h diary noting time and voided volume to determine the maximum volume, or the rapid oral fill, where the child ingests a oral water load approximately $20 \, \text{ml kg}^{-1}$ over 1 h and asking the child to hold his or her urine for as long as possible and then to measure the volume. These values are the estimated functional bladder capacity and can be compared to age-appropriate nomograms as discussed prior. This can be performed in conjunction with an uroflow measurement to identify children with a slow stream, and bladder ultrasounds to measure postvoid residuals.

Monosymptomatic vs. Polysymptomatic Enuresis

At the end of the history, physical examination, and initial laboratory and radiographic imaging, a decision is made whether the child has monosymptomatic or polysymptomatic enuresis. Any child with findings on the review of symptoms and physical examination suggestive of neurologic or anatomic abnormalities, or persistent positive laboratory studies needs to be referred for further urologic evaluation which may include voiding cystourethrography and bladder ultrasonography to evaluate the lower urinary tract and renal ultrasonography to evaluate the upper urinary tract for aberrant anatomy. More recently, magnetic resonance imaging has become a powerful imaging tool to evaluate for genitourinary anomalies. A complete urodynamic test to elucidate abnormal physiology of voiding may be required. The child may require surgical intervention and reconstruction and the discussion is reviewed elsewhere.

Treatment

Once a decision has been made that the bedwetting may not spontaneously resolve, children need to take an active role in treating enuresis. Children should begin treatment only if they are interested and committed. A child unwilling to invest time and energy, regardless of parental concern, is unlikely to respond to therapy. We generally institute treatment at 7–8 years of age. Treatment can be frustrating for parents and children and taxing on physicians. Rates of relapse can be significant and parents need to be made aware and have realistic expectations. Age-appropriate norms should be reviewed. Given the benign nature of the condition, it is also extremely important to implement measures that have virtually no side effects and a risk no greater than that of treatment failure. We also stress the effect of the placebo which shows that treatment is measurably more effective when the patient perceives it as being personally and individually administered by a committed physician rather than through an impersonal protocol. Here we review both behavioral therapy and medical management with pharmacotherapy (**Table 2**). Ultimately, multiple treatment modalities may be employed to achieve a balanced program with the goals of a significant improvement in the number of wet episodes.

Table 2 The common classes of behavioral and pharmacological treatments for nocturnal enuresis

Behavioral	Pharmacological
Fluid intake regulation	
Bladder training	Desmopressin
Bed-wetting alarm	Imipramine
Motivational therapy	Anticholinergic drugs
Hypnotherapy	Acupuncture

Behavioral

Behavioral therapy for enuresis is safe, effective, and often used in conjunction with medical therapy. Traditional therapies include regulating fluid intake, bladder training, and an enuresis alarm. Recently, developments in motivational therapy and hypnotherapy hold promise in the treatment of nocturnal enuresis.

Fluid intake

Although fluid restriction is often recommended, it has not been shown to be effective, and could place the child at risk for dehydration. More effective is a redistribution of fluid intake to decrease nocturnal polyuria. The child's fluid requirements are calculated using the approximation of $100 \, ml \, day^{-1}$ for the first 10 kg body weight, 50 ml day^{-1} for the second 10 kg, and $25 \, ml \, day^{-1}$ for every additional kilogram body weight. The child is instructed to consume approximately 40% of total fluid intake in the morning, 40% in the afternoon, and 20% in the evening. We never ask children to restrict fluid intake. This 'redistribution' helps to promote healthy drinking habits while seeking to decrease urine production at night. Caffeine is eliminated from the diet.

Bladder training

Retention-control training strives to increase the functional bladder capacity of enuretic children with decreased functional capacity. Bladder retention training involves increasing bladder capacity by asking children to hold urine for successively longer intervals after first sensing an urge to void. Voiding diaries are kept to document frequency and voided volumes. The largest volumes are plotted reflecting functional bladder capacity, and compared to calculated age-appropriate bladder capacity. Although results have been variable, mean bladder capacity can be increased over twofold in some studies with cure rates estimated up to 35%. When retention training is combined with other modalities, the results can be impressive. We stress the importance of increasing functional bladder capacity prior to pharmacotherapy with antidiuretic hormone desmopressin acetate (DDAVP).

Alarms

Bladder alarms originate back to 1902, and are arguably the most effective behavioral therapy. Initial models consisted of a detector pad on which the child slept that was activated by urine and awakened the child with an alarm. Current models use transistor technology and consist of a battery-operated device attached to the collar or wrist with an audible alarm or vibrator that is connected to a thin wire attached to the child's underclothes, resembling a small pager in a self-contained unit. A few drops of urine activate the system. The alarm acts as a conditional stimulus that awakens the child when micturition occurs. The mechanism by which the alarm paired with bedwetting is not fully understood. One theory is the alarm conditioned patients to wake up when the bladder is full. However, when using the alarm, many children learned to sleep throughout the night without waking or wetting, with findings of increased functional bladder capacity over the treatment course. This suggested that the alarm may condition the inhibition of the detrusor muscle allowing increased bladder capacity to compensate for bladder fullness.

Randomized, controlled trials showed the enuresis alarm system to be quite effective with a 40–80% response rate, and a relapse rate of only 20–40% and minimized with retreatment. Compared to other behavioral treatments and medical management of nocturnal enuresis, the alarm has the best long-term efficacy. Treatment duration is usually stopped after four dry weeks are achieved with interval usage possibly decreasing the rate of relapse. However, the conditioned response can be a lengthy process and may disrupt the family more than is acceptable with an average of 16 weeks of therapy required. Some families will not tolerate the frequent night waking or the alarm may not wake the child, or may wake other siblings. Success improves with motivation of the child and parents willing to get up with their children at night.

Motivational and hypnotherapy

Motivational therapy promotes behavior modification by making the child responsible for his or her enuresis and crediting for their successes. The therapy requires that the parents and child develop a positive relationship with respect to enuresis and a good rapport between the physician and the family. Although it is difficult to assess the success of motivational therapy, it has been estimated to be as high as 25%. If the child does respond to therapy, a low rate of relapse can be expected.

In hypnotherapy, the patient is first induced to enter a hypnotic state, and then the therapy begins by suggesting that the child will wake up if he or she needs to urinate during the night, that the bladder will be able to hold more urine, and that the child will be able to control his or her urination. A clinical trial has shown that three 30 min sessions of hypnotherapy had similar immediate response rates compared to imipramine, but with improved response rates at 6 months of 68% compared to 24%, respectively. Case series have shown response rates of 60–70%. These two modalities will need to be studied further but reveal the promise of positive suggestions in the treatment of nocturnal enuresis.

Scheduled voiding

In addition to punishment, there are a number of practices that parents should be discouraged from employing. Picking up a child during the night to allow urination without fully awakening the child or waking the child at night to void before wetting has occurred has not been shown to resolve bedwetting. The time of night when a child wets is variable and these practices may teach the child to empty without fully awakening. Also, prolonged use of diapers or pull-ups is inappropriate because it encourages regressive behavior.

Medical Management

Pharmacotherapy for enuresis targets the proposed physiologic alterations contributing to nocturnal enuresis, mainly altered AVP secretion and bladder instability. These medications include DDAVP, imipramine, and oxybutynin. Promising reports on the use of acupuncture will also be discussed in this section.

Desmopressin acetate

The newest medication approved for enuresis appears the most promising. In 1990, the (FDA) Food and Drug Administration approved DDAVP for the treatment of nocturnal enuresis. A synthetic analog of vasopressin with a long half-life, DDAVP decreases urine output by retaining water at the level of the distal tubules. It theoretically functions by reducing the nocturnal urine output below the functional bladder capacity and may be most effective in the approximately 25% of children who do not demonstrate the normal diurnal increases in AVP secretion. Its efficacy is maximized once children regulate their fluid intake and have normalized their functional bladder capacity. A review of randomized, controlled trials using DDAVP showed that 10–40% of patients became totally dry with a mean of 25%. Unfortunately, relapse rates have been as high as 60%, suggesting a symptomatic control of enuresis.

DDAVP is available as a nasal spray or tablet. The nasal spray is started at 20 μg and titrated up to 40 μg daily, while the oral tablet is started at 0.2 mg daily at bedtime and can be titrated up to 0.6 mg daily. Treatment is continued for 3–6 months with a gradual taper of the medication. Side effects are rare with the most common complaint of nasal irritation for the nasal spray formulation, abdominal discomfort, nausea, and headache. The most severe, yet rare side effect is hyponatremia, with no reports occurring in controlled clinical trials.

Imipramine

The tricyclic antidepressant imipramine was first shown to improve bedwetting in 1960. It is still the most widely prescribed in its class although other family members have been used. Imipramine has multiple effects, with a weak anticholinergic activity and an α-adrenergic activity on the internal urethral sphincter to promote continence. Imipramine has also been shown to stimulate ADH secretion. Results with imipramine are variable with cure rates reported up to 50%. However, high relapse rates (up to 60%) with long-term cure rates of only 25% after discontinuation of the medicine suggest a predominant role in the symptomatic control of enuresis.

We recommend an initial 2-week trial, and if a child responds, continuing a 2-month course with gradual weaning by decreasing dosage and frequency. If the patient relapses, therapy is continued with trial cessation at 3-month intervals. Imipramine is taken once per day, usually before bedtime, at $0.9–1.5\,\text{mg}\,\text{kg}^{-1}\,\text{day}^{-1}$. Average doses given for children 5–8 years old are 25 mg with 50 mg given to older children and adolescents. Side effects are generally uncommon and include nervousness, sleep disturbance, and gastrointestinal irritability. However, the largest risk is in children who accidentally ingest the drug in large quantities with toxic overdose leading to cardiac arrhythmias, conduction block, hypotension, convulsions, and death. Parents must secure and control the drug carefully.

Anticholinergic Drugs
Anticholinergic Drugs such as oxybutynin have been found to be largely ineffective in children with monosymptomatic nocturnal enuresis with a partial response rate ranging from 5% to 40% in bedwetting reduction, which was no better than placebo. In children with polysymptomatic nocturnal enuresis with documented bladder instability by urodynamics, oxybutynin may be effective in decreasing symptoms of daytime urgency, frequency, and diurnal incontinence. However, recent studies investigating combination therapy with oxybutynin plus imipramine, and oxybutynin plus desmopressin, suggested a synergistic effect with combinatorial therapy more effective than monotherapy with either agent along.

Acupuncture
Several case series have shown impressive results for the use of acupuncture in the treatment of nocturnal enuresis with 73–98% cure rates, requiring anywhere from one to more than 40 sessions. Although one randomized controlled trial showed similar responses compared to desmopressin, further investigation in the effect and number of treatments needs to be performed for this promising alternative therapy.

Conclusion

Nocturnal enuresis is a common childhood urinary condition that has a high rate of spontaneous cure, but its prolongation can interfere with socialization and raise anxiety for children and their families. Multiple etiologies contribute to nocturnal enuresis including physiological and behavioral conditions. Proper diagnosis is critical and identifying signs of complicated or diurnal enuresis in the initial evaluation warrants further investigation and studies. We recommend seeking therapy when primary monosymptomatic nocturnal enuresis persists at 7–8 years of age. Behavioral therapies including altering fluid intake, bladder training, and motivational therapy are benign and have shown positive results. The conditioned response from enuresis alarms have proved to be the most efficacious treatment, while pharmacological therapy with desmopressin has demonstrated significant responses with minimal side effects. No one treatment modality has a 100% response rate; thus, combinatorial therapy tailored to the individual child and family proves the most expedient solution to resolution of primary nocturnal enuresis.

See also: Endocrine System.

Suggested Readings

Blum NJ (2004) Nocturnal enuresis: Behavioral treatments. *Urologic Clinics of North America* 31: 499–507.
Jalkut MW, Lerman SE, and Churchill BM (2001) Enuresis. *Pediatric Clinics of North America* 48: 1461–1488.
Koff SA and Jayanthi VR (2002) Nocturnal enuresis. In: Walsh PC, Retik AB, Vaughan DE, and Wein AJ (eds.) *Campbell's Urology*, 8th edn., pp. 2273–2283. Philadelphia, PA: W.B. Saunders.
Mammen AA and Ferrer FA (2004) Nocturnal enuresis: Medical management. *Urologic Clinics of North America* 31: 491–498.
Rushton HG (1989) Nocturnal enuresis: Epidemiology, evaluation, and currently available treatment options. *Journal of Pediatrics* 114: 691–696.

Relevant Websites

http://www.bedwettingstore.com – Bedwetting Store.
http://www.pottypager.com – Potty Pager.

Birth Complications and Outcomes

D L Smith, The Children's Hospital, Denver, CO, USA

Glossary

Bronchopulmonary dysplasia – A chronic lung condition that is caused by tissue damage to the lungs, is marked by inflammation and scarring, and usually occurs in immature infants who have received mechanical ventilation and supplemental oxygen as treatment for respiratory distress syndrome.
Cerebral palsy – A nonprogressive central nervous system disorder characterized by abnormal development of movement and posture that results in impaired motor activity and coordination.

Extremely preterm infant – An infant born at less than 28 completed weeks of gestation.

Hydrocephalus – An abnormal increase in the amount of cerebrospinal fluid within the cranial cavity that is accompanied by expansion of the cerebral ventricles and enlargement of the skull.

Hypoxic ischemic encephalopathy (HIE) – A clinical condition in newborn infants characterized by damage to the central nervous system resulting from an inadequate supply of blood and oxygen to the brain.

Ischemia – Deficient supply of blood to a body part (heart or brain) that is due to obstruction of the inflow of arterial blood.

Necrotizing enterocolitis (NEC) – A gastrointestinal disease that mainly affects premature infants characterized by infection and inflammation of the bowel wall that can lead to irreversible damage and destruction.

Perinatal asphyxia (also known as intrapartum asphyxia) – An interruption in placental blood flow during labor that is significant enough to cause decreased oxygen delivery to the infant.

Preeclampsia – A serious condition developing in late pregnancy that is characterized by a sudden rise in blood pressure, excessive weight gain, generalized edema, proteinuria, severe headache, and visual disturbances.

Preterm infant – An infant born at less than 37 completed weeks of gestation.

Retinopathy of prematurity (ROP) – A disease of premature infants that is caused by abnormal growth and development of retinal blood vessels that can lead to permanent damage to the retina and vision loss.

Very preterm infant – An infant born at less than 32 completed weeks of gestation.

Introduction

There are roughly 4 000 000 infants born in the US each year and the vast majority of these babies do well. However, about 10% of these newborn infants will be sick enough to require care in the neonatal intensive care unit (NICU). Of those infants cared for in the NICU, a small percentage will sustain injury significant to produce long-term morbidities that include neurodevelopmental impairment. There are a number of reasons that infants are admitted to the NICU and a number of conditions that result in long-term impairment. This article focuses on the two most common identifiable causes of neurodevelopmental delay and cerebral palsy (CP): premature birth and perinatal asphyxia.

Premature Birth

Premature birth is a significant problem in the US that has a major impact on the development of infants and children. Despite major advances in the care of pregnant women and premature infants, premature birth remains a leading cause of infant mortality and childhood disability. This section offers an overview of the risk factors and causes of preterm birth. The mortality and morbidity associated with prematurity are then described in detail with a focus on long-term outcome. Specific therapeutic interventions that have significantly altered the outcome of premature infants are also discussed.

Gestational Age and Birth Weight

Preterm birth is defined as delivery of an infant at less than 37 completed weeks of gestation. Premature infants are further classified as 'very preterm' and 'extremely preterm' because the complications associated with preterm birth vary based on the infant's gestational age. Infants can also be classified based on their birth weight. The definition of a low birth weight (LBW) infant is an infant weighing less than 2500 g (5.5 lb) at delivery. Very low birth weight (VLBW) is defined as a weight of less than 1500 g (3.3 lb) and extremely low birth weight (ELBW) is a weight of less than 1000 g (2.2 lb).

In general, there is agreement between gestational age and birth weight. Most infants born at less than 28 weeks, gestation weigh less than 1000 g and are therefore extremely preterm and ELBW. However, only two-thirds of all LBW infants are born preterm. The remaining third of LBW infants are born at term but are small for their gestational age. In addition, premature infants can also be small for their gestational age and these infants are at risk for additional complications.

It is important to recognize the distinction between gestational age and birth weight when reviewing studies about preterm infants. These two classifications are not interchangeable. For example, two infants may be born weighing 1300 g but one infant is an appropriately sized 31 week preterm infant and the other is a small for gestational age 34 week preterm infant. These two infants should not be treated the same, either in clinical practice or in research studies.

Epidemiology of Preterm Birth

The percentage of preterm births in the US in 2004 was 12.5%, which is equal to one in eight infants being born preterm. The incidence of preterm birth has steadily increased since the early 1980s (9.4% in 1981). The percentage of infants born very preterm in 2004 was approximately 2%, which has been relatively stable since about the mid-1990s. The rate of LBW infants was 8.1% in 2004, which is the highest level since 1970. One reason for the increase in preterm and LBW infants is the increase in multiple births in the US. The risk of preterm delivery is six times greater for a multiple birth than for a singleton pregnancy. In addition, approximately half of all multiple births are LBW infants.

The incidence of preterm delivery varies with maternal age and maternal race. Women under 20 and over 40 years of age have the highest rates of preterm delivery. In addition, black women have a significantly higher rate of preterm delivery compared to all other racial and ethnic groups. The disparity in preterm birth between black and white women has been persistent over a number of years and the reasons for the differences are not completely known. This increased risk of preterm birth is not fully explained by differences in socioeconomic status or access to prenatal care. The rate of preterm birth is higher for black women compared to nonblack women for all educational levels.

Etiology of Premature Birth

Table 1 lists the common causes of preterm delivery. Preterm birth is a heterogeneous condition and there are important differences in outcomes based on the cause of delivery and associated complications. The most recent data from the US show that approximately 50% of preterm deliveries occur after the spontaneous onset of preterm labor. The cause of spontaneous pre-term labor remains unclear but there is substantial evidence that infection plays an important role in the etiology of preterm birth. In addition, perinatal infection and inflammation is associated with increased morbidity for the infant and is an important risk factor for later neurodevelopmental impairment. Pregnancies complicated by premature rupture of membranes are also at increased risk of infection and corresponding neurological deficits.

Roughly 40% of preterm infants are the result of medically indicated preterm delivery. Indications for preterm delivery can be either fetal compromise (poor growth or poor placental perfusion) or maternal medical conditions (severe hypertension or intrauterine infection).

Table 1 Causes of pre-term delivery

Spontaneous pre-term labor
Multiple gestation
Cervical incompetence
Uterine malformations
Pre-term premature rupture of membranes
Medically indicated pre-term delivery
   Pregnancy induced hypertension/preeclampsia
   Intrauterine growth retardation
   Antepartum hemorrhage
   Fetal distress

There has been a significant increase in the number of medically indicated preterm deliveries in the US over the 1990s. This increase in medically indicated preterm deliveries was associated with a decrease in perinatal mortality and stillbirths over that same time period. It should be viewed as a success of the advances made in obstetrical and neonatal care. Many infants with significant intrauterine compromise are now delivered prematurely and have an excellent prognosis, especially if delivered after 32 weeks, gestation. However, there is still a need to decrease the incidence of spontaneous preterm delivery as this remains a leading cause of infant mortality and morbidity.

Mortality Associated with Premature Birth

The incidence of both mortality and major morbidity increases with decreasing gestational age and birth weight. Infants born between 23 and 26 weeks, gestation are at the highest risk for death or major disability. **Figure 1** shows a summary of the current survival rates for very preterm infants. Data from large network studies show that the chance of surviving to hospital discharge for an infant born between 23 and 24 weeks, gestation is only 30%. The rate of survival steadily increases after 24 weeks, gestation from 50% survival at 24 weeks, to 80% survival at 26 weeks, completed gestation. Survival is generally good for infants born after 27 weeks, gestation, with 90% being discharged home from the hospital. Mortality is uncommon for infants delivered after 31 weeks, gestation and greater than 95% of those infants survive.

The Centers for Disease Control and Prevention states that preterm birth is a leading cause of infant mortality in

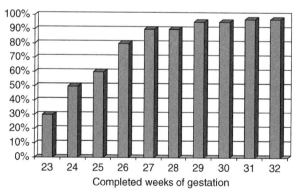

Figure 1 Likelihood of survival based on gestational age. Summary of data from: Bolisetty S, Bajuk B, ME A, *et al.* (2006) Preterm outcome table (POT): A simple tool to aid counseling parents of very preterm infants. *Australian and New Zealand Journal of Obstetrics and Gynecology* 24: 189; Jones HP, Karuri S, Cronin C, *et al.* (2005) Actuarial survival of a large Canadian cohort of preterm infants. *BMC Pediatrics* 5: 40; and Lorenz JM (2001) The outcome of extreme prematurity. *Seminars in Perinatology* 25: 348–359.

the United States, accounting for over 30% of the infant deaths reported in 2002. Premature birth was second only to birth defects as a cause of death in the first year of life. The majority of premature infants who died in the 2002 study were born at less than 32 weeks, gestation with birth weights less than 1500 g. The number of infant deaths attributed to preterm delivery was highest at 23 weeks, gestation and decreased steadily as gestational age increased. The majority of the infants died soon after birth, with two-thirds dying within the first 24 h of life.

The mortality reported above are population-based statistics that can be used as general guidelines when discussing the likelihood of survival of infants born at a given gestational age. There are a number of additional factors, however, that must be taken into account when discussing the expected survival of a particular infant. Both the race and gender of the infant have been shown to affect survival. These differences are most pronounced at earlier gestational ages. For infants born at less than 28 weeks, gestation, there appears to be a slight survival advantage for black infants over white infants. In addition, female infants have a survival advantage when compared to male infants regardless of race. Another important determinant of the infant's chance of survival is birth weight. Infants who are growth-restricted have an increased mortality compared to appropriately grown infants of the same gestational age. Just like race and gender, the effect of birth weight on mortality is most pronounced for infants delivered at less than 28 weeks.

Care at the Limits of Viability

Infants that are born between 22 and 24 weeks, gestation are often referred to as being at the threshold of viability. There continues to be active debate on whether or not these patients should receive aggressive obstetrical and neonatal care. There are significant gaps in knowledge concerning the care of pregnant women at risk for delivering between 22 and 24 weeks and how to best care for the newborn infant. It is safe to say that most neonatologists consider intensive care therapy at 22 weeks, gestation to be of no benefit to the infant. Many neonatologists even consider therapy at 23 weeks, gestation to be of questionable benefit. These conclusions are based on the very poor survival rate for these infants despite intensive care. In addition, of the infants that do survive, the majority will have severe disabilities in childhood. These disabilities include CP, mental retardation, and blindness.

Given the uncertain benefit of therapy for this population, many obstetricians and neonatologists do not recommend aggressive obstetrical management, such as Cesarean section delivery, or active resuscitation for infants born at less than 24 weeks, gestation. Despite the overall poor prognosis of these infants, some parents request that everything be done on behalf of their baby.

In these cases it is appropriate to offer resuscitation and aggressive intensive care. The care of the infant must be decided on a case-by-case basis and cannot be generalized for all patients.

It is imperative that the healthcare team be aware of the most current data on the survival and outcomes of these infants in order to help the parents make an informed decision about how to best care for their child. Whenever possible there should be a joint discussion with the obstetrical and pediatric team. Unfortunately, most of these conversations occur under suboptimal circumstances when a mother presents with an acute complication and the parents are asked to make difficult decisions in a short amount of time. If the parents do not elect to provide aggressive resuscitation for their infant, the baby should receive comfort care and the parents offered ongoing emotional support.

Morbidity Associated with Premature Birth

The majority of complications associated with premature delivery occur in the 1–2% of infants that are born before 32 weeks, gestation, in particular those babies born at 28 weeks or less. The two most significant morbidities associated with premature birth are lung disease and neurodevelopmental delay. Other less common, but potentially devastating, morbidities include retinopathy of prematurity (ROP), necrotizing enterocolitis (NEC), and infection.

Respiratory distress syndrome and chronic lung disease

One of the most common complications experienced by preterm infants is respiratory distress syndrome (RDS). RDS and the resulting respiratory failure is the leading cause of death in premature infants and infants born at less than 28 weeks, gestation are at greatest risk. RDS results from a lack of surfactant in the newborn's lungs. Surfactant is a chemical that is normally produced by the lungs between 34 and 37 weeks, gestation. The main role of surfactant is to reduce the surface tension of the small air sacs (alveoli) in the lung and prevent their collapse. Premature babies born with surfactant deficiency have significant respiratory distress and hypoxia which requires mechanical ventilation. In addition to a lack of surfactant, extremely premature infants are born with structurally very immature lungs that have both a decreased number of alveoli and incomplete development of the alveoli that are present. These infants are at very high risk to develop significant lung disease in the neonatal period which may have long-term implications.

There have been two significant advances since the late 1980s that have altered the incidence and severity of RDS. These therapies are worth discussing in detail because they have allowed for the increased survival of extremely premature infants. The first intervention is the administration of steroid therapy to the mother before delivery. Corticosteroids given to the mother in anticipation of pre-term delivery have been shown to decrease early neonatal mortality, RDS, and the need for mechanical ventilation. Despite the fact that antenatal steroid therapy does reduce the incidence and severity of RDS, the majority of infants born before 28 weeks will still require assisted ventilation at delivery. Some of these infants will then go on to develop chronic lung disease.

In addition to antenatal steroid therapy, infants routinely receive exogenous surfactant after delivery. Surfactant therapy immediately after birth decreases the severity of lung disease. Numerous studies from 1980 on have demonstrated that surfactant therapy rapidly improves oxygenation and leads to decreased ventilator support. There have also been several observational studies that show increased survival of VLBW infants after the introduction of surfactant into routine practice. These studies give further evidence of its beneficial effects. Unfortunately, there are no consistent data that surfactant decreases the incidence of chronic lung disease. This is because the pathophysiology of lung disease in extremely premature infants is more than a lack of surfactant. There is also a component of abnormal alveolar development. These infants' lungs demonstrate injury from oxygen toxicity and trauma that results from the mechanical ventilation of structurally immature alveoli. The remodeling that results from this injury has long-term consequences for pulmonary function.

Chronic lung disease, also known as bronchopulmonary dysplasia, remains a common long-term complication of babies born at less than 28 weeks, gestation. The exact incidence in preterm infants is hard to determine since there is no universal definition used in the literature but most studies report that between 30% and 40% of infants born before 28 weeks, gestation develop chronic lung disease. Chronic lung disease is relatively uncommon in babies born after 30 weeks or with a birth weight greater than 1200 g.

The morbidity associated with chronic lung disease includes a greater likelihood of re-hospitalization in the first 2 years of life with up to 50% of infants being re-admitted to the hospital for respiratory illnesses. Although hospitalizations decrease after the age of 4–5 years, these children continue to have a greater frequency of chronic respiratory symptoms such as recurrent wheezing and cough. In addition, infants with chronic lung disease have a worse developmental outcome compared to premature infants who do not develop chronic lung disease. The association between chronic lung disease and impaired neurodevelopment is complex and not completely understood. It is likely that the same conditions that predispose to developing chronic lung disease, namely inflammation and infection, also predispose to developmental delay.

Neurodevelopmental disability

The second common morbidity associated with prematurity is neurodevelopmental disability. The first two questions a parent of a premature infant asks are whether their baby will survive and be normal. The risk of neurologic impairment for premature infants is well known. The following sections offer an overview of the current information available concerning the neurodevelopmental outcomes of premature infants and describe factors that adversely affect outcome.

Numerous studies have looked at the changes in outcomes of VLBW and ELBW infants over the 20 years between the 1980s and the 1990s. The most consistent finding in all of these studies is that although survival of these infants has increased, rates of neurodevelopmental disability have remained stable. Some studies have even shown an increased rate of disability in this population over time. As obstetrical and neonatal intensive care has improved over the past two decades many of the smallest and youngest infants are able to survive, but they are still at great risk for complications that lead to long-term neurodevelopmental impairment.

When reviewing the literature on neurodevelopmental outcomes in premature infants some common limitations need to be discussed. The first is the length of follow-up. The majority of studies reporting developmental outcomes of preterm infants only follow children up to the age of 2 or 3 years. This is particularly true in studies that are evaluating a particular therapeutic intervention in the nursery. Developmental outcomes in early childhood do not always accurately predict outcomes in later childhood, for example, school performance. In general, a severe disability that is identified in early childhood is predictive of significant disability throughout childhood. However, there are a number of children who have severe disabilities and limitations at school age that are not predicted by an evaluation in early childhood.

Another limitation of these outcome studies is the number of patients who are lost to follow-up and unable to be evaluated. The authors should clearly state whether the patients that were unavailable for follow-up differed in any way from the patients who were evaluated. In this way the reader is aware of any potential bias of the study. One final potential limitation of an outcome study is the reference or control group that is being compared to the premature infant population. Studies can show different rates of neurodevelopmental impairment depending on whether the reference population is contemporary full-term classmates or the mean of a standardized test.

Neurodevelopmental outcome of premature infants

Using the data available from large multicenter studies it is possible to make some general statements about the likelihood of neurodevelopmental impairment in premature infants. Most studies focus on infants born before 28 weeks, gestation or less than 1000 g because this is the most-at-risk population. The two most commonly reported adverse outcomes are CP and developmental delay. CP is a term for a number of related conditions that are characterized by abnormal development of movement and coordination. CP results from central nervous system injury in fetal life or early infancy and does not progress over time. The diagnosis of CP covers a wide spectrum of disorders ranging from impaired coordination to an inability to walk independently.

The prevalence of CP between 18 and 24 months of age is between 10% and 15% in infants born before 28 weeks. This is compared to less than 0.5% in full-term infants. The prevalence of developmental delay in this same group of infants at 18–24 months of age is greater than 20%, compared to less than 3% in full-term infants. Other studies have looked at functional impairment during early childhood as a primary outcome measure for pre-term infants. Using these criteria, roughly half of VLBW infants who survive will have some functional disability and one-quarter of these children will have severe impairments. Keep in mind that even in this group of extremely preterm infants the rate of major disability varies based on gestational age. Infants born at less than 25 weeks have a significantly worse outcome than infants born at 27 weeks.

Studies evaluating these high-risk infants at school age show a high degree of cognitive impairment and need for special education. Large, international, population-based studies have shown that only about half of these infants have IQ scores in the normal range between the ages of 8 and 11 years and that up to one-quarter of children evaluated have an IQ of at less than 70. Up to 50% of children born at less than 1000 g require special education services or have repeated a grade. The special needs of these children are substantial for both the family and the education system. Families should be counseled about these outcomes in early childhood so they have a realistic expectation about the challenges their child is likely to face.

Factors that adversely affect neurodevelopmental outcome

Just as the likelihood of survival is impacted by conditions specific to each individual baby, there are a number of complications that can occur in the neonatal period that significantly increase the risk of poor neurologic outcome. These complications include both central nervous system injury and systemic conditions.

Intraventricular hemorrhage (IVH), also known as germinal matrix hemorrhage, is the most common intracranial hemorrhage in the neonatal period and seen almost exclusively as a consequence of prematurity. It can be a devastating injury and is a major cause of both mortality and long-term disability. Premature infants are at increased risk for IVH because of their inability to regulate cerebral blood flow and cerebral blood pressure. Fluctuations in cerebral blood flow can lead to rupture of the immature and friable blood vessels in the premature infant's brain. This causes bleeding into the fluid-filled spaces in the brain, called ventricles. IVH may also be complicated by hemorrhage in the brain tissue, also known as the parenchyma, surrounding the ventricles. Hemorrhage into the brain parenchyma is associated with permanent brain injury. This type of IVH is often referred to as a hemorrhagic infarct.

IVH is graded from I to IV based on the appearance of the bleed on head ultrasound. An ultrasound is an imaging study that uses sound waves to generate a picture of the infant's brain and the fluid-filled ventricles. Grade I and II IVH are small bleeds that are considered mild. A grade III IVH is often referred to as a moderate hemorrhage and is complicated by enlargement of the ventricles. The ventricles can continue to enlarge over time and lead to an increased accumulation of fluid in the brain, a condition known as hydrocephalus. The most severe IVH is a grade IV bleed which is a hemorrhagic infarct of the brain tissue surrounding the ventricle. The incidence of IVH varies among nurseries, but on average is between 15% and 20% of extremely premature infants born in the US. The incidence of moderate-to-severe IVH is as high as 30% for infants born at 23 weeks, gestation and decreases to 10% for infants born at 26 weeks. Significant IVH is rare in infants born after 30 weeks, gestation with an incidence of only 1%.

The extent of neurologic damage associated with IVH depends on the size of the hemorrhage, whether or not there is involvement of the brain parenchyma, and the development of hydrocephalus. Grade I and II IVH do not lead to serious neurologic impairment but studies have shown that premature infants with mild IVH do have deficits that can be seen on specific cognitive tests when compared to premature infants without IVH. Infants with grade III and grade IV IVH are at increased risk of neurologic impairment with rates of CP and developmental delay that approach 50%.

In addition to IVH the premature infant is also at increased risk for developing periventricular leukomalacia (PVL). PVL is an injury of the white matter adjacent to the lateral ventricles. Like IVH it is seen almost exclusively in premature infants and the injury is thought to occur in the perinatal period. PVL is diagnosed by the presence of cysts in the white matter surrounding the lateral ventricles seen on ultrasound. It is often bilateral and the ultrasound findings appear 4–6 weeks after birth. The most common clinical outcome is CP.

The presence of PVL on ultrasound is currently the best predictor of poor neurodevelopmental outcome in preterm infants. However, the absence of PVL on ultrasound does not ensure a normal long-term outcome.

A number of infants with normal head ultrasounds in the neonatal period will go on to develop neurological deficits in childhood. The reason for this is presumed to be that ultrasound only identifies the most severe form of white matter injury and many premature infants have sustained significant injury that goes undetected. Recently, magnetic resonance imaging (MRI) of the brain has been used to define white matter injury in preterm infants better. MRI studies done at 40 weeks-corrected gestational age have detected both white matter and gray matter abnormalities in very premature infants. These abnormalities have been shown to predict adverse outcomes in early childhood. As more data becomes available on the ability of MRI findings to predict neurodevelopmental outcome it is likely that this will become a valuable tool for identifying those pre-term infants most at risk for poor outcomes before they leave the nursery.

In addition to the clear relationship between IVH and white matter injury with long-term impairment, there has been an increasing awareness of the role of infection as a major contributor to poor neurodevelopmental outcome. The relationship between infection and adverse neuro-developmental outcome is complex. Intrauterine infection, either clinical or subclinical, is estimated to be involved in nearly half of all preterm deliveries and the lower the gestational age at delivery the greater the likelihood of infection. It is generally accepted that pre-term infants born to mothers with intrauterine infection, also known as chorioamnionitis, have an increased risk of PVL and CP. In fact, the timing of delivery for women with premature prolonged rupture of membranes, a con-dition with a significant risk of intrauterine infection, is often dictated by the desire to avoid infection.

In addition to intrauterine infection, infection in the nursery also increases the infant's risk of neuro-developmental impairment. A large study performed by the National Institute of Child Health and Human Development Neonatal Research Network demonstrated that two-thirds of ELBW infants had at least one infection documented during their stay in the nursery. Infants who had infections in the neonatal period had a significant increase in the incidence of CP and developmental delay when evaluated at 2 years of age. More research is clearly needed to define further the association between infection and adverse neurodevelopmental outcome, in particular the mechanism underlying brain injury that results from inflammation and infection. The prevention of infection remains a major goal of the obstetrical and neonatal team caring for premature infants.

Retinopathy of prematurity

Another common morbidity seen in premature infants, in addition to chronic lung disease and neurodevelopmental impairment, is retinopathy of prematurity (ROP). ROP is an abnormality of the vascular development of the retina that is seen exclusively in premature infants. It is a major cause of visual impairment and blindness in children. Development of the retinal blood vessels begins at 16 weeks, gestation and is essentially complete by 36 weeks. Preterm delivery causes an arrest of normal vascular development and incomplete vascularization of the retina. This incom-plete vascularization leads to hypoxia, which induces new, but abnormal, vessel growth. If this process continues it can result in progressive damage of the retina and ultimately retinal detachment.

The incidence of ROP varies among institutions but it is diagnosed in roughly two-thirds of infants born at less than 1250 g. The rate of severe ROP that threatens vision and requires surgical therapy is between 25% and 35%. Although the overall incidence of ROP has not increased since the mid-1980s, the incidence of severe ROP has increased. This is due to the increased survival of extremely premature infants who have the greatest risk of developing ROP.

Therapy for ROP has focused on prevention, universal screening for at-risk infants, and surgical laser therapy. ROP cannot be completely prevented because it is a natu-ral consequence of premature birth; however, we can try to decrease the incidence and severity of the disease. There is a clear relationship between oxygen toxicity early in life and the subsequent development of ROP. It appears that sudden and wide fluctuations in oxygen saturations are associated with an increased severity of ROP. Many nur-series have developed protocols to maintain the oxygen saturation of premature infants at a constant level to try and reduce the incidence of ROP. Another mainstay of therapy for ROP is universal screening of all infants born at less than 1500 g to identify those high-risk infants likely to need surgery. The current standard for treating severe ROP is laser therapy to prevent retinal detachment. Despite aggressive attempts to prevent and treat ROP, it remains an important morbidity among premature infants.

Necrotizing enterocolitis

The last common complication associated with prematu-rity that can result in an adverse long-term outcome is necrotizing enterocolitis (NEC). NEC is the most com-mon acquired intra-abdominal emergency in newborns. It affects approximately 10% of all VLBW infants and has significant mortality and morbidity. NEC is characterized by inflammation of the bowel wall that progresses to necrosis (tissue death) that may lead to intestinal perfora-tion in the most severe cases. NEC may involve an isolated segment of bowel or it may involve multiple areas of the intestine. Although full-term infants can develop NEC, 90% of cases are seen in premature infants and infants with birth weights below 1500 g are most at risk. The majority of cases are sporadic but epidemics of NEC are well described in the literature which has suggested a role for infection in the etiology of NEC.

The cause of NEC is not clearly known, despite decades of research. It is thought to be the result of a combination of factors including a susceptible premature intestine which lacks normal integrity and defense mechanisms, ischemia or compromised blood flow, and bacterial overgrowth. The only risk factor clearly associated with NEC is prematurity. Other conditions thought to be associated with NEC are severe growth restriction, significant perinatal hypoxia or asphyxia, congenital heart disease, and certain medications. The relationship between feedings and NEC is the focus of many research studies. Enteral feedings are strongly associated with NEC because greater than 90% of infants that develop NEC have been fed. However, feeding an infant is clearly not the only cause of NEC because the majority of premature infants that are fed do well. It is hypothesized that the presence of milk feedings places additional stress on an already compromised intestine that can lead to local hypoxia and tissue necrosis.

NEC is a serious complication of prematurity with a mortality ranging from 10% to 30% despite aggressive management. The mainstay of therapy for NEC is supportive medical care and antibiotics. Approximately one-third of patients will require abdominal surgery to remove necrotic bowel. In a small number of babies the amount of intestine lost leads to an inability to tolerate feedings and prolonged dependence on intravenous nutrition, a condition known as short bowel syndrome. For those infants who do survive, NEC has been shown to be an independent risk factor for poor neurodevelopmental outcome and, therefore, can have lifelong implications.

Summary

Premature delivery remains a common cause of death and disability in infants in the US despite years of research and advances in perinatal care. The most vulnerable infants are those born before 28 weeks, gestation or at less than 1000 g. These infants have a high mortality and commonly experience complications related to their prematurity. The morbidities associated with preterm birth are numerous and often have lifelong consequences. We have seen an increase in adverse long-term outcomes as more ELBW infants are surviving the newborn period and early childhood. The morbidity associated with preterm delivery exerts a large burden on the child and his or her family as well as the heathcare and public education systems.

Perinatal Asphyxia and Hypoxic Ischemic Encephalopathy

Perinatal asphyxia refers to an interruption in blood flow and oxygen delivery to the infant which occurs during labor and delivery. One possible consequence of perinatal asphyxia is hypoxic ischemic encephalopathy (HIE). HIE is a clinical term used to describe a newborn infant with neurologic abnormalities resulting from an interruption of blood flow to the brain. The combination of perinatal asphyxia and HIE is often referred to as perinatal hypoxic ischemic brain injury.

Perinatal hypoxic ischemic brain injury is one of the most common identifiable causes of long-term neurodevelopmental disability and CP. It occurs in one to two out of every 1000 term infants. This means that a hospital with a moderate size delivery service is likely to have at least one case each year and a large tertiary care NICU will see several cases a year. This is most often an unexpected outcome of an otherwise uncomplicated pregnancy and is devastating for families. Despite advances in obstetrical care, the incidence of long-term disability associated with perinatal hypoxic ischemic injury has not changed since the late 1970s. Up until the early 2000s, the only therapy we had to offer these infants was supportive care. There are now promising new therapies being developed that may actually prevent ongoing injury and therefore improve outcome.

Mechanism of Injury

The brain injury associated with HIE occurs in two phases. The primary injury occurs as a consequence of decreased cerebral blood flow most often caused by an interruption in placental blood flow. This interruption in blood flow is often called perinatal asphyxia. The interruption in placental blood flow can be caused by acute umbilical cord compression, rupture of the uterus, a sudden separation of the placenta from the uterus (abruption), or maternal cardiovascular compromise. The decrease in cerebral blood flow and oxygen delivery results in a series of metabolic changes in the brain that will eventually lead to neuronal cell death. If, however, the infant is delivered and successfully resuscitated in the delivery room, cerebral blood flow is restored. After a brief recovery period a second phase of neuronal injury begins which has been called reperfusion injury.

Reperfusion injury is a term that refers to the damage that occurs after blood supply is restored to a tissue or organ after a period of ischemia. The return of blood flow leads to an influx of oxygen and inflammatory white blood cells that causes local oxidative damage and inflammation. The result is ongoing cell damage and cell death despite an adequate blood supply. This second phase of injury lasts from 6 to 48 h after the initial insult. Recent therapies for HIE that have been investigated are designed to alter the second phase of injury in an attempt to preserve as much function as possible.

Risk Factors for Asphyxia

Table 2 lists common conditions that increase an infant's risk of suffering from perinatal asphyxia. Asphyxia can be the result of an acute and severe interruption in blood

Table 2   Factors associated with increased risk of perinatal asphyxia

Maternal medical conditions	Obstetric complications	Fetal medical conditions
Pregnancy-induced hypertension/preeclampsia	Placental abruption	Intrauterine growth retardation
Diabetes mellitus	Umbilical cord compression/prolapse	Prematurity
Collagen vascular disease	Multiple gestation	Infection/septic shock
Substance abuse	Premature rupture of membranes	Congenital anomalies
Hemorrhage	Prolonged labor	
Acute cardiorespiratory collapse	Prolonged pregnancy (>41 weeks)	

flow, such as compression of the umbilical cord. It can also occur from a less severe compromise in blood flow in a susceptible fetus. For example, severely growth-restricted infants are chronically hypoxic and even the transient decrease in blood flow that can occur during labor can lead to significant asphyxia. Obstetricians are well aware of the potential for asphyxia in these patients and will often choose to deliver at-risk infants by Cesarean section to avoid labor.

Clinical Markers of Asphyxia

One critical aspect in caring for infants with hypoxic ischemic brain injury is to identify those infants who are most at risk for adverse outcomes. This is important for targeting therapy that may be neuroprotective. Individual clinical markers of perinatal asphyxia are not well defined and do not readily correlate with long-term developmental outcome. It is the combination of factors that is most helpful for identifying infants at risk for neurologic injury.

Fetal heart rate tracings are used routinely during labor and delivery to monitor fetal wellbeing and tolerance of labor. However, fetal heart rate tracing abnormalities do not predict neonatal or long-term outcome. This has been demonstrated by the fact that the widespread use of fetal heart rate monitoring during labor has not significantly altered the incidence of CP in term infants since the 1970s. Fetal acidemia is another clinical marker used for asphyxia. At the time of delivery a blood gas can be measured from the umbilical cord to measure fetal acid–base status. If the umbilical cord blood gas shows evidence of severe acidosis this is suggestive of significant hypoxia and increases the risk of adverse neurologic outcome. Fetal acidemia alone, however, does not always predict poor outcome. In fact, the majority of infants do well in the newborn period and only a small number develop evidence of significant injury.

Another marker that has been used for predicting adverse outcomes in neonates is the Apgar score. The Apgar score is a universally used assessment tool in the delivery room to evaluate newborn infants. It is based on a scale of 0 to 10 and encompasses five easily measured clinical features. These include heart rate, respiratory effort, muscle tone, color, and response to irritating stimuli. A sore

of 7 or above indicates an infant in good or excellent condition. The Apgar score is given at 1 and 5 min after birth and the 5 min score is most predictive of outcome. A low 5 min Apgar score, defined as 3 or less, is associated with increased neonatal mortality and long-term neurologic morbidity. A persistently low Apgar score at 10 and 20 min after delivery indicates a poor response to resuscitation and an even greater increase in mortality and morbidity.

The Apgar score was created to predict the likelihood of survival during the neonatal period and not as a marker for asphyxia. However, many clinicians use the 5 min Apgar score as an indicator of perinatal hypoxia or asphyxia. This is incorrect because there are a number of factors that can cause a low Apgar score, such as congenital anomalies and maternal medications, which are not a consequence of asphyxia. The American Academy of Pediatrics and the American College of Obstetricians and Gynecologists clearly state that "Apgar scores alone should not be used as evidence that neurologic damage was caused by hypoxia..."

The infant's overall clinical condition at delivery is probably the most helpful predictor of the degree of asphyxia and the extent of injury. The need for cardiopulmonary resuscitation in the delivery room increases the risk for adverse neurologic outcome. This relationship is particularly true in the face of significant fetal acidemia. The combination of fetal acidosis and cardiorespiratory failure at birth indicates an infant who has suffered profound hypoperfusion and is likely to have sustained central nervous system injury. Asphyxiated infants can also show evidence of renal failure, liver injury, cardiac dysfunction, or hematologic abnormalities.

In summary, there is no single clinical marker that indicates perinatal asphyxia significant enough to result in lifelong impairment. However, the more risk factors that an infant exhibits, the worse the overall prognosis. A joint statement by the American Academy of Pediatrics and the American College of Obstetricians and Gynecologists summarizes it this way: "A neonate who has had asphyxia proximate to delivery that is severe enough to result in acute neurologic injury should demonstrate all of the following: profound metabolic or mixed acidemia (pH <7.00) on an umbilical cord arterial blood sample, if obtained; an Apgar score of 0 to 3 for longer than 5 minutes; neonatal neurologic manifestations, e.g., seizures, coma, or hypotonia; and multisystem organ dysfunction, e.g., cardiovascular, gastrointestinal, hematologic, pulmonary, or renal system."

Hypoxic Ischemic Encephalopathy

Neonatal HIE is a clinical description of a combination of neurologic abnormalities that may include altered consciousness, abnormal muscle tone and reflexes, inability to feed, and seizures. It should be clearly stated that not all infants with HIE go on to develop permanent neurologic impairment, but neurologic abnormalities present shortly after birth are one of the best predictors of long-term outcome. The most widely used classification system for neonatal encephalopathy is the Sarnat staging system. This classifies infants into three groups based on level of consciousness, activity, muscle tone, reflexes, and the presence of autonomic dysfunction. Infants with mild encephalopathy do very well and should be considered to have a normal neurologic outcome. Infants presenting with moderate encephalopathy are described as lethargic with decreased muscle tone and poor sucking behavior. Between 20% and 25% of these infants will have an abnormal neurodevelopmental outcome. Infants with severe encephalopathy are comatose and flaccid with no spontaneous activity and commonly have seizures in the first 24 h of life. These infants have a poor outcome, with essentially all patients that survive having significant impairment.

An infant's neurologic examination is likely to evolve over time and most infants who survive will demonstrate some degree of improvement in the nursery. The degree and timing of recovery can be helpful in providing information about the infant's long-term prognosis. For example, infants who recover quickly and are able to leave the nursery on full nipple feeds have a better prognosis than infants who have prolonged hospitalizations and difficulty feeding.

In addition to the neurologic examination, special imaging studies of the brain can be done to better define the prognosis for an infant. MRI provides a detailed picture of the brain and is very helpful in defining the location and extent of injury. Hypoxic ischemic injury has a distinct appearance on MRI that changes over time. Therefore, MRI can also be used to describe the timing of injury. This is important in determining if an injury occurred during delivery or some time remote from the delivery.

In addition to an MRI, an electroencephalogram (EEG) is routinely performed on any infant with significant HIE. An EEG is a noninvasive test that measures the electrical activity of the brain recorded by electrodes placed on the scalp. The EEG can be used to document seizure activity, which can sometimes be difficult to assess clinically in newborns. In addition, the EEG can provide prognostic information on the severity of long-term deficits. A severely and persistently abnormal EEG indicates a very poor prognosis of either death or severe long-term disability. In contrast, a moderately abnormal EEG that normalizes over the first week of life is associated with a more positive prognosis.

Therapy for Hypoxic Ischemic Encephalopathy

Up until the past few years there has been little to offer an infant with HIE except supportive medical care. Immediate intervention includes resuscitation in the delivery room and correction of acidosis as well as cardiovascular support to maintain adequate perfusion. The use of moderate hypothermia has been the first therapy since the 1970s that has shown the potential to improve the outcome of these infants by decreasing the extent of central nervous system injury. Animal studies have shown that hypothermia initiated soon after hypoxic ischemic brain injury decreases neuronal loss and cell injury. The degree of neuroprotection is dependent on the severity of injury and the timing of hypothermia. The more severe the injury and the later hypothermia is initiated, the less effective the therapy. Hypothermia must be initiated within 6 h of injury to demonstrate neuroprotection.

Moderate hypothermia has now been studied in newborn infants and has been demonstrated to be safe without clinically significant adverse effects. Two large multicenter trials have recently been published evaluating whether moderate hypothermia can reduce the incidence of death or neurologic impairment in infants with moderate-to-severe HIE. The two studies used two different methods to produce hypothermia. One study evaluated whole body hypothermia using a cooling blanket to maintain core body temperature at 33.5 °C (92.3 °F). The other study evaluated selective cooling of the head with a cooling cap along with mild whole body hypothermia, keeping the body temperature between 34 °C (93.2 °F) and 35 °C (95.0 °F). These two studies showed promising results in that infants with moderate HIE who underwent 72 h of hypothermia had improved outcomes at 18 months of age. There was no significant benefit, however, for infants who presented with severe encephalopathy.

Despite the initially promising results, hypothermia is not recommended for the routine therapy of infants with perinatal asphyxia and HIE. There are a number of questions that still must be answered to determine which infants would benefit the most from hypothermia and which is the most effective method of hypothermia. In addition, long-term follow-up studies are needed to determine if the neurologic benefits seen at 18 months continue as these children go through childhood.

Summary

Perinatal asphyxia and resulting HIE is one of the most common identifiable causes of CP and poor neurologic outcome in full-term newborns. The clinical assessment of perinatal asphyxia is based on a specific combination of criteria that identify those infants most likely to have suffered acute injury. There are a number of maternal and fetal conditions that can predispose to HIE, but the underlying etiology is decreased cerebral blood flow. The infant's neurologic examination, MRI findings, and EEG results are used to offer a prognosis about long-term neurologic impairment. Modest hypothermia is a promising new therapy that has been shown to be neuroprotective and improve the outcome of infants with moderate HIE.

See also: Birth Defects; Cerebral Palsy; Developmental Disabilities: Cognitive; Developmental Disabilities: Physical; Intellectual Disabilities; Obesity; Reflexes.

Suggested Readings

Bolisetty S, Bajuk B, ME A, *et al.* (2006) Preterm outcome table (POT): A simple tool to aid counseling parents of very preterm infants. *Australian and New Zealand Journal of Obstetrics and Gynecology* 24: 189.

Committee on Fetus and Newborn, American Academy of Pediatrics and Committee on Obstetric Practice, American College of Obstetricians and Gynecologists (1996) Use and abuse of the Apgar score. *Pediatrics* 98: 141–142.

Higgins RD, Delivoria-Papadopoulos M, and Raju NK (2005) Executive summary of the workshop on the border of viability. *Pediatrics* 115: 1392–1396.

Hoyert DL, Mathews TJ, Menacker F, Strobino DM, and Guyer B (2006) Annual summary of vital statistics: 2004. *Pediatrics* 117: 168–183.

Jones HP, Karuri S, Cronin C, *et al.* (2005) Actuarial survival of a large Canadian cohort of preterm infants. *BMC Pediatrics* 5: 40.

Lorenz JM (2001) The outcome of extreme prematurity. *Seminars in Perinatology* 25: 348–359.

Marlow N, Wolke D, Bracewell MA, and Samara M (2005) Neurologic and developmental disability at six years of age after extremely preterm birth. *The New England Journal of Medicine* 352: 9–19.

Msall ME (2006) The panorama of cerebral palsy after very and extremely preterm birth: Evidence and challenges. *Clinics in Perinatology* 33: 269–284.

Recchia FM and Capone A (2004) Contemporary understanding and management of retinopathy of prematurity. *Retina* 24: 283–292.

Saigal S, Ouden L, Wolke D, *et al.* (2003) School-age outcomes in children who were extremely low birth weight from four international population-based cohorts. *Pediatrics* 112: 943–950.

Speer M and Perlman JM (2006) Modest hypothermia as a neuroprotective strategy in high-risk term infants. *Clinics in Perinatology* 33: 169–182.

Vannucci RC (2002) Hypoxia-ischemia: Clinical aspects. In: Fanaroff and Martin RJ (eds.) *Neonatal–Perinatal Medicine,* 7th edn., pp. 867–878St. Louis: Mosby.

Volpe JJ (2001) Intracranial hemorrhage: Germinal matrix-intraventricular hemorrhage of the premature infant. In: Volpe JJ (ed.) *Neurology of the Newborn,* 4th edn., pp. 428–496. Philadelphia: Saunders.

Relevant Website

http://www.marchofdimes.com – March of Dimes – Saving babies, together.

Birth Defects

D Adams and M Muenke, National Institutes of Health, Bethesda, MD, USA

Published by Elsevier Inc.

Glossary

Anterior – The front of the body, for example, the heart, is anterior to the shoulder blades.

Association – A set of medical conditions and/or physical features that occur together more often than would be expected by chance.

Deformation – Unusual forces acting on otherwise normal tissue to cause an alteration in structure.

Disruption – Destruction of otherwise normal tissue to cause an alteration in structure.

Distal – Further from, for example, the hand is more distal to the shoulder than the elbow.

Dorsal – An anatomic term, used for some embryonic structures, meaning the back of the structure. For instance, the dorsal surface of the hand is the back of the hand.

Dysmorphology – The study of variants in anatomic structure, specifically those variants that are associated with significantly impaired function and/or cosmesis.

Dysplasia – The abnormal organization of a tissue.

Embryopathy – A general term for a disease or other process that has an adverse effect on a developing embryo.

Idiopathic – A problem (pathology) of unknown cause, for example, idiopathic pulmonary fibrosis, is pulmonary fibrosis for which the underlying cause is unknown.

Malformation – The abnormal formation of a tissue.

Posterior – The back of the body, for example, the shoulder blades are posterior to the heart.

Proximal – Closer to, for example, the elbow is more proximal to the shoulder than the hand.

Syndrome – A set of medical conditions and/or physical features that occur together more often than would be expected by chance. In addition, the word syndrome implies a common causation or small set of causations.

Teratogenic – A teratogenic event is one in which the fetal environment is changed in, manner that causes an alteration in normal fetal development. The word teratogen is often used when referring to a drug with potential teratogenic effects.

Ventral – An anatomic term, used for some embryonic structures, meaning the front of the structure. For instance, the ventral surface of the hand is the front of the hand.

Introduction

The term birth defect describes a large and complex field of study. For most measurable characteristics, there is a broad range of normally functioning states. The March of Dimes defines a birth defect as, "An abnormality of structure, function or metabolism 'body chemistry' that results in physical or mental disabilities or death." This definition is designed to be inclusive but illustrates some of the difficulties inherent in the term. An example of a newborn with medical pathology who would not be described as having a birth defect is an otherwise healthy newborn emerging from a difficult delivery. He might need medical intervention only during the first hours of life. Abnormalities of metabolism are certainly present, but are transient and will not cause permanent disability. A second newborn may have a DNA change that will predispose her to an adult-onset illness. This is a structural and functional problem in a molecular sense, but does not present an immediate health threat and may not be recognized in the newborn period. The Centers for Disease Control and prevention (CDC) provide a narrower definition. To be named a birth defect, a condition must be:

1. present at birth;
2. the result of a malformation, deformation, or disruption in one or more parts of the body; and
3. characterized by serious, adverse effects on health, development, or functional ability.

This definition may be overly restrictive. First, as we will see, the terms malformation, deformation, and disruption have specific, yet imprecise meanings in the context of

congenital (present at birth) abnormalities. A newborn may have features that do not easily fit into those definitions. The truth is likely somewhere in between, including those conditions that generally come to attention in the newborn period, have serious/prolonged health (including social) consequences, and are due to some deviation from the range of normal embryogenesis.

Birth defects are extremely variable. One only need consider the complexity of a process that allows a single cell to transform into a newborn baby to appreciate the scope of things that could go awry. Even 'normal' embryogenesis results in a range of features 'minor variations' that have no functional significance. These can include small skin tags around the ear and variation in the patterning of palm creases. Sometimes, particular patterns of minor variations can be used to identify a more severe underlying condition. 'Major variations' are those that, by themselves, cause an alteration in the functioning of the individual. Examples include some cardiac defects, severe anomalies of the hands and feet, and clefts in the lip and palate. Major variations are detected in 2–3% of pregnancies. Whether or not a variation is 'normal' may also be a function of cultural context. The particular shape, color, or size of a part of a body part may have cultural significance (positive or negative) that is not accompanied by any change in physical function. Other conditions, such as some congenital heart defects, are clearly present at birth, but do not manifest until days, weeks, or years later. The large range of possible birth defects makes their study both interesting and daunting.

Birth Defects: General Principles

As with any major field of study, the initial understanding of a phenomenon is based on simple observation. Ancient statues and paintings depicted conjoined twins and persons with achondroplasia, a specific form of short stature. Religion and mysticism were often convoluted together with birth defects such that an unusual baby was considered to be a consequence or sign of supernatural agency. As the medical profession grew to embrace the principles of scientific investigation, a systematic approach understanding birth defects arose. 'Dysmorphology' (the study of abnormal form) is a medical field of study concerned with the relation between external physical features, for instance, the shape of a nose or a fingerprint pattern, and health. Birth defects are often first recognized by suggestive physical features, thus creating a use for dysmorphology in the diagnosis of birth defects. Dysmorphologists initially relied on the combined clinical experience to ascertain patterns of features that were associated with health implications. As more and more individuals with a given pattern were recognized, summed clinical experience could be used to devise rational approaches to diagnosis, family counseling, and treatment. It was soon recognized that many (although not all) birth defects had a component of heredity. The alliance of dysmorphology with the study of the health implications of inheritance gave birth to a medical specialty, medical genetics.

Early on, the efforts of medical geneticists were complicated by a number of characteristics possessed by inherited traits, both pathogenic and normal. Such characteristics included genetic heterogeneity, defined as an inherited trait that has multiple genetic causes (more than one gene). Variable expressivity is defined as a trait that has different manifestations in different individuals. Penetrance is defined as the likelihood that an individual who has an inherited trait shows any associated characteristics of the trait. Penetrance values less than 1.0 indicate that a fraction of the population of people who carry the trait gene will show no characteristics. Beyond inheritance, many birth defects arise solely or partly because of nongenetic environmental factors. Given an insufficient number of characteristic physical features, a lack of evidence of a known heritability pattern, or a lack of a known environmental etiology, the root cause of many birth defects remains unknown.

The most important advances in our ability to understand the etiology of birth defects have come in the form of progress in research pertaining to cell biology, molecular (DNA-related) biology, and development. Progress in those fields is yielding an expanding understanding of how disruptions to normal development can lead to birth defects.

Epidemiology and Social Impact

Birth defects are common. The CDC estimates that approximately 120 000 (1 in 33) newborns are born with birth defects each year. Birth defects are the number one cause of infant mortality in the US. Despite rapid advances in our understanding of the causes of birth defects, 70% occur for unknown reasons.

A recent research report released by the CDC attempted to quantify some of the financial impact of birth defects. They noted that birth defects account for 20% of the total infant deaths in the US. They calculated that the associated hospital costs alone exceeded $2.5 billion.

Variability

As discussed in the introduction, the term 'birth defect' covers a wide variety of variation present among newborns. Variability in severity is exemplified by hand malformations. At one end of the spectrum is postaxial polydactyly type B, which manifests as a skin tag on the on the fifth-digit side of the hand. Such skin tags are common and do not cause any functional impairment (**Figure 1**). At the family's

request, skin tags can be removed in the newborn nursery using a simple procedure. In contrast, split-hand/split-foot malformation (SHFM) can cause significant functional impairment (**Figure 2**). Multiple, complex surgeries may be required to achieve usable function. SHFM is an example of genetic heterogeneity as it can be cause by several different genes.

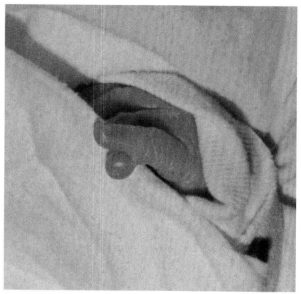

Figure 1 Cutaneous postaxial polydactyly. The fifth finger of the hand of this newborn has an attached extra digit. The digit is partially formed and is not likely to contain any bones. Often such digits are even simpler and do not have a partially formed fingernail as this example does. Such digits are easily removed with a minor surgical procedure.

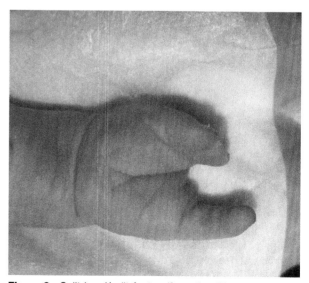

Figure 2 Split-hand/split-foot malformation. The pictured hand of a newborn infant shows anterior/posterior clefting and digit separation. Existing digits are not fully forme.

Causation

Inherited factors

Birth defects can be caused by genetic factors – generally changes in the affected individual's DNA sequence. Some genetic changes arise for the first time in the affected individual, while others are inherited from either affected or unaffected ('carrier') parents. Some inherited birth defects are transmitted through families across multiple generations. Some conditions are so severe that affected children do not live long enough to produce offspring. Other birth defects are mild enough that they have little impact on reproduction.

Craniosynostosis, the premature fusion of the sutures of the skull, occurs in 1/2500 live births. Craniosynostosis syndromes, a subset of all craniosynostosis, show varying severity in the newborn period. Apert syndrome (**Figure 3**) is a rare condition that includes abnormal shape of the skull bones and abnormalities of the hands and feet. Apert syndrome is caused by changes in the fibroblast growth factor receptor 2 (*FGFR2*) gene and most (>90%) of new cases arise as new mutations in the affected child. The manifestations of Apert syndrome make the condition universally diagnosable at birth. In contrast, another craniosynostosis syndrome, Crouzon syndrome, also caused by mutations in *FGFR2*, may not be diagnosed in the first affected individual in a family. Some mildly affected

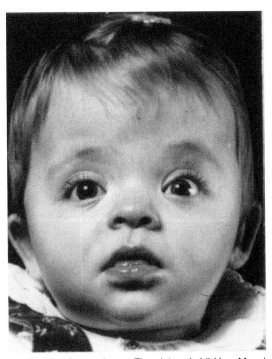

Figure 3 Muenke syndrome. The pictured child has Muenke syndrome with several facial dysmorphisms including facial asymmetry. Muenke syndrome can be considered in patients with craniosynostosis leading to a tall and wide forehead. Because of the wide spectrum of findings, some children with Muenke syndrome may not be diagnosed in the newborn period.

individuals are themselves diagnosed when they have an affected child. Newborns with oculocutaneous albinism are often recognizable at birth by skin and hair coloration that is markedly lighter than other family members. Most forms of albinism do not reduce the individual's ability to have children later in life.

Environmental factors
Teratogens

The process of embryonic development is susceptible to disruption by a number of environmental factors including a woman's use of prescribed or nonprescribed drugs during her pregnancy. Certain drugs may be known to affect pregnancies most severely at early or late gestational dates (**Table 1**). Drugs that are approved for medical use are classified by a system that rates their potential averse affects on a fetus (**Table 2**).

One of the most infamous teratogens is the medication thalidomide, marketed widely in the 1950s as a treatment for pregnancy-associated nausea. A dramatic increase in the incidence of severe congenital malformations of the arms and legs (phocomelia) was eventually attributed to the use of thalidomide during pregnancy. The drug was taken off the market for several decades until it was discovered that it was uniquely useful for the treatment of some of the symptoms present in a few uncommon diseases including leprosy. Today, the drug is once again available for use; however, strict monitoring requirements are in place in an attempt to prevent its use during pregnancy. Debate continues as to whether the benefits of the drug outweigh the risk that further cases of phocomelia might occur.

Infections

Certain infectious diseases are known to cause birth defects. One example is German measles (rubella), a viral illness. In healthy children and adults, rubella causes a usually mild, self-limited illness with a rash, swollen lymph nodes, and achy joints. If a pregnant woman becomes infected, there is a

Table 1   Examples of teratogens and times of maximal gestational sensitivity

Maximal sensitivity	Example agents
First trimester	Androgens (virulization)
	Carbamazepine (malformations)
	Ethanol (fetal alcohol syndrome)
	Thalidomide (days 34–50, limb reduction)
Second and/or third trimester	Coumadin (embryopathy)
	Iodides (fetal hypothyroidism)
	Tetracyclines (tooth enamel changes)

Summarized from http://www.uspharmacist.com/ (accessed on April 2007).

Table 2 FDA use-in-pregnancy ratings

A	Adequate, well-controlled studies in pregnant women have not shown an increased risk of fetal abnormalities to the fetus in any trimester of pregnancy.
B	Animal studies have revealed no evidence of harm to the fetus, however, there are no adequate and well-controlled studies in pregnant women. Or animal studies have shown an adverse effect, but adequate and well-controlled studies in pregnant women have failed to demonstrate a risk to the fetus in any trimester.
C	Animal studies have shown an adverse effect and there are no adequate and well-controlled studies in pregnant women. Or no animal studies have been conducted and there are no adequate and well-controlled studies in pregnant women.
D	Adequate well-controlled or observational studies in pregnant women have demonstrated a risk to the fetus. However, the benefits of therapy may outweigh the potential risk. For example, the drug may be acceptable if needed in a life-threatening situation or serious disease for which safer drugs cannot be used or are ineffective.
X	Adequate well-controlled or observational studies in animals or pregnant women have demonstrated positive evidence of fetal abnormalities or risks. The use of the product is contraindicated in women who are or may become pregnant.

risk that the virus will be transmitted to her developing child causing a potentially severe embryopathy. Birth defects that can result from rubella infection include growth retardation, cognitive impairment, cataracts, deafness, and cardiac defects. Immunization for rubella during childhood has decreased the frequency of the disease in the general population, and subsequently, the frequency of rubella embryopathy.

Maternal illness

Some noninfectious maternal illnesses can cause birth defects. Elevated maternal blood sugar during pregnancy, such as that which can occur with diabetes mellitus, is a well-known cause of congenital abnormalities. The risk of a major malformation among all newborns is approximately 2–3%; among children of diabetic mothers, it is 6–9%. Diabetes-related birth defects can cause abnormalities in lower extremity development (caudal regression) in addition to spinal, brain, and cardiac malformation. Careful control of blood sugar levels during pregnancy is critically important for women with diabetes.

Mixed factors

Holoprosencephaly (HPE) is the result of the failure of the developing brain to divide into two separate hemispheres. HPE is associated with structural abnormalities of the mid-face. HPE demonstrates significant variation in severity and manifestations (variable expressivity), meaning that two people with the same genetic predisposition to HPE can have significantly different physical features. At the mild end of the spectrum is the presence of a single central incisor (one upper front tooth rather than the usual two). At the severe end of the spectrum, newborns present with a single central eye (cyclopia) and related facial abnormalities. Intermediate manifestations often include a cleft lip. **Figure 4** shows examples of the wide variation in the condition. Around 25% to 50% persons with HPE have a microscopically visible chromosomal abnormality, while 20–25% of persons with normal chromsomes have detectable defects in one or more of the genes known to be associated with HPE. In addition to any genetic susceptibility, however, environmental factors are thought to play a role in determining how the condition manifests in a given individual. The most convincingly related environmental factor is maternal diabetes although other factors, including cholesterol metabolism and cholesterol-lowering drugs, are under investigation as possible contributors.

Screening and Detection

The current standard of care for pregnancies in the US, and some other industrialized countries, is to offer screening for common pregnancy complications. Many such complications have the potential to produce children with birth defects. Although the exact protocols for such screening are evolving, the following section outlines the general categories of techniques in use. At the time of birth, routine examination of the newborn may reveal malformations that are either diagnostic or suggestive of a birth defect. Often, further medical workup is required to make a definitive diagnosis. Even with the best available resources, the root cause of a number of congenital malformations is never discovered. In such cases medical issues must be addressed as they arise.

Social/Psychological Impact

The diagnosis of a birth defect during pregnancy, or at the time of delivery, is an unwelcome event for any family. Even if a clear-cut diagnosis can be made expeditiously, the family often has to make difficult decisions about whether to continue an affected pregnancy, how to cope with a special needs child, and how to prepare for a different life than they were expecting. The family may have to simultaneously proceed with grieving and face the financial and time-related hardships of a prolonged hospitalization. Many parents find that a particularly difficult aspect of a birth defect diagnosis is that they have to communicate unexpected news to other family members. It is said that parents of a newborn with birth defects must "grieve the loss of the child they were expecting before they can accept the child they have."

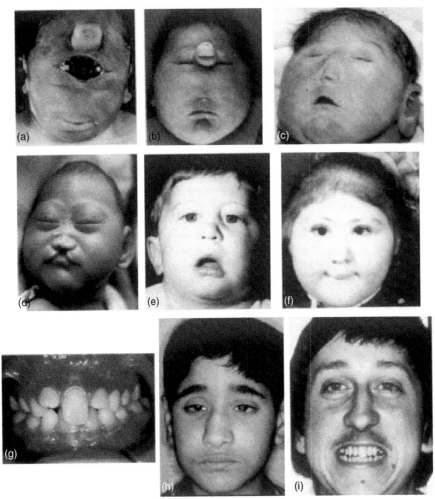

Figure 4 The spectrum of holoprosencephaly (HPE). Wide variation in holoprosencephaly ranges from malformations that are incompatible with life to suble changes in otherwise health individuals. The fetus in the upper part shows severe lack of midline development including a single, unseparated eye (cyclopia) and a severely underdeveloped nose (the fleshy tube, or proboscus, on the forehead). The mildly affected person in the lower right corner has HPE manifestations limited to a single central incisor.

Birth Defect Mechanisms and Classification

Classical Nosology

A general framework exists for categorizing and naming birth defects. Historically, the framework was useful when little biochemical or molecular understanding of the origins of congenital malformations was available. It is currently useful both as an educational framework and as a set of diagnostic anchors that can help an experienced clinician to narrow the field of potential diagnoses.

Categories of dysmorphic mechanisms

Smith's Recognizable Patterns of Human Malformation by Dr. Kenneth Lyons Jones is a classic dysmorphology text-book. It defines several types of structural defects. **Figure 5** describes the relations between the defined types.

Malformations

Malformations encompass dysmorphic features that are the result of the abnormal formation of a particular tissue. Malformation sequences describe the situation when a malformation causes a cascade of subsequent events that affect other, related tissues. SHFM, described above, is an example of a malformation.

Pierre Robin sequence is an example of a malformation sequence. In the classic description of Pierre Robin, a small (micrognathic) or posteriorly positioned (retrognathia) jaw is the initiating malformation. The malpositioning of the jaw causes an elevated position of the tongue, which in turn interferes with the joining of the shelves of tissue that become the palate. At birth, the child has micrognathia or retrognathia, a malpositioned tongue that can interfere with breathing, and a cleft palate (**Figure 6**).

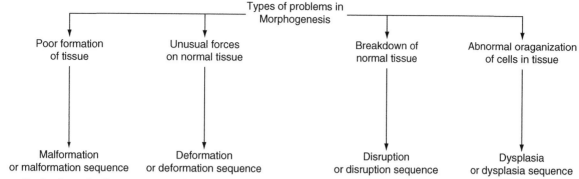

Figure 5   A scheme for the general classification of the causes of birth defects. See text for further explaination. Modified from Jones KL (1988) *Smith's Recognizable Patterns of Human Malformation*, 4th edn. Toronto: W.B. Saunders.

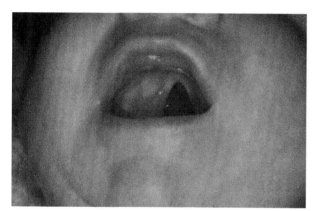

Figure 6   A cleft palate malformation in a newborn. One cause of cleft palate is the Pierre Robin sequence described in the text.

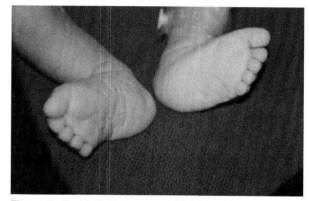

Figure 7   Feet in Potter sequence. The feet of this a newborn child are abnormally positioned secondary to the lack of adequate interuterine space during gestation.

Deformation

A deformation results from external (to the fetus) forces acting on otherwise normal tissue. As with malformation, subsequent consequences can be grouped with the initial deformation to form a deformation sequence. A syndrome that is often used to illustrate the principle of a deformation is the Potter sequence. In the Potter sequence, an inadequate amount of amniotic fluid results in a restrictive intrauterine space. The resulting fetal compression results in deformation of the face, hands, and feet (**Figure 7**).

Disruption

A disruption birth defect occurs when normal tissue is destroyed as the result of external forces acting on it. For instance, amniotic banding is a type of birth defect in which a child is born with missing limbs, or other body parts. An otherwise normal looking limb will appear as if it were amputated at some point along its length. Sometimes, a small residual remnant (hand, foot) will be visible past the site of the apparent amputation. One theory to explain this phenomenon is that the limb gets tangled in folds of amniotic tissue at some point during fetal development. The fold then cuts off blood supply to the distal

part of the developing limb, destroying it, and causing a disruption birth defect (**Figure 8**).

Dysplasia

Dysplasia is defined as the abnormal organization of a tissue. As an example, the large family of 'skeletal dysplasias' includes many different conditions. Osteogenesis imperfecta, for instance, is often called 'brittle bone disease' and features easily broken bones. The fragility of the bones in affected individuals is caused by the abnormal production of collagen, a protein that gives bending strength to bone. Achondroplasia, another type of skeletal dysplasia, is caused by a specific DNA change in the fibroblast growth receptor gene (*FGFR3*) that disrupts normal bone development. One characteristic feature of achondroplasia, and some other skeletal dysplasias, is a short upper arm bone, or humerus (**Figure 9**).

Categories of grouping

The fact that the study of birth defects arose from a descriptive science is reflected in the use of grouping terms that attempt to convey the frequency with which constellations of congenital variations are seen in the same individual. The word 'syndrome', for instance, conveys a greater degree of

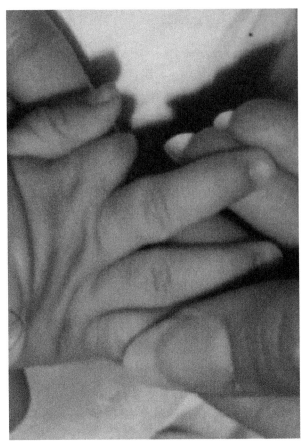

Figure 8 Terminal reduction. The second (index) finger of this child's hand is shortened and missing distal elements such as the fingernail and some joints.

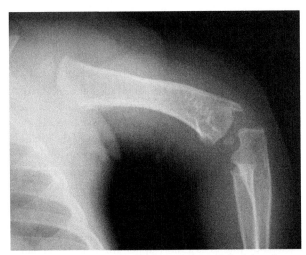

Figure 9 Short humerus. The X-ray photograph pictured shows the bone of the upper arm (the humerus) in an infant. In this case, the humerus is significantly shorter than expected relative to its width and the size of the other bones.

unifying causation than the word 'association'. The term 'developmental field defect' was used to describe birth defects that occur in a group of tissues that are near one another during fetal development. Our growing molecular understanding of the causes of birth defects is having a dramatic and ongoing affect on how birth defects are grouped.

An example of the evolution of birth defect naming is a group of conditions related to the chromodomain helicase DNA-binding protein (*CHD7*) gene. What is now known as the CHARGE syndrome was originally called an association. CHARGE is an acronym for 'coloboma' (an eye defect), 'heart defects', 'choanal atresia' (a defect of the skull and upper airway), 'retarded growth and development', 'genital abnormalities', and 'ear anomalies'. Component members of the association were grouped together because they often appeared together in individuals. Although the etiology for CHARGE was not known initially, the use of a grouping ('association') allowed for the accumulation of clinical experience with affected children. It is now known that many persons who were diagnosed with the CHARGE association (~2/3) have changes in the *CHD7* gene. The presence of a unifying molecular etiology prompted a change in the name from CHARGE association to CHARGE syndrome. The function of the *CHD7* gene is not well understood. However, it bears strong resemblance to other members of the *CHD* family. Genes in the *CHD* family are thought to be involved in the control of chromatin maintenance during embryogenesis. Specifically, *CHD* genes may have the ability to control the tightness with which DNA is wound. Unwound regions of DNA are readable; tightly round regions of DNA are generally not readable. Therefore, *CHD* genes may help to determine which regions of the DNA are available for reading. The general nature of the proposed *CHD* activity is consistent with a the finding that many systems are affected in CHARGE syndrome.

Grouping by embryonic age

Birth defects may occur during characteristic periods of embryogenesis. Teratogens, for instance, are often categorized according to when maximum sensitivity to the agent occurs during gestation (**Table 2**). By noting the timing of a drug exposure during pregnancy, the possible origins of a birth defect may be refined.

Birth Defects: Diagnosis and Treatment

Birth defects may be diagnosed during gestation, at birth, or at any time after birth. The timing of diagnosis depends on whether the diagnostic tools being used (e.g., prenatal ultrasound or physical examination) are capable of detecting the manifestations of the birth defect, and, the extent to which the severity of the consequences of the birth defect prompt further investigation and medical workup. Some conditions are routinely screened for both during pregnancy and in the neonatal period. Such screening provides increased sensitivity for birth defect detection and increased opportunities for utilizing any available therapeutic interventions.

Screening and Testing of Pregnancies

Routine pregnancy care includes a number of screening tests. Blood glucose screening, fetal ultrasound, and fetal growth monitoring can all provide evidence of increased risk for a birth defect. Genetic testing and/or screening are offered for pregnancies that are identified as being at elevated risk. Selected techniques are discussed in the following section.

Ultrasound

Fetal ultrasound is used for a variety of purposes including the verification of gestational age. The sensitivity of ultrasound to find signs of a birth defect generally increases with gestational age. At-risk pregnancies can be monitored by serial ultrasounds so as to monitor the growth of portions of the body associated with specific fetal anomalies. Femur length, for instance, can be used to screen for certain types of skeletal dysplasia. A deficient rate of head growth is suggestive of a deficiency in brain growth. Ultrasound is not 100% sensitive, however. In Down syndrome, a chromosomal abnormality associated with a number of minor and major malformations (see below), the sensitivity of prenatal ultrasound is only 50%.

Screening for chromosomal aneuploidy – Down syndrome

Women who are found to be at elevated risk for birth defects may be offered diagnostic testing if it is available. The distinction between a screening test and a diagnostic test is critical to understand. A screening test produces a revised estimate of the probability of a particular outcome. For instance, the risk for a birth defect might be 1/10 before a screening test and either 1/5 or 1/1000 afterward. A diagnostic test gives a definitive diagnosis, yes or no, within the limitations of the sensitivity and specificity of the test. The principles of pregnancy screening and diagnosis are illustrated by the chromosomal condition Down syndrome.

Some birth defects are the result of an abnormal number of chromosomes (aneuploidy). Many chromosomal changes, both aneuploidy and nonaneuploid, result in a spontaneous premature termination of gestation. The most common aneuploidy to survive to birth is Down syndrome, caused by an extra copy of chromosome 21. At birth, individuals with Down syndrome have variable degrees of characteristic facial features and other minor and major malformations. Many individuals with Down syndrome survive to adulthood, although all have some degree of cognitive impairment and other, usually manageable, medical issues.

The likelihood of a Down syndrome pregnancy increases with increasing maternal age, being approximately 0.05% at the age of 35 years and 20% in the late 40s. Screening for Down syndrome is routinely offered to women 35 years old or older. The technology for screening is evolving, but generally involves a combination of blood tests and specialized ultrasound-based fetal measurements. As noted above, the result of screening is a modification of a risk estimate based on the age of the woman carrying the pregnancy. Once the revised risk estimate becomes available, the pregnant woman might elect to undergo diagnostic testing. Diagnostic testing can be done using chorionic villous sampling (CVS) or amniocentesis. CVS is a technique whereby pregnancy-associated nonfetal tissue is sampled using either a needle passed through the abdominal wall or a thin tube inserted through the vagina and cervix. Amniocentesis samples amniocytes shed from the fetus into the amniotic fluid, also using a needle passed through the abdominal wall. In either case, the exact configuration of the fetal chromosomes can, within the limitations of tests, be ascertained and a diagnosis made.

Pregnancy screening and diagnostic procedures can also detect some other aneuploidies.

Molecular screening

Sometimes direct measurements of material or fetal DNA are the best option for detecting whether a fetus is at risk of, or affected by, a heritable illness. DNA testing for illness is termed 'molecular testing' by tradition. Most of the common molecular testing used during pregnancies does not relate to illnesses that present as birth defects. However, if a family has had a previous pregnancy affected by a birth defect, molecular testing may have a role. If the birth defect was attributable to a specific, known DNA change, subsequent pregnancies can be tested to see if a similar DNA change is present. The rapid rate at which specific illnesses are being linked to specific DNA changes suggests that scope of molecular screening and testing will continue to expand.

Birth Defects Newly Diagnosed at Birth

When a birth defect is first recognized at the time of birth, a larger range of diagnostic and therapeutic interventions are possible. The scope and number of such procedures is large; only selected topics are discussed here.

The first step in dealing with an unexpected birth defect is to address the immediate health implications for the affected child, which may range from incompatibility-with-life to nonexistent. Once medical stabilization is underway, an organized process of diagnostic thinking follows. Some birth defects can be diagnosed by characteristic sets of features visible during physical examination. Individually, the features may be relatively common in the general population. For instance, a single palmar crease can be used along with other physical features to make a diagnosis of Down syndrome. By itself, however, single palmar creases can be found in individuals with no other related medical issues (**Figure 10**).

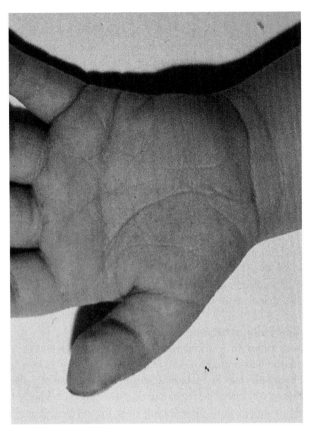

Figure 10 Single palmar crease. The prominent horizontal crease on this child's hand streches across then entire palm. Any cause of reduced fetal movement may cause this pattern and it is present among many, otherwise normal individuals.

If an exact diagnosis is not possible with examination alone, further testing can often narrow the diagnostic possibilities. It should be remembered that many physical anomalies present at birth are 'idiopathic' and a cause is never identified. Initial testing should be tailored to the findings at hand, but may have to be broad if the available evidence does not allow the field of possibilities to be successfully narrowed. For birth defects that involve multiple sites or organ systems, a genetic screening procedure such as karyotyping or microarray analysis is usually included in the workup. Karyotype analysis may show a microscopically visible difference from normal chromosome structure. Major organ systems such as the heart, brain, and kidneys are often evaluated to look for diagnostic clues that are not externally visible, and to rule out structural abnormalities with health implications. A careful examination of the eyes, face, and extremities can often provide valuable information.

Unexpected cleft lip and palate provides an example of how birth defects are evaluated. Assuming that no other physical anomalies have been discovered, and that the infant is stable (breathing and swallowing issues have been assessed and addressed), the diagnostician will consider the following information.

Cleft lip plus cleft palate (CL/P) is fairly common, occurring in approximately 1/700 births. The formation of the palate and upper lip occur by day 60 of fetal development, so the origins of the observed defect can be attributed to a particular span of time during pregnancy. The textbook *Principles and Practice of Medical Genetics* by Emery and Rimoin notes that approximately 70% of cases of CL/P are nonsyndromic meaning that there is no known causes and no other associated abnormalities. Of those that are syndromic, The Online Mendelian Inheritance in Man database lists more than 400 conditions in which CL/P is a feature. Alterations in many different genes can produce CL/P, some of them producing syndromes with subtle characteristic features that might not have been detected during an initial examination. Van der Woude syndrome, for instance, is associated with clefting and may produce lip pits. A repeat examination may be useful in detecting subtle clues.

A thorough pregnancy history is taken to exclude exposure to teratogens and pregnancy complications. Smoking, alcohol use, and some prescription drugs are under investigation or known to increase the risk of CL/P. A family history is taken to ascertain whether clefting or evidence associated with clefting-related syndromes has been seen in other family members.

Once all of the available information has been collected, a diagnostic plan will be implemented. If no diagnostic leads have been unearthed, common CL/P-associated conditions, including Stickler syndrome and DiGeorge syndrome, may be tested. Cardiac echocardiography may be considered due to the fact that some of the syndromes that produce clefting may also produce structural cardiac anomalies. A karyotype will likely be obtained to look for evidence of mosaic trisomy 13 (a chromosomal aneuploidy associated with clefting) or other microscopically visible chromosome anomaly. A counseling strategy will be defined and implemented to help the family to cope with the unexpected finding and to plan for future workup. Follow-up with a multidisciplinary team specializing in CL/P will be arranged. Although simplified, the presented CL/P example highlights some of the processes by which unexpected birth defects are evaluated and diagnosed.

Preventing Birth Defects

The prevention of disease is always better than the curing of disease. Most known birth defects are not preventable with current medical technology. However, particularly in industrialized countries, there have been some notable prevention successes. The prevention of iodine and folic acid deficiencies of pregnant women has had dramatic impacts on congenital hypothyroidism and neural tube defects (NTDs), respectively. Universal immunization has reduced the rate of birth defects due to some transmissible diseases. The careful treatment of women with phenylketonuria, while they are pregnant, reduces the likelihood of birth defects in their offspring. Further research in other areas, including diabetes, holds promise for additional improvements in prevention.

The story of folic acid supplementation is illustrative of a success in birth defect prevention. NTDs are a subclass of birth defects that involve the development of the spine during embryogenesis. Spina bifida, where the vertebrae fail to close over the spinal cord in one or more places, is an example of an NTD. NTDs are not rare, occurring as often as 1/1000 pregnancies. In the 1950s, it was observed that NTDs were more common among women of low socioeconomic status. That finding suggested that some environmental factor might have a role in NTDs. Further support for an environmental theory included the fact that most women who have children with NTDs do not have a family history of NTDs themselves, making a genetic cause less likely. In the 1960s, it was discovered that folate deficiency caused birth defects in animal models. In 1991, a landmark British study showed that folic acid supplementation reduced the risk that a woman with a history of an NTD-affected pregnancy would have a subsequent NTD-affected pregnancy. In 1992, the FDA recommended that folic acid be given to all women of childbearing age, and, that folic acid be added to certain grain-based foods including some types of flour, rice, and bread. In 1998, the Food and Drug Administration (FDA) mandated folic acid supplementation in these foods. The consensus among researchers and epidemiologists is that folic acid therapy has been a success. For instance, a 2001 Cochrane Library meta-analysis examined the data regarding the success of folic acid supplementation in preventing NTDs. The authors found the following: "Periconceptional folate supplementation reduced the incidence of neural tube defects (relative risk 0.28, 95% confidence interval 0.13 to 0.58)."

Birth Defects Research

Biomedical research has had a profound effect on our understanding of birth defects. What was once described by appearance alone can now be understood in terms of specific developmental mechanisms. In addition, advances in surgical technique are showing promise for interventions that may prevent or mitigate the effects of some birth defects. The following two examples demonstrate how an understanding of cellular and molecular mechanisms, and the use of pioneering therapies, are improving what medicine has to offer to families affected by birth defects.

Three-Dimensional Limb Patterning

The development of a limb from a few embryonic cells to a complex adult structure requires a highly coordinated set of cell interactions. One aspect of limb development that lends itself to a discussion of the relations between research and birth defects is limb patterning (**Figure 11**). The upper extremity (arm, forearm, and hand) is an asymmetric structure. Anatomical terms are used for orientation. The proximal portion of the upper extremity is that closest to the shoulder; the distal most portions are the tips of the fingers. The dorsal part of the upper extremity includes the back of the hand, the back of the forearm, and, roughly, the outside of the arm; the ventral parts include the palm, the inside of the forearm, and the inside of the arm. Finally, the anterior portion is the thumb, the radial side of the forearm, and the 'front' of the arm; the posterior portion is the fifth finger side of the hand, the ulnar side of the forearm and the 'back' of the arm. The hand provides a ready example of the asymmetry of the upper extremity – the thumb is a significantly different structure than the fifth finger. Given that the upper extremity starts fetal life as a small lump of cells, specific cellular machinery must direct the patterning of the growing limb. Furthermore, it would be

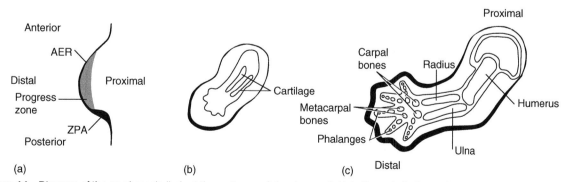

Figure 11   Diagram of the an ebryonic limb at three stages of development. Note the anterior/posterior and proximal/distal orientation of the limb as referred to in the text. The dorsal/ventral orientation (palm and back of hand) are not labeled. Specific cellular pathways, outlined in the text, control the pattering of the limb as is develops.

expected that defects in such developmental processes would have specific consequences for the fully developed extremity. A partial schematic of the structural and molecular signaling mechanisms in the developing limb will be used to highlight how a molecular understanding of limb development can be used to understand birth defects.

Anterior–posterior patterning

The earliest recognizable upper-extremity limb structure in a developing embryo is the approximately paddle-shaped limb bud. Early in embryogenesis, several recognizable structures are present. The edge of the limb bud that is furthest away from the fetal body forms an apical ectodermal ridge (AER). The edge of the limb bud that is closest to the tail contains a group of cells that form a zone of polarizing activity (ZPA). The ZPA cells generate a signal (comprising a molecule called sonic hedgehog or Shh) that defines the posterior aspect of the growing limb. On the other side of the limb bud, Shh signaling is repressed by a second molecule, Gli3, defining the anterior edge of the limb. These and other cellular signals are used to define the differential development of the anterior and posterior structures of the upper extremity.

Proximal–distal patterning

The AER remains at the tip, or distal end, of the limb as it grows. Experimental removal of the AER in model organisms will halt the lengthening of the limb. An important group of molecules involved in AER signaling are the fibroblast growth factors (FGFs). As the limb grows, cascades of signaling interactions form a pattern of gene expression that differs from the proximal to distal portions of the limb. One set of genes involved in forming this pattern is the homeobox, or *Hox* genes.

Dorsal–ventral patterning

As with the other developmental patterning axes, dorsal-ventral (DV) patterning is mediated by complex cascades of cell-signaling molecules. One such molecule that defines the dorsal portion of the limb is Wnt7a. Wnt7a acts on specific embryonic tissues to promote the expression of Lmx-1b, which in turn promotes a dorsal character to local tissues. On the ventral side of the limb, the molecule 'engrailed' En-1 inhibits Wnt7a, which in turn downregulates expression of Lmx1b. The result is a default, ventral limb surface.

Pallister–Hall syndrome

Dorsal–ventral, anterior–posterior, and proximal–distal limb patterning mechanisms interact during development to create a fully formed upper extremity. Genetic changes to the gene's coding for the involved signaling processes have the potential to disrupt normal limb formation.

Pallister–Hall syndrome (PHS) results from a subset of mutations of the *GLI3* gene. PHS includes several congenital abnormalities including polydactyly (extra fingers), upper airway abnormalities, and specific brain tumors. Relevant to limb development, PHS can cause postaxial polydactyly, a defect in anterior–posterior limb development. PHS is an example of the general rule that developmental signaling molecules are involved in the development of numerous systems throughout the body. Polydactyly can be caused by a number of inherited conditions and is often not attributable to any known cause. Making a diagnosis of PHS in a child with polydactyly allows clinicians to use the historical experience with PHS to design strategies for counseling and therapy.

Nail Patella syndrome

Nail patella syndrome (NPS) classically includes abnormalities of the finger/toenails, knees, elbows, and pelvic bones. In addition, a substantial number of individuals will have kidney and eye involvement, often appearing later in life. NPS is caused by mutations in the *LMX1B* gene, and is therefore categorized as a defect of dorsal–ventral patterning. Several classic NPS features make intuitive sense as disruptions of dorsal–ventral patterning including the nail abnormalities and the presence of abnormal or missing kneecaps (both dorsal structures). Making a diagnosis based on congenital abnormalities allows for screening for later manifestations of the disease.

Retinoic acid embryopathy

Retinoic acids are chemically related to vitamin A. Some types of retinoic acid are used medicinally, including the severe acne treatment Isotretinoin. Isotretinoin use in pregnant women is contraindicated because of an association with a well-described set of birth defects. Retinoic acids normally formed in the body participate in the regulation of limb development and interact with other signaling systems such as the *Hox* genes. It is not surprising, therefore, that some cases of retinoic acid embryopathy include limb reduction defects – a disruption of proximal–distal patterning.

Three-dimensional limb patterning: Conclusions

Research into the molecular underpinnings of development continues. Further insight into the mechanisms by which normal development proceeds will continue to improve our ability to understand how and why specific birth defects occur.

Fetal Surgery

Another area of research focuses on the prenatal treatment of birth defects. Fetal surgery involves gaining surgical access to the fetus, usually through the mother's abdominal wall and the wall of the uterus. Once the fetus is exposed, surgery on the fetus is performed, followed by repair of the mother's uterine and abdominal incisions. Often a conservative surgical approach is taken, whereby a minimal set of interventions is designed to help the fetus survive to birth. After birth, additional medical and surgical treatments may be necessary. For instance, in 1981, a pioneering surgery performed by Dr. Michael Harrison involved a fetus that had a congenital blockage of urinary bladder outflow called a posterior urethral valve. A shunt was placed, allowing the passage of urine and decompressing the dangerously expanded bladder. After birth, the congenital anomaly was definitively repaired and the child developed normally. Similar, and more complicated, surgeries are being developed to treat a number of amenable conditions.

Summary

The term birth defect encompasses a wide variety of birth anomalies resulting from deviation in normal embryogenesis. There is a continuum of variation among newborns, including some variation that has detrimental health consequences for the child. Medical geneticists and other specialists evaluate children with birth defects in an attempt to classify them as an aid in counseling and treatment. Although the number of recognized mechanisms for birth defects is growing, the root cause of the majority of birth defects is unknown. Birth defects continue to pose a large medical and economic burden on individual families and on society. Biomedical research is expanding our ability to diagnose and treat birth defects.

See also: Birth Complications and Outcomes; Developmental Disabilities: Cognitive; Developmental Disabilities: Physical; Down Syndrome; Intellectual Disabilities; Teratology.

Suggested Readings

Epstein CJ, Robert PE, and Wynshaw-Boris A (2004) *Inborn Errors of Development.* Oxford: Oxford University Press.

Jones KL (1988) *Smith's Recognizable Patterns of Human Malformation,* 4th edn. Toronto: W.B. Saunders.

Jones KL (2005) *Smith's Recognizable Patterns of Human Malformation,* 6th edn. Philadelphia, PA: W.B. Saunders.

Martin JA, Kochanek KD, Strobino DM, Guyer B, and MacDorman MF (2005) Annual summary of vital statistics – 2003. *Pediatrics* 115(3): 619–634.

Rimoin DL, Connor JM, Pyeritz RE, and Korf BR (2006) *Emery and Rimoin's The Principles and Practice of Medical Genetics.* Oxford: Elsevier.

Robbins JM, Bird TM, Tilford JM, *et al.* (2007) Hospital stays, hospital charges, and in-hospital deaths among infants with selected birth defects – United States, 2003. *Morbidity and Mortality Weekly Report* 56(2): 25–29.

Relevant Websites

http://www.cdc.gov – Centers for Disease Control and Prevention – Basic Facts About Birth Defects (accessed 18 September 2007); Birth Defects: Frequently Asked Questions (21 March 2006).

http://marchofdimes.com – March of Dimes Foundation.

C

Cerebral Palsy

M L Campbell, A H Hoon, and M V Johnston, Kennedy Krieger Institute, Baltimore, MD, USA

Glossary

Associated disorders – Other medical conditions that are seen in individuals with cerebral palsy.

Birth asphyxia – Asphyxia is a condition of severely deficient supply of oxygen to the brain, which, if prolonged, will result in metabolic acidosis and shutdown of body functions. The diagnosis of birth asphyxia is based on several criteria, including signs of fetal distress, serious brain dysfunction affecting breathing, movement, swallowing, as well as seizures in newborn infants.

Brain malformation – An abnormality in brain formation occurring early in fetal development, which is permanent, and which may be caused either by a genetic factor or by prenatal event(s) that are not genetic. It is a common cause of cerebral palsy.

Cerebral palsy (CP) – CP describes a group of disorders of the development of movement and posture, causing activity limitation, that are attributed to nonprogressive disturbances that occurred in the developing fetal or infant brain. CP may be categorized into spastic, extrapyramidal, and mixed forms. It is the result of underlying medical disorders or risk factor(s), which result in abnormal brain formation or injury.

Dyskinetic – Impairment in the ability to control movements; an alternative term to extrapyramidal CP.

Dystonia – A neurological movement disorder characterized by involuntary muscle contractions, which force certain parts of the body into abnormal, sometimes painful, movements or postures. Dystonic CP is a type of extrapyramidal cerebral palsy.

Etiology/risk factors – Underlying contributing or causal factors leading to the development of a medical condition such as CP.

Extrapyramidal – Refers to central nervous system structures (i.e., outside the cerebrospinal pyramidal tracts) that play a role in controlling functions.

Intellectual disability (mental retardation) – Mental retardation is a disability characterized by significant limitations both in intellectual functioning and in adaptive behavior as expressed in conceptual, social, and practical adaptive skills. This disability originates before age 18 years. The term mental retardation is being replaced by 'intellectual disability.'

Low birth weight – Birth weight of less than 2500 g.

Magnetic resonance imaging – an imaging tool used to identify structural abnormalities. It is very helpful in determining the underlying medical diagnosis in children with CP.

Management – A comprehensive approach to care including medical, rehabilitative, and alternative therapies that reflects the needs of the person. It is lifelong and changes over time with the person.

Mental retardation – See Intellectual disability above.

Periventricular leukomalacia – White matter injury in the developing brain, often occurring between 24–34 weeks of gestation in children with CP.

Prematurity – The current World Health Organization definition of prematurity is a baby born before 37 weeks of gestation, counting from the first day of the last menstrual period.

Spasticity – An involuntary increase in muscle tone (tension) that occurs following injury to the brain or spinal cord, causing the muscles to resist being moved.

Very low birth weight – Birth weight of less than 1500 g.

Introduction

Cerebral palsy (CP) describes a group of lifelong neurological disorders that affects muscle tone, posture, mobility, and hand use. CP is the most common cause of motor disability in childhood. It affects approximately 2/1000 children, with about 8000 young children diagnosed yearly in the US. Functional limitations vary in severity from isolated gait disturbance to an inability to move, and may change over time. Many children have associated problems with speech, cognitive processing, seizures, eye movements, and swallowing, as well as orthopedic deformities. The majority grow into adulthood, and can lead successful lives with appropriate supports.

CP is a clinical diagnosis that serves to identify the child as needing specific rehabilitative services, as well as a commonly understood term for families to use with others to describe their children, that is, "My child has cerebral palsy." From a medical perspective, CP results from a wide range of genetic or acquired risk factors and disorders that disrupt developing areas of the brain that control movement (**Table 1**). While muscles are secondarily affected, it is not a primary disorder of either muscle or nerve. Clinicians work to establish the underlying medical diagnosis that results in CP. This knowledge is useful in determining treatment, prognosis, and recurrence risk, as well as in allaying feelings of parental guilt or responsibility.

Knowledge of normal brain development as well as of the effects of deleterious genetic and environmental factors is beneficial in understanding developmental disabilities such as CP, as well as mental retardation (MR) and autism. When the disruption affects developing motor pathways, the result is CP; and when it affects cognitive parts of the brain, the result may be intellectual disability (MR), autism, or learning disabilities.

Effective management requires a thorough understanding of the causes, manifestations, and management options for children with CP. Maintaining open lines of communication between a wide variety of medical, rehabilitative, and social practitioners who treat the myriad of presentations and variable patterns of clinical expression is also required (**Table 2**). Early identification of CP as well as associated disorders facilitates the establishment of effective management plans. Inclusion of children and their families in decision making is critical to optimizing function.

Progress in brain imaging and epidemiology has provided new insights into underlying causes, while advances in medical care such as therapeutic botulinum toxin (Botox) and intrathecal baclofen (ITB) offer improved treatment options. In the past, interventions such as rubella immunization and Rhogam to Rh-negative women have eliminated CP from these causes. Important areas of current research focus on the prevention of prematurity/low birth weight as well as strategies to treat brain injury in high-risk newborns.

Table 1   Risk factors for cerebral palsy

Maternal factors
- Maternal age (<20 years or >35 years)
- History of infertility
- Previous pregnancy loss or neonatal death
- Prior-born child (elder sibling) with CP
- Thyroid disease
- Diabetes

Pregnancy complications
- Maternal infection (e.g., chorioamnionitis)
- Preclampsia
- Prolonged rupture of membranes
- Placental abruption
- Placental insufficiency

Infant attributes
- Prematurity/low birth weight
- Multiple gestation
- Male gender
- Growth retardation
- *In vitro* fertilization

Neonatal morbidities and interventions
- Genetic disorders
- Congenital brain malformations
- Hyperbilirubinemia (kernicterus)
- Perinatal stroke
- Chorioamnionitis (placental infection)
- Birth asphyxia
- Postnatal steroids
- Pneumothorax
- Prolonged exposure to mechanical ventilation
- Prolonged hypocarbia

In childhood
- Brain infections (i.e. bacterial meningitis, viral encephalitis)
- Vascular episodes (stroke)
- Brain injury-accidental, nonaccidental

History

The cause(s) of CP has been vigorously debated for 150 years. In 1862, Sir William Little attributed CP to problems with childbirth, which has had ongoing effects in the legal arena to the present. In 1897, Sigmund Freud offered an alternative view point, suggesting that the cause of CP was of prenatal origin. ("Difficult birth, in certain cases … is merely a symptom of deeper effects that influence the development of the fetus.") Sir William Osler added the broader overview of the combination of brain anatomy, etiology, and extremity involvement in the diagnosis and classification of CP.

The modern view of CP is concordant with the views of Freud and Osler, emphasizing prenatal antecedents in the majority of affected children. This understanding has been supported by the work of Dr. Karin Nelson from the National Institutes of Health (NIH). In the 1980s Dr. Nelson and colleagues, in a study examining mothers and newborns to determine the cause of CP, found that

Table 2 Associated disorders

	Spastic diplegia	Spastic quadriplegia	Hemiplegia	Extrapyramidal	Hyptonia/ataxia
Tone	Spasticity	Spasticity	Spasticity	Rigidity	Hyptonia
Extremity	involvement UE = LE	LE > UE	LE = UE	Unilateral	UE > LE
Movement disorders	Clonus, spasms, toe walking	Clonus, spasms	Clonus, spasms	Dystonia, chorea, athetosis	Ataxia
Speech/ swallowing	Mild impairment	Impaired	Intact	Impaired or absent speech	Variable
Cognitive impairment	Mild–moderate, learning disorders	Moderate–severe	Intact to mild	Intact to moderate	Variable
Associated problems	Strabismus, orthopedic deformities	Orthopedic deformities, epilepsy	Epilepsy	Orthopedic deformities, genetic–metabolic disorders	Undiagnosed genetic–metabolic disorders

LE – lower extremities; UE – upper extremities; Clonus – movements characterized by alternate contractions and relaxations of a muscle, occuring in rapid succession. Clonus is frequently observed in conditions such as spasticity (from website WE MOVE); Athetosis – involuntary, relatively slow, writhing movements that essentially flow into one another. Athetosis is often associated with chorea, a related condition characterized by involuntary, rapid, irregular, jerky movements (from website WE MOVE).
From Hoon AH and Johnston MV (2002) Cerebral palsy. Asbury AK, McKhann GM, McDonald WI, Goadsby PJ, and McArthur JC (eds.) *Diseases of the Nervous System*, 3rd edn., pp. 568–580. Cambridge: University Press. Associated disorders refers to other medical conditions a child with CP may have.

the majority of cases were due to prenatal factors, which were often unknown. Current understanding has built on Nelson's research, to shift the focus from single causes to the recognition that in many affected children, there is a cascade of contributory factors acting along causal pathways, with the challenge being the identification of these pathways.

Classification

Movement requires the coordinated passage of simultaneous messages through different tracts in the brain, and then onto the spinal cord, peripheral nerves, and finally to the muscles themselves. CP type is related to the location(s) in the brain of white or gray matter injury or abnormal formation (**Figure 1**). One of the tracts, the cortical spinal tract (CST) or pyramidal tract, sends messages for motor movement to the spinal cord. If this tract is injured during brain development, a person will often develop spastic CP. Recent information indicates that pathways in the brain involved in processing sensory information may also lead to spastic CP.

A second motor control pathway tract in the brain provides messages for the control of movement. This pathway runs in a loop from the cortex of the brain through the basal ganglia/thalamus and back to the cortex, thereby regulating movement. If this tract is injured during brain development, a child may develop extrapyramidal CP, often with dystonia. Injury to this tract may

be caused by problems with oxygen, increased jaundice at birth, or genetic diseases.

CP may be classified on the basis of neurologic examination, limb involvement, or degree of functional impairment. Each classification system has strengths and limitations that should be considered in selection and use.

A commonly employed classification with clinical implications for treatment is that based on examination into spastic, extrapyramidal, and mixed forms (**Figure 2**). Spastic CP is characterized by increased muscle tone (resistance similar to that felt in opening a clasp knife), greater leg than arm involvement, and increased risk for orthopedic deformities including hip dislocation and scoliosis. Seventy per cent of affected children have primarily spastic or spastic/mixed forms of CP, which can be subcategorized into diplegia, quadriplegia, and hemiplegia. Diplegia refers to primary lower extremity involvement; quadriplegia to four limb involvement; and hemiplegia when one side of the body is affected. It should be noted that the causes of hemiplegia differ significantly from other types of CP in which both sides of the body are affected.

Extrapyramidal forms constitute the remaining 30%, and include dystonic, rigid, choreic, ataxic, and hypotonic subtypes. Another term used is dyskinetic CP, which refers to an impairment in the ability to control movements. Dystonia refers to sustained muscle contractions associated with involuntary twisting or repetitive movements, and is seen rather than felt on examination. Rigidity refers to increased tone similar to the sense of pulling taffy, and is

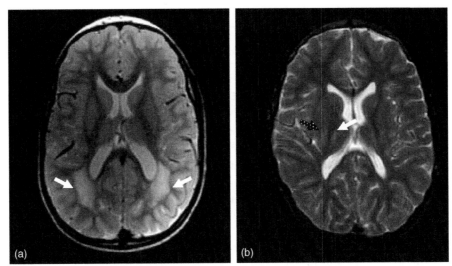

Figure 1 Brain MRI in two children with CP. (a) The MRI is from a child with spastic diplegia associated with preterm birth. The arrows point to areas of injury in white matter ('brain wiring'). (b) The MRI is from a child with dystonic CP associated with hypoxic–ischemic injury (low oxygen) in an infant born at term. The black speckled arrow shows injury in the putamen and the white arrow in the thalamus.

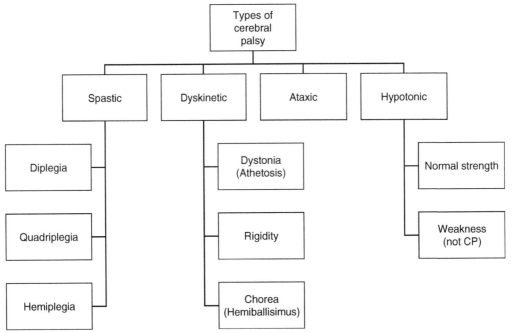

Figure 2 Neurological classification of cerebral palsy. Please see Section 'Classification' for description of terms.

related to muscle co-contraction. Chorea can be thought of as the opposite of dystonia, and is characterized by jerky, irregular, and rapid involuntary movements. Ataxia refers to abnormalities in balance and coordination. Hypotonia refers to decreased muscle tone. Children with extrapyramidal CP often have underlying genetic disorders.

Mixed forms manifest both spasticity and extrapyramidal signs. With careful examination, many children have mixed signs. In these cases, medical treatment is often determined by the primary neurological finding(s).

As highlighted in the recent WHO publication, *The World Health Organization International Classification of Functioning, Disability and Health*, it is important to characterize the functional consequences of disorders such as CP. To classify ambulation, the gross motor function classification system (GMFCS) is often used, with five levels based on functional mobility or activity limitation. The manual ability classification system (MACS) is a recently described instrument with good reliability to classify upper extremity function. These instruments serve as a basis for discussion of clinical characteristics among healthcare professionals as well as in research studies of treatment interventions.

Causes

Prenatal genetic and environmental risk factors are linked in 70% of children with CP, while birth asphyxia plays a role in 10–20%. Risk factors which have been linked to CP include prematurity, low birth weight, multiple gestation, maternal thyroid abnormalities, intrauterine viral infection, male gender, hereditary disorders of clotting, placental abnormalities, hypoxia–ischemia, and signs of intrauterine infection/inflammation.

Using brain magnetic resonance imaging (MRI) as the primary diagnostic tool, children with CP can be categorized into four groups, based on the timing of the underlying etiological factors: (1) disorders of early brain formation, (2) injury associated with prematurity, termed periventricular white matter injury or periventricular leukomalacia (PVL), (3) disorders presenting in the term infant, and (4) a heterogeneous group of disorders occurring in early childhood. Although there is variability in the developing and developed world, approximately 30% are associated with brain malformations, 40% with prematurity, 20% in term infants, and 10% to postnatal causes.

Diagnosis

A careful history and neurological examination remain key components to diagnosis. Symptoms may appear soon after birth or during early childhood. Risk factors in infants include significantly increased or decreased muscle tone, difficulty with head control, delay in rolling, sitting, crawling, standing, or early preferential hand use.

A minority of children, including those with genetic disorders, may appear normal and then manifest motor delay later in infancy or early childhood. A well-recognized example of this is the genetic disorder glutaric aciduria, type 1. In this condition, infants or young children develop normally until metabolic stress such as chickenpox or dehydration leads to acute signs of neurological injury, which progresses to extrapyramidal forms of CP.

In addition to a thorough physical examination looking for findings suggesting a genetic cause, a careful head measurement of head circumference (i.e., too small (microcephaly) or too large (possible hydrocephalus)), and neurological examination of eye movements, tone, and reflexes is important. Infants have reflexes such as the Moro (a quick body movement leading to arm movements that resemble an embrace), which normally disappear by 3–6 months of age. Persistence of this and other infant reflexes are neurological signs of possible CP. Tone

abnormalities as described above are also concerning findings. Additionally, if an infant favors 1 hand or side of his/her body strongly before 1 year of age, this may be of a sign of hemiplegic CP.

If the history suggests that the child is losing abilities, or the examination shows unusual findings such as muscle weakness, this may represent one of a wide variety of other neurological disorders of childhood that do not fall under the diagnosis of CP. Referral to a pediatric neurologist is strongly recommended in this situation. In some cases, it may take several examinations to determine whether the findings are consistent with CP or represent another type of neurological condition.

Brain scans using ultrasound, computed tomography (CT), and MRI provide images of the brain structure. In children with CP, MRI has revolutionized understanding of the underlying cause in many children, with abnormalities seen in 70–90% of children with CP. MRI findings can serve to guide additional diagnostic testing, including blood and urine studies.

Management

The overall management of children with CP is directed toward optimizing function and quality of life. This is accomplished by improving muscle strength and endurance, enhancing academic success, facilitating personal hygiene, treating associated disabilities, and preventing medical complications such as slow growth, joint problems, and reduced bone mass/fractures.

The human brain grows rapidly from conception through early childhood. During this time connections between the brain and white matter pathways that make up the central nervous system are forming. During childhood approximately half of these connections are maintained due to stimulation through activity, and half are eliminated. This concept is called plasticity. This is the underlying medical basis of early intervention.

Early identification of motor delay or CP is important in establishing effective treatment. In this regard, the federal law IDEA (Individuals with Disabilities Education Act) provides the framework for eligibility and service delivery. This law has two important components, the Infants and Toddlers Program for children 0–3 years of age, and the Child FIND program for those aged 3–21 years. There are three ways to qualify for the free, home-based services in the Infants and Toddlers Program: grater than 25% delay in developmental abilities, high probability for developmental delay (e.g., Down syndrome), and atypical development. To qualify for Child FIND, a diagnosis such as CP, learning disability, or MR must be established.

Therapy and treatment options are key in successfully managing CP. A multidisciplinary team approach provides the best management strategy, leading to optimal outcome. A team may variably include a developmental pediatrician, pediatric neurologist, physiciatrist, orthopedic surgeon, physical therapist (PT), occupational therapist (OT), speech pathologist, social worker, and a psychologist. Collectively, this team focuses on an individual treatment plan for each child. Prior to beginning an intervention, treatment goals should be clearly established between the family and careproviders. For example, these goals might include ease of care, improved function, decreased risk for orthopedic problems, or reduction in pain/spasms.

Children with CP develop to their full potential when treatment programs optimize motor capabilities, minimize orthopedic deformities, and address associated impairments. Management can be divided into rehabilitative, medical, and surgical components, and may include physical/occupational therapy, therapeutic botulinum toxin, oral medications, and orthopedic and neurological surgery (**Figure 3**). Physical and occupational therapists provide the backbone of management for the child, in addition to providing education and guidance for family members.

In children with CP, there is a small but growing number of genetic disorders, including dopa responsive dystonia, glutaric aciduria type 1, and methymalonic acidemia, which may significantly improve or be ameliorated with appropriate medical therapy. Clinicians involved in diagnosis should maintain an eye of vigilance for these conditions.

Physical and Occupational Therapy

PTs and OTs provide initial and ongoing treatment for children with CP. From early infancy and throughout life, PT and OT services are important in treatment. PTs focus on optimizing functional abilities and preventing orthopedic deformities, using a variety of individually tailored approaches, including stretching, strength training, bracing, gait training, and equipment, including wheelchair, walker, and prone stander. OTs evaluate and treat oromotor/swallowing dysfunction, as well as upper extremity use in the context of activities of daily living and also address occupational/vocational opportunities.

Therapeutic Botulinum Toxin

Therapeutic botulinum toxin is used to for treating focal spasticity and dystonia. For this therapy, affected muscle groups are isolated and injected with a small amount of botulinum toxin. The toxin binds to the nerve endings and weakens the isolated muscle group. Balance can then be re-established with other muscles across the affected joint(s). It often works best when combined with casting or splinting. This therapy lasts for about 3 months and may be repeated. Botulinum toxin injection is relatively safe and can be used in the upper extremities, lower extremities, and neck.

Oral Medications

Medications such as baclofen (Lioresal), diazepam (Valium), trihexyphenidyl (Artane), and carbidopa/levodopa (Sinemet) can be used to treat CP (**Table 3**). Oral medications are variably used to improve function; decrease spastic, rigid or dystonic hypertonicity; as well as to decrease muscle spasms in certain situations (e.g., diazepam use after orthopedic surgery).

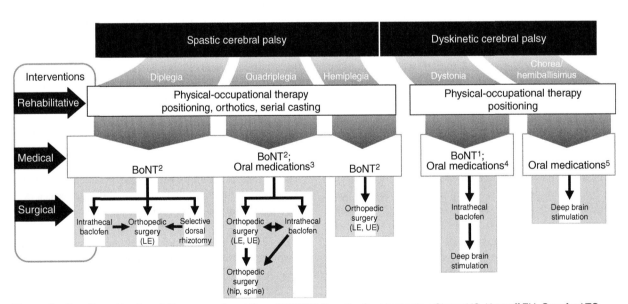

Figure 3 Algorithm of treatment. Puscavage A and Hoon AH (2005) Spasiticy/cerebral palsy. Singer HS, Kossoff EH, Crawford TO, Hartman AL (eds.) *Treatment of Pediatric Neurologic Disorders*, p.17. New York: Dekker. LE, lower extremities; UE, upper extremities.

Table 3   Medications that have been used for cerebral palsy and other motor disorders

Oral medication	Drug class	Spasticity	Rigidity	Athetosis	Dystonia	Chorea	Hemiballismus	Epilepsy
Baclofen	GABAergic	X	X	X	X			
Carbamazepine	Neuronal stabilizer					X	X	X
Clonazepam	Benzodiazepine	X				X		X
Clonidine	α2 agonist	X						
Dantrolene	Direct muscular	X	X		X			
Diazepam	Benzodiazepine	X	X	X	X			X
Levodopa	Dopaminergic	X			X			
Reserpine	Dopamine depleter					X		
Resperidone	Neuroleptic					X	X	
Tiagabine	GABA agonist	X						X
Tizanidine	α2 agonist	X						
Trihexyphenidyl	Anticholinergic			X	X			
Valproate	Neuronal stabilizer					X	X	X

Oral medications that are commonly prescribed in treating cerebral palsy and other childhood motor disorders.

When using oral medications, the functional benefits for the person must outweigh the side effects of the medication. Often these medications have unwanted side effects that need to be monitored to make sure they are not interfering with functional outcomes. Furthermore, abrupt withdrawal of these oral medications may also cause unwanted effects as children become accustomed to these medications and must be weaned off slowly. Finally, these medications should periodically be tapered off to see if any recognized, positive effects are medication-related.

Orthopedic Surgery

A baseline evaluation from an orthopedic surgeon experienced in the management of children with CP is of benefit both for recommendations on nonsurgical treatment as well as for planning potential, later surgical interventions. Despite all efforts, some children with spastic forms of CP will require orthopedic surgery. The orthopedic management of spasticity is directed toward reducing deformity and thereby facilitating function, utilizing tendon lengthenings/transfers, bony osteotomies, and joint fusion procedures. The current approach is often multilevel soft tissue procedures initially, with later bony procedures as required. Computerized gait analysis for preoperative planning may be of benefit.

Intrathecal Baclofen Pump

For people with severe spastic or dystonic CP, for whom other less-invasive approaches have not been beneficial, ITB may be a treatment option. Children, adolescents, and adults who are interested in this treatment should be initially evaluated in a clinic with expertise in ITB management. After a small test dose of baclofen given by spinal tap to assess effectiveness, a pump is placed in the abdomen and connected to a catheter threaded into the intrathecal cerebrospinal fluid-filled space around the spinal cord. The pump works by pumping tiny amounts of baclofen directly into the cerebrospinal fluid, which is then absorbed in the spinal cord reducing spasticity. Instead of using milligrams of baclofen orally, the ITB system uses micrograms of baclofen. As it is targeted more directly to the nervous system, it is often more effective than oral baclofen for people with severe CP. After the pump is installed, it is refilled every 2–6 months. Dosing can be increased or decreased at any time painlessly with a special programmer. A pump can last for 7–9 years before the battery runs down, requiring replacement.

Selective Dorsal Rhizotomy

Selective dorsal rhizotomy (SDR) is a permanent neurosurgical treatment option for children with spastic diplegic cerebral palsy, most commonly associated with prematurity and PVL. During surgery, 30–50% of sensory nerve fibers that run in the lower part of the spinal cord (lumbar/sacral area) are selectively cut. By cutting these nerve fibers, leg spasticity is reduced and function improves. As with ITB, initial evaluation should be made by a team with experience in SDR, including the necessary postoperative rehabilitation.

Complementary and Alternative Therapies

When conventional approaches do not lead to the anticipated improvements, families may explore other treatment options, including complementary and alternative medicine (CAM). CAM includes acupuncture, cranio-sacral therapy, myofascial release, therapeutic taping, diet and herbal remedies, electrical stimulation, constraint-induced training, chiropractic treatments, massage and hyperbaric oxygen therapy (HBOT). While there are individual reports and testimonials of dramatic improvements with various alternative therapies, some carry risk such as middle-ear dysfunction requiring PE tubes with HBOT. Furthermore, rigorous studies have not been conducted to assess efficacy. As with any treatment, families and clinicians should consider cost, efficacy, and potential side effects before embarking on one of these approaches.

Living Considerations

Accessibility

While the American Disabilities Act (ADA) passed in 1993 has significantly improved accessibility, it may still be a continuing problem for individuals with CP and other disabilities. Accessibility concerns may range from housing, to transportation, or using the bathroom. Parents of a child with CP need to be prepared for the ever-changing accessibility needs as their child grows. Working with local agencies can assist in addressing these issues. As children with CP grow, movement may begin to decrease and mobility options may change. These changes will affect accessibility.

People with CP are often assumed to have MR, recently termed intellectual disability. This is not always true. Having CP does not mean the person is mentally retarded or intellectually disabled. People with CP can have normal intelligence. Sometimes a person with CP cannot vocally communicate, but they are able to understand what is going on around them. Evaluations by both psychologists and speech language pathologists can be of great benefit in assessing cognitive abilities and recommending approaches to optimize communication.

As mandated by the federal law IDEA, children with CP and other disabilities should have educational opportunities in a least restrictive environment. There is an extensive list of rights that parents have in protecting their child's right to an appropriate education. An individualized education plan (IEP) is often used in education planning for children with CP. This plan is created with the assistance of a local school system. An IEP planning team must have a chairperson, special educator, and general educator. Parents should and are often invited to participate in the planning and must be given 10 days notice before the IEP meeting is to happen. Depending on the services provided in the IEP, input from a PT, OT, and/or speech language pathologist may be required. Parents have to approve the IEP which are reviewed minimally once a year. The IEP team can also suggest assistive technology to continue the child's access to education. Also, as the child with CP grows and is cognitively capable, he/she should be a part of the IEP planning process.

Another option in education is a 504 plan. A 504 plan is a legal document provided for children who have a physical and/or mental impairment that substantially interferes with one or more major life activities. Impairments can include attention deficit hyperactivity disorder, asthma, diabetes, and problems with speech, reading, and vision. Specialized accommodations are given to assist the child in the learning environment. Examples are scribe, proximal seating, extended time for daily classroom activities, and repetition of directions. A child may have either an IEP or a 504 plan.

Adult Outcome

As children with CP now live longer, as adults they face new challenges, including medical care, accessibility, and vocational opportunities. The risks for ischemic cardiac disease, cerebrovascular disease, cancer, and trauma are increased compared to the general population. While medical care is well established for children with CP, it is more fragmented for adults. Some adult medical practitioners are not familiar with management in CP and do not know how to integrate the care these persons have previously received into customary adult care.

Adults with CP should look for practitioners experienced in the care of chronic disorders, and who provide the additional time that may be required for evaluation. They also need to recognize the importance of preventive care, and report any changes in neurological function, as they may represent new impairments secondary to the underlying motor disorder.

Mobility as well as the ability to perform activities of daily living should be carefully monitored, as some adults will experience slow declines over time. Cognitively intact individuals should be provided with instruction in practical matters such as hiring quality personal aids and caregivers, as well as in self-advocacy and in seeking employment opportunities.

Conclusions

Individuals with CP often seek the same opportunities for employment, living, marriage, families, and recreation/leisure as others in their communities. Dramatic innovations in diagnosis using MRI and new treatment modalities offer improved quality of life, treatment options, and educational opportunities. The challenge is providing these opportunities in a changing medical environment, where a premium is not always placed on coordination of care.

See also: Birth Complications and Outcomes; Developmental Disabilities: Cognitive; Developmental Disabilities: Physical; Intellectual Disabilities.

Suggested Readings

Bax M, Murray G, Peter R, *et al.* (2005) Proposed definition and classification of cerebral palsy. *Developmental Medicine and Child Neurology* 47: 571–576.
Elaine G (1998) *Children With Cerebral Palsy: A Parents' Guide,* 2nd edn. Bethesda, MD: Woodbine House.
Eliasson AC, Krumlinde – Sundholm L, Rosblad B, *et al.* (2007) Using the MACS to facilitate communication about manual abilities of

children with cerebral palsy. *Developmental Medicine and Child Neurology* 49: 156–157.

Freeman M and Steven B (1998) *Cerebral Palsy: A Complete Guide for Caregiving.* Baltimore, MD: The Johns Hopkins University Press.

Hoon AH and Johnston MV (2002) Cerebral palsy. Asbury AK, McKhann GM, McDonald WI, Goadsby PJ, and McArthur JC (eds.) *Diseases of the Nervous System*, 3rd edn., pp. 568–580. Cambridge: University Press.

Jane FL, Sherri C, and Margaret M (1997) *Keys to Parenting a Child With Cerebral Palsy (Barron's Parenting Keys).* New York: Barron's Educational Series.

Keogh JM and Badawi N (2006) The origins of cerebral palsy. *Current Opinions in Neurology* 19: 129–134.

Krigger KW (2006) Cerebral palsy: An overview. *American Family Physician* 73: 91–102.

Mark L and Batshaw MD (2002) *Children with Disabilities,* 5th edn. Baltimore, MD: Paul H Brookes.

Nelson KB and Ellenberg JH (1986) Antecedents of cerebral palsy. Multivariate analysis of risk. *New England Journal of Medicine* 315: 81–86.

Palisano R, Rosenbaum P, Walter S, *et al.* (1997) Development and reliability of a system to classify gross motor function in children with cerebral palsy. *Developmental Medicine and Child Neurology* 39: 214–223.

Puscavage A and Hoon AH (2005) Spasiticy/cerebral palsy. Singer HS, Kossoff EH, Crawford TO, Hartman AL (eds.) *Treatment of Pediatric Neurologic Disorders* p.17. New York: Dekker.

Relevant Websites

http://www.aamr.org – American Association on Mental Retardation (AAMR).
http://www.eparent.com – Exceptional Parent.
http://idea.ed.gov – IDEA (The Individuals with Disabilities Education Act).
http://www.ucp.org – United Cerebral Palsy (UCP).
http://www.wemove.org – WE MOVE (Worldwide Education and Awareness for Movement Disorders).

Colic

D R Fleisher, University of Missouri School of Medicine, Columbia, MO, USA
R Barr, University of British Columbia, Vancouver, BC, Canada

Introduction

The term 'colic' implies abdominal pain of intestinal origin. However, it has never been proved that colicky crying is caused by pain in the abdomen or anywhere else. Although infant colic is not considered to be a functional gastrointestinal disorder, the abdominal pain attribution persists and pediatric gastroenterologists receive referrals of babies with refractory colic or infants who cry excessively due to unsuspected colic. Therefore, familiarity with the 'colic syndrome' is necessary for the avoidance of diagnostic and therapeutic misadventures.

Definition

Colic has been described as a behavioral syndrome of early infancy involving large amounts of crying, long crying bouts, and hard-to-sooth behavior. Although colic-like crying may occur in infants who are sensitive to cow's milk proteins, by definition, infant colic is not caused by organic disease. Infant colic was defined heuristically by Wessel as "paroxysms of irritability, fussing or crying lasting for a total of more than three hours per day and occurring on more than three days in any one week." Crying bouts start and stop suddenly without obvious cause and are more likely to occur late in the day. Colicky crying tends to resolve spontaneously by 3–4 months

of age or, in the case of babies born prematurely, 3–4 months after term.

Normal infants cry more during the early months of life than at any age thereafter. T. Berry Brazelton studied crying in normal infants and found that, on average, crying peaks at about 6 weeks and then steadily diminishes by 12 weeks of age. Ronald Barr, another researcher in this field, confirmed Brazelton's data and concluded that the normal 'crying curve' of healthy infants is not the result of pain. Colic "is something infants do, rather than something they have," according to Dr. Barr.

Epidemiology

About 20% of infants are perceived by their mothers to be colicky by Wessel's criteria. However, the prevalence of infant colic is influenced by parents' perceptions of the intensity and duration of crying bouts, the method by which data on crying are collected, the psychosocial well-being of the parenting couple and culturally determined infant care practices. Barr found, in his study of caregiving practiced by Kung San hunter-gathers of the Kalahari Desert, that the frequency of onsets of crying conform to the Brazelton–Barr 'crying curve', but the amount of crying was much less than in Western cultures. This may be due to the almost continuous contact between mother and infant and the consistently prompt comforting responses provided to the infant within the family group. Apparently, babies around the world start to cry with similar frequency, suggesting that an inherent trigger for crying is 'built-into' all babies, regardless of their cultural origin. What varies is the length of crying after of onset of fussiness and the comforting response patterns from culture to culture and between parents within a cultural group.

Clinical Evaluation

Many disorders cause irritability and crying that can mimic colic, including cow's milk protein intolerance, fructose intolerance, maternal drug ingestion during pregnancy causing withdrawal irritability in the infant, infantile migraine, gastroesophageal reflux disease (GERD), and anomalous origin of the left coronary artery with meal-induced angina. The colicky crying pattern results from organic disease in 10% or less of colicky babies. Behaviors associated with colicky crying, for example, prolonged bouts, unsoothable crying, crying after feedings, facial expressions of pain, abdominal distention, increased gas, flushing, and legs over the abdomen, are not diagnostic clues indicative of pain or organic disease but they do explain and justify parents' concerns.

A presumptive diagnosis of colic can be made in any infant under 4–5 months of age whose crying has the temporal features of infant colic, who has no signs of central nervous system (CNS) or intrinsic developmental difficulties, is normal on physical examination, and has normal growth patterns. If necessary, it is reasonable to apply a time-limited therapeutic trials appropriate for each of the causes most frequently suspected. Switching to a predigested (hypoallergenic) formula or omitting milk and milk products from the diet of the mother who breastfeeds should result in a rapid and sustained remission of colic-like crying due to cow's milk protein sensitivity. A similarly time-limited trial of medication that suppresses the production of stomach acid should relieve crying caused by acid reflux. If these diagnostic possibilities are correct, an unequivocal improvement should occur within 48 h.

The satiated infant's response to nonanalgesic, nonnutritive soothing maneuvers (such as rhythmic rocking and patting 2–3 times per second in a quiet, nonalerting environment) may quieten the baby. The soothing may work for as long as it goes on, but the infant may resume crying as soon as it is stopped. Repeatedly demonstrating such an 'off–on–off–on' sequence caused by stimulation that could not eliminate pain but does quieten colicky crying has great diagnostic and therapeutic value. Similarly, some colicky infants are quieted during rides in a car. Parents report what has been called the 'red light–green light' phenomenon in such babies: the car rolls and the baby is quiet; the car stops for a red light and the baby starts to fuss; the light turns green, the car moves, and the baby quiets down again. Parents have reported that they approach distant red lights with deliberate slowness when their colicky baby is in the car. 'Off–on' and 'red light–green light' phenomena would not be expected to affect crying caused by bodily pain or hunger.

Physiologic Features

Significant differences have been found in comparisons of colicky infants and infants who did not cry excessively, such as increased muscle tone, heart rates during feedings, ease of falling asleep and soundness of sleep, stool patterns, postprandial gallbladder contraction, and other features. However, none of these findings have been shown to be more than epiphenomena or have provided a basis for successful treatment in 90% or more of babies with colic syndrome. In addition, no differences between colicky and noncolicky infants were found with respect to the activity of the gastrointestinal tract, indicators of intestinal disease, amounts of gas within the intestines, or the frequency of flatulence.

Current evidence suggests that colicky crying is behavior originating in the brain rather than the gastrointestinal tract. Colicky babies have been shown to have different temperament characteristics. Another hypothesis for the genesis of colic is based on differences in infants' reactivity (i.e., the excitability and/or arousability of behavioral and physiologic responses to stimuli) and infants' inherent ability to self-regulate responses to stimuli and benefit from externally applied soothing procedures. Colicky infants seem to have more difficulty with state transitions. For example, a noncolicky baby may feel sleepy, be put down, perhaps fuss briefly, but easily makes the transition from being sleepy to being asleep. A noncolicky infant may feel hungry, fuss briefly, be offered a bottle, feed well, and enter a state of calm satiety. A colicky infant, by comparison, may feel hungry, fuss, and be offered a bottle; he begins to suck, but soon stops, stiffens, arches, and begins crying. He is still hungry and likes his food, but he cannot make the transition to comfortable feeding and relief of hunger. Colicky infants may be difficult to feed, especially if feeding is attempted in an environment that has distracting sights and sounds or by a feeder who is exhausted and tense. Infants with 'active temperaments' are keenly receptive and intensely reactive to stimuli in their environment and this characteristic makes transitions to states of greater comfort more difficult for them as indicated by 'crying for no good reason'.

Psychologic Features

Understanding infant colic requires an appreciation of the subject experience and development of the infant, the mother, their dyadic relationship, and the family and social milieu in which they exist.

At about 2–3 months of age, normal infants become more attentive, socially responsive, and aware of the distinction between 'self' and 'other'. They become better able to sooth themselves and interact and give pleasure to their caregivers. This developmental shift occurs at about the age that colic subsides. These developmental advances are smoother if the infant's temperament is easy, the mother is caring, intuitive, and self-confident, and if the dyadic relationship between them proceeds with smooth reciprocity.

Parents usually have conscious and unconscious ambivalence toward their infant. If the infant is not fussy or difficult to regulate, and if the circumstances of their lives are pleasant, positive feelings predominate and family life is happy. However, if the infant is colicky, resentful feelings may rise to the surface of the mother's awareness. Recognition of angry feelings toward her own infant triggers anxiety and guilt which may prompt her to intensify her efforts at being 'a good mother'. If she is unsuccessful at controlling her baby's crying, her guilty anxiety and her reaction to it may develop into a vicious cycle causing profound physical and emotional exhaustion. This is made more likely when the mother's relationship with her partner is unsupportive. This stressful state impairs her ability to sooth her infant and causes her to doubt her competence as a mother. The emergence of adversarial or alienated feelings toward the unsoothable infant lowers the threshold for abuse. Infant colic may then present as a clinical emergency. Even in noncritical cases, excessive crying may be associated with transient developmental delay in the infant and family dysfunction 1–3 years after the infant's birth.

Table 1 Elements to consider in helping parents of a colicky infant

- A painstaking history that elicits a detailed picture of the baby's symptoms is important; superficial assessment and casual reassurance are not helpful to worried parents. A clinical interview can explore conditions of family life, past, and present, that may impair coping.
- Although colicky crying is seldom caused by disease, it is valuable to acknowledge the severity and importance of the stress that parents experience and how disruptive the crying is to family life.
- It is helpful to schedule a consultation during a time when the infant is likely to be fussy so that the clinician can experience first hand what the parents have been going through. This is also an opportunity to observe parents' attempts at soothing as well as the infant's soothability as he/she attempts to quieten the baby.
- A thorough, gentle physical examination by a diligent, open-minded physician is necessary to search for organic disease (the parent's chief concern).
- Consider 'an alternative to the pain hypothesis' for colicky crying, namely, that crying is a manifestation of normal development in infants with active temperaments who have more difficulty with 'state transitions' during the early months of their lives.
- A colicky baby taxes even the most experienced, devoted parents who fail to sooth because of their own state of exhaustion. Infants sense parents' tension and react to it with more crying. Parents need to know this, especially if they are attempting to double and re-double their efforts while ignoring their own needs for sleep and respite.
- If the infant is healthy, confirm it unequivocally to the parents, along with the realistically optimistic outlook for subsidence of colic by 3–5 months of age.
- It is crucially important to identify methods for calming the infant, at least temporarily. Review and demonstrate the list of common techniques, such as rocking and patting, secure swaddling, rhythmic rolling back and forth in a pram, car rides, pacifiers, or monotonous noise. Because crying bouts gain momentum rapidly, they are easier to stop if soothing maneuvers are applied promptly.
- Management must be individualized. Find out what has worked in the past and what is easiest for each family. Then, support them in doing it their easy way. Avoid stock recommendations regarding feeding, burping, or holding techniques, especially if they may increase the infant's or the mother's stress. For example, burping after every ounce is a recommendation based on the unsubstantiated notion that swallowed air causes colic. Actually, such repeated interruptions make feedings frustrating for both infant and mother.
- Parents of colicky babies often experience feelings of hostility and rejection toward the baby they love and want, whether they are aware of them or not. The more conscientious the parent, the more prone he or she is to self-reproach. The clinician should reflect upon 'irrational parental guilt', how 'normal', if not unavoidable, it is, and (in the words of Dane Prugh) "incise and drain it!"
- Parents' needs must be recognized. Many minimize or deny their anguish and fatigue. They need 'time off', that is, scheduled times when they can withdraw from caring for their infant, leave the house, indulge in rest or recreation, and return to their baby refreshed. Such free time is helpful provided it is scheduled in advance and a competent surrogate caregiver is available. In addition, mothers need a 'rescue' arrangement, a pre-arranged contingency plan whereby a trustworthy relative or friend can promptly take over, should the mother suddenly feel overwhelmed. The more confident the parents are that help is accessible, the less vulnerable they feel and the less likely they will need a rescue. Parents of nocturnal criers need sleep. They might divide the night into two 4 h shifts. The parent who is 'off' can continue sleeping and the parent who is 'on' knows that, when his or her shift is over, sleep is guaranteed. Four hours of guaranteed sleep is likely to be more restful than 8 h of apprehensive dozing in anticipation of the next crying bout.
- The physician's promise to remain available enables parents to continue to cope with their colicky infant without turning to unnecessary diagnostic medical procedures or false 'cures'. They need to know that some intercurrent ear infection has not supervened, or if it has, that it will be treated without delay.

Management

Any measure that parents perceive as definitely helpful is worth continuing, provided it is harmless. If there is a question of milk intolerance or acid reflux as causes of crying, a time-limited therapeutic trial of a hypoallergenic formula or medication to suppress stomach acid production is warranted. Relief in such cases should become apparent within 48 h. However, in more than 90% of cases, management consists not of 'curing the colic', but of helping parents get through this challenging period in their infant's development. There are at least 12 elements to consider in helping parents of a colicky infant, as shown in **Table 1**.

A problem that has been given too little attention is 'persistent colic', for example, the 9-month-old who has not grown out of colicky crying and is still difficult to feed and keep asleep. The following hypothesis is offered as an explanation. An overwrought infant during the first 3 months needs help in developing self-regulation. Responsive soothing prevents the onsets of fussing from progressing to hours-long periods of crying. Parents expect colic to subside by about 3 months and when it does, expectations are fulfilled and the care of their infant becomes a lot less arduous. In the case of the 9-month-old infant who still does colicky crying, the infant is mature enough to be capable of self-regulation. However, his parents are exhausted, somewhat desperate, and fearful that something potentially tragic affects their baby because he is still crying months beyond the age it should have ceased. By this time, the parents' interaction with their infant is dyssynergic, that is, the reciprocal quality of their interaction has been lost and caregiving tends to increase, rather than relieve tension. The author has hospitalized such infants in a quiet private room devoid of colorful or noisy or otherwise distracting stimuli. The mother is relieved of having to care for her baby by herself so that she can rest or recreate herself away from her baby for at least some of the time. Feeding and other infant care procedures are done by a sensitive, comfortable, nonjudgmental nurse. Although the infant is responded to promptly, he is allowed to sleep and is protected from procedures that cause pain of frustration. Usually, a surprising change becomes apparent within 24–48 h in the form of much less crying and easier feeding. Diagnostic interviews with the parents are carried out to elucidate sources of stress in their family life and to dismantle the tendency to self-blame. If this hypothesis is correct, it implies that young colicky babies need very attentive holding and other comforting maneuvers, while persistently colicky older babies benefit from being shielded from overly attentive holding during times they need the peace and quiet that permits them to regulate themselves and relax.

See also: Feeding Development and Disorders.

Suggested Readings

Barr RG (2001) 'Colic' is something infants do, rather than a condition they 'have': A developmental approach to crying phenomena, patterns, pacification and (patho)genesis. In: Barr RG, St. James-Robert I, and Keefe MR (eds.) *New Evidence on Unexplained Early Infant Crying: Its Origins, Nature and Management*, pp. 87–104. Johnson & Johnson Pediatric Institute.

Barr RG, Konner M, Bakeman R, and Adamson L (1991) Crying in !Kung San infants: A test of the cultural specificity hypothesis. *Developmental Medicine and Child Neurology* 33: 601–610.

Brazelton TB (1962) Crying in infancy. *Pediatrics* 29: 579–588.

Fleisher DR (1998) Coping with colic. *Contemporary Pediatrics* 15(6): 144–156.

Liebman W (1981) Infant colic: Association with lactose and milk intolerance. *JAMA* 245: 732–733.

Murray L and Cooper P (2001) The impact of irritable infant behavior on maternal mental state: A longitudinal study and a treatment trial. In: Barr RG, St. James-Roberts I, and Keefe MR (eds.) *New Evidence on Unexplained Early Infant Crying*, pp. 149–164. Johnson & Johnson Pediatric Institute.

St. James-Roberts I (1997) Distinguishing between infant pussing, crying, and colic: How many phenomena? In: Sauls HS and Redfern DE (eds.) *Colic and Excessive Crying – Report of the 105th Ross Conference on Pediatric Research*, pp. 3–14. Columbus, OH: Ross.

Stifter CA and Bono MA (1998) The effect of infant colic on maternal self-perceptions and mother-infant attachment. *Child: Care, Health, and Development* 24: 339–351.

Treem WR (1994) Infant colic, a pediatric gastroenterologist's perspective. *Pediatric Clinics of North America* 41: 1121–1138.

Depression

J Luby, M M Stalets, and A Belden, Washington University School of Medicine, St. Louis, MO, USA

Glossary

Affect – The observable manifestations of a subjectively experienced emotion.
Anaclitic – A term coined in 1946 by psychiatrist Rene Spitz to refer to children who became depressed after being separated from their mothers during the second 6 months of life.
Anhedonia – The experience of having an inability to derive pleasure in normally pleasurable acts.
Dysphoria – A mood of general dissatisfaction, restlessness, depression, and anxiety; a feeling of unpleasantness or discomfort.
High-risk state – Being more likely than the general population to experience a disorder, on the basis of certain characteristics or conditions.
Mood – One's predominant emotion or state of mind.

Introduction

Depression is a clinical mental disorder characterized by a constellation of dysphoric emotional and behavioral symptoms lasting for 2 weeks or longer. Sad or irritable mood and anhedonia, the inability to experience pleasure and joy, are the core symptoms of depression but physiological changes, known as 'vegetative signs' that include changes in sleep or appetite, are also known to occur. A clinical depressive episode is distinct from a sad mood or a transient grief reaction and is not a normative phenomenon. The prevalence rate of the disorder in adults varies with age and gender but depression stands as a major public health problem worldwide. However, the recognition and treatment of the disorder varies by culture and socioeconomic conditions. Women in the childbearing years are at the highest risk with an estimated 10% prevalence rate while there are lower (approximately 2%) prevalence rates in males and prepubertal females. Therefore, the majority of the population will never experience a clinical depressive state even when faced with significant losses and/or stresses. While the exact etiology of this disorder remains unclear, numerous research groups have established the finding that the onset of the disorder is based on both genetic and psychosocial risk factors. Along these lines, it appears that individuals with a genetic vulnerability to the disorder are at highest risk for an episode of depression when they experience stressful life events. However, it is also possible to have a depressive episode without a prior family history of the disorder although this is less common.

Historically, a distinction between 'reactive' or psychosocially based vs. 'endogenous' or biologically based depression was made in adults. However as more data about the etiology of the disorder has been ascertained, this distinction no longer appears to be valid or clinically useful. Despite findings from numerous studies demonstrating that there is a neurobiological basis to depression, there is currently no medical test that can be used to confirm or disconfirm the diagnosis. The diagnosis of depression is made based on clinical interview and mental status examination of the patient. For an adult, this involves an 'interview' in which thought content and predominant feeling states are assessed among other things. For young children, this includes interviewing parents or caregivers to obtain a detailed history about key emotions and behaviors and also requires direct observation of the child and the parent/child dyad to assess play skills and interests as well as psychosocial and relationship functioning. A 'mental status' examination of a young child should involve observations of play behavior and developmental skills and abilities within a dyadic context.

The Concept of Depression Arising in the Very Young

Depression has been recognized as a mental disorder in adults as early as the late nineteenth century or perhaps earlier. For decades after its discovery, developmental theorists asserted that it would be developmentally impossible for a child to experience a depressive episode. This was based on the notion that prepubertal children would be cognitively and emotionally too immature to experience the complex negative emotions, such as shame and guilt, known to be integral to a depressive state. In contrast, the clinical observations of Rene Spitz (described below) and the theoretical work of psychiatrist John Bowlby documented infantile depression and had an impact on some areas of mental health and public policy. However, despite these descriptions, mainstream child mental health clinicians suggested instead that children would manifest 'masked' symptoms of depression, such as somatization or aggression, in lieu of the typical depressive affects and this presumption was widely accepted in clinical practice despite the absence of empirical evidence.

Subsequently, in the early 1980s child psychiatrist investigators, Dennis Cantwell and Gabrielle Carlson, provided empirical data demonstrating that children as young as 6 years of age could display typical symptoms of depression similar to those that characterize the adult disorder. In their landmark paper entitled 'Unmaking masked depression in children and adolescents' they noted that while 'masked' nonspecific symptoms such as stomach aches, were also observed in depressed children, the 'typical' symptoms known in depressed adults and described in the standard diagnostic manual used to define diagnoses in psychiatry, the Diagnostic and Statistical Manual (DSM), were also the most common and specific markers of the disorder in children. These findings and the findings from many other studies that followed replicating and expanding these data revolutionized public health as it opened the doors to the recognition and treatment of depressive disorders in children.

One reason why the discovery of a depressive syndrome in children was so delayed is perhaps related to the underlying idea and wish that childhood should be a joyful time of life. It is unpleasant and difficult to imagine a depressed child. Based on this historically, and to a surprising degree still currently, there is a great deal of social resistance to the idea that depression can arise in childhood. Following this pattern of thought, the idea of depression arising even earlier in life, during the infancy and preschool period, is particularly difficult to imagine or accept. As will be reviewed in this article, there is now empirical evidence demonstrating that depression can arise in children as young as 3 years of age when developmentally adjusted symptom manifestations are assessed. While empirical studies of clinical depression have not yet been conducted in infants and toddlers, clinicians have observed and described infant depression for some time. Numerous high-risk studies demonstrating that the infants of depressed mothers had a greater tendency for negative affect and depressed mood (described below) have also provided support for the idea that depressive affects could occur much earlier in life than previously recognized. These data on early alterations in emotion development set the stage for an exploratory study of clinical symptoms of depression in children between the ages of 3 and 6 years. However, to date there are no available controlled studies that have investigated the question of whether children under the age of 3 years can experience a clinical depressive syndrome.

Theory and Early Observations of Infant Depression

Psychoanalyst Melanie Klein was perhaps the first to elaborate on the idea that a form of depressed affect arose in infancy. She postulated that infants experienced a normative and transient 'depressive position' at approximately 8 months of age. Klein proposed that this very early affective experience represented feelings of guilt that emerged as a result of the infant's aggressive impulses toward the caregiver. This theory has had little clinical application or utility in the practice of mainstream mental health and was never empirically tested. Current developmental data demonstrating that the capacity for guilt does not arise until approximately 3 years of age would suggest that this theory does not represent a valid phenomenon. Therefore, Klein's 'depressive position', which postulates a nonclinical developmental form of depressive experience, is now of interest as a unique historical developmental theory.

The first published observations of depressed affect arising in infants date back to the mid-1940s when psychoanalyst Rene Spitz provided compelling reports of withdrawal, apathy, depressed mood, and failure to thrive in institutionalized infants. He suggested that these infants who had been separated from their primary caregivers and placed in institutional settings were displaying a syndrome he referred to as 'anaclitic depression'. This name was based on the idea that this was a depression that arose secondary to separation from the caregiver with whom the infant was developing a close relationship to and was dependent upon. Even more astonishing, these infants who were deprived of the opportunity for primary caregiving relationships displayed failure to thrive despite adequate nutrition and physical care. Remarkably, these delays were found to diminish significantly after the child and primary caregiver were reunited. Spitz also described 'hospitalism' in which infants institutionalized very early in life, prior to the development of a close relationship with a caregiver, displayed more severe delays, which were thought to be largely irreversible. Despite how remarkable this finding of depressed affect and physical growth retardation arising from psychosocial deprivation was, Spitz's observations had little impact on the practice of mainstream child psychiatry for decades (despite impact in other areas of public health).

High-Risk Studies of Infants of Depressed Mothers

Numerous empirical studies since the mid-1980s have shown that maternal depression is a risk factor for a range of poor developmental outcomes in children. Maternal depression that extends beyond the transient experience of 'baby blues' and crosses the threshold into a clinical postpartum depression, or a more chronic major depressive syndrome, has been shown to be associated with impairments in caregiving capacities. Findings indicate that overall depressed mothers are less responsive, display less positive affect, and gaze at their infants less than nondepressed mothers. Other findings suggest that mothers experiencing chronic depression had difficulty providing an adequate level of social stimulation for their babies. Depressed mothers touched their babies less, engaged in fewer games, and participated in fewer activities with their infants compared to nondepressed mothers. Depressed mothers have also been found to talk to their infants less than nondepressed mothers do. Further, studies show that instead of reciprocating their infants' smiles, depressed mothers are more likely to look sad and anxious while interacting with their infants. Importantly, these alterations in parenting have been associated with a range of negative emotional developmental outcomes in infancy and early childhood.

These 'high-risk' studies focusing on the mood and affective responses of the infant offspring of depressed mothers have produced converging evidence demonstrating that maternal depression occurring early in a child's development may have adverse effects on the emotional development of infants. Observational paradigms in which infants' facial expressions and motor activity in response to evocative events are observed and systematically rated have been designed so that inferences about the emotional states of infants can be made. Such indirect measures are necessary due to the infant's inability to make his/her feeling states clear. Jeffrey Cohn and Edward Tronick are two developmental psychologists who were among the first to design such a paradigm to test the emotional states of 6-month-old infants in response to their mother's varying emotional expressions. These investigators designed a paradigm known as the 'still face' during which the infant is seated directly facing their mother. Mothers are instructed to respond to their infants and then to behave in an artificial emotionally unresponsive fashion in an effort

to simulate a depressed and withdrawn affect, similar to what might be seen during a depressed state.

The response of the infant to their mother's lack of reciprocal emotional response has been shown to vary significantly depending upon the infant's past experience of parenting. Studies utilizing this paradigm in healthy vs. depressed mothers and their infants have indicated that infants of depressed mothers are less active, more withdrawn, and display less positive affect than infants of nondepressed mothers at baseline. Of key importance was that in response to mother's expression of a 'still face' these infants displayed less protest than the infants of nondepressed mothers. These behaviors suggested that infants of depressed mothers are accustomed to maternal nonresponse and do not protest or experience this as an unusual event. These findings were among the first to demonstrate the sensitivity of very young infants to the emotional states of their caregivers. The implications of this are very important as they confirm that early interpersonal and environmental factors may have a material impact on key aspects of development in the infant and very young child.

Maternal Depression and Its Influence on Infants' Psychobiological Processes

In addition to inferring differences in infants' emotional responses based on their facial expression or bodily movements, investigations that look at other physiological markers of reactivity, such as brain activity and heart rate variability, are important for understanding influential factors of emotion development during the infancy period. Specifically, developmental researchers use electroencephalogram recordings to trace connections between electrical activity in the brain and ongoing thoughts as well as emotions being experienced by infants. Records from an EEG are obtained from a series of electrodes that rest on the scalp allowing participants to move freely, making this technique especially useful for infants. Richard Davidson is a psychologist who was among the first researchers to show that the left side of the frontal area is associated with approach-type emotion reactions, which are positive emotions, such as joy in adults. These same researchers also demonstrated decreases in left frontal brain activity in depressed adults. Withdrawal and inhibitory emotion reactivity, such as fear, have been traced to the right side of the brain. Numerous studies using both adults and very young infants have found that asymmetries in frontal lobe activation and function are related to discrete emotions. That is, results indicate that right frontal lobe activations are more likely to occur during crying and sadness, whereas relatively stronger left frontal lobe activation occurs during happiness.

Psychologist Geraldine Dawson proposed that differences in individual children's frontal lobe activation might be a result of life experience as opposed to innate biological factors. The significant role that parents play in infants' emotion development capacities (e.g., regulation, expression, and understanding), undoubtedly accounts for some of the difference in children's frontal brain activity. Empirical findings indicate that during pleasurable and playful interactions with their primary caregivers, infants typically show greater activation in the left frontal area. Dawson and colleagues found that infants of depressed mothers show no difference in left and right activation of the frontal area, indicating that infants of depressed mothers may not find mother–child interactions highly pleasurable. These results support the notion that caregiver socialization can influence frontal asymmetries. One of the critical questions to be answered by future longitudinal studies is whether measures of frontal lobe activity and asymmetry can predict vulnerability for emotional disorders both concurrently as well as later in life.

Overall, these developmental studies provided key evidence for the previously unrecognized relative emotional sophistication of infants and very young children. That is, these data demonstrated that infants were aware of and sensitive to emotional factors and events in their environments at very early stages in development. Such findings opened the door to the idea that early alterations in mood and affect could occur and might be early markers of risk and/or signs of clinical depressive syndromes. There now is an established body of evidence pointing to the emotional sensitivity of young children. This literature was reviewed by a group of scholars in 2000 resulting in the conclusion that "all children are born wired for feeling" and that the quality of early environments and relationships sets the stage for later emotional health.

Empirical Studies of Preschool Depression

Several clinical reports of depression occurring in preschool children were published in the 1970s, but little systematic study of the disorder was conducted until the 1980s when Javid Kashani and colleagues published a series of papers examining the existence of depression in preschoolers using standard diagnostic criteria. These studies identified several children from community and clinical samples who met the widely accepted adult Diagnostic and Statistical Manual (DSM)-III criteria for major depressive disorder (MDD), providing further evidence for the existence of preschool depression. However, the disorder defined by the DSM criteria for adults was found to occur less frequently in preschool children compared to the prevalence rates in older children, adolescents, and adults. In addition to children who met full diagnostic DSM-III MDD criteria, larger numbers of children who displayed concerning depressive symptoms, but failed to meet diagnostic criteria were also identified. These findings led to the suggestion that due to their immature development, preschool age children may manifest symptoms differently than how they were described in the DSM system. These authors therefore suggested that modifications to DSM criteria to identify depressed preschoolers should be explored.

Using age-appropriate diagnostic measures that assessed for age-adjusted symptoms of depression, data from two independent samples of preschoolers in the St. Louis metropolitan area have demonstrated that preschool children can manifest a clinical depressive syndrome. An example of a developmental adjustment would be a focus on negative or sad themes in play, instead of focusing on the emergence of this in thought as would be done in adolescents or adults. Based on the preschool child's more limited verbal abilities, the content of play themes is the best representation of the young child's mental preoccupations. Developmental modifications to the standard DSM criteria, which were developed largely for application to adults, are outlined in **Table 1**.

Symptoms of preschool depression have been found to cluster together and to differentiate depressed preschoolers from those with other psychiatric disorders.

Similar to Cantwell and Carlson's findings with older children mentioned earlier, depressed preschooler children exhibited higher rates of 'typical' depressive symptoms rather than 'masked' symptoms. Thus, age-adjusted

Table 1   Diagnostic criteria for MDD adapted for preschool age

1. Depressed, sad, or irritable mood for a portion of the day for several days, as observed (or reported) in behavior.
2. Markedly diminished interest or pleasure in all, or almost all, activities or play for a portion of the day for several days (as indicated by either subjective account or observations made by others).
3. Significant weight loss or weight gain (not explained by normal growth) or decrease or increase in appetite nearly every day.
4. Insomnia or hypersomnia nearly every day.
5. Psychomotor agitation or retardation nearly every day (change that is observable by others).
6. Fatigue or loss of energy nearly every day.
7. Feelings of worthlessness or excessive or inappropriate guilt (that may be only evident as persistent themes in play).
8. Diminished ability to concentrate on a task, or indecisiveness, for several days (either by subjective account or as observed by others).
9. Recurrent thoughts of death (not just fear of dying), recurrent suicidal ideation without a specific plan, or a suicide attempt or a specific plan for committing suicide. Suicidal or self-destructive themes may be evident only as persistent themes in play.

typical symptoms serve as the best clinical markers even in this very young age group. One distinction between depressive episodes arising in children compared to adults is that the symptom of irritability may present instead of the symptom of sadness. For this reason the DSM system has one adjustment in the formal criteria for depression for children and it is that irritability may present instead of sadness. The symptom of anhedonia, or the inability to experience pleasure, emerged as a key and highly specific symptom of depression in young children. This means that the presence of this symptom serves as a specific marker of depression and can distinguish this from other psychiatric disorders. In the young child, anhedonia may manifest most typically as an inability to enjoy activities and play. Because joyfulness and the experience of pleasure in play is a key focus of the young child's life, it stands to reason that the absence of this is a marker of an aberrant developmental process. Depressed preschooler children who demonstrate anhedonia appear to have a more severe and biologically based subtype of depression. While the presence of this symptom is cause for concern, it alone does not mean that the child is depressed. If this symptom arises and endures over a period of several days to weeks, referral to a mental health clinician is warranted.

One issue that arises when considering psychiatric diagnoses for very young children is the prevailing attitude that most children 'grow out' of their difficulties and therefore they are of little clinical consequence. However, available evidence indicates that this is not true for many preschool-onset mental disorders. Along these lines, there is evidence that preschool depression is stable over a 6-month period, which is a considerable span of time considering the rapid development that occurs in the preschool period. Further, depressed preschoolers appeared impaired both developmentally and functionally when compared to normally developing peers. These findings indicate that preschool depression is of significant consequence to the young child as it affects their general functioning and development and therefore warrants intervention. Further, evidence of impairment is especially important in establishing the validity of preschool depression, as impairment is a key marker of a clinically significant mental disorder according to the DSM system.

In addition to a specific and stable symptom constellation, other key markers of diagnostic validity have been found in depressed preschoolers. Similar to findings of studies of older depressed children and adults, depressed preschoolers have a greater family history of depression and similar disorders than comparison groups. Biological markers, specifically changes in stress hormone reactivity, have been found in depressed preschoolers lending additional support for the validity of the disorder.

As recognition of the existence and clinical characteristics of depression arising during the preschool period is relatively new, little information is currently available regarding the prevalence of the disorder. However, the most recent and most diagnostically and developmentally specific data indicate that 1.4% of preschoolers exhibit depressive symptoms consistent with DSM-IV criteria. As there are over 6 000 000 children between 3 and 6 years of age in the US, as many as 84 000 preschoolers in the US may be experiencing clinically significant depressive symptoms and it is reasonable to speculate that the vast majority of these children are not identified as depressed or offered treatment to target depressive symptoms.

Given findings supporting the validity and clinical importance of preschool depression, continued investigations of the characteristics and antecedents of this early-onset disorder are warranted. Longitudinal studies following depressed preschoolers through school age would provide important information about the longer-term outcome of these children. Biological correlates of depression, including differences in the size and shape of specific brain regions have been found in depressed compared to healthy adults. A study in which depressed preschoolers and healthy control children undergo structural brain imaging is currently underway and may provide additional support for the validity of preschool depression and clues to the neurobiological mechanisms that underlie the disorder. An important area of investigation is the determination of factors that place preschoolers at risk for depression. Information relating to family history of psychiatric disorders, history of stressful events, and the quality of the parent–child relationship is being investigated and may ultimately allow for early identification of those preschoolers at greatest risk.

Depression in Infants and Toddlers

Although empirical investigations of clinical depression in infants and toddlers are not yet available, an alternative developmentally sensitive diagnostic system entitled the 'Diagnostic classification of mental health and developmental disorders in infancy and early childhood' has outlined diagnostic criteria and symptom descriptions designed for application to this younger group. This diagnostic system is based on the experience and clinical observations of a multidisciplinary group of mental health clinicians and has also been informed by the available empirical database; a revised edition was published in the year 2005. A section on depression of infancy and early childhood outlines proposed developmental translations of depressive symptoms that encompass two diagnostic categories: major depression and depressive disorder not otherwise specified (NOS). These categories are designed to apply to infants and toddlers and may provide a useful framework for future empirical investigations. In addition, the DC:0–3R includes a unique category entitled 'Prolonged bereavement/grief reaction' that addresses the more transient depressed affect that may arise after the loss of a primary caregiver.

Numerous compelling clinical observations of depressed infants and toddlers, as well as the findings of alterations of affect in infants at high risk for mood disorder previously described, suggest that a clinical depression can arise at this earlier point in development. However, at this point in time controlled investigations of clinically significant depression among children younger than 3 years of age have not yet been conducted. Therefore, this is an area in which empirical studies are needed to inform diagnostic classification and clinical identification.

Treatment

As preschool depression has only recently been recognized and efforts to validate the disorder are still in progress, treatment studies have not yet been done. Therefore, there are currently no empirical treatment studies to guide clinical practice for depressed preschool children at this time. However, in general, psychotherapeutic treatments for preschool-aged children are conducted in a dyadic context. That is, the preschooler and their primary caregiver are seen together as a 'couple' and the relationship becomes the focus of the treatment. This is based on the idea that the young child cannot be viewed as an independent entity and is inextricably dependent upon the caregiver for emotional and adaptive functioning. Therefore, a primary focus of treatment is on helping the caregiver to meet the emotional needs of the young child better and to facilitate positive development. It should be noted that the dyadic focus does not imply that the etiology or cause of mental problems in young children is based on relationship problems. Rather, because the primary caregiver plays such a key role in the young child's life they are in a unique position to facilitate healthy development.

In keeping with the importance of the dyadic relationship in the treatment of early onset psychopathology, the DC:0–3 system includes a unique relationship axis. This represents an addition to the multiaxial diagnostic system as it is outlined in the DSM system that focuses on the quality of the caregiver–child relationship and considers that disorders may be specific to relationships in young children. In addition to consideration of this issue, the objective is for the clinician to assess the caregiver–child relationship and consider this not only as a potential source but also as the context in which the child's symptoms arise and therefore may be ameliorated.

When considering specific treatments for preschool depression, lessons learned from treatment studies of older school-age depressed children might be highly applicable and informative. Early treatment studies of depressed children using antidepressant medications, known as tricyclic antidepressants, demonstrated that these medications, known to be effective in adults and adolescents, did not show the same efficacy in depressed children. Specifically, outcomes of children treated with tricyclic antidepressants were no better than those taking a sugar pill or placebo. This finding had a profound impact on our understanding of the treatment of childhood mental disorders overall, suggesting that children could not be viewed as miniature adults and that the treatments and pathophysiology of childhood mental disorders may be unique and certainly worthy of independent study.

More recently, new medications for the treatment of depression have been developed. This class of medicines, so-called selective serotonin reuptake inhibitors or SSRIs, have proved to be very useful in the treatment of adult depression as they have proved efficacy and a more favorable (well-tolerated) side-effect profile. One double-blind, placebo-controlled study of an SSRI medication in children demonstrated that it was efficacious for the treatment of childhood depression. Concerns about this class of medication and the potential for increasing suicidality has resulted in the Food and Drug Administration (FDA) issuing stronger warning labels and therefore have mitigated clinical enthusiasm for their use in child populations. Whether increases in suicidal ideation or behavior arise as a result of the medication or the underlying illness remains unclear and is the subject of investigation.

In addition to medication, psychotherapies have also proved effective in the treatment of depression. In particular, two therapeutic modalities have been the subject of empirical investigation. Cognitive-behavioral therapy (CBT) is one modality that has been well tested and proved effective in adults. CBT focuses on identifying and correcting the negative cognitive distortions known to occur in depression. This means that depressed individuals are known to perceive events in a more negative way than how those without depression might perceive the same events. Several studies have demonstrated efficacy of CBT in adolescent as well as school-age children. Its application to younger preschool-age children may be limited by immature cognitive development. Another form of psychotherapy called interpersonal psychotherapy (IPT) has also demonstrated efficacy in the treatment of depression in adults and adolescents. Studies of its use and adaptation in school-age children are now underway. This modality focuses on the impairments in interpersonal functioning that arise as a result of depressed mood. The application of these psychotherapeutic treatments to even younger preschool-age children has not yet been explored but may be promising.

Due to the lack of necessary empirical data exploring the safety and efficacy of antidepressant medications in young children, the first line of treatment for preschool depression should be psychotherapeutic. Parent–child relational therapies have been developed for the treatment of other preschool disorders and efforts are underway to adapt and test some of these techniques for application to depression. While it seems clear that parenting and other key aspects of the psychosocial environment are important mediators of outcomes for young children, studies that address the effects of interventions in these domains are needed.

Clinical Vignette

Identifying depression in a preschool-aged child is difficult and not immediately obvious even to the well-trained child mental health clinician. Depressed preschoolers often do not have an obvious sad or withdrawn mood as is often true of severely depressed adults. Therefore, detailed questions about the child's pattern of behavior and play are essential and may be highly informative. A line of questioning that focuses on negative mood, affect, and internalizing symptoms is important as caregivers tend to pay less attention to these behaviors and instead focus on behaviors that are disruptive. Because of this, it is not uncommon for these symptoms to be present but not spontaneously reported by the parent/caregiver. The following is a case example that highlights some of the features that are typical markers of depression arising at the preschool age.

RK is a 4.2-year-old Caucasian male who was referred by his mother due to concerns about frequent episodes of extreme irritability. Mother reported that RK often seemed to "wake up on the wrong side of the bed." That is, he often would appear angry, irritable, and withdrawn for no apparent reason. Further questioning revealed that during these times RK also did not seem interested in his favorite play activities. One fall, this symptom was so severe that he did not want to go trick-or-treating for Halloween, a holiday he typically enjoyed greatly and looked forward to participating in. Mother also reported upon specific questioning that RK's play involved very negative themes in which dangerous events were taking place and/or harm was befalling the play character. This seemed to be a recurrent play preoccupation and not just a transient interest. In addition, he had a restless sleep pattern characterized by multiple night awakenings. He also did not seem to enjoy his favorite foods such as pizza during these periods. RK did not express feeling sad directly but did endorse this symptom when it was approached as "not feeling as happy as your siblings or other kids seem to feel."

This case underscores the importance of irritability as a marker of depression in early childhood. It also highlights the central feature of the symptom of anhedonia as was evidenced in the child's lack of interest in Halloween festivities. The absence of clear and overtly expressed sadness is also an important issue as depressed preschoolers tended to report themselves as 'less happy' rather than 'sad' on an age-appropriate puppet interview. In addition, the presence of vegetative signs such as disturbances in sleep and changes in appetite were also evident.

Conclusion

Depression is a serious clinical disorder that has long been recognized in adults, has been recognized in school-age children for more than 20 years but has only more recently been recognized as occurring in early childhood during the preschool period. Early case reports suggested that some preschool children meet standard diagnostic criteria for MDD, despite the fact that these criteria were developed primarily for application to adults. Two independent studies utilizing symptom criteria adjusted to reflect the developmental level of the preschool child have identified groups of depressed preschoolers. Among these depressed preschoolers, the symptom of anhedonia, or the inability to experience pleasure or enjoyment of activities and play, emerged as a clinically significant and specific symptom. These studies also found important markers supporting the validity of the disorder similar to those found in studies of depressed older children and depressed adults, including a stable symptom constellation, greater family history of affective disorders, and physiological correlates. Although systematic studies of depression in infants and toddlers are not yet available, a compelling body of case reports and clinical experience suggest the disorder can arise at this even earlier stage of development. Given that preschool depression has only recently been the subject of systematic investigation, little information is available regarding effective treatment of the disorder when it onsets during the preschool period. Information available from the treatment of other preschool-age disorders indicates that treatment should target the parent–child relationship. Studies of early intervention may be particularly important as early intervention in mental disorders may represent a window of opportunity for more effective treatment. Additional study of the risk factors and treatment of this disorder are therefore warranted both for the benefit of preschool children as well as for their implications on the lifelong trajectory of the disorder.

See also: Mental Health, Infant; Parental Chronic Mental Illnesses; Postpartum Depression, Effects on Infant.

Suggested Readings

Downey G and Coyne JC (1990) Children of depressed parents: An integrative review. *Psychological Bulletin* 108: 50–76.
Kashani JH and Carlson GA (1987) Seriously depressed preschoolers. *The American Journal of Psychiatry* 144(3): 348–350.

Luby JL (2000) Depression. In: Zeanah ChL (ed.) *Handbook of Infant Mental Health,* 2nd edn., pp. 382–396. New York: The Guilford Press.

Luby JL, Heffelfinger AK, Mrakotsky C, *et al.* (2002) Preschool major depressive disorder: Preliminary validation for developmentally modified DSM-IV criteria. *Journal of the American Academy of Child and Adolescent Psychiatry* 41(8): 928–937.

Luby JL, Heffelfinger AK, Mrakotsky C, *et al.* (2003) The clinical picture of depression in preschool children. *Journal of the American Academy of Child and Adolescent Psychiatry* 42(3): 340–348.

Luby JL, Mrakotsky C, Heffelfinger AK, *et al.* (2003) Modifications of DSM-IV criteria for depressed preschool children. *American Journal of Psychiatry* 160(6): 1169–1172.

Developmental Disabilities: Cognitive

S L Pillsbury, Richmond, VA, USA

R B David, St. Mary's Hospital, Richmond, VA, USA

Glossary

Echolalia – The repetition of that which is said.

Etiology – The origin or cause of a medical disease or condition.

Language pragmatics – the set of rules governing the use of language in context. This includes factors such as intention; sensorimotor actions preceding, accompanying, and following the utterance; knowledge shared in the communicative dyad; and the elements in the environment surrounding the message.

Prosody – The element of language which concerns intonation, rhythm, and inflection.

Semantics – The study of meaning in language, including the relations between language, thought, and behavior.

Syntax – The way in which words are put together in a sentence to convey meaning.

Verbal auditory agnosia – The inability to understand spoken words; pure word deafness.

Verbal dyspraxia – Also referred to as childhood apraxia of speech; a nonlinguistic sensorimotor disorder of articulation characterized by the impaired capacity to program the speech musculature and the sequencing of muscle movements for the volitional production of phonemes (sounds).

Introduction

Developmental delay is the failure to achieve developmental skills at are appropriate for the age of the child. This article will concern itself with developmental disabilities in the area of higher-order cognition, as seen in preschoolers.

It is universally agreed that early recognition of developmental disability is key in optimizing functioning of the child. The age at which identification is possible varies with the nature of the developmental disability. For example, some disabilities at occur relatively infrequently, but which carry high morbidity (such as cerebral palsy, severe degrees of mental retardation, sensory impairments (blindness, deafness), lower-functioning autism spectrum disorders (ASD), and severe communication disorders), are more likely to be diagnosed in the preschool years. In contrast, disabilities at occur much more frequently but which carry lower morbidity (such as learning disabilities, mild-to-moderate mental retardation, attention deficit hyperactivity disorder (ADHD), higher-functioning ASD, Asperger's syndrome, and higher-order language disorders) often will not be diagnosed until school age. Early identification, with appropriate referrals and interventions, permits counseling for families and planning for the child's future. The child's progress is monitored over time, and interventions are modified as needed. In the very young child, there is obviously a great deal of uncertainty, both in diagnosis and prognosis. The passage of time allows greater diagnostic precision and therefore better targeted therapies.

Not all children subsequently diagnosed as having developmental disabilities will have any identifiable risk factors at birth, and many causes of developmental disability are unknown. When risk factors are present from birth or early infancy, they may be isolated or multiple, and they may interact in complex ways. Multiple risk factors can have an additive effect. However, the absence of risk factors does not guarantee typical development. Risk factors present from birth or early infancy may include:

- genetic syndromes (patterns of malformation), chromosomal abnormalities, malformations of the central nervous system (CNS);
- prematurity (although prematurity alone is a weak risk factor; its effect is probably mediated by those complications that are seen commonly in low birth weight infants such as metabolic disturbances like

hypoglycemia, severe chronic lung disease, CNS hemorrhage, sepsis, and infections of the CNS);

- conditions in pregnancy that interfere with uteroplacental circulation, oxygenation, or nutrition, which may lead to premature delivery or intrauterine growth retardation (a baby who is significantly smaller than would be predicted for his gestational age). Among these are pregnancy-induced hypertension, chronic maternal disease (such as hypertension, renal disease, and cyanotic congenital heart disease), maternal smoking, and maternal drug abuse;
- congenital infections (including cytomegalovirus, rubella, HIV, herpes, congenital syphilis, congenital toxoplasmosis);
- adverse prenatal and perinatal events such as hemorrhage from placenta previa or placental abruption, severe maternal disease (e.g., infections, seizures, trauma), anoxia (especially when the newborn is symptomatic in the immediate neonatal period with seizures, hypotonicity, and feeding problems); and
- sociocultural factors including poverty, poor access, to or underutilization of, medical care, lower maternal educational levels, physical or mental illness in the mother or other caregivers, abuse, and neglect.

Imagine the complex interplay of factors when an infant is delivered prematurely to a young, single mother who has a history of mental illness and substance abuse, and infant neorate intensive care unit (NICU) with multiple medical needs.

The pediatrician is the professional in the best position to identify the infant at increased risk for developmental disability. A careful developmental history should be obtained for milestones in the entire range of development (gross motor, fine motor, language, social, and adaptive). Parent histories may be influenced by the level of their knowledge of typical child development, and also by their readiness to acknowledge delays or atypicalities when present. The physician must, therefore, supplement the history by observation of the child's acquired skills in the office. When indicated, formal standardized screening instruments may be administered. The Denver Developmental Screening Test has been popular for many years because of its ease of administration. Another such tool, the Cognitive Adaptive Test/Clinical Linguistic and Auditory Milestone Scale (CAT/CLAMS), yields a developmental quotient (DQ) which correlates well with the 'mental development index' of the more labor-intensive Bayley Scales of Infant Development, at least in healthy children without risk factors for developmental delay. Developmental progress should be tracked over time, as the outcomes will be markedly different depending on whether the infant has suffered the consequences of a prenatal or perinatal event without ongoing insult, vs. an ongoing risk factor such as abuse or neglect, vs. a neurodegenerative disease, for example.

Earliest indicators of developmental disability may include abnormalities of tone, feeding problems, and poor response to stimuli. As the child's neurological development normally progresses from primitive reflexes and postural responses to volitional movement patterns, the persistence of primitive reflexes may be an early sign of developmental atypicality, as are asymmetries and tone abnormalities (both hypertonicity and hypotonicity). Motor delays later in the first year, such as delays in sitting and crawling, may be noted. Language and behavioral abnormalities are commonly noted in the second and third years of life. Indicators of ADHD and learning disability may be seen by the time the child is ready to enter kindergarten.

Significant progress has been made in the area of early identification and intervention for infants with developmental disabilities and those at high risk over the years since 1975, when the Education for All Handicapped Children Act (EHA) was passed. Public Law 94-142 mandated "free and appropriate education in the least restrictive environment" for children with disabilities. In 1977, this was extended to include ages 3–21 years (although coverage from ages 3 to 5 years was optional). PL 99-457 in 1986 added coverage for infants and toddlers below age 2 years with disabilities. It provided for Individual Family Service Plans (IFSPs) for the delivery of individualized services to the families of these infants and toddlers. The EHA was reauthorized in 1991; PL 101-476 gave the new title of Individuals with Disabilities Act (IDEA). Its key components were: (1) identification of children with learning-related problems; (2) evaluation of the health and developmental status of the child with special needs, determining present and future requirements for intervention, with the formulation of a plan to address each area of need with appropriate services; (3) provision of those services, both educational and related services; and (4) guaranteed due process. Under PL 101-476, it was now assured that children with disabilities and their parents were as entitled to a free and appropriate education as were those without disabilities. Children from birth to age 3 years continued to have a written plan of service known as the Individual Family Service Plan (IFSP). From age 3 to 21 years, this written plan is known as an IEP or Individual Education Plan. Autism and traumatic brain injury (TBI) were included for special education coverage by PL 101-476.

As reauthorized in 1997 in PL 105-17, so-called 'Part C' called for the provision of early intervention services for all infants and toddlers with disabilities through the creation of statewide, coordinated, multidisciplinary, interagency programs. This law did not mandate these services, but did provide partial reimbursement for their cost. Currently, all 50 states have established early intervention services for children from birth to age 3 years, addressing developmental issues in the physical, communicative, cognitive, and psychological realms, as well as self-help skills, with the goals of minimizing disability and enhancing the ability of families to meet their children's special needs. It was hoped that early intervention would also decrease the costs for special education services once they reached school age. It was left to the states to define developmental delay for the purposes of establishing eligibility for services. Services are provided both to children with demonstrated delays and to those with biological conditions that place them at high risk for delays. The states may provide services to children at risk due to environmental factors, at their discretion. At the heart of 'Part C' of PL 105-17 is its focus on family involvement and family support. Evaluation, assessment, and planning are all subject to the approval and participation of the family. Likewise, intervention services are optional. When provided, these services are rendered in the most natural setting possible, such as in the home or the day care center. Follow-up surveys of families who have been involved in early intervention services under 'Part C' have shown a generally high level of parent satisfaction with their access to services, and also their perception of optimism for the future and their own competence in caring for and advocating for their children (although less positive outcomes were seen in minorities, in families with children with complex medical needs, and in single-parent families). Another important component of PL 105-17 was the extension of coverage to include ADHD.

Any child who presents to the physician with developmental delays should receive a thorough general and neurological examination. Particular attention should be paid to growth abnormalities, congenital anomalies which may suggest a genetic syndrome or chromosomal abnormality, a congenital CNS disorder, or intrauterine infection. Abnormal skin markings may be seen in genetic disorders as well as congenital infections. Abnormalities of the eyes, heart, limbs, and abdominal organs should also be noted. As the number of physical anomalies increases, the likelihood of a genetic disorder also increases. Neurological examination should especially include measurement of head circumference, examination of the cranial nerves, and assessment of tone. Persistent primitive reflexes and any asymmetries should be noted. Testing of hearing and vision should next be undertaken, using tools that are appropriate for the age and developmental level of the child. Other tests may be obtained, as clinically indicated, and may include genetic studies, imaging of the brain using magnetic resonance imaging (MRI), electroencephalogram, and others. Specialists from pediatric neurology, cardiology, orthopedics, genetics, psychology, or psychiatry may be consulted. However, referral to the early intervention program need not be delayed pending the results of these evaluations. The early intervention interdisciplinary team includes evaluation by occupational therapists, physical therapists, speech and language pathologists, and social workers. With the establishment of the IFSP (or IEP),

services may then be initiated with the cooperation of the families, with systematic monitoring of the progress of the child and his family.

Cognitive disorders in infancy and early childhood fall into three fundamental domains: disorders of communication, disorders of socialization, and visual–spatial disabilities. Within each domain, there is a continuum of severity and complexity. There is also considerable overlap among the identified domains.

Individual variations in cognitive style and temperament include activity level, rhythmicity, approach to new stimuli, adaptability, intensity, mood, perseverance, distractibility, and threshold to stimulation. Areas of concern may include withdrawal from novel stimuli, slowness to adapt, intensity of response, a predominantly negative mood, shyness, and withdrawal. While these are not considered disorders in the infant and preschool children, they may predispose the child to problems later in life.

Disorders of Communication: Developmental Language Disorders

Normal Language Development

There is a large degree of variability in the rate at which language is acquired (first words anywhere from 6 to 30 months), as well as variability in the rate of acquisition of different linguistic components, such as phonology, lexical retrieval, and syntax. For example, many normal children concentrate their early acquisition of new words to nouns, while others add verbs and adjectives at a similar pace. There is no explanation at present for these differing styles of learning, and both groups of children are normal. The wide variability in so-called normal children can make it difficult to distinguish children with developmental language disability from those normal children with an idiosyncratic initial delay who will eventually catch up. Typically, developing children have good receptive language by 2 years of age, with an expressive vocabulary of 50 words or more and some two-word phrases. A general rule of thumb suggests that, after children develop a 50-word expressive language repertoire, other individual words, as well as phrases and sentences, will generally follow quickly. Expressive language is usually well-developed by 3 years of age.

There is clear evidence that children with developmental language disorders (DLDs) are at risk for a variety of social–emotional problems in older childhood and in adult life. There are certain 'red flags' for DLDs. Children with DLDs may demonstrate early problems relative to other oral functions such as sucking, swallowing, and chewing. Infants who fail to vocalize to social cues or to vocalize two syllables by age 8 months are suspect. Slightly older children are at risk if they acquire new words only slowly and with great difficulty, if they rely too much on contextual cues for understanding of language, if their social interactions are limited to getting their needs met, if they produce few or no creative utterances of three words or more by age 3 years, and if they show little attention and interest for language-related activities such as book reading, talking, or communicating with peers. By age 3 years, typically developing children have developed symbolic, imaginative play.

Currently available tools for assessment of early language development can result in both underdiagnosis and overdiagnosis of DLDs. As many as 40% of children identified as having DLDs in the first 2 years of life may no longer retain that diagnosis at age 3 or 4 years. Ten per cent of these children are 'normal' at school age, while others have had their diagnoses refined to mental retardation, ASD, and others. It is preferable in the very young child to overidentify DLDs, as delay in diagnosis and treatment may have long-term social, behavioral, and educational implications.

Children at Risk

Risk factors for DLDs include parental mental retardation or a family history of DLDs. Premature and small-for-gestational-age infants are also at greater risk. There is a higher concordance rate in monozygotic vs. dizygotic twins, suggesting that environmental influences alone are insufficient to explain the occurrence of DLDs. A number of gene loci have been identified, implicating 13q, 16q, and 19q as candidate genes for further study. An autosomal dominant mode of inheritance is frequently seen, but there is variability in penetrance as well as in expressivity. For the purposes of this discussion, children with significant hearing loss and those who have identifiable brain lesions have been excluded.

Subtypes of Developmental Language Disorders

DLDs are described based on the linguistic area which is most significantly disturbed.

Articulation and expressive dysfluency disorders

Phonologic (pure articulation) disorders. Most children will speak intelligibly by 2 years of age. By age 3 years, fewer than 15% of children have unintelligible speech. Minor articulation defects, such as a distortion of the "th" and "r" sounds may persist with little consequence. Phonologic awareness, however, is critically important in the acquisition of normal reading skills, and children with delayed phonologic acquisition are at greater risk for developmental reading disorders at school age.

Dysfluency (stuttering and cluttering). Some degree of dysfluency is common as language skills develop, particularly as the mean length of utterance reaches six to eight words between 3 and 4 years of age. Some children with dysfluency may be relatively fluent for days or weeks at a time, then experience a protracted interval of relative dysfluency. Both stuttering and developmental dysfluency may be influenced by factors such as the complexity of the thought to be expressed and by being rushed or when excited, happy, or angry. Between-word dysfluencies include interjecting 'um' in a sentence, repeating a phrase, or revising the sentence structure in midstream. Within-word dysfluencies include repetitions of individual sounds or syllables, prolongations of sounds, and blocks. Stuttering is a disorder in the rhythms of speech, in which an individual produces a disproportionately large frequency of within-word dysfluencies compared to normally fluent peers, particularly at grammatically important points in the sentence. It often is a genetic trait, and occurs more frequently in children with other DLDs as well as with mental retardation. It is equally common in boys and girls at its onset, but is three times more likely to persist in males. Associated behaviors such as head, torso, or limb movement, audible exhalation or inhalations immediately prior to the dysfluency, and visible muscle tension in the orofacial region are signs that the child is becoming aware that talking is difficult. In younger children, the earliest and most frequently observed associated behaviors involve the eyes (such as blinking, squeezing the eyes shut, side-to-side movements of the eyes, and consistent loss of eye contact with the listener). These behaviors are seen in stutterers and usually not in children who are simply developmentally dysfluent. Most children who begin to stutter at preschooler age will recover without specific therapy, especially those with onset prior to age 3 years, if family history is either negative or characterized by spontaneous resolution, and if there are no coexisting speech and language or learning problems. Cluttering, by contrast, is characterized by echolalia, palilalia (compulsive repetition in increasing rapidity and decreasing volume), incomplete sentences, perseveration, poor articulation, and stuttering, seen in children with fragile X syndrome.

Verbal dyspraxia. This condition, in which children are extremely dysfluent, as often been called 'dilapidated speech'. Language is produced only with great effort. Phonology is impaired, including omissions, distortions, and substitutions. Language comprehension is preserved, and intelligence is normal.

Disorders of receptive and expressive language

Each of these disorders has a receptive component. While receptive language is heavily dependent upon attentional factors, reception may be impaired independently. Reception is dependent upon spoken rate, register, and dialect. It is a mistake to assume that the child who appears to be paying attention also understands what is said to him. In an emotionally charged context, reception breaks down further.

Phonologic syntactic syndrome. This condition, which is very common, is characterized expressively by disturbances in phonology, particularly in consonant sounds and consonant clusters in all word positions. The child is extremely difficult to understand, and grammatical forms are atypical. Semantics, pragmatics, and prosody are normal. Associated neurological problems are particularly common in this DLD, as are problems with feeding (sucking, swallowing, and chewing).

Verbal auditory agnosia (VAA). Children with VAA do not understand meaningful language, despite normal hearing. VAA may be seen as a DLD, or may be acquired in association with a form of epilepsy in which the epileptogenic portion of the brain involves the receptive language areas of the temporal lobe. The prognosis for this disorder is generally poor, although better in children with the acquired variety.

Higher-order language syndromes

Lexical syntactic syndrome. This common disorder is characterized by dysfluent speech, the consequence of word-finding difficulties, and a deficiency in syntactic skills. In the absence of finding the appropriate word, the child may 'talk around' the word in what are referred to as paraphasias. Speech is intelligible because phonology is normal. The child's language production is better for repetition than for spontaneous speech. Comprehension is normal except when the child is required to process very complex utterances.

Semantic pragmatic syndrome. Children with this condition are fluent, even verbose, but their large vocabularies belie the difficulty they have with meaningful conversation and informative exchange of ideas. Their chatter and often formal style may give the impression of a high intelligence quotient (IQ). Speech in this disorder has been described as stilted, pedantic, or professorial; the speech quality may be mechanical, monotonous, or 'sing-song'. Children with this disorder are often unable to respond to 'who', 'what', 'where', 'when', or 'why' questions, but may appear to exhibit great eloquence in subject matters of their interest or fixation. Comprehension is impaired. This syndrome is often seen in high-functioning autistic children.

Outcome for Children with Developmental Language Disorders

Preschool language skills predict later reading ability. DLDs are associated with problems such as ADHD, behavioral and emotional problems, and academic under-achievement. While articulation and fluency problems may be the most obvious, more subtle disorders of comprehension may be misdiagnosed as conduct disorders or oppositional-defiant disorder, owing to the emotional 'meltdowns' in the child who is chronically unable to understand the intentions and expectations of others, both peers and adults. These communication problems

may persist into adulthood in more than half of these children, impairing both social interactions and career success. The effect of speech and language therapy on outcome, particularly in the more significantly affected children, is still a matter of debate. This therapy is labor intensive, and may need to continue for prolonged periods of time. Continued association with more normally conversant children in the daycare or preschool setting is helpful.

Autism Spectrum Disorders

The clinical presentation (phenotype) of autism is highly variable, as is its natural history. There are several hypotheses regarding the essential cognitive deficit in ASD. The theory of mind blindness is related to the theory of mind; it implies that individuals on the autism spectrum lack the capacity for understanding or sensing another individual's state of mind. In other children with ASDs, the ability to solve problem, to shift sets, and to plan to reach a goal are deficient. A third theory suggests that children on the autism spectrum fail to integrate information, and are deficient in Gestalt ('big picture') formulations.

ASDs are characterized by the triad of impaired socialization skills, impaired verbal and nonverbal (body language) communication skills, and restricted areas of activity and interests.

Classic autism, as originally described by Leo Kanner in 1943, is estimated to occur in approximately 1 in 1000 individuals. ASD occurs in a wide degree of severity in an estimated 1 in 150 individuals (2007). Fifty to seventy per cent of autistic individuals can be determined to have demonstrated impairments since birth (e.g., using, scoring of the infant's interpersonal interactions on home videos). There is a subtype of ASD children, 30–50%, who evidently were typically developing children until language/autistic regression occurred at a mean age of 21 months (range 12–36 months) under the influence of unknown triggers (including potentially infectious, immunologic, or psychosocial stressors).

Etiology

There is strong evidence for a genetic (probably multigenic) basis for ASD, including a recurrence risk of 4.0–9.8% in subsequent children in a family with one autistic child. In fact, the recurrence rate would certainly be higher but for the stoppage rule, that is, parents with one severely affected child often do not have more children. Lower-functioning autistic adults commonly lack the social skills that lead to successful interpersonal relationships, decreasing their likelihood of becoming parents. Males predominate at a rate of approximately four to one. There is a high concordance rate in monozygotic twins, approximately 90%. Several candidate genes have been identified. In addition, children with certain identified genetic disorders (including fragile X syndrome, phenylketonuria, tuberous sclerosis, Angelman's syndrome, and Cornelia de Lange syndrome) may demonstrate autism symptoms.

Future genetic studies may demonstrate that, for the autism spectrum, there are indeed many specific genotypes, as opposed to a single defective gene. In addition, confusion may arise, since there are many other conditions overlap with ASDs, including obsessive–compulsive disorder, Tourette's syndrome, and ADHD. Elements of these disorders are often found within ASDs. Future research depends upon standardization of diagnostic criteria to a research level of certainty.

The recent 'epidemic' of individuals identified to be on the autism spectrum is believed by most in the scientific community as being a manifestation of increased awareness and better identification, although research is also ongoing in the areas of possible environmental triggers, especially for those children who have appeared to undergo autistic and/or language regression in the second year of life.

Diagnosis

The diagnosis of autism is based upon the presence of specific criteria. The meeting of these criteria represents an analysis of phenotype, as opposed to genotype. It is currently possible to make a reliable diagnosis of ASD at age 24–36 months in many cases, with stability of the diagnosis up to 9 years later. The DSM-IV criteria are less useful in younger toddlers, below 24 months of age, and it is not yet well understood how early symptoms map onto later symptoms. Research is ongoing to develop reliable markers as young as 6 months of age, using the lack of joint attention as the operational definition of infantile autism. (Joint attention is a platform for language development, closely linked to abstract rule-learning, which is measured by three-point gaze shifts and following the look and point gestures of others.) Children subsequently diagnosed with 'congenital' ASD typically demonstrate language delays by 14 months of age, slower than normal language development from 6 to 36 months, and decreased initiation of communication for social or instrumental purposes. Because most children who present early are identified due to delays in acquisition of language skills, the first specialist consulted is commonly the audiologist. Sixty per cent of 14-month-olds later diagnosed with ASD, and 90% of 24–36-month-olds with ASD, were seen to have stereotyped patterns and interests. In endeavoring to make the diagnosis early, the clinician is challenged to differentiate the child with early signs of autism from the range of normal variability in development.

Tools to aid in early diagnosis of autism include detailed questionnaires, specific interview techniques, and blinded reviews of home videotapes. Using such tools, it can be seen that a subset of autistic children underwent global regression prior to 24 months of age. Most studies have shown that the majority of these children with autistic regression had minor impairments prior to the onset of the regression, however. This phenomenon is well described but poorly understood. It is crucial to assess the hearing of all children with language impairment, using, when necessary, brainstem auditory evoked responses (BAERs, otherwise known as auditory evoked potentials). This will distinguish those children who are language impaired or on the autism spectrum from those who are severely hearing impaired. (Although there are children who are severely hearing impaired who also meet criteria for ASD, in general, children who are hearing impaired alone do not manifest the degree of social impairment seen in autism. However, It can be very difficult to diagnose ASD in the deaf child with significant behavior problems such as severe ADHD.) The skilled evaluation of a speech and language pathologist is also mandatory. The gamut of language disorders described earlier in this article can be seen in ASD individuals, and severely language impaired children may also present diagnostic confusion with autism, especially, again, when behavior is abnormal. Seventy to eighty-five per cent of children with ASD are mentally retarded on standard testing; this group has a generally poorer prognosis. In contrast, many other children on the autism spectrum are above average, or even superior in intellectual functioning. It should be borne in mind that measurable mental retardation does not always translate to functional retardation. Many ASD adults may take advantage of their relatively well-preserved or even enhanced abilities in the visual–spatial domain, performing such repetitive functions as data entry. Preschool children with ASD may demonstrate excellent skills in puzzle construction, for example.

Core Deficits

Social competence

Social incompetence is the hallmark of ASD. It represents a lack of intuitive social skills. Children on the autism spectrum are unable to sense the emotional state of others. The 'theory of mind' refers to the concept that autistic individuals demonstrate a lack of awareness of the internal state of others. Their play is often parallel rather than interactive, with little symbolic play. When they do engage in interactive play, they generally take a passive role. At the extremes, they may be socially unavailable, aloof, or with an intense stranger anxiety, but there are also those autistic children who are socially impaired by virtue of being 'too social', with a dramatic lack of apprehension of strangers, and a willingness to go off with anyone, even those who are totally unknown to them.

Most autistic children are withdrawn and exclude themselves (and their idiosyncrasies lead their peers to exclude them as well, thus reducing their opportunities to pattern social behaviors and language on typically developing peers). Autistic individuals may exhibit difficulties with personal space, which may be represented as a reluctance to have their own individual space invaded, with no corresponding reluctance to invade the personal space of others. Lack of eye contact was thought at one time to be the hallmark of ASD, but this is not necessarily the case. Children on the autism spectrum may look at, through, or beside others. There is, for the most part, an impairment in the quantity or quality of eye engagement. Children with ASD demonstrate a lack of interest in the human face, and are more likely to concentrate on the mouth or other parts of the correspondent, rather than his eyes. (Brain imaging in adults has shown differences from normals in the cortical areas involved in the perception of facial emotion.) Sharing and turn-taking are almost always impaired. Verbal autistic children give the impression of talking 'at' others (see the discussion of language impairments in ASD, below). Socially impaired children who are also nonverbal are often hyperactive, inattentive, and aggressive. Tantruming and uncontrollable screaming – what parents often refer to as 'meltdowns' – are common, especially in the children under age 3 years. These children may be inconsolable. Sleep is often disturbed. Bowel and bladder training are difficult and often significantly delayed. Self-injurious behavior may be present, particularly in lower-functioning children. Many consider the difficulties in the domain of social cognition to be the most essential feature of ASDs.

Language impairment

Verbal and nonverbal communication deficits are an essential part of the autism triad. Language generally parallels intelligence. Echolalia, while occasionally seen as a brief developmental interlude in normal children, and infrequently seen in persistent fashion in pure DLDs, is common in children on the autism spectrum. (Echolalic speech often portends the development of more fluent speech, and therefore it is not necessarily a bad sign.) As previously stated, a thorough assessment of hearing and the evaluation of a skilled speech and language pathologist are essential. In low-functioning children, verbal auditory agnosia, phonologic-syntactic, and lexical–syntactic language disorders are seen. In higher-functioning children, pragmatic and semantic deficits are characteristic. This includes deficits in who/what/where/when/how questions and in language turn-taking. In addition, prosody is frequently impaired, such that these children speak in monotone rather than in well-modulated speech. Hyperactivity and inattention relate inversely to language competence in autistic children under the age of 3 years. It is the consensus that language competence at 5 or 6 years of age quite accurately predicts long-term prognosis, since language, as suggested earlier, determines intelligence, which then relates to functionality. Chances for a child who remains nonverbal at the age of 8 or 9 years becoming linguistically competent are very poor.

Restricted range of behaviors, interests, and activities

ASDs are characterized by behaviors that are, from the viewpoint of the observer, odd or idiosyncratic. Activities such as toe-walking, twirling, licking, flapping, rocking, opening and closing doors, and manipulating light switches are seen. Again, there is variability, and these stereotyped behaviors may appear only for a brief period of time, only to be replaced by another oddity. Motor stereotypies are repetitive actions which are complex, involuntary, and purposeless, which are carried out with predictable form, amplification and location, in the autistic individual. They usually have their onset prior to the age of 2 years. Although tics may also be seen not uncommonly in ASD individuals, these brief, uncomplicated movements usually have onset after 6 or 7 years of age. Inattention and hyperactivity may be seen in ASD, thus overlapping with ADHD. Children with ASD may have great difficulty with transitions, and may become overfocused on certain activities, especially in the visual–spatial realm, such as assembling puzzles. As mentioned earlier, preschool children with ASD behavioral idiosyncrasies serve to accentuate their social isolation.

Treatment

There have been no long-term studies comparing those individuals who received early intervention vs. those who did not. Nevertheless, it is a good presumption that early intervention can improve eventual outcomes. Of the treatment modalities currently available, those that use an operant conditioning approach appear to be the most efficacious. While all use an applied behavior analytic approach (operant conditioning), individual protocols may vary widely. There is currently no way to compare protocols.

Pharmacologic treatment is presently limited to helping with related problems (such as stimulants for hyperactivity, medications to help with sleep, anticonvulsants for coexisting seizures, etc.). Speech and language therapies and social skills training may also be of benefit.

Visual–Spatial Disabilities

Visual–spatial disabilities (VSDs) involve perceptual organization, memory, and imagery. The literature on visual–motor and spatial disabilities in young children is very limited, but impairments in this domain will significantly impact future academic success. For example, the preschooler child's ability to copy geometric shapes has predictive value for reading and math in elementary school. Motor execution is the fundamental medium for expression of function or dysfunction in the visual–spatial areas. While there are motor-free tests for perceptual dysfunction, more commonly VSDs are grouped with related disorders of motor execution as perceptual–motor disabilities, and it can be difficult to consider one without the other.

Traditional IQ tests demonstrate VSDs by the discrepancy between verbal and performance IQ. Subtests include those of design copy and memory, picture memory, and mental rotation. Other easily administered tests include requesting a child to draw or copy shapes, or to draw a human figure. There are age-related norms for both these tasks.

The etiology of visual–spatial and motor deficits in the preschooler is in the right hemisphere of the brain, as evidenced in studies comparing the copying and drawing skills and the ability to create spatial arrays of toys in children with known injury (e.g., stroke) involving the right vs. the left hemisphere.

A long-term follow-up study of premature babies demonstrated that the inability to copy a circle and a low score of sorting blocks (by shape, color, and size) at age 4 years correlated with hyperactivity and an abnormal neurological examination (so-called 'soft signs') at age 7 years. The 30% of children in the same study who showed poor execution of copying of a cross had a higher rate of diagnosis of learning disabilities and also of neurological soft signs. Poor performance on a maze task correlated with learning disabilities, ADHD, and abnormal neurological examination. Conversely, those children who demonstrated proficiency in the copying of a square at age 4 years, and who had high scores on block-sorting tasks, were actually at decreased risk for learning disabilities and hyperactivity.

Referral to occupational therapy is important for the preschooler with suspected visual–spatial and motor disability. Treatment using perceptual training programs has been reported to be helpful. Disability in this realm may seriously impair the child's perception of the world. Understanding the relationship between visual–spatial and motor disability and subsequent learning disabilities may aid in earlier recognition and special education for learning disabilities and nonverbal learning issues.

A related issue which will be discussed elsewhere in this encyclopedia merits mention here. Disorders of motor planning and execution are difficult to separate from disorders in the visual–spatial and motor realm. Disorders of motor execution can accompany paralysis, spasticity (most forms of cerebral palsy), and movement disorders, but there are also a variety of disorders of motor execution that do not result in apparent alterations in strength, tone, or posture, but rather manifest themselves by clumsiness and inadequate performance of motor acts. The true incidence of higher-order motor deficits in first graders in regular schools is estimated at somewhere between 2% and 12%. These

higher-order motor abnormalities are best detected if age-appropriate sequences of individual motions are performed under an examiner's observation. These disorders of motor execution frequently occur concurrently in children diagnosed with ADHD or learning disabilities. It is a mistake, however, to consider disorders of motor execution only in the context of other conditions, because impairments in this realm are disabling in themselves.

Historically, these children often will not have met gross motor milestones such as independent walking (usually met by 10–15 months of age), climbing stairs by themselves (normally 14–24 months), riding a tricycle (2–3 years), and riding a bicycle (4–6 years). They may also have failed to meet fine motor milestones, including holding a cup (10–14 months), executing buttons and snaps (3–4.5 years), printing their own name (4.5–6 years), and tying shoe laces (4.5–6 years). On examination of gait, their walking, running, skipping, tandem gait, hopping on one foot, and climbing stairs are clearly impaired. Upper extremity functions, including finger-tapping, wrist-turning, button-pressing, finger-nose-finger, copying, drawing, and writing are also impaired. The ability to imitate nonsense gestures (dyspraxia), to pantomime to command, and to use actual objects are similarly impaired. There are age-standard normative values for performance on the Purdue Pegboard and the subtests of Kaufman that relate to hand movements and spatial memory.

In the vernacular, a clumsy child is the classic 'klutz'. The purely clumsy child exhibits slow and inaccurate fine or gross motor performance deficits. The abnormality does not pertain to impairment of strength or tone, but rather to speed and dexterity. Clumsiness is a primary cause of school failure in early grades where the demands for motor task performance are great.

Synkinesis is an involuntary movement of voluntary musculature that occurs during the course of a voluntary action. One test that can elicit this, the Fog test, requires that a child walk on the sides of his feet, either on the insides or the outsides of the sole. When the child performs this maneuver, especially when a narrow base is demanded, the arms and hands frequently enter into distorted postures. Of synkinetic movements, mirror movements are the most commonly appreciated form of synkinesis. In a finger-tapping test, mirror movements commonly occur. The demonstation of synkinetic movements can be a part of normal developmental variation, but it is abnormal in children older than 6 years. Clumsy children often exhibit synkinetic movements as well.

Dyspraxia represents a characteristic failure in a complex, voluntary act, which is more easily recognizable when the child attempts to learn more complex motor sequences. Because dyspraxia is generally not evaluated apart from clumsiness or synkinesis, it is often not described, therefore, in preschool children. The failure to appreciate the presence of dyspraxia may result in a child being regarded as lazy, oppositional, or unintelligent, and this can result in poor self-esteem, poor motivation, and poor conduct. These children may demonstrate delays in self-care skills such as dressing and grooming themselves. Their specific problems may relate to buttoning, snapping, zipping, dressing, tying shoe lace, manipulating combs, toothbrushes, and particularly scissors. They may manifest as refusing to attempt tasks such as writing and coloring, at the same time that gross motor skills may be age appropriate. Most children with dyspraxias have no identifiable brain abnormality. Dyspraxias can be elicited by asking younger children to pantomime, for instance, blowing a kiss, or waving goodbye. A child can also be asked to fold a piece of paper, fit it into an envelope, or roll up a paper to use as a pretend telescope. Practice has a significant influence in children with dyspraxia as well as in clumsy children. Unlike the clumsy child, successful performance of the task by the dyspraxic child does not improve when extra time is allotted. It is particularly important in preschoolers to note that clumsy children and children with dyspraxia are more likely to injure themselves, and parents may be wrongly accused of abuse.

Other disorders of cognitive functioning that will be seen in the older child are not well studied in preschoolers. These include deficits in memory and in executive function. Executive function refers to the ability to maintain an appropriate set of procedures for problem solving, to attain a future goal. It involves the intention to inhibit a response to defer it, to formulate a sequential, strategic plan of action, and to encode relevant material in memory for future use. Preschoolers developmentally do not demonstrate significant skills in such future-oriented behavior, but some difficulties may be noted with self-regulation, selective attention, and vigilance.

Summary

Cognitive disorders in infancy and early childhood may have long-term consequences, for learning, for social success, and for employment. Cognitive limitations and the child's frustrations related to them may lead to significant behavior problems as well. The goal of early identification and early intervention is to recognize those children at risk, as well as those children demonstrating signs of cognitive disabilities. Appropriate consultations and therapeutic regimens may then be utilized to optimize the outcomes for the child and his family. The challenge for future research is to develop the tools for practitioners to aid in early recognition. Greater precision in diagnosis will also aid in the understanding of the natural history of cognitive disabilities, and also their causes. Longitudinal studies will be helpful in comparing the outcomes of varying educational and other treatment modalities.

See also: ADHD: Genetic Influences; Autism Spectrum Disorders; Birth Defects; Learning Disabilities; Vision Disorders and Visual Impairment.

Suggested Readings

Nass R and Ross G (2005) Disorders of cognitive function in the preschooler. In: David RB (ed.) *Child and Adolescent Neurology*, 2nd edn., pp. 486–510. Oxford: Blackwell.

Rapin I (ed.) (1996) *Preschool Children with Inadequate Communication: Developmental Language Disorder, Autism, Low IQ.* Cambridge: Cambridge University Press.

Tuchman R and Rapin I (eds.) (2006) *Autism: A Neurological Disorder of Early Brain Development.* Cambridge: Cambridge University Press.

Developmental Disabilities: Physical

R R Espinal and M E Msall, University of Chicago, Chicago, IL, USA

Glossary

Acute lymphoblastic leukemia (ALL) – The most common type of childhood leukemia and the most common childhood cancer.

Antifolate – A substance that blocks the activity of folic acid. Antifolates are used in chemotherapy for cancer, since folate is necessary for the production of new cells.

Antineoplastic – Acting to prevent, inhibit, or halt the growth of tumors.

Arabinoside – A chemotherapeutic agent.

Ataxia – Unsteady and uncoordinated movements of limbs or torso due to cerebellar dysfunction.

Cerebral palsy (CP) – A disorder of movement and posture due to central nervous system impairments with associated impairments often occurring in vision, audition, communication, learning, manipulation, perception, and neurobehavioral control.

Clean intermittent catheterization – Technique to manage neurogenic bladder.

Congenital heart disease – Structured malformations of the heart that impact on cardiac structure or function.

Conotruncal cardiac abnormalities – Abnormalities of the outflow of the heart and great vessels. The entities include tetralogy of fallot, transposition of the great arteries, truncus arterisois, and higher interrupted aortic arch.

Cranial radiation therapy (CRT) – Treatment targeted to destroy leukemic or tumor cells in the brain.

Creatine phosphokinase (CPK) – A chemical found in muscle fibers that is released into the bloodstream when the muscles undergo damage and breakdown.

Deep hypothermic circulatory arrest (DHCA) – Specialized procedure during cardiac surgery to stop the heart so as to carry out safe surgical repair.

Dexamethasone – A steroid medication given to cancer patients undergoing chemotherapy to counteract side effects.

Dysphagia – Difficulty swallowing.

Dystrophin – A rod-shaped cytoplasmic protein that connects the cytoskeleton of a muscle fiber to the surrounding extracellular matrix through the cell membrane. Its gene's locus is Xp21.

Encephalopathy – Disorders caused by the impairment or damage of the brain.

Endothelium – Inner lining of blood vessels.

Excitotoxic neuronal death – Mechanism of cell death through predominance of excitatory neurotransmitter amino acids and small molecules.

Extrapyramidal – Organization of the basal ganglia, thalamus, and cerebellum for motor control of fine, balance, and precision movements.

Extremely low birthweight (ELBW) – <1000 g at birth.

Factor 5 leiden mutations – One of the family of proteins responsible for hemostasis (when bleeding is stopped).

Fludarabine – A chemotherapy drug commonly used to treat a type of leukemia known as chronic lymphocytic leukemia.

Focal calcifications – Abnormalities on comarter tomography in specific brain regions.

Glucocorticoid – A steroid with anti-flammatory properties.

Hematopoiesis – Development of blood cells.

Hemiplegia – A condition where paralysis is present in the vertical half of the patient's body (i.e., right arm and right leg, or left arm and left leg).

Homocysteine – A type of amino acid.

Hydrocephalus – Abnormal accumulation of cerebrospinal fluid (CSF) in the brain.

Hypoplastic heart syndrome – A cardiac malformation resulting in an underdeveloped left heart.

Hypoxemic–ischemic–reperfusion injury – Inability of impaired brain regions to tolerate the metabolic demands of restored blood flow.

Intensification (or consolidation) therapy – A type of high-dose chemotherapy often given as the second phase (after induction therapy) of a cancer treatment regimen for leukemia.

Interrupted aortic arch – Abnormalities in the ascending aorta.

Intrapatrum asphyxia – Interference with blood–gas exchange during labor and delivery that occurs with a major sentinel event and meets the criteria specified by the American College of Obstetricians and Gynecologists, which can lead to cerebral palsy.

Intrathecal chemotherapy – Receiving chemotherapy through the spinal canal.

Leukoencephalopathy – A rare side effect caused by methotrexate and/or radiation on the central nervous system of leukemia patients. Chemotherapy and/or radiation cause the destruction of the myelin sheaths covering nerve fibers, which results in motor and cognitive impairment.

Magnetic resonance imaging (MRI) – A procedure that allows imaging of internal organs. Cranial MRI allows visualization of the central nervous system.

Meninges – Membrane that covers the central nervous system.

Merosin – Biochemical that is part of stabilizing muscle cells.

Microangiopathy – Abnormal disease process affecting small blood vessels.

Necrosis – Accidental death of living cells and tissues brought on by injury, infection, cancer, and inflammation.

Necrotizing enterocolitis – Infection and gangrene of the neonatal intestine.

Nelarabine – A chemotherapeutic agent.

Nucleoside analogs – An artificially made nucleoside that interferes with the replication of DNA and RNA of viruses.

Oligodendroglia – A type of central nervous system cell.

Pentostatin – A chemotherapy drug commonly used to treat types of leukemia.

Perioperative hypoxemia – Abnormally low blood oxygen level during surgery which meets the criteria specified by the American College of Obstetricians and Gynecologists (ACOG) standard.

Periventricular leukomalacia – White matter injury in brain tracts near the ventricles.

Quadriplegia – A condition where decreased voluntary movement is present in all four limbs.

Remission-induction therapy – Initial treatment with anticancer drugs to decrease the signs or symptoms of cancer or make them disappear.

Secondary ventricular dilation – Increased ventricular size after intraventricular hemorrhage (IVH).

Sepsis – Bacterial infection of the blood.

Synkinesia – Symmetric overflow movements.

Systemic lupus erthematosis – An autoimmune disease.

Tetralogy of fallot – A cardiac malformation.

Truncus arterisois – Abnormalities of the aortic and pulmonary blood vessels resulting from a common trunk.

Velo-cardio-facial syndrome (VCFS) – A cleft palate, heart defect, and facial malformation syndrome.

Ventriculoperitoneal (VP) shunt – A catheter that redirects cerebrospinal fluid from the inner space of the brain (ventricles) to the abdominal cavity (peritoneum).

Very low birthweight (VLBW) – <1500 g at birth.

Introduction

Over the past 20 years, major advances in maternal–fetal medicine, neonatology, and translational developmental biology have resulted in unprecedented survival rates for very preterm (29–32 weeks' gestation) or extremely preterm (≤28 weeks' gestation) infants. These very low birthweight (VLBW; 1001–1500 g) and extremely low birthweight infants (ELBW; ≤1000 g) who received neonatal intensive care currently have survival rates of 90% and 80%, respectively, and include over 50 000 US children per year. In addition, with advances in pediatric cardiology and oncology, over 90% of children with congenital heart disease and over 90% of children with leukemia are surviving. These children number over 30 000 in the US per year. Although increasing numbers of these children with life-threatening disorders are surviving, they face neurodevelopmental disabilities as a result of their treatments affecting systems that contribute directly or indirectly to brain structure and function. We focus on prematurity as a model disorder for understanding

several important pathways of the cerebral palsy (CP) syndromes of diplegia, hemiplegia, and quadriplegia. These neurodevelopmental motor impairments remain a substantial sequelae in 30% of infants weighing <500 g, 15–20% of infants weighing <750 g, and 10% of infants weighing 750–1499 g. These rates of functional motor disability contrast with 3–5% rates among infants weighing 1501–2499 g and 0.2–0.5% in infants weighing >2500 g. In addition, the developmental consequences of CP impact on children's vision, hearing, perception, communication, learning, and neurodevelopmental process are high. We also highlight advances in leukemia as this malignancy has significant lessons for how chemotherapy or radiation therapy in early childhood impact the developing brain. Major advances in congenital heart disease will also be examined due to the increased attention to neuroprotection during cardiac surgery. The management of muscular dystrophy (MD) and spina bifida (two of the most common causes of physical disability in children) is also discussed. These five groups of pediatric physical disability can help us to understand the critical importance of a biopsychosocial, functional, and family ecological approaches to pediatric physical disability.

The International Classification of Functioning Model Applied to Early Childhood Disability: Cerebral Palsy after Prematurity, Leukemia, Congenital Heart Disease, Muscular Dystrophies, and Spina Bifida

One key framework for understanding child disability is the International Classification of functioning (ICF) model, proposed by the World Health Organisation (WHO) in 2001. This model describes a child's health and wellbeing in terms of four components: (1) body structures, (2) body functions, (3) activities, and (4) participation. Body structures are anatomical parts of the body such as organs and limbs, as well as structures of the nervous, visual, auditory, and musculoskeletal systems. Body functions are the physiological functions of body systems, including psychological functions such as being attentive, remembering, and thinking. Activities are tasks done by children and include walking, climbing, feeding, dressing, toileting, bathing, grooming, communicating, and socially interacting. Participation means involvement in community life, such as playing with peers, preschool education experiences and attending family activities such as visiting relatives, attending religious services, or going shopping. The ICF model also accounts for contextual factors in a child's life, including environmental facilitators and environmental barriers as well as personal factors. Environmental facilitators include family leave policies, daycare and early education accessibility, and comprehensive health insurance. Environmental barriers include negative attitudes of others, lack of legal protections, and discriminatory practices. Personal factors include age, gender, interests, and sense of self-efficacy, and these can be facilitators or barriers. **Table 1** illustrates application of the ICF model to a 3-year-old girl with diplegic CP after extreme prematurity, a 4-year-old with hearing loss and communicative delays after leukemia, a 5-year-old with hyploplastic left heart repair who developed hemiplegia and attention deficit hyperactivity disorder (ADHD) after an embolic cerebral vascular accident (CVA), a 5-year-old boy with Duchenne's muscular dystrophy (DMD), and a 6-year-old girl with spina bifida.

Table 1   ICF model scenarios in preschool children with physical disability

Dimension	Girl, 3 years	Boy, 5 years	Girl, 4 years	Boy, 5 years	Girl, 6 years
Pathophysiology Molecular/ cellular mechanisms	800 g, 27 weeks' gestation, periventricular leukomalacia	Left CVA after staged hypoplastic heart repair	Hearing loss and communicative delays, leukemia in remission	DMD; absence of dystrophin	Meningomyelocele with Ventriculoperitoneal shunt
Body structures and body functions Organ structure/ function	Asthma Spastic diplegia Speech delays	Hemiplegia; neurobehavioral and adaptive delays	Speech and adaptive delays, 50 db sensory hearing loss bilaterally	Speech delay	Perceptual and learning delays, neurogenetic bladder, decreased sensation of feet
Activity (functional) strengths Ability to perform essential activities: feed, dress, toilet, walk, talk	Indoor walking with AFOs; drinks with straw; likes to pretend play with dolls	Climbs slide and goes down easily; loves talking books	With hearing aides, can carry on conversation. Speech understood by mother 50% of time	Knows colors; counts to 5	Able to decode words; independent in dressing
Activity (functional) limitations Difficulty in performing essential activities	Unable to climb steps; unclear speech unless repeats	Difficulty with fasteners, difficulty waiting and transitioning; impulsive	Inattentive in large groups; speech not understood by peers	Cannot run; speech understood by his mother 50% of time	Cannot run or peddle 2 wheel bicycle; wears pull-up diapers
Participation Involvement in community roles typical of peers	Plays in parallel with peers	On T-ball baseball team	Loves to dance and skate	Loves to swim	Enjoys singing
Participation restrictions Difficulty in assuming roles typical of peers	Misses day care due to asthma; uses supplemental nutrition products	YMCA will not let him use play-ground because he falls too much	No audiological consultation available to rural school	Cannot play ice hockey with brother	Excluded from YMCA swimming because of diapers
Contextual factors: environmental facilitators Attitudinal, legal, policy, and architectural facilitators	Has asthma care plan; participates in Hanen speech therapy group	Mother unable to attend pediatric stoke support groups because of her work hours	Community speech therapist works closely with teacher and school therapist	Community pool does not require climbing stairs	Active wheel chair sports leagues at YMCA
Contextual factors: environmental barriers Attitudinal, legal, policy, and architectural	Loves to watch brother age 5 use computers; on waiting list for speech therapy	Denied life insurance policy	Kindergarten has signing as only education option	Kindergarten class on 2nd floor	No nurse at school to supervise CIC

CVA, cerebral vascular accident; AFO, ankle-foot orthosis; DMD, Duchenne's muscular dystrophy; VP, Ventriculoperitoneal; CIC, Clean intermittent catheterization.

Understanding Cerebral Palsy

Of the 4 000 000 children born each year in the US, 2 per 1000 will go on to have one of the CP syndromes. These syndromes include spastic diplegia, hemiplegia, and quadriplegia as well as dyskinetic (extrapyramidal) disorders. Advances in epidemiology, neuroimaging, and habilitiative interventions have included a revised consensus definition of CP, application of noninvasive neuroimaging modalities that allow examination of central nervous system (CNS) structure, and a gross motor and manual ability functional classification systems. The epidemiological advances have reinforced what was initially discovered the 1960s in the US Collaborative Perinatal Project. In this prospective study, approximately 50 000 pregnant women were recruited between 1959 and 1966. Their children were prospectively followed from birth to age 7 years. Fewer than 10% of the children who went on to have a confirmed diagnosis of CP had intrapatum asphyxia. Major etiological contributions to CP included CNS dysgenesis, (e.g., microcephaly and holoproencephaly), non-CNS malformations (e.g., congenital heart disease), and congenital infections (e.g., rubella, Cytomegalovirus, and toxoplasmosis).

The value of neuroimaging in understanding the timing of CP was recently highlighted in the European Cerebral Palsy cohort of children born between 1996 and 1999. This population-based sample involved children from London, Edinburgh, Dublin, Lisbon, Stockholm, Tubingen, and Helsinki. Almost one in three children had the diplegic pattern of CP, one in four had hemiplegia, and one in five had quadriplegia. In addition, one in five had extrapyramidal CP with either ataxia or dyskinesia. White-matter abnormalities were present in 43% overall. However, this abnormality of white matter was present in 71% of children with diplegia, 33% of children with hemiplegia, and 33% of children with quadriplegia. These white-matter lesions highlight a critical window of timing in that the period of vulnerability is maximal between 24 and 34 weeks' gestation. Currently, extensive research efforts are occurring to understand the complex causal pathways of inflammation and infection and their role in oligodendroglia vulnerability.

In the European cohort, malformations were as common as cortical–subcortical damage and occurred at the frequency of 9%. The latter abnormality is the most common lesion associated with term infants with neonatal encephalopthy. This selective vulnerability of cortical and subcortical areas reflects the complex metabolic demands of these regions in term infants. Of children with basal ganglia and thalamic injury, 76% had dystonia manifested by involuntary movements, difficulty with fine motor skills, and difficulty with oral-motor control. Of children with hemiplegic CP, 27% had focal infarcts, reflecting a

neonatal stroke. It is in this group that maternal disorders of coagulation need to be investigated comprehensively. These disorders include maternal systemic lupus erythematosis that can cause clotting to a critical brain region and biochemical genetic factors (factor 5 Liden mutations and protein C abnormalities).

Advances in neuroimaging have helped in the understanding of timing and extent of lesions in children with CP. However, almost one in eight children with CP have a normal magnetic resonance imaging (MRI) scan. This group awaits the promise of neurogenetic technologies. Among the term and near-term children with CP, approximately 20% have the MRI abnormality of cortical–subcortical or basal ganglia injury. Since a large number of this population had emergency cesarean section deliveries, fewer than 10% of infants have had CP because of delayed obstetrical interventions. These 1996–1999 estimates are similar to the Collaborative Perinatal Project outcome data as well as data from the Western Australian CP registry for children born between 1975 and 1980.

In summary, ongoing population data, coupled with neuroimaging and functional measures, have helped advance our knowledge about the complexity of CP syndrome. Several lessons emerge from this.

1. More than half of the children with CP continue to be term gestation.
2. Multiple pregnancy increases the risk of CP.
3. Poor intrauterine growth increases the risk of CP.
4. Children born at 28–36 weeks' gestation contribute the largest numbers of CP preterms. Fewer than 10% of children with CP are less than 28 weeks of gestation. However, these children have high rates of communication, cognitive, and adaptive delays.
5. Approximately 10% of the children born in Europe with CP were born at less than 28 weeks of gestation.
6. Children with CP have high rates of recurrent seizures and sensory impairment. More than one in four children experience epilepsy, and more than one in three experience strabismus, restricted visual fields, and refractive errors. Seven per cent experience hearing impairment.
7. The majority of CP is not severe. Approximately three in five children have hemiplegia or diplegia. These children with two limb involvement can be considered as having less challenges in performing motor and functional skills compared with children with quadriplegia and four limb involvement. Overall, children with hemiplegia and diplegia have an excellent prognosis for ambulation. One hundred per cent of children with hemiplegia and 90% of children with diplegia are able to walk.
8. Quadriplegia is the least common, but most severe form of CP. The majority of children with quadriplegia have sitting challenges, manipulative challenges, and

communicative difficulties as well as comorbidities of dysphagia, seizures, and recurrent pneumonia. Only 9% of children with quadriplegia can walk. In addition, there are multiple severe neurodevelopmental functional challenges, medical frailty, and high rates of caregiver stress.

From a population standpoint, reducing the prevalence of CP requires understanding pathways of the CP syndromes in term infants, improved understanding and management of moderately preterm infants, and reducing CP in survivors of multiple births. More than 750 000 children and adults in the US have a CP syndrome. Their lifetime medical cost is estimated at $1 million per individual. In this respect, disproportionate attention to perinatal hypoxemic–ischemic encephalopathy in term infants and neurodevelopmental complications in extreme prematurity lead to the erroneous perception that these two risk groups of children account for the majority of cases of children with CP.

Current advances in developmental medicine highlight pathways of risk and protection for specific groups of children with one of the CP syndromes. These pathways include twins and higher-order multiples, children with intrauterine growth restriction, children with malformations, children undergoing congenital heart surgery, and children with neonatal seizures and encephalopathy. Major neuroscience research has focused on mechanisms of white-matter injury in preterm infants and neuroprotection of term infants with severe encephalopathy. It is critically important that all health, education, and rehabilitation professionals understand that a substantial number of term and near-term children do not have a simplistic cause for their motor disability. In this way, families can be helped and the general public can understand the need for addressing shortcomings in current knowledge. Most importantly, health and educational professionals can work together to optimize functioning, learning, and participation of children with CP.

Understanding Leukemia

Childhood cancers result in neurodevelopmental disabilities related to tumors, complications of surgical resection, or exposure to chemotherapy or cranial irradiation. Leukemias and brain tumors account for over one-half of all new childhood cancers. About one-third of childhood cancers are leukemias. Of the leukemias, acute lymphoblastic leukemia (ALL) is the most common, affecting 2400 children annually in the US. ALL accounts for 75% of all pediatric leukemia cases. In the 1990s the 5-year event-free survival rates for childhood ALL ranged from 70% to 83% and the overall survival exceed 90%. The current understanding of ALL has led to intensive treatment based on phenotype, genotype, and risk. Specific treatment approaches differ but consistently emphasize: (1) remission–induction therapy to eliminate greater than 99% of the initial tumor burden, (2) intensification (or consolidation) therapy, and (3) continuation treatment to eliminate residual leukemia. Primary treatment modalities include systemic or intrathecal chemotherapy, cranial irradiation, and bone marrow transplantation. Therapy directed at the central nervous system (CNS), which starts early in the clinical course, is given for varying lengths of time. These interventions depend on the child's risk of relapse, the intensity of systemic treatment, and whether cranial irradiation is used. Research over the last 20 years has demonstrated that CNS treatment with radiation and/or chemotherapy frequently results in neurocognitive dysfunction. Difficulties in memory, attention, information processing speed, visuospatial skills, and executive functioning result from these side effects. Challenges to both preschool developmental and school-age academic output can also occur. There is evidence that the incidence of severe cognitive impairment is decreasing with the diminished use of craniospinal irradiation. Intrathecal chemotherapy for CNS prophylaxis is the current preferred intervention that is used to prevent CNS relapse. The disease and treatment appear to have little impact on the brain structures and processes that are in place prior to onset of disease and treatment. The younger the child, therefore, the more global and severe the delayed effects will be. Factors predictive of increased risk for late effects are younger age at the time of CNS prophylaxis, female gender, high radiation dose, treatment with dexamethasone, and a history of CNS relapse.

Mechanisms of Central Nervous System Injury in Childhood Cancer

The principal mechanisms responsible for delayed neurotoxic effects are white-matter damage, disruption of the blood–brain barrier, vascular insults, and calcifications. Regions with greater myelin density, such as the right frontal lobe, are particularly vulnerable. The distribution of white-matter density may explain why some neurocognitive functions are affected and others relatively spared. The developing brain may be more susceptible to damage, because newly synthesized myelin has higher metabolic activity that makes it more susceptible to the toxic effects of therapy. Leukoencephalopathy may be detected by MRI in over 20% of patients after therapy for ALL. Correlation between these neuroradiographic findings and a neuropsychological injury has been inconsistent. However, a recent study demonstrated that smaller white-matter volumes were directly associated with challenges in attention, intelligence, and academic performance.

Cranial Radiation Therapy

Cranial radiation therapy (CRT) prophylactically is given to all patients to prevent leukemic cells from infiltrating the CNS and consists of CNS chemotherapy alone or in combination with cranial irradiation. Multiple studies demonstrate that of anticancer treatments, CRT appears to have the greatest impact on demyelination and therefore on delayed neurocognitive effects. CRT is also linked to necrosis with secondary ventricular dilation, vascular compromise, and focal calcifications in the basal ganglia and periventricular region. There is ongoing controversy between dose of CRT and risk for neurotoxic effects. Initial studies noted significant declines in intellectual functioning, especially in younger children. A meta-analysis of 30 studies of cognitive function conducted before 1988 concluded that those completing CRT experience on average a 10-point decline in intelligence quotient (IQ). Decreased rates of neurotoxic effects were noted when CRT was reduced from 2400 to 1800 cGy. There is no consensus on a safe dose. Cranial irradiation has largely been replaced by intrathecal or systemic chemotherapy. In most clinical trials, cranial irradiation is still recommended for those with a high risk for relapse such as initial CNS leukemia, T-cell ALL, or high tumor burden. The combination of CRT and chemotherapy results in the most severe neurotoxic effects and is attributed to injury to the blood–brain barrier.

Chemotherapy

Three classes of chemotherapeutics are most responsible for late neurotoxic effects: nucleoside analogs, glucocorticoids, and antifolates.

Nucleoside Analogs

The antineoplastic effect of nucleoside analogs depends on their inhibition of DNA and RNA synthesis. Agents in this class include cytosine, arabinoside, pentostatin, fludarabine, and nelarabine. Irreversible neurotoxicity and leukoencephalopathy may be evident weeks to months after exposure to these agents. The mechanism of action for the neurotoxic effects is unclear but appears to be related to duration rather than dose or dose intensity.

Glucocorticoids

Glucocorticoids may induce transient mental status, changes, confusion, or disturbances of sleep, affect, or memory. Their mechanism of action is through their action on the hippocampus, which is the brain structure with the highest concentration of glucocorticoid receptors.

Glucocorticoids inhibit glucose utilization by neurons and glia, increase the concentration of glutamate in the hippocampal synapse, and lead to excessive stimulation of postsynaptic receptors and excitotoxic neuronal death. Dexamethasone has a longer half-life and better penetration into the cerebrospinal fluid than prednisone or prednisolone. As a result, dexamethasone is used more frequently in induction and continuation therapies.

Antifolates

The primary antifolate is methotrexate (MTX). As their name implies, antifolates function as antineoplastic agents by interfering with folate-dependent biochemical systems. Steady-state cerebral spinal fluid (CSF) folate concentrations are two to three times those of serum values. The high concentration of folate in the CNS is essential for cell replication and to establish and maintain axonal myelination. MTX given intravenously at high doses decreases hematologic, testicular, and CNS relapses. All patients treated with MTX are at risk for delayed neurocognitive effects. The risk of late effect is related to individual dose and cumulative exposure to high-dose ($>500\,\mathrm{mg\,m^{-2}}$) intravenous therapy. Chronic MTX exposure is thought to deplete folate in the brain and thereby increase homocysteine levels. Homocysteine is toxic to the endothelium promoting occlusive vascular disease and microangiopathy, which results in focal neurological deficits. Homocysteine and its metabolites are excitotoxic amino acids and may contribute to the development of seizures. The disruption of folate-dependent systems may lead to demyelination and subsequent neurological manifestations such as developmental delay, intellectual disability, depression, seizures, or leukoencephalopathy.

Leukemia: Neurocognitive and Academic Outcomes

Declines in cognitive functions and academic performance are extensively described in the literature on long-term outcomes of childhood leukemia. However, the long-term educational and social outcomes of childhood cancer survivors have not received the same attention. Initially, the Canadian Late Effects Study examined parent-reported educational and social outcomes among child and adolescent survivors of childhood cancer and compared these survivors to a population-based control group with no cancer history. Significantly, more survivors than controls experienced poorer educational outcomes as measured by attending a learning-disabled program (19% vs. 7%), a special-education program (20% vs. 8%), or failing a grade (21% vs. 9%). Similarly, data from the Childhood Cancer Survivor Study (CCSS) described the self-reported utilization and factors associated with the use of special education services. The CCSS identified 12 430 English- or Spanish-speaking patients under the age of 21 years at time of cancer diagnosis from 25 sites across the US and Canada between January 1970 and December 1986. All children in this study had survived 5 years from the date of diagnosis. Younger ages at initial diagnosis were associated significantly with higher needs for special education services. Among children with leukemia, the odd ratios (ORs) for special education services were 4.40 (3.75–5.16) in preschool, 3.30 (2.66–4.00) at 6–10 years, and 1.70 (1.26–2.24) at 11–15 years. Although all academic subjects were affected, mathematics, English, and science were the most impaired. In a study of 593 survivors of ALL and 409 sibling controls from the Children's Cancer Group, there was a 3.6-fold increase in risk for special education services. Importantly, survivors had the same likelihood as their siblings of completing high school and entering college (93.6% vs. 92.4%). The likelihood of entering college (51.9% vs. 57.2%) and earning a bachelors degree (56.6% vs. 54.2%) were also similar among survivors and their siblings. However, a more recent study revealed that survivors of childhood leukemia were 60% more likely to complete high school and 30% more likely not to complete college than their siblings regardless of their treatment modality. In addition, the survivors enrolled in special education services were as likely to complete high school as those enrolled in special education without a history of cancer. The implication of these data is that with appropriate intervention, many survivors of childhood leukemia can complete high school. However, many are at continued risk for school failure and educational underachievement. Treatment modality may offer insight into the differences in educational outcomes. The OR of not finishing high school was 2.50 (1.76–3.67) for those who received only CRT; 1.0 (1.33–2.42) for those who received both intrathecal MTX and CRT; 1.60 (1.11–2.18) for those who received intrathecal MTX only.

Social Outcomes

There is increasing interest in the social and emotional outcomes of long-term cancer survivors. As the number of survivors have increased, it is increasingly important to understand the impact of cancer survival on personal sociobehavioral and emotional adjustment. Young adult survivors of childhood cancer are more likely to be underemployed and have lower income. Parents of survivors were more likely to report that their child did not have close friends or use friends as confidants. Children with leukemia often miss many days of school that may contribute to difficulties with social integration. The emotional adjustment of childhood cancer survivors may be measured in terms of overall functioning, self-esteem, anxiety, and depression. In 2001, Stam and colleagues reviewed several studies that addressed emotional adjustment of cancer survivors and reported that overall emotional adjustment of cancer survivors as a group was within normal limits. A closer look at the components of emotional adjustment revealed that on measures of self-esteem, cancer survivors felt better about their intellectual and academic status, behavior, and overall happiness than controls. A limitation of these studies is their reliance on self-report measures of general psychological functioning such as anxiety and depression rather than on measurement of the stress of a chronic illness. However, one in five of young adults with a history of cancer meet criteria for post-traumatic stress disorder (PTSD) as compared to one of the 10 abused adolescents and one in 20 typical adolescents.

Developmentally adolescents strive to become independent and define an identity. The adolescent cancer patient, however, is faced with a life-threatening illness that results in pain, physical changes, and forces them to depend on others. The degree to which late effects of cancer affect the quality of life of the increased number of long-term survivors of ALL needs to be better addressed. Strategies that augment supportive care services, increase patient's network size and reliance on formal and informal social ties will enhance long-term survivor's quality of life.

Understanding Congenital Heart Disease

Congenital heart disease occurs with a frequency of 7 per 1000 livebirths and are the leading cause of death between ages 1 month and 1 year. Early postoperative CNS sequelae such as stroke and seizures occurs in a small percentage of children with congenital heart disease. Since cardiovascular and neurologic systems develop in tandem during the first trimester, a variety of genetic etiologies often accompany congenital heart disease. These include well-known disorders of chromosome number (Trisomy 21,18,13) contiguous gene disorders (e.g., Williams syndrome and DiGeorge syndrome), and syndromes with multiple congenital malformations (e.g., CHARGE and VACTERL). Microdeletions of the 22nd chromesome (22q11) are associated with conotruncal cardiac abnormalities, including tetralogy of fallot, interuped aortic arch, or truncus arterisois. This contiguous gene disorder includes branchial arch abnormalities that impact facial structure, endocrine, immunological, and auditory systems including the DiGeorge phenotype. Other individuals with complex genetic abnormalities in this chrosomal region have the velo-cardio-facial syndrome with an associated range of communicative, learning, and behavioral impairment.

Early Childhood Outcomes

The study of preschool outcomes of children with congenital heart disease receiving open heart surgery in infancy took place in Montréal, Boston, and Philadelphia. Children with hypoplastic heart syndrome were excluded. In a cohort of 118 survivors, 83% were followed at 18 months and adaptive behavior was measured by using either the WeeFIM or the Vineland Scales. Children demonstrated functional limitations in self-care, mobility, and social cognition. Only 21% of the cohort was functioning in basic skills similar to peers. Moderate functional disability was noted in 37%, and severe functional disability in 6%. On the Vineland Scales, functional difficulties in daily living skills were documented in 40%, with more than half of the children having poor socialization skills. Factors enhancing the risk for functional disabilities included perioperative neurodevelopmental status, microcephaly, length of deep hypothermic circulatory arrest (DHCA), length of stay in the intensive care unit, age at surgery, and maternal education. This study demonstrates that there were high prevalence rates of functional limitations that significantly impacted development and community care. In addition, there are opportunities for prospectively examining supports that enhance parent management skills involving some of these functional challenges.

The mechanisms of CNS injury in children with congenital heart disease are complex. Up to 25% of neonates with congenital heart disease have periventricular leukomalacia before surgery. Other mechanisms for CNS vulnerability include perioperative hypoxemia and hypotension, cardiac arrest, hypoglycemis or hyperglyncemiia, hyperventilation, and hyperthermia. Bellinger and colleagues described the developmental and neurological status of children at 4 years of age after DHCA or low-flow cardiopulmonary bypass (CPB). With circulatory arrest the risk to the CNS is through hypoxemic–ischemic–reperfusion injury. With low-flow CPB, embolic complications are associated with increase time of extracorporeal circulation as happened in our illustrated third case. At the age of 4 years, the mean IQ was 93 with no difference in treatment groups. At the age of 8 years, more than one in three required special education services and one in 10 had repeated a grade. Compared to children without cardiac disorders, there were higher rates of speech, developmental, learning, and attention problems. In particular, there were significant challenges in visual spatial, visual motor, executive functioning, working memory, sustained attention, and higher-order language skills. In addition, there was difficulty with hypothesis generation and coordination skills. The DHCA group did worse on motor and speech functioning while the low-flow CPB had worse impulsivity and behavioral disorders.

Model Multicenter Studies for Understanding Mechanisms Impacting on Central Nervous System Structure and Function after very low birthweight and extremely low birthweight

Several recent studies have examined postneonatal processes that might be amenable to interventions that decrease risks for long-term CNS dysfunction. One study in the US Neonatal Network examined neurodevelopmental impairments among 6093 survivors who weighed between 401 and 1000 g and were born between 1993 and 2001. Among those without infection, 29% had neurodevelopmental impairments. Approximately 50% of infants with sepsis, sepsis and necrotizing enterocolitis, or meningitis had neurodevelopmental impairments. One of the disquieting outcomes of this study was in the high rate of early cognitive developmental disability. This intellectual disability occurred in one in five of infants without infection and in as many as two in five of those with infection. One mediator of this effect was brain growth at 36 weeks postmenstrual age. In children with infection, 40–60% had acquired microcephaly (e.g., head circumference of less than 10% on standardized premature infant charts). In contrast, only 25% of children without infection had acquired microcephaly.

A different approach was undertaken in a randomized clinical trial of inhaled nitric oxide (INO) to reduce death and chronic lung disease in very preterm infants in respiratory failure. In this study the children receiving INO had lower rates of death, chronic lung disease, severe intraventricular hemorrhage (IVH), and perviventricular leukomalacia. In addition, the risk of neurodevelopmental disability in the survivors at the age of 2 years who had received INO was 53% less than controls. This occurred predominantly by decreasing cognitive developmental disability. Thus, current studies are now underway to determine neuroprotective properties of INO in preterm infants.

Kindergarten Functional Status, School Function and 10-Year Health-Related Quality of Life

Children with severe neonatal retinopathy of prematurity (ROP) are the sickest, tiniest, and most medically fragile of VLBW and ELBW infants. Functional assessment of daily living skills in mobility, self-care, and social cognition was used at age 5.5 years to over 1000 children less than 1250 g enrolled in the National Institutes of Health (NIH) sponsored multicenter randomized trial of cryosurgery for ROP. Overall, 88% of these children were followed across 23 centers. As severity of retinopathy increased, functional status declined, and severe disability in social roles increased. The complexity and severity of disability was worse in the children with severe ROP and unfavorable visual acuity compared to children with severe ROP and favorable visual acuity. The former group had a rate of motor limitations of 43% compared to 5% for the latter group; a rate of self-care limitations of 78% compared to 25%; a rate of continency limitations of 51% versus 4.5%; and a rate of communicative/cognitive limitations of 67% vs. 22%. Functional limitations in children without ROP were low: motor – 4%, self-care – 7%, continency – 4%, and communicative/cognitive limitations – 8%. Multiple logistic regression analysis revealed that favorable visual status, and favorable 2-year neurologic score predicted functional status at age 5.5 years. The favorable 2 year neurological score included the absence of microcephaly, seizures, and/or hydrocephalus. Access to health insurance and African-American race also contribute to better functional status at age 5.5 years. At the age of 8 years, the group that had the most severe retinopathy of prematurity was examined with respect to developmental and educational outcomes. Favorable visual and functional status at kindergarten entry and higher socioeconomic status were associated with significantly lower rates of special education services and below grade level educational achievement. Factors that were significantly associated with an increased risk for special education services included minority status, poverty, lack of access to a car, and supplemental social security income because of disability and poverty. In multivariate regression analysis the key predictors of special educational services at the age of 8 years were unfavorable visual status and unfavorable functional status at 5.5 years.

Additional studies at the age of 10 years involved parental assessments with the Health Utilities Index (HUI) for Health Related Quality of Life (HRQOL). The proportion of sighted children with limitations in four or more HUI attributes of mobility, speech, dexterity, cognition, emotion, pain, or hearing was 6.4% compared to 47% in children with blindness or low vision. The median HUI score was 0.87 for sighted children compared to 0.27 for blind/low-vision children ($p < 0.001$) with scores of 1 indicating perfect health and scores of 0 reflecting death. Thus, this series of outcomes at ages 5.5 years, 8 years, and 10 years revealed the value of both functional assessment and health-related quality of life for children receiving new technologies. Both the pathways that lead to more severe ROP and the processes that allow for preservation of some visual functioning after threshold ROP are involved in the severity of neuromotor, adaptive, and communicative disability at kindergarten entry. In addition, understanding mechanisms involved in extreme prematurity that result in the absence of retinopathy are critically important for preserving CNS neuromotor, higher cortical integrity, and participating with peers.

Understanding Muscular Dystrophy and Neuromuscular Coordination

MD is not one single disorder, but a collection of over 30 genetic/hereditary disorders with progressive degeneration of skeletal muscles. Many of these conditions have onset in childhood (including Duchenne's (DMD), Becker's (BMD), and congenital muscular dystrophy (CMD)) while others do not begin showing symptoms until adulthood or middle age (distal MD, myotonic MD, and oculopharyngeal dystrophy). Some, such as DMD, eventually lead to paralysis and death of the young adult in teenage years due to respiratory and/or cardiac muscle failure. However, for several MDs (such as myotonic MD), the progress of the disorder can be very slow and can span several decades before the adult becomes severely disabled. It is no surprise, therefore, that treatment and prognosis varies depending on the type of the disorder. To date, no effective treatment or cure has been found for MD. In this section, we examine the four most common types of MD and their impact on child health and development.

Duchenne's Muscular Dystrophy

DMD is an X-linked recessive disorder due to a mutaton on the *Xp21* gene. This gene is one of the largest known genes and has greater chance for mutation or deletion compared to other smaller genes. DMD occurs in 1 in 3500 live male births and is the most common form of MD. Onset of symptoms occurs in the preschool years. Early symptoms include delay in learning to walk, waddling gait, difficulty running, climbing stairs, or rising from the floor. By the ages 3–4 years, the child is not able to keep up with his peers. By age 12 years, the vast majority of children with DMD requires wheelchairs for mobility and can be community independent with the use of electric motor chairs. On average, boys with DMD tend to have a lower IQ with increased rates of, slow learning (IQ 70–85), and mild intellectual disability (IQ 55–69) than their healthy counterparts. The child's muscles, including the heart, becomes progressively weaker, and life expectancy is shortened to late teens or early 20s.

Apart from clinical examinations during early childhood (from characteristic pattern of weakness in limbs such as lordotic gait), DMD can be identified through series of tests such as measuring the creatine phosphokinase (CPK) level, ultrasound of the muscles, and muscle biopsy. Patients with high level of CPK in their blood, and a deficiency in dystrophin in their muscle can be confirmed as having DMD. Prenatal tests (such as chorionic villus sampling, amniocentesis, placental biopsy, and fetal blood sampling) can also be used to determine if the child has MD prenatally. DNA analysis can provide definite diagnosis, carrier detection, and prenatal diagnosis.

Although support and treatment are available through physical therapy, surgery (to treat scoliosis), and rehabilitation engineering, deterioration of both respiratory and cardiac muscles lead to death in young adulthood.

Congenital Muscular Dystrophy

The term CMD refers to a group of inherited disorders. Unlike DMD, muscle weakness for CMD patients is present at birth, and children of both genders are affected. Six forms of CMD have been identified to date: three without structural brain abnormalities, and three with structural brain change. In the latter case, significant intellectual disability can accompany severe muscle weakness.

A significant number of children with CMD without intellectual disability have either reduced or absence of merosin in their muscle tissue. Infants with merosin-deficient CMD often have severe weakness, decreased muscle tone, floppiness, congenital contractures, as well as breathing and swallowing problems. Although some children learn to stand or walk with supportive devices, the majority of children with merosin-deficient CMD achieve sitting unsupported as their best motor skill. Elective surgeries should be performed with great caution as there is high risk for pneumonia or ventilator dependence.

Spinal Muscle Atrophy

Spinal muscle atrophy (SMA) is a motor neuron disease where the degeneration of anterior horn cells of the spinal cord impact on voluntary muscle strength and control. SMA affects proximal muscles (muscles closest to the trunk – i.e., shoulders, hips, and back) than the distal muscles. SMA is an autosomal-recessive genetic disorder, and for a child to be affected by SMA, both parents must be carriers. There are four types of SMA: type 1 (severe SMA, also known as Werdnig–Hoffman disease), type 2 (intermediate SMA), type 3 (mild SMA, also known as Kugelberg–Welander disease), and type 4 (adult onset).

The age of onset for type 1 SMA is often prenatal, with mothers reporting decreased movements in the last trimester. Infants with type 1 SMA show symptoms of severe hypotonia and weakness, difficulty in sucking and swallowing, as well as respiratory problems immediately after birth. Infants adopt a frog-like posture, have paucity of movement, poor head control, bell-shaped chest, diaphragmatic breathing (appearing to breathe with their stomach muscles because of weak intercoastal muscles), weak cry, absent of tendon reflex, and internal rotation of arms. These infants struggle to lift their heads against gravity or accomplish motor milestones. They are unable to roll or sit unsupported. Infants with type 1 SMA are prone to respiratory infections, and the majority die of pneumonia and respiratory failure in the first year of life.

The age of onset for type 2 SMA is usually between 6 and 12 months with diagnosis before the age of 2 years. Children with type 2 SMA exhibit symptoms of weakness of legs and inability to stand or walk. Although some may sit unsupported when placed in a seated position, many are not able to sit upright by themselves without assistance. Typical clinical signs of type 2 SMA are inability to take full weight on legs, symmetrical weakness of legs and hypotonia, fasciculation of tongue, tremor of hands, absence of deep tendon reflexes, and various respiratory problems. Children with type 2 SMA have normal facial movements, as well as normal-to-above-average intelligence. Their muscle weakness is not progressive, and some children show signs of functional improvement, although many have long-term disability.

Type 3 SMA has more variable onset and age of presentation, from the second year of life to adolescence. Most children are diagnosed in the preschool years. Children are able to stand and walk without assistance, but generally have difficulty in running, climbing steps, and jumping. They also fall more frequently and have difficulty in getting up from sitting on the floor or a bent over position. Hand tremors and tongue fasciculation can be present with varying degrees of severity. Children with type 3 SMA have a very good chance at long-term survival, given preventive pulmonary care, nutrition supports, and rehabilitation intervention.

Myotonic Dystrophy

Myotonic dystrophy (also known as Steinert's disease) affects about 1 in 8000 people worldwide. The age of onset can be anywhere from birth (congenital myotonic dystrophy) to 80 years, and muscle problems can range from none to severe. Two main muscle symptoms of myotonic dystrophy are weakness and inability to relax a muscle grip. Patterns of muscle weakness include weakness of face and jaw muscles, droopiness of the eyelids (ptosis), weakness of neck, hands, and lower leg muscles, as well as thighs, shoulders, and trunk. This leads to loss of facial expression, indistinct speech, difficulty in writing, lifting, and fine movements, as well as clumsiness and unsteadiness. One of the common characteristics of myotonic dystrophy is the difficultly in relaxing hand muscles, resulting in the inability to quickly let go after a hand shake.

Although myotonic dystrophy can potentially be debilitating, deterioration is not rapid, and the disorder rarely changes its rate of progression if the onset was in adulthood. Most children and adults with myotonic dystrophy will not require a wheelchair during their lifetime. This is because large muscles needed for weight bearing and walking are only moderately affected. However, myotonic dystrophy can cause distressing symtoms including irregular heartbeat, frequent respiratory infections, choking, difficulty in swallowing, constipation, poor vision due to cataracts, and daytime sleepiness.

Congenital myotonic dystrophy, in contrast, has serious consequences. Infants born to mothers with myotonic dystrophy have severe hypotonia at birth, facial weakness, and a wide range of breathing and swallowing difficulties. It is believed that the infant is affected in the uterus, with mothers noting poor movements during the second and third trimester. From birth, infants display muscle weakness with floppiness, poor sucking, difficulty swallowing, respiration insufficiency, severe hypotonia, facial weakness, and weakness of limbs. Although early childhood respiratory insufficiency may be life threatening, once the child survives infancy, respiratory problems improve, as do swallowing difficulties and hypotonia. However, children with congenital myotonic dystrophy often have delay in communicative and cognitive milestones.

While many physicians rely on family history to diagnose myotonic dystrophy, there are several tests that can be performed to confirm the diagnosis. The myotonic dystrophy gene and the level of muscle protein creatine kinase level can be detected through blood tests. Muscle tests include biopsy and electromyography (EMG).

Early Childhood Outcomes of Muscular Dystrophy

MD is a collection of a wide range of inherited muscular disorders with varying degrees of symptoms, management and, treatment. However, few children with MD lead an independent life or hold a job without assistance. Management includes physical therapy, orthopedic surgery to manage deformity and scoliosis, occupational therapy to enhance the use of electronic switches, special education supports to optimize academic and social participation, nutrition supports, cardiac care for cardiomyopathy, and respiratory care (especially noninvasive ventilators).

Understanding Spina Bifida

Spina bifida (also known as meningomyelocele) is a birth defect that occurs during the first month of pregnancy. One or more vertebral laminae fail to fuse in the midline. The defect usually occurs in the midback (thoracic), lower back (lumbar), or at the base of the spine (sacral). There are three types of spina bifida, depending on the severity of the condition: spina bifida occulta, meningocele, and meningomyelocele.

Spina bifida occulta is the mildest and the most common form of spinal bifida. Although the bones of the spine are incomplete and the spine therefore is incomplete, the malformation (i.e., opening of the spine) is covered by a layer of skin. Children with spina bifida occulta rarely have neurological symptoms or have any developmental or medical complications. This condition does not require neonatal surgery.

Meningocele is the bulging of meninges of the spinal cord through an opening in the vertebrae; thus, the baby is born with a sac protruding from its back. However, no spinal cord is present in the sac and few nerves are affected. Surgery is needed to repair the affected area. Some minor neurological sequelae can be present.

Meningomyelocele is the most serious type of spina bifida where the sac protruding from the infant's back contains spinal cord and nerve tissues. There is no skin covering the malformation, which means that the spinal cord is exposed to amniotic fluid that has open communication with the external environment; therefore, meningitis can occur. The infants require surgery at 24–48 h of birth in order to enclose the CSF and the damaged nerves surrounding the malformation. Children with meningomyelocele have neurological symptoms including muscle weakness, sensory loss, and neurogenic bowel and bladder.

Early Childhood Outcomes of Spina Bifida

As with any congenital malformations, childhood outcomes of spina bifida depend on various factors, namely, the level of the lesion, how early treatment is administered, how soon or often rehabilitation services are received, constant monitoring from caregivers and teachers, and experience healthcare professionals.

One of the most serious consequences of spina bifida is hydrocephalus, secondary to the Arnold Chiari malformation. In order to prevent additional neurological damage from increased intracranial pressure, ventricular–peritoneal shunting is performed. Although the effects of shunt treatments on cognitive and motor abilities are still under debate, several studies suggest that children with spina bifida who did not require the aid of shunts performed better in intelligence tests than patients with spina bifida who underwent shunt treatments. This reflects a decreased risk from increased intracranial pressure. However, without shunts, children with hydrocephalus can have increased impaired mobility, seizures, and cognitive decline. Children with meningomyelocele and hydrocephalus, are more likely to experience difficulty in fine motor and visual perceptual skills. For this group, the severity of the motor impairment and/or cognitive performance depends largely on the location of the lesion: the higher the lesion, the more severe the impairment.

Upper extremity incoordination is common in spina bifida. It includes fine motors difficulties such as use of hands and fingers for grasping and manipulation of objects, as well as speed and strength during bilateral hand use and motor planning ability. These impairments can lead to the child having challenges with grooming, dressing, bathing, and toileting. However, it is important to note that lack of dexterity of movement in children with meningomyelocele can be the result of limited opportunity to use their hands for manipulation, play, or everyday activities.

See also: Cerebral Palsy; Intellectual Disabilities; Learning Disabilities; Mental Health, Infant.

Suggested Readings

Bellinger DC, Wypij D, Kuban KC, *et al.* (1999) Developmental and neurological status of children at 4 years of age after heart surgery with hypothermic circulatory arrest or low-flow cardiopulmonary bypass. *Circulation* 100(5): 526–532.

Biggar WD (2006) Duchenne muscular dystrophy. *Pediatrics in Review* 27(3): 83–88.

Dickerman JD (2007) The late effects of childhood cancer therapy. *Pediatrics* 119(3): 554–568.

Doherty D and Shurtleff DB (2006) Pediatric perspective on prenatal counseling for myelomeningocele. *Birth Defects Research Part A, Clinical Molecular Teratology* 76(9): 645–653.

Krageloh-Mann I and Horber V (2007) The role of magnetic resonance imaging in elucidating the pathogenesis of cerebral palsy: A systematic review. *Developmental Medicine and Child Neurology* 49(2): 144–151.

Msall ME and Tremont MR (2002) Measuring functional outcomes after prematurity: Developmental impact of very low birth weight and extremely low birth weight status on childhood disability. *Mental Retardation and Developmental Disabilities Research Reviews* 8: 258–272.

Msall ME, Phelps DL, Hardy RJ, *et al.* (2004) Educational and social competencies at 8 years in children with threshold retinopathy of prematurity (ROP) in the CRYO-ROP multicenter study. *Pediatrics* 113: 790–799.

Skinner R, Wallace WH, and Levitt G (2007) Long-term follow-up of children treated for cancer: Why is it necessary, by whom, where and how? *Archives of Disease in Childhood* 92(3): 257–260.

Wernovsky G, Shillingford AJ, and Gaynor JW (2005) Central nervous system outcomes in children with complex congenital heart disease. *Current Opinion in Cardiology* 20(2): 94–99.

World Health Organization (2001) *International Classification of Functioning Disability and Health.* Geneva: WHO.

Diarrhea

J A Rudolph, Children's Hospital Medical Center, Cincinnati, OH, USA
P A Rufo, Children's Hospital Boston, Boston, MA, USA

This article is reproduced from the *Encyclopedia of Gastroenterology*, volume 1, pp 585–593, 2004; © Elsevier Inc.

Glossary

Acute diarrhea – A diarrheal illness of less than 14 days duration. Acute diarrheal disease in children is most often the result of self-limited viral infections. Management includes prompt assessment and repletion of hydration status. Evaluation for an etiologic process is generally not warranted unless there is an associated finding such as blood in the stool or systemic symptoms.

Chronic diarrhea – A diarrheal illness of greater than 14 days duration. Chronic diarrhea in children can be due to either infectious or noninfectious processes. Evaluation for a specific etiology is indicated. Management of comorbid conditions such as poor growth or malnutrition is essential.

Colitis – Any inflammatory process affecting the colon. Colitis usually presents clinically as bloody diarrhea, abdominal cramping, and tenesmus.

Congenital diarrhea – A group of diarrheal illnesses that are present from birth. Congenital diarrhea can be the result of either a specific genetic defect in a secretory or absorptive pathway or abnormal intestinal development.

Gastroenteritis – A diarrheal process that affects the upper gastrointestinal tract and presents most typically as an acute watery diarrhea. Gastroenteritis usually denotes an acute diarrhea that is infectious and self-limiting.

Hemolytic uremic syndrome – A sequela of *Escherichia coli* O157:H7 colitis. This toxin-mediated microangiopathy results in a triad of hemolytic anemia, thrombocytopenia, and renal failure. The occurrence of the syndrome is generally limited to children under 10 years of age.

Inflammatory diarrhea – A diarrheal illness in which the predominant pathologic finding is an invasion of the intestinal epithelium by immunocytes. This type of diarrhea can be the result of either a normal immune response to an abnormal environment, as in infection, or an abnormal immune response to a normal environment, as in inflammatory bowel disease.

IPEX syndrome (Immunodysregulation, polyendocrinopathy, and enteropathy: X-linked) – An inherited X-linked syndrome that results from a mutation in the *FOXP3* gene in humans. It is characterized by autoimmune enteropathy and multiple endocrinological abnormalities including diabetes mellitus, hypothyroidism, and hemolytic anemia.

Osmotic diarrhea – A diarrheal illness that is driven by osmotic forces that promote a net flux of water out of the interstitium and into the intestinal lumen. A stool sodium level of mEq l^{-1} and an osmotic gap of greater than 100 mosm l^{-1} suggest an osmotic diarrhea.

Secretory diarrhea – A diarrheal illness that is driven by the active secretion of salt and water by intestinal epithelial cells. A stool sodium level of greater than 70 mEq l^{-1}, an osmotic gap of less than 100 mosm l^{-1}, and a failure of the diarrhea to respond to a controlled fast suggest a secretory diarrhea.

The frequency and consistency of stool can vary considerably from individual to individual, as well as in the same individual over time. There has therefore remained a lack of a consensus as to how diarrheal illness should be defined. Investigators have employed a number of qualitative and quantitative dimensions of stool output to address this issue in the past. For the most part, children pass between one and three stools, or approximately 5–10 ml of stool per kilogram of body weight per day. As such, investigators have begun to use these benchmarks as the upper limits of normal in their identification of subjects in studies addressing acute or chronic diarrheal disease.

Regulation of Intestinal Fluid Secretion and Absorption

The mucosa lining the gastrointestinal tract must reconcile daily a seemingly contradictory array of physiologic tasks. These conflicting responsibilities include the maintenance of a tight barrier against potentially virulent bacterial and viral pathogens in the intestinal lumen, while at the same time presenting a selectively permeable interface through which to carry out immune surveillance and nutrient absorption. In this context, intestinal fluid secretion can serve both defensive (flushing away pathogens and toxins) and homeostatic (maintenance of mucosal hydration necessary to facilitate enzymatic digestion) purposes.

Stool output in humans is a composite of ingested, secreted, and absorbed fluid intermixed with residual dietary matter and cellular debris. Adults typically ingest approximately 2 l of fluid per day and produce an additional 9 l in the form of salivary, gastric, small intestinal, and pancreato-biliary secretions, to complete the process of digestion. The small intestine and colon have evolved highly efficient intercellular and transcellular pathways for the reabsorption of the vast majority (approximately 99%) of this intestinal fluid, and the average adult will pass only approximately 200 g of stool per day. This balance between fluid secretion and absorption is therefore quite tight. Any microbiologic, dietary, pharmacologic, or hormonal input that affects cell membrane transporters and/or the intercellular tight junctions responsible for fluid absorption can tip this net fluid balance in favor of secretion (or reduced absorption) and thereby trigger the increased stool output observed in patients with diarrheal illnesses.

The cellular basis for salt and water secretion in the intestine, as well as in other hydrated mucosal surfaces in the body, depends upon a vectorial transport of Cl^- ions by specialized epithelial cells. Intestinal crypt epithelial cells use basolateral membrane Na^+/K^+-ATPase pumps as well as the Na^+- and K^+-coupled cotransporter NKCCl to accumulate Cl^- ions above their electrochemical gradient (**Figure 1**). The subsequent opening of Cl^- channels located in the apical membrane of enterocytes permits sequestered Cl^- ions to move down their electrochemical gradient and into the intestinal lumen. The parallel

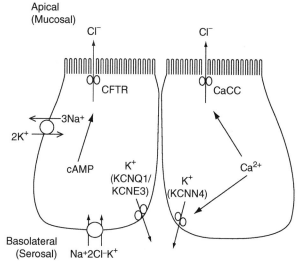

Figure 1 Intestinal crypt epithelial cells use basolateral membrane Na^+/K^+-ATPase pumps as well as the Na^+- and K^+-coupled cotransporter NKCCl to accumulate Cl^- ions above their electrochemical gradient. The subsequent opening of Cl^- channels located in the apical membrane of enterocytes permits sequestered Cl^- ions to move down their electrochemical gradient and into the intestinal lumen. The parallel activation of plasma membrane K^+ channels conduct K^+ outside, thereby sustaining the inside-negative cell membrane potential that is necessary to initiate and maintain a Cl^- secretory response.

activation of plasma membrane K^+ channels conducts K^+ outside, thereby sustaining the inside-negative cell membrane potential that is necessary to initiate and maintain a Cl^- secretory response.

Fluid secretion in the intestine is tightly regulated by endocrine as well as neuroenteric mechanisms that utilize either cyclic nucleotides ($3',5'$-monophosphate (cAMP) or cyclic GMP (cGMP)) or Ca^{2+} as second messengers. Cyclic nucleotide-dependent agonists initiate Cl^- secretion through the parallel activation of the apical membrane Cl^- channel CFTR (the cystic fibrosis transmembrane receptor) as well as the basolateral membrane K^+ channel KCNQ1/KCNE3. In contrast, agonists utilizing Ca^{2+} as a second messenger activate the apical membrane Cl^- conductance CaCC in concert with the basolateral membrane K^+ channel IKl (KCNN4). The net movement of Cl^- ions into the intestinal lumen imparts a transiently negative charge to this extracellular compartment and positively charged Na^+ ions move via paracellular pathways in response. The osmotic force generated by transported Cl^- and Na^+ ions pulls water molecules along to effect net fluid secretion. The activity of CFTR is regulated primarily by cAMP- and cGMP-dependent protein kinases. In contrast, Ca^{2+}-dependent Cl^- secretion in the intestine conducted by CLCA appears to be limited by the generation of the intracellular down-regulatory intermediates inositol-3, 4,5,6-tetrakisphosphate, and phosphorylated extracellular signal-regulated kinase.

Whereas Cl^- secretion drives intestinal fluid secretion, fluid absorption is mediated primarily by the vectorial transport of Na^+ ions out of the intestinal lumen and into the interstitium. Na^+ transport can be electrogenic (as in the case of apical Na^+ channels), Na^+-coupled, or electroneutral. The accumulation of absorbed Na^+ ions in the tissue interstitium favors the subsequent movement of Cl^- ions and water molecules out of the intestinal lumen via transcellular and paracellular pathways, thereby effecting salt and water uptake. Na^+ channels have been identified in the apical membrane of the epithelium of the gastrointestinal tract. By acting in a coupled fashion with basolateral membrane Na^+/K^+- ATPase pumps, these channels permit lumenal Na^+ ions to move down their electrochemical gradient and into the cell. The favorable Na^+ gradient established by Na^+/K^+ pumps has also been exploited by the small intestine to promote nutrient absorption. SGLT1 is the Na^+-coupled glucose transporter expressed along the apical membrane of enterocytes. Similarly, Na^+ uptake in the small intestine is effected through Na^+-coupled amino acid transporters that are present along the enterocyte brush border. Finally, the Na^+/H^+ exchanger NHE-3, expressed in the apical membrane of enterocytes, appears to mediate electroneutral Na^+ transport in the intestine.

The tasks of intestinal fluid secretion and absorption are separated spatially along the length of the crypt–villus axis through a segregation of relevant plasma membrane channels and transporters. Cells newly differentiated at the crypt base display a primarily secretory phenotype and express high levels of CFTR. As these cells mature and migrate up the axis to take up more villous positions, they express increasing numbers of absorptive proteins including NHE-3 and Na^+-coupled glucose and amino acid transporters. Stool output is therefore the net product of intestinal fluid secretion originating in crypt cells (which occupy approximately one-third of the crypt–villus axis) and fluid absorption from villus cells (which take up the remaining two-thirds of the crypt–villus axis). Any disorder damaging surface villi, and thereby decreasing the villus/crypt ratio, will selectively decrease mucosal absorptive potential and cause increased stool output. This explains the increased stool output observed in patients with celiac disease, postviral syndromes, and giardiasis.

Approach to the Child with Diarrhea

Diarrhea can be classified on the basis of several descriptive factors (acute vs. chronic, inflammatory vs. noninflammatory, infectious vs. noninfectious, secretory vs. osmotic) that aid in the diagnostic approach. These include the duration of the illness, the existence of a secretory or osmotically driven mechanism, the presence or absence of a pathogen, and the degree of mucosal inflammation. Although the pathogenesis of diarrheal disease can be explained by a discrete process in some patients, increased stool output is more often the result of a combination of factors. As such, patients with inflammatory diarrhea can present with a secretory component due to the local release of endogenous secretagogues. Clinical diagnosis rests on an understanding of the close interplay between environmental and host factors in these patients.

Central to the diagnosis of a diarrheal illness is the clinical context in which it presents. Characteristics of the individual, such as age, are often the first clue in determining an etiology. This is most apparent in the case of congenital diarrheas, which present exclusively within the first few days of life. Components of the child's overall health, such as atopy or immunodeficiency, can also suggest a particular etiology. Environmental factors, including diet, must also be taken into consideration in the diagnostic approach to the pediatric patient with diarrhea. In the setting of infectious diarrhea, an exposure history such as an ill contact at home or in daycare, a recent travel history, or contact with a pet or animal, can sometimes provide useful epidemiologic information when attempting to understand how a pathogen may have been acquired.

The character of the stool itself is often helpful when arriving at a specific diagnosis. Stool that is both watery and voluminous in nature suggests an abnormality in the absorptive or secretory function of the small intestine. In contrast, crampy abdominal pain, tenesmus, and the presence of frank blood in the stool suggest colitis or large bowel disease.

Several aspects of diarrheal disease in children merit special consideration. Children, and most especially infants, are more susceptible to dehydration than their adult counterparts. This is due both to their greater overall body surface area relative to their weight and to a dependence on caregivers, who may be less likely to offer fluids to or feed a child who is vomiting or appears ill. Poor growth and malnutrition can also become a factor in children when diarrhea is chronic in nature. During infancy and early childhood, a large proportion of caloric intake is devoted to growth. Diarrheal disease, resulting in inadequate intake or poor nutrient absorption during this critical developmental period, can alter weight gain and, in severe cases, result in stunted linear growth.

The scope of the remaining article will discuss the causes, evaluation, and treatment of diarrheal disease in infants and children. By convention, the discussion will be segregated into infectious causes and noninfectious causes with a special reference to age of onset where appropriate.

Infectious Diarrhea in Children

Infectious diarrhea is usually of acute onset in a previously healthy child. Fortunately, most causes of infectious diarrhea are self-limited and require only symptomatic care. However, if left untreated, acute diarrheal illness can progress to chronic diarrhea in some patients. Fever is a common associated symptom of infectious diarrhea and vomiting is not unusual, especially if the infection occurs in the upper gastrointestinal tract (i.e., gastroenteritis). In general, infectious diarrheas are secretory or mixed secretory/osmotic in character. Toxin production, pathogen adherence, or frank tissue invasion all can contribute to increased Cl^- secretion by affected epithelial cells. When pathogenic invasion of the epithelium occurs, there is usually an inflammatory component to the diarrhea as well. Pathogens that cause diarrhea can be viral, bacterial, or parasitic.

Viruses are the most common cause of acute infectious gastroenteritis in children (**Table 1**, part A). There are several reasons for the preponderance of cases of viral diarrheas. The naive immune system of an infant has not been exposed to many of the viral pathogens present in the environment. In addition, daycare provides group settings that facilitate the transmission of enteric and respiratory viral diseases.

Table 1 Etiology of pediatric diarrhea

Infectious diarrhea	Noninfectious diarrhea
A. Viral pathogens	D. Inflammatory
Rotavirus	Inflammatory bowel disease
Adenovirus	Celiac disease
Norwalk agent	Allergic enteropathy
Calicivirus	Autoimmune enteropathy
Astrovirus	Graft-vs.-host disease
Coronavirus	E. Noninflammatory
B. Bacterial pathogens	Congenital diarrheas
Campylobacter spp.	Congenital chloride
Salmonella spp.	diarrhea
Shigella spp.	Congenital sodium
Escherichia coli	diarrhea
Enterotoxigenic	Microvillus inclusion
Enteropathogenic	disease
Enterohemorrhagic	Tufting enteropathy
(shigatoxin producing)	Carbohydrate transporter
Enteroadherent	defects
Enteroinvasive	Dissacharidase deficiency
Yersinia spp.	Amino acid transporter
Vibrio spp.	defects
Aeromonas spp.	Pancreatic insufficiency
Plesiomonas spp.	Bile acid transport defects
Clostridium difficile	Abetalipoproteinemia
C. Parasitic pathogens	Acquired diarrheas
Giardia lamblia	Toddler's diarrhea
Cryptosporidia	Short bowel syndrome
Cyclosporidia	Small bowel overgrowth
Entamoeba histolytica	Antibiotic-associated
Nematodes	diarrhea
Cestodes	Münchausen's syndrome
(tapeworms)	Secondary lactase
Trematodes	deficiency

Rotavirus is the most common viral pathogen. All children exposed to rotavirus, regardless of whether or not they manifest symptomatic diarrhea, will develop circulating antibodies to this pathogen. The decreasing incidence of rotavirus in adults is thought to be due to the protective effect of these antibodies. Rotaviruses are small, wheel-shaped viruses approximately 70 nm in diameter. Of the four major groups (A, B, C, and D), type A viruses are the most important in children. The virus invades the epithelium and promotes an inflammatory response that ultimately contributes to the destruction of the villous surface. However, the frequency and severity of stool output in these patients does not correlate closely with the degree of intestinal damage observed endoscopically or histologically. This has led to the speculation that there are other pathogenic mechanisms that contribute to the malabsorption and net fluid losses observed in these patients. Although villous destruction can be severe in rotaviral disease, recovery is rapid in most patients and symptoms typically resolve in 2–7 days.

Caliciviruses, including the Norwalk and Norwalk-type agents, are the second leading cause of pediatric viral diarrheas. This group of viruses presents in a similar fashion to rotavirus, with the exception that the diarrhea is usually milder. Astroviruses are similar to calciviruses and are a common cause of diarrheal illness. Adenovirus (serotypes 40 and 41) is a well-established cause of viral diarrhea and has a slightly longer incubation period and a longer course than rotaviral disease. More recently, Torovirus has been implicated as a potential cause of diarrhea in children. However, more definitive epidemiologic data concerning this pathogen are currently lacking.

Bacterial infections can also cause diarrheal disease in infants and children (**Table 1**, part B). As in the case of viral diarrhea, the onset of bacterial illness is usually acute and presents with fever and sometimes vomiting. Because the most common forms of bacterial diarrhea are invasive, bloody diarrhea is often reported in these patients. Specific types of bacterial illness have been reported to occur more commonly in specific age groups. *Campylobacter jejuni*, for instance, has a bimodal distribution of onset with the first peak occurring in children from 1 to 5 years old and a second peak in adolescents. Nontyphoid *Salmonella enteritidis* can cause a bacteremia in infants and in immunocompromised hosts. *Shigella* species can be found in the toddler age group, but is not a commonly isolated pathogen in the US. *Clostridium difficile*, an important cause of antibiotic-associated diarrhea in adults, is not usually a pathogen in infants. *C. difficile* toxin can be found in up to 10% of healthy newborns and is even more prevalent in neonatal intensive care units. The reason for the inability of this organism to cause diarrhea in infants remains unclear. Based on animal studies, it is thought that the receptor for this toxin is developmentally regulated and absent in early infancy. *Vibrio cholerae* causes a prototypical bacterial secretory diarrhea. It produces a toxin composed of two subunits. The B, or binding, subunit displays a pentameric form that binds selectively to the ganglioside GM_1. The A, or active, subunit is internalized by intestinal epithelia, alters signal transduction, and leads to increased production of cAMP and Cl^- secretion. Other forms of toxin-producing organisms include enterotoxigenic *Escherichia coli*, the pathogen responsible for traveler's diarrhea, and organisms responsible for acute food poisoning such as *Staphylococcus aureus* and *Bacillus cereus*. *E. coli* O157:H7 is an important pathogen in children. This enteropathic *E. coli* adheres to the intestinal lumen and produces a toxin that is absorbed and causes the hemolytic–uremic syndrome.

Parasitic disease causing diarrhea is far less common in industrialized countries (**Table 1**, part C). One notable exception is *Giardia lamblia*, which is especially prevalent in the daycare setting. *Giardia* can present as an acute diarrheal illness or as a more chronic process. The mechanism by which this organism causes diarrhea is not fully understood. There is no gross alteration in intestinal architecture or evidence of a significant immunologic response. There are multiple other parasites that can cause diarrheal disease in children. However, these occur much less commonly and will not be discussed further.

Noninfectious Diarrhea in Children

Occasionally, a child will present with a diarrheal illness that is not self-limiting. Fever may or may not be present and other comorbidities, such as growth failure and malnutrition may be prominent. Stool cultures are negative. The etiology of diarrheal disease in these patients can be broadly classified as being inflammatory or noninflammatory in nature, based on clinical history, physical examination, and biochemical workup. Similar to patients with infectious diarrhea, the increased stool output observed in these patients is typically the result of a combination of pathogenic mechanisms.

Inflammatory Diarrhea

The intestine displays a tremendous capacity to generate an immune response based on the presence of numerous effector immunocytes that lie within the intestinal mucosa and submucosa. More recent data have demonstrated that intestinal epithelial cells themselves also possess the ability to process lumenal antigens and present them to the underlying immune cells. The intestinal epithelium is in constant contact with the external environment. It is subsequently in a constant state of low-grade inflammation (often referred to as 'physiologic inflammation') that is the result of the epithelium playing its role in the surveillance of and response to the broad array of dietary, microbiologic, and toxigenic stimuli present within the intestinal lumen. When the degree of mucosal inflammation is severe enough to affect the absorptive and secretory function of the intestine, diarrhea ensues.

A number of immune defects or imbalances can affect the intestine (**Table 1**, part D). Inflammatory bowel disease is example of an inflammatory diarrhea that is likely the result of a genetically driven dysregulated immune response to the lumenal environment. It is also likely that genetic predisposition may leave some individuals vulnerable to an exaggerated immune response to dietary antigens that are usually not perceived to be a threat to intestinal function. This may explain the incidence of allergic enteropathies in some children. In patients with celiac disease, or gluten-sensitive enteropathy, there is an immune-mediated response to a protein present in wheat and related grain products. Although these patients can show marked diarrhea, they more commonly present with a failure to thrive precipitated by the introduction of wheat-containing solid foods between 6 and 9 months of age.

Autoimmune disease can target the intestinal epithelium itself and antibodies directed against enterocytes contribute to the severe inflammation and tissue destruction observed histologically in these patients. The IPEX syndrome is an X-linked autoimmune enteropathy that is associated with polyendocrinopathy and results in high morbidity and mortality. The gene defect is thought to lie within the *FOXP3* gene and it has been shown to encode the protein scurfin, a regulator of T-cell function in mice. The important role played by lymphocytes in maintaining intestinal barrier function can be appreciated in the context of bone-marrow transplant recipients. Diarrhea is a major feature of graft-vs.-host disease, a clinical condition in which donor lymphocytes recognize host intestinal epithelial cells as being foreign. Activated immunocytes subsequently initiate a destructive process that is manifest histologically as increased epithelial cell apoptosis and clinically as a secretory or inflammatory diarrhea.

Noninflammatory Diarrheas

Children can also suffer from diarrhea that is neither infectious nor inflammatory in nature. These diarrheal illnesses can be broadly categorized into congenital or acquired forms (**Table 1**, part E). Congenital diarrheas are most often the result of abnormal gene expression, resulting in a clinical presentation within the first week of life. Congenital chloride diarrhea is caused by a mutation in the down-regulated in adenoma (*DRA*) gene, thought to be a colonic chloride transporter. This disease presents uniformly *in utero* with polyhydramnios. Severe diarrhea and abdominal distension appear shortly after birth and profound electrolyte disturbances can occur in these patients if not resuscitated promptly. In contrast, the cause of congenital sodium diarrhea is not known but is thought to be due to a functional uncoupling of sodium and hydrogen exchange in the intestine. No mutations have been described in the known Na^+/H^+ exchangers in the intestine to date. The clinical presentation of congenital sodium diarrhea is similar to congenital chloride diarrhea with the exception that stool chloride levels in these patients are typically lower and the stool pH tends to be more alkaline. In addition to defects in ion transporters, there have been a number of diseases that have been described with altered transport of glucose, galactose, and amino acids. Gastrointestinal symptoms vary from defect to defect. Amino acid transport defects often have extraintestinal manifestations whose consequences far outweigh changes in bowel patterns.

Congenital diarrheas can also be caused by genetic defects that result in the malabsorption of the products of digestion such as carbohydrates and fat. Congenital disaccharidase deficiencies are rare and result in an osmotically driven diarrhea. Much more common are the transient and secondary deficiencies in mucosal disaccharidase levels that result from small intestinal injury or inflammation. Fat malabsorption can also present with diarrhea of variable severity. Congenital fat malabsorption can be the result of pancreatic insufficiency, seen in patients with cystic fibrosis, or due to specific genetic defects such as abetalipoproteinemia. Fat malabsorption is characterized by varying degrees of greasy and malodorous stools. Finally, congenital disorders of the intestinal architecture can lead to diarrhea. Microvillus inclusion disease is a rare autosomal recessive disease that is characterized by severe watery diarrhea at birth. Diagnosis is based on a histologic demonstration of marked or complete villous atrophy and electron microscopic evidence of intracellular microvillus inclusions and absent or rare microvilli.

There are multiple acquired forms of pediatric diarrhea that can be characterized as being noninfectious and noninflammatory in nature. Often, these diarrheas result from a predisposing insult that diminishes the ability of the intestinal mucosa to absorb nutrients, thereby contributing to an osmotic diarrhea. The most common example of this is toddler's diarrhea or chronic nonspecific diarrhea of childhood. There is no underlying inflammatory or biochemical abnormality that drives the increased stool output seen in these young children. In many cases, these patients will respond to a reduced dietary intake of fruit juices. Because many of these juices contain large amounts of sorbitol, an indigestible carbohydrate, they can induce an osmotic diarrhea. As such, the diarrhea will resolve in most patients within a few days after removal of the offending juice. Other examples of acquired and primarily noninflammatory diarrheas that fall into this category include antibiotic-associated diarrhea, short bowel syndrome, and small bowel bacterial overgrowth. Additionally, Münchausen's syndrome-by-proxy must always be considered in children with diarrhea and no predisposing factors.

Laboratory Evaluation of Diarrhea

Laboratory evaluation of the pediatric patient with diarrhea varies with the suspected cause and is dictated by the clinical picture. Any suspicions about potential inflammation or bacterial infection should be addressed immediately. Evaluation of acute diarrhea is usually limited to cases in which a given patient is presenting with systemic symptoms or comorbidities. Chronic diarrhea must always be evaluated, especially in the context of poor growth or malnutrition. An evaluation that proceeds in a logical and stepwise manner generally results in the most expedient and cost-effective diagnosis.

The first step in the evaluation process is to determine whether or not the presenting patient's symptoms are most consistent with an inflammatory or noninflammatory process. This can be done by an examination of the stool for gross or occult blood or the presence of fecal leukocytes. Previous studies have also demonstrated the sensitivity and specificity of biochemical assays for fecal lactoferrin, a constituent of neutrophil granules. Patients with infectious or inflammatory diarrhea will typically present with rectal bleeding or overt (positive fecal leukocyte smear) or biochemical evidence (lactoferrin) of fecal white blood cells. In contrast, these studies should be negative in patients with noninflammatory (viral, osmotic, or secretory) diarrheal disease. Nonetheless, although these markers may increase the yield of sending stool cultures, they do not exclude intestinal inflammation and any final decision about pursuing an infectious workup must be made on clinical grounds.

If there is clinical or biochemical evidence of an inflammatory process, then routine stool cultures remain the gold standard in the search for a bacterial cause of diarrhea. Most hospital-based laboratories have a standard panel of cultures associated with common pathogens including *Campylobacter*, *Shigella*, *Salmonella*, and *Yersinia enterocolitica*. Many hospitals also routinely screen for *E. coli* O157:H7. The identification of some pathogens relies on the detection of a particular toxin that is produced by the bacteria and released into the stool. *C. difficile* is perhaps the best recognized pathogen in this class.

The diagnosis of parasitic disease is most often made by a close microscopic evaluation of the stool for ova and parasites. The identification of *Giardia* and Cryptosporidia has been further facilitated by the development of enzyme-linked immunosorbent assay (ELISA)-based stool tests. It is imperative to know a specific laboratory's capabilities and limitations prior to interpreting the results of any stool, toxin, or parasitic studies.

Most 'noninflammatory' diarrheal disease is viral in nature. However, routine evaluation of stool for viral pathogens is not often useful because of the self-limiting nature of the disease process in the vast majority of patients, the specialized nature of obtaining viral cultures, and the expense of detecting specific viral pathogens. One notable exception is the rotavirus stool antigen test. This commercially available ELISA-based test provides relatively rapid results that can assist both in patient care and in making decisions about the need for isolation of hospitalized patients. Other viral stool tests include polymerase chain reaction-based screening for viral DNA in the case of adenovirus. However, these more costly and specialized tests are typically reserved for the evaluation of immunocompromised patients, in whom targeted supportive or antiviral therapy is much more critical.

Characterization of the stool can be helpful for determining the nature of noninflammatory diarrheal illness. Stool evaluation for fat, pH, and reducing substances is important in determining whether or not there is an underlying malabsorptive process. The presence of 'neutral' fat in the stool suggests some deficiency in the production or delivery of pancreatic (lipase) or hepatic (bile acid) secretions into the intestinal lumen. An increase in 'split' fat in the stool indicates a primary inability of enterocytes to perform fat absorption. Reducing substances are the result of undigested carbohydrates making their way into the large intestine. The presence of these fecal sugars can be readily assessed with commercially available colorimetric strips or test solutions. It must be remembered that sucrose is a nonreducing sugar. As such, stool must first be pretreated with an acid solution to make this nonreducing sugar detectable. Undigested carbohydrates, as well as dietary fiber, are consumed by bacteria in the large bowel and generate short-chain fatty acids. Carbohydrate malabsorption can therefore also be assessed by a fall in stool pH.

Stool electrolytes can help to determine whether or not a diarrheal process is secretory in nature. In general, a stool Na^+ concentration of greater than $70\,mEq\,l^{-1}$ is indicative of a secretory process. The stool osmotic gap, calculated by:

$$([Na^+] + [K^+]) \times 2 - \text{stool osmolarity}$$

where $[Na^+]$ = concentration of Na and $[K^+]$ = concentration of K are useful in distinguishing between osmotic and secretory diarrheal disease. An osmotic gap greater than $100\,mosm\,l^{-1}$ are suggests an underlying osmotic process. Similarly, whereas osmotic diarrhea will typically respond to a dietary fast, secretory diarrheal diseases are driven by processes that are independent of exogenous (dietary or pharmaceutical) factors.

The ability to study the large and small intestine of patients using videoscopic endoscopy has greatly advanced the ability to diagnose and treat diarrheal disease in pediatric and adult patients. Clinicians are now able to assess the gross appearance of the lining of the small and large intestine, obtain biopsy samples for histologic examination, measure directly mucosal disaccharidase levels, collect pancreatic and biliary secretions, and sample fluid from the small intestine for quantitative culture.

Blood tests can often prove to be useful adjuncts to stool studies. Peripheral eosinophilia may point to an underlying allergic disease. Decreased serum albumin levels can suggest malnutrition or a protein-losing enteropathy. Specialized serum tests such as the detection of antibodies directed against tissue transglutaminase are highly predictive of celiac disease. However, for most patients, blood work plays a supportive role in the workup of diarrheal disease. Results from serologic studies most often suggest an etiology that will need to be confirmed by more definite stool or endoscopic studies.

Treatment of Diarrheal Disease

The treatment of pediatric diarrheal disease can be divided into symptomatic and curative therapies. First and foremost in the treatment of any child with diarrhea is a prompt assessment of hydration status. For most cases of mild to moderate diarrhea, oral rehydration solutions are the first line of therapy. When oral intake is limited secondary to an altered mental status or when severe dehydration or shock is present, intravenous replacement of fluid and electrolytes can be lifesaving. Once the patient is adequately hydrated, the diet may be readily advanced. The provision of adequate calories is critical to maintain an anabolic state that will provide the metabolic fuel necessary to promote epithelial restitution. The advantages of enteral supplementation should not be overlooked as lumenal contents have been shown to be trophic to the intestinal epithelium. A transient lactose intolerance may occur in either acute or chronic diarrhea. This can be addressed using soy, rice-based, or lactose-free milk products. High-fructose and sorbitol-containing drinks are palatable, but should be avoided due to the increased osmotic load they place on an already compromised epithelial lining. Other supportive measures that have been used include antisecretory agents, antimotility agents, and resin binders. These agents decrease overall stool output by slowing intestinal transit. Although clinically beneficial in most cases, clinicians must be wary of the possibility that these agents can contribute to third-spacing of body fluid in distended and pharmacologically atonic intestinal loops.

Specific therapies that are designed to treat the underlying cause of diarrhea can be employed. This includes antibiotic use in certain forms of infectious diarrheas. In general, however, antibiotics should be avoided in patients with diarrheal disease unless there are systemic consequences of the diarrhea, such as that observed with *Salmonella* infections in infants and the elderly. Inappropriate antibiotic use can lead to resistant organisms or prolong the carrier state. Notable exceptions include infectious diarrheas that may become chronic if left untreated, such as diarrhea caused by *C. difficile* and *G. lamblia*.

Other specific therapies for diarrheal disease in pediatric patients include the following: immunosuppression in the immunologically mediated diarrheas such as inflammatory bowel disease or autoimmune enteropathy; specific replacement of electrolytes in the case of the congenital chloride and sodium diarrheas; or enzyme replacement therapy in patients with pancreatic insufficiency or lactose intolerance. Removal of an offending agent, such as gluten-containing foods in celiac disease, lactose in lactase deficiency, or specific dietary antigens in congenital or acquired protein intolerances, can be critical in certain diarrheal illnesses.

Summary

The intestine is a site of competing physiologic processes including salt and water secretion, nutrient absorption, and immune surveillance. Stool output is subsequently the net product of opposing secretory and absorptive capacities that are separated geographically along the length of the intestine as well as along the length of the crypt–villus axis. Any disruption of these tightly regulated homeostatic processes can lead to altered stool formation and the development of pathologic diarrhea. In most cases, these illnesses are self-limited in nature and respond favorably to supportive measures. Nonetheless, pediatric diarrheal diseases remain a significant cause of morbidity and mortality worldwide.

The diagnostic approach to diarrheal disease in children differs substantially from that pursued in other age groups. Consideration must be given to congenital or developmental etiologies not seen in adult populations. Moreover, because children are still growing, the impact of chronic diarrheal processes on linear growth and physical development must also be addressed. Evaluation of diarrheal disease in pediatric patients should proceed in a stepwise fashion that begins with an indepth clinical history and includes a limited number of microbiologic and biochemical tests. Physicians with a firm grasp of the epidemiology and pathogenesis of diarrheal illness in children will be better positioned to pursue a rational approach to the diagnosis and management of their pediatric patients with these common and potentially debilitating illnesses.

See also: Immune System and Immunodeficiency.

Suggested Readings

American Academy of Pediatrics. Provisional Committee on Quality Improvement, Sub-committee on Acute Gastroenteritis (1996) Practice parameter: The management of acute gastroenteritis in young children. *Pediatrics* 97: 424–435.
Corrigan JJ and Boineau FG (2001) Hemolytic–uremic syndrome. *Pediatrics in Review* 22: 365–369.
Fuller CM, Ji HL, Tousson A, Elble RC, Pauli BU, and Benos DJ (2001) Ca(2+)-activated Cl(−) channels: A newly emerging anion transport family. *Pfluger's Archive* 443: S107–S110.
Guandalini S (2000) Acute diarrhea. In: Walker WA, Drurie PR, Hamilton JR, and Watkins JB (eds.) *Pediatric Gastro-Intestinal Disease*, pp. 28–38. Lewiston, NY: B. C. Decker.
Jensen BS, Strobaek D, Olesen SP, and Christophersen P (2001) The Ca^{2+}-activated K$^+$ channel of intermediate conductance: A molecular target for novel treatments? *Current Drug Targets* 2: 401–422.
Keely SJ and Barrett KE (2000) Regulation of chloride secretion: Novel pathways and messengers. *Annals of New York Academy of Sciences* 915: 67–76.
Ramaswamy K and Jacobson K (2001) Infectious diarrhea in children. *Gastroenterol. Clinics of North America* 30: 611–624.
Rudolph JA and Cohen MB (1999) New causes and treatments for infectious diarrhea in children. *Current Gastroenterology Reports* 1: 238–244.
Sandhu BK (2001) Practical guidelines for the management of gastroenteritis in children. *Journal of Pediatric Gastroenterology and Nutrition* 33: S36–S39.

Schroeder BC, Waldegger S, Fehr S, *et al.* (2000) A constitutively open potassium channel formed by KCNQ1 and KCNE3. *Nature* 403: 196–199.

Sellin JH (1993) Intestinal electrolyte absorption and secretion. In: Feldman M, Sharshmidt BF, and Sleisenger MH (eds.) *Gastrointestinal and Liver Disease.* pp. 1451–1471. Philadelphia, PA: W. B. Saunders.

Sicherer SH (2002) Food allergy. *Lancet* 360: 701–710.

Vanderhoof JA (1998) Chronic diarrhea. *Pediatrics in Review* 19: 418–422.

Velázquez FR, Matson DO, Guerrero ML, *et al.* (2000) Serum antibody as a marker of protection against natural rotavirus infection and disease. *Journal of Infections Diseases* 182: 1602–1609.

Wildin RS, Smyk-Pearson S, and Filipovich AH (2002) Clinical and molecular features of the immunodysregulation, polyendocrinopathy, enteropathy, X linked (IPEX) syndrome. *Journal of Medical Genetics* 39: 537–545.

Down Syndrome

D J Fidler, Colorado State University, Fort Collins, CO, USA

Glossary

Attachment – An enduring bond between a child and his or her caregiver.

Autism – A neurodevelopmental disorder that is manifested in terms of deficits in core social relatedness, language and communication deficits, and narrow/repetitive interests.

Behavioral phenotype – The observable expression of behavioral traits; in this case a profile of behaviors associated with a specific genetic disorder.

Genotype – The genetic make-up, manifested in the form of genes on chromosomes, of an organism.

Joint attention – The use of verbal or nonverbal communicative forms (eye contact, gesture, vocalization) to direct and focus a partner's attention on an object or an event with the purpose of social sharing.

Nondisjunction – When paired homologs fail to migrate to different cells during cell meiotic division.

Nonverbal requesting – The use of verbal or nonverbal communicative forms (eye contact, gesture, vocalization) to regulate another's behavior in order to obtain object, initiate action.

Phenotype – The observable expression of traits, based on genetic make-up and environmental influences.

Introduction

Down syndrome is a genetic syndrome, occurring in from 1 in 650 to 1 in 1000 live births. In 95% of cases, Down syndrome is caused by nondisjunction during cell division, resulting in an extra chromosome 21 (trisomy 21). Most cases of Down syndrome involve a nondisjunction during the first meiotic cell division, with mothers contributing the extra chromosome in 85% of cases. When nondisjunction occurs after fertilization, this leads to mosaic Down syndrome, where one line of cells in the developing fetus contains the extra copy of chromosome 21 and a second line of cells in the developing fetus does not. In a small percentage of cases, Down syndrome is caused by a translocation of genetic material on chromosome 21. Risk for Down syndrome is associated with maternal age. The pathways from genotype to phenotype in Down syndrome are currently not well characterized. However, current studies aim to identify how the additional chromosomal material on chromosome 21 impacts upon the developmental process.

Down syndrome was first described in the 1860s by John Langdon Down, who observed the clustering of specific physical and psychological features in a subgroup of individuals with cognitive impairments in medical settings. At that time, an unfortunate association was made between the craniofacial appearance of individuals with this clustering of symptoms and the physical features of specific ethnic groups. Modern genetic research has completely dispelled any a link between ethnic origin and Down syndrome. The discovery of the chromosomal cause of Down syndrome (trisomy 21) was made in 1959 by Jerome LeJeune. Since then, many notable advances have been made in this population, including increases in the life expectancy of individuals with Down syndrome (average life expectancy in the late 50s), as well as improvements in developmental outcomes and quality of life.

Though Down syndrome can be diagnosed clinically, a chromosome analysis is still considered necessary in order to confirm the clinical impression and to identify the underlying type of chromosome disorder. Common physical features associated with Down syndrome include a distinctive craniofacial structure, brachycephaly (abnormally wide head shape), short neck, congenital heart defects, anomalies of the extremities, muscular hypotonia, and musculoskeletal hyperflexibility. Most individuals with Down syndrome are born with a unique craniofacial appearance that includes palpebral fissures, epicanthal folds, Brushfield spots, flat nasal bridge, dysplastic ear, and a high arched palate.

Medical Issues in Early Development

Thorough physical examinations are recommended throughout the neonatal period, with careful monitoring of the systems that are most frequently impaired in this population. Approximately 50% of individuals with Down syndrome are born with congenital heart disease, with atrioventricular defects most commonly observed. Because of these vulnerabilities, examination by a pediatric cardiologist is recommended shortly after birth and monitoring is recommended throughout childhood. Cardiac anomalies are the main cause of death in children with Down syndrome, especially within the first 2 years of life. Beyond heart-related issues, routine screening for errors of metabolism and compromised thyroid function are recommended though the first few years of life. Children with Down syndrome are also vulnerable to congenital abnormalities of the gastrointestinal tract. A small number (3–4%) of infants with Down syndrome are born with congenital cataracts, which should be corrected with glasses or contact lenses.

Behavioral Features in Young Children with Down Syndrome

Beyond these health issues, there is evidence that Down syndrome predisposes children to a distinct behavioral phenotype (profile of behavioral outcomes). Research findings since the late 1960s suggest that individuals with Down syndrome are predisposed to relative strengths in visual processing, receptive language, and some aspects of social relatedness. Relative deficits have been reported in the areas of verbal processing, expressive language, and some aspects of motor functioning (see **Table 1**). More

recent studies have also explored how Down syndrome impacts the development of problem-solving skills and personality motivation as well. It is important to note that not every individual with Down syndrome will show all aspects of the behavioral profile. Rather, the likelihood that individuals with Down syndrome will show this pattern of outcomes is elevated relative to other children with developmental disabilities.

This article focuses on the manifestations of these phenotypic outcomes in early childhood. While a great deal of research has been conducted on older children, adolescents, and adults, existing research on early development in Down syndrome has shed light on how these phenotypic outcomes emerge and develop over time. Rather than considering these areas of strength and weakness as static outcomes in middle childhood and adulthood, the developmental approach can offer a picture of the early manifestations of later, more-pronounced outcomes. Identifying these early pathways gives researchers and practitioners a critical opportunity to target these early pathways before they develop and become more pronounced in later ages.

Cognition

Overall Intelligence Quotient

The majority of children with Down syndrome score in the mild (55–70) to moderate (40–55) range of cognitive impairment, though the range of outcomes includes mild-to-profound impairments. Over the first few years of life, most children with Down syndrome make steady gains in mental age, but they do not make these gains at the same rate as other children without disabilities. Thus, their Intelligence Quotient (IQ) scores tend to become gradually lower throughout childhood. Longitudinal studies report mean IQs in the 60s or 70s in children under the age of 3 years and mean IQs in the 40s and lower 50s in children aged 5–7 years. By the time children are between 9 and 11 years, studies report average IQs in the upper 30s and lower 40s. Two points should be noted. First, children with idiopathic mental retardation do not show this pattern of decline. Thus, this developmental trajectory appears to be somewhat specific to children with Down syndrome. Second, these IQ declines do not

Table 1   Phenotypic outcomes associated with Down syndrome

Developmental domain	Phenotypic outcome
Cognition	Visual > verbal processing; deficits in instrumental thinking; cognitive slowing
Speech, language, and communication	Receptive > expressive language; strengths in joint attention; deficits in nonverbal requesting
Social functioning	Strengths in core social relatedness; higher rates of insecure attachment
Motor development	Hypotonia; hyperflexbility; deficits in motor planning
Maladaptive behavior	Increased risk for comorbid autism spectrum disorder
Personality, motivation	Decreased persistence; inconsistent performances
Families/parenting	Lower levels of family stress than other disabilities; maternal directiveness

reflect a loss of skills or developmental regressions in Down syndrome. Rather, children with Down syndrome appear to be making gains at increasingly slower pace; thus, the differential between their performance and those performed by typically developing children becomes more pronounced over time. There is some controversy regarding whether children with Down syndrome are following a delayed or deviant pathway of development. Nonetheless, in most cases, children with Down syndrome will continue to show a differential between their chronological and developmental ages throughout their lives.

Instrumental thinking and problem solving

Older children with Down syndrome show atypical performance on goal-oriented problem-solving tasks in laboratory settings, like puzzle completion. But in young children with Down syndrome, more subtle evidence of an emerging deficit in problem solving can be observed with close examination. Two early components of problem solving will be considered: the ability to represent goals, and the ability to chain behaviors together strategically in order to achieve those goals. While there is relatively little evidence that children with Down syndrome show difficulty with the ability to represent goals, young children with Down syndrome may show delays in the foundational skills related to strategizing.

In studies of sensorimotor development, infants with Down syndrome have been shown to develop competently in some areas, with sequences and structures observed as similar to development in typically developing infants, albeit in a delayed fashion. However, in the area of means–end thinking, infants with Down syndrome have been shown to develop more slowly, and there is evidence that they demonstrate unusual developmental structures in this area as well. For example, unlike typically developing children, milestones in the area of means–end performance early in infancy in Down syndrome are statistically unrelated to milestones achieved later in infancy. In addition, infants with Down syndrome take longer to transition from one stage to the next in the area of means–end thinking than they do in other areas of sensorimotor development. These difficulties seem to persist beyond infancy, as toddlers with Down syndrome show shorter goal-directed chains of behavior and poorer-quality strategies on problem-solving tasks. Instrumental thinking deficits may also be observed in the early communicative profile of young children with Down syndrome, who tend to show difficulties with nonverbal requesting, an instrumental communicative behavior that is associated with means–end thinking.

Information Processing

Research on information processing in older individuals with Down syndrome suggests that visual processing is an area of relative strength and verbal processing is an area of distinct challenge. While there is only limited information on functioning in these domains during early development, infants with Down syndrome may show subtle evidence of this profile in some ways as well. Competence in the area of visual imitation and some components of visual memory have been reported in some studies, while other areas, such as visual acuity, visual exploration, and the development of eye contact, seem to be relatively delayed. Early auditory/verbal processing appears to already be impaired, as atypical auditory brainstem responses have been reported in infants with Down syndrome, and poor vocal imitation (not visual; see below) has been reported in this population as well.

It is important to note that these findings are modest evidence for early manifestation of later phenotypic outcomes, and it may be that the true early forms of this profile only become evident later in development. Furthermore, while these findings have been reported in studies of specific areas of functioning in isolation, studies that attempt to compare early performances in auditory and visual processing in infancy and toddlerhood do not report pronounced dissociations at these early stages of development. This may be because the split is truly not evident at this early stage of development, or these findings may be related to the measures selected, which may confound the measurement of visual performances with other receptive skills.

Speech, Language, and Communication

Speech and language skills are delayed relative to nonverbal abilities in young children with Down syndrome. In terms of speech and expressive language, atypical vocalizing is already evident in infants with Down syndrome from 2 to 12 months, who produce atypical prelinguistic phrases compared to those produced by typically developing infants. In contrast with the relatively strong visual imitative competence in young children with Down syndrome, vocal imitation is attenuated. Decreased vocal imitation in Down syndrome has been shown to be associated with lower expressive and receptive language skills.

In the first 6 months of life, infants with Down syndrome also produce more nonspeech-like sounds than speech-like sounds, which may negatively impact the later development of normal vocal behavior. Additionally, delays in age of onset of canonical babbling have been found in some studies of development in infants with Down syndrome. The early development of canonical babbling is linked to later communication milestones, as the age of onset of canonical babbling is correlated with later performances on measures of early social communication in toddlerhood. Several factors may contribute to delayed babbling in Down syndrome, including maturational delay, hypotonia, and conductive hearing loss in infancy.

Nevertheless, other aspects of prelinguistic vocal development seem to be on par with typically developing infants, including the amount of vocalization produced, developmental timetable of vocalizations, and characteristics of consonants and vowels produced during babbling. The rhythmic organization of babbling in infancy in Down syndrome is similar to patterns observed in typically developing infants; however, infants with Down syndrome generally take longer to finish a prelinguistic phrase. These slower, longer vocal turns may contribute to the increased rates of conversational 'clashes' with a parent, a finding often observed in parent–infant dyads in this population.

Children with Down syndrome generally show delays in the transition from prelinguistic communication to meaningful speech. Studies report an average productive (signed or spoken) vocabulary of 28 words at 24 months, 116 words at 36 months, 248 words at 48 months, and 330 words at 72 months. Other studies that include only spoken (not signed) vocabulary words report that only 12% of 1-year-olds with Down syndrome have produced their first words, and only 53% of 4-year-old children have vocabularies larger than 50 words, a level that would be on par with a typically developing 16-month-old child. This profile appears to be delayed even when compared to children with other developmental disabilities at the same overall developmental level.

There is some debate regarding whether children with Down syndrome have the same 'vocabulary spurt' observed in typically developing children. Some researchers have reported that vocabulary growth in Down syndrome does follow an exponential trajectory, but it takes place later in development than would be expected based on overall mental age. Others argue that only some children with Down syndrome show such a vocabulary spurt, but vocabulary acquisition does not follow the exponential trajectory of a vocabulary spurt in many other individuals with Down syndrome.

Despite showing pronounced delays in expressive language, receptive language seems to develop with relative competence in Down syndrome, with the majority 0–5-year-old children showing mental-age-appropriate receptive language skills. While the majority, but not all, children with Down syndrome show a profile of receptive over expressive language, there may be different pathways leading to this outcome. One group of children with Down syndrome may show expressive language impairments from the onset of first words, while other children may only begin to show pronounced lags when the morphosyntactic (grammatical) demands of more complex language become a factor.

Most children with Down syndrome begin to generate two and three word utterances by the time they are 3 or 4 years old. In general, these utterances are similar to the early word combinations observed in typically developing children. Early grammar develops slowly and is related to vocabulary size, while more complex grammar is specifically delayed relative to vocabulary. Some have noted the paradox that while children with Down syndrome do not have difficulties with word order in simple utterances, many have difficulties with more complex morphosyntactic forms (third person, past tense) later in development.

It has also been noted that children with Down syndrome often opt to use short, telegraphic sentences rather than more complex syntactic forms, a finding that has been linked to both atypical language development and motivational/persistence issues in this population. Young children with Down syndrome produce fewer grammatical words (e.g., prepositions) than would be expected for their developmental level, a finding that persists throughout development. Case reports in the literature describe slow and steady syntactic development until roughly 5 years of age, after which children may hit a plateau. Yet, though children with Down syndrome may show less-complex morphosyntactic forms as they develop, it has been noted that they use language in pragmatically appropriate ways for their mental age. Thus, early in development, children with Down syndrome appear to be using language to achieve the same types of interpersonal goals as other children without Down syndrome at the same developmental level.

In terms of early communicative competence, some areas seem to be intact while others are impaired. Referential pointing in young children with Down syndrome emerges prior to the production of referential language, a sequence observed in typically developing children. Young children with Down syndrome show mental age-appropriate levels of nonverbal joint attention according to most studies. In addition, despite deficits in expressive language development, the early use of gestures in children with Down syndrome seems to be intact, with some reports of relatively stronger gestures in young children with Down syndrome compared with controls matched for word comprehension. Children with Down syndrome have been shown to use more advanced gestures than expected based on their general language development levels, and a wider repertoire of functional, symbolic, and pretending gestures than typically developing children at the same language level.

Yet, even in the context of these communicative strengths, other aspects of early communicative competence seem to be impaired. In particular, young children with Down syndrome show deficits in nonverbal requesting behaviors, or the use of eye contact, gesture, or vocalization for instrumental purposes. Rates of nonverbal requesting across a structured social communication assessment are associated with the quality of strategies performed by children with Down syndrome on a nonverbal problem-solving task. This suggests that deficits in nonverbal requesting may stem primarily from difficulties with early instrumental thinking, and not difficulties with early pragmatics or nonverbal communication.

Social–Emotional Development

There is evidence that infants with Down syndrome follow a typical pathway in the development of visual imitation in infancy. Some 1- and 3-month-old infants with Down syndrome have been found to imitate facial displays (tongue protrusions and mouth openings), as typically developing infants do. It is argued that these skills enable young infants with Down syndrome to engage dyadically with a caregiver in competent ways that establish the origins of social relatedness.

Later into infancy, increased looking directed at parents has been observed in studies of infants at 4, 6, and 9 months of age. Increased looking in infants with Down syndrome has also been shown in ambiguous situations, but not in social referencing contexts. Infants with Down syndrome also produce more vocalizations (emotional, melodic) when interacting with people rather than objects. Toddlers and preschoolers with Down syndrome display relative strengths in certain types of nonverbal social interaction including more reciprocal turn taking and other social initiations (object shows, invitations) when compared with typically developing children.

While very young children with Down syndrome show less exploratory behavior with toys, their trajectory of play development is similar to that observed in typically developing children. As they develop, children with Down syndrome spend less time engaging in functional play with objects and increase the amount of time they spend engaged in sociodramatic and symbolic play. When they do reach the symbolic play stage, children with Down syndrome show pattern of themes and language usage in their play similar to those observed in typically developing children.

In terms of attachment, conflicting accounts of outcomes have been reported. Some studies suggest that children with Down syndrome and MA-matched children without Down syndrome show similar attachment behaviors during Ainsworth's strange situation. In addition, a typical positive association between distress intensity and contact maintenance, and a negative association between distress intensity and distance interaction is observed in this population, suggesting that the organization of attachment behavior in Down syndrome is structured in similar ways to the organization of attachment in typically developing children.

Other reports suggest that attachment in Down syndrome is unlike attachment in typically developing children. Children with Down syndrome show less intense and shorter duration separation distress than children at similar mental and chronological ages. They also show less proximity seeking, contact maintenance, and resistance than other children. In terms of attachment quality, the frequency of insecure attachments in Down syndrome may be elevated compared to other children with disabilities at similar developmental levels. According to some reports, roughly 45% of children with Down syndrome are rated as type B (secure) in their attachment. Another large percentage of children are classified as type D (insecure unclassifiable), a finding that has been attributed to diminished negative reactivity in young children with Down syndrome. As a result, some suggest that the strange situation may not be an appropriate measure of attachment in this population. Others argue that increased numbers of category D classifications is attributed to hypotonia, ataxia, abnormal motoric responses in children with Down syndrome, and as a result, it is suggested that motor atypicalities be considered in the larger picture of attachment classification in this population.

The emotional displays of young children with Down syndrome were first described as muted relative to typically developing infants. Subsequent studies conducted with more objective coding systems reported that frequent low-intensity smiling in young children with Down syndrome occurred in the context of typical rates of other emotional displays, including high-intensity smiling. In addition, young children with Down syndrome are also more likely to send ambiguous nonverbal signals that are more difficult for adults to interpret than the signals of other children at similar developmental levels.

Two important issues should be considered in the exploration of early social development in Down syndrome. While early social skills seem to be developing with some measure of competence in young children with Down syndrome, it is important to acknowledge that such strengths may not persist later in development, as the demands of social interactions become more sophisticated and cognitively mediated. In addition, emerging relative strength in social functioning may interact with other areas of development that are lagging behind. There is evidence that from 12 to 30 months, young children with Down syndrome make greater gains in the area of social development than in the areas of motor development and cognitive development. It may be that young children with Down syndrome come to rely on their strengths in social functioning and adopt social strategies at times when other instrumental strategies may be more effective or appropriate. A discussion of this profile is presented in the following section.

Temperament, Personality, and Motivation

Studies of temperament in young children report no temperament differences between infants with Down syndrome and typical infants in early infancy (at 2 months), and later at 12–36 months. Other studies, however, report that toddlers with Down syndrome are rated as of more positive mood, more rhythmic, and less intense than CA-matched children. These findings echo the findings of increased predictability, increased positive mood, and decreased persistence in older children with Down syndrome. However, nearly one-third of young children with Down syndrome show signs of difficult temperament as well, a possible precursor to stubbornness and other behavior problems.

There may also be a connection between problem solving and motivational orientation in Down syndrome, where children with poor problem-solving skills may abandon challenging tasks more readily than children who can strategize more effectively. When faced with cognitive challenges, many children with Down syndrome avoid the tasks with both positive and negative behaviors. In young children, these behaviors can include refusing to look at a task, struggling out of a chair, or sudden crying behavior. Older children may use their relative strengths in social functioning to engage the experimenter and distract them from the task at hand. These behaviors may contribute to inconsistent performances observed over time in children with Down syndrome, who may select appropriate or inappropriate behavioral strategies as a function of motivation related to a given activity.

Poorer mastery motivation continues to be evident throughout early development in Down syndrome. Preschooler children show lower levels of task persistence and higher levels of off-task behavior during simple play tasks than MA-matched comparison group children. Toddlers with Down syndrome show increased rates of toy rejection, indicating that 'quitting out behaviors' still impact performance at this point in development. Children with Down syndrome also show lower levels of causality pleasure, exhibiting fewer positive facial displays during goal-directed mastery behaviors than developmentally matched typically developing children.

Yet, other findings suggest that by the time they reach 3–4 years of age, most children with Down syndrome place great value on success during goal-directed tasks. Compared with developmentally matched children, preschool-aged children with Down syndrome show higher rates of pride-related displays during laboratory tasks. Children with Down syndrome show more positive affect, more frequent pauses to regard their finished product, and increased referencing of their caregiver upon successfully completing their task than other children at similar developmental levels. This suggests that though children with Down syndrome may have greater difficulty reaching desired goals, they are no less rewarded by the experience of having achieved their goals than other children.

Motor Development

Motor development is an area of pronounced delay in many children with Down syndrome. Atypical development of reflexes, low muscle tone, and hyperflexibility are often observed in infancy. As a result of hypotonia, infants with Down syndrome often show unusual postures and leg positions. The achievement of important motor milestones is also delayed during early development in Down syndrome:

the average age for rolling over in Down syndrome is 8 months (typical = 5 months); sitting without support happens on average at 9 months (typical = 7 months); walking with support happens on average at 16 months (typical = 10 months); standing alone happens on average at 18 months (typical = 11 months); and walking alone happens on average at 19 months (typical = 12 months).

Later in early childhood, children with Down syndrome show difficulty with the development of motor planning, in the form of reaching and other essential skills. Children with Down syndrome have been shown to exhibit poorer-quality reaching strategies on an object-retrieval task, where children must reach for a desired object through the one side opening of a clear box. In order to reach efficiently, rather than coordinating eye gaze and reach, many children with Down syndrome use less optimal strategies such as looking through the open side of the box, straightening up, and then reaching for the desired object. This type of motor planning is essential for the development of efficient day-to-day adaptive skills, and thus, targeting these skills in early development may have downstream effects on important skills for later independent functioning.

Maladaptive Behavior

While children with Down syndrome show lower levels of maladaptive behavior than children with other developmental disabilities, rates of behavior problems and comorbid psychiatric diagnoses are still elevated relative to typically developing children. Disruptive disorders is the most common category of psychiatric diagnosis in individuals with Down syndrome under age 20 years (6% attention deficit disorder, 5% conduct/oppositional disorder, 6% aggressive behavior). In contrast, the most common diagnoses in adults with Down syndrome over the age of 20 years are major-depressive disorders (6%) and aggressive behavior (6%).

While temperament at 12 months is a predictor of maladaptive behavior outcomes at 45 months in children with other developmental disabilities, no such association has been observed in children with Down syndrome. The lack of association between infant temperament and later behavior problems suggests that young children with Down syndrome may make a more pronounced shift in the development of behavior problems than do typically developing children and children with other developmental disabilities. This may impact the parenting experience, as parents of children with Down syndrome may observe changes in their child's behavior that are more unexpected during early childhood, which may necessitate different parental supports to adjust to the changing needs of the child.

There is an increasing awareness of the subgroup of individuals with Down syndrome who also meet criteria for autism spectrum disorders (ASDs). Current estimates of comorbidity prevalence range between 3% and 10% of children with Down syndrome meeting criteria for autism or ASD. However, diagnosing these two disorders, especially in early childhood, remains a complex task. To meet criteria for comorbid autism or ASD and Down syndrome, problems in core social relating must be evident, not attributable to alternative explanations (such as very low cognition, very poor motor skills, or depression and mood problems) and persistent (across a variety of contexts and functioning levels). It may be that existing standardized assessments of autism symptoms may overidentify children with Down syndrome as having autism or ASDs if they function below 18 months cognitively, exhibit signs of depression, irritability, and extreme mood lability, and/ or show significant impairment with regard to initiation of motor movements. Thus, obtaining an accurate diagnosis of the presence or absence of an ASD in children with Down syndrome must be performed by a clinician with both an expertise in autism and an understanding of the complex manifestation of autism in individuals with Down syndrome.

Families of Children with Down Syndrome

Parenting Behavior

Atypical patterns are observed from the earliest measures of parent–infant interaction in Down syndrome. The establishment of eye contact is delayed by several weeks and the amount of eye contact increases at a slower pace over the first few months of life. However, once infants with Down syndrome have reached a peak level of eye contact with their caregiver, they engage in higher levels of mutual eye contact than typically developing infants. Most typically developing infants experience a decline in the amount they gaze toward their caregiver by 5 or 6 months. In contrast, some studies report infants with Down syndrome at these ages and beyond who are focused overwhelmingly on their caregiver's face, and in particular, their eyes. This higher level of eye contact is maintained throughout much of early development in Down syndrome. Mothers of infants with Down syndrome have been shown to use more tactile and kinesthetic stimulation than mothers of typically developing infants on laboratory interaction tasks. Infants with Down syndrome have also been shown to be less distressed and responsive to the still-faced paradigm than typically developing infants in laboratory settings.

During toddlerhood, parent–child relations in Down syndrome also have some unique features. Mothers of toddlers with Down syndrome make significantly more frequent unsuccessful invitations to their child for interaction. Mothers of toddlers with Down syndrome are also found to be more directive and less child-dependent

during their interactions with their children. Along these lines, mothers of children with Down syndrome have been found to take longer and more frequent turns during their parent–child interactions than other mothers. They also tend to change the topic of conversation more frequently than other mothers when interacting with their child, and they show increased rates of verbal clashing, where both mother and child speak at the same time.

However, maternal directiveness does not appear to be associated with a lack of maternal sensitivity, and maternal stimulation behaviors are associated with child's developmental level, suggesting that these strategies may be adaptive given the child's disability. In addition, maternal sensitivity has been linked to other factors, including education level and family income. In intervention studies where mothers have been taught techniques to improve their responsivity to their child, increased responsive behavior and a less intrusive style can be successfully fostered. In addition, certain child factors may impede a parent's ability to be responsive, including hypotonia, ambiguous emotional signaling, temperament, and distractibility.

Parents of preschool-aged children with Down syndrome give more praise to their children during goal-directed tasks. During laboratory tasks, parents of preschool-aged children with Down syndrome have been shown to use higher rates of praise than parents of developmentally matched typically developing children, perhaps in order to encourage their child to stay on task. In contrast, there are some reports that parents of children with Down syndrome use less positive verbalizations during naturalistic settings. Instead, in these naturalistic environments, mothers of children with Down syndrome have been found to do more explaining, modeling and demonstrating, labeling, and questioning for the purpose of teaching some concept, as well as more frequent attempts to assist their child complete tasks of daily living.

Yet other features of parenting behavior, such as parent input language, are similar across groups. For example, parents of children with Down syndrome give similar levels of language input (e.g., grammatical complexity; type of information) as mother of children at similar developmental levels without disabilities. In addition, some parenting behaviors that are considered more beneficial for typically developing children are also more beneficial for children with Down syndrome. For example, as observed in typically developing children, higher rates of joint attention in parent–child dyads are associated with greater gains in child receptive language in children with Down syndrome, too.

In general, mothers of children with Down syndrome report different goals in their interactions with their children. More often than in typically developing children, mothers of children with Down syndrome report that they feel a need to use interactions as a chance to teach their child a new skill or practice an existing one. Rather than enjoying interaction as a time to play with their time, mothers are more likely to request that their child produce higher-level behaviors than those they are producing spontaneously. This may be an adaptive parenting response given the child's developmental delays, but it may also lead to a different parenting style than observed in the general population.

Family Stress

Many parents experience life disruption and elevated stress upon receiving a diagnosis of Down syndrome for their child. This may be related to the quality of the interaction they experience with the diagnosing clinician, who may not have the counseling skills or the specific knowledge based to provide information to new parents of young children with Down syndrome. In one study, 60% of parents reported dissatisfaction with the experience of receiving their child's Down syndrome diagnosis, citing issues related to a lack of sympathy on the part of the healthcare professional, the inability of the professional to share information that would reduce anxiety, and delays in receiving information.

However, after an initial period of adjustment, families of children with Down syndrome report lower levels of stress and higher levels of rewardingness than families of children with other developmental disabilities. Some studies show similar patterns of cohesiveness and adaptation in families of children with Down syndrome and families of typically developing children. Lower levels of stress have been attributed to several possible factors: lower levels of behavior problems observed in children with Down syndrome relative to other children with disabilities, perceived maturity in Down syndrome, social relatedness in Down syndrome, age and higher socioeconomic status of parents of children with Down syndrome, and the support networks available for families of children with Down syndrome in their communities.

While cross-sectional studies of outcomes in families of children with Down syndrome have shed much light on the family experience, it may also be important to explore how the family experience changes over time. There is evidence that families of young children with Down syndrome may experience a different stress trajectory than families of other children with disabilities, starting out with lower levels of maternal stress at 1 year of age, but showing equivalent stress levels when the child reaches preschool age. Since family responses are closely associated with specific child characteristics, it may be the case that as the child's behavioral profile changes during development, and phenotypic characteristics become more pronounced, family stress responses shift.

Conclusion

Children with Down syndrome are predisposed to a specific profile of strengths and weaknesses in development, which include strengths in visual processing and social relatedness, and deficits in verbal processing, motor planning, and expressive language. Parents of children with Down syndrome are also likely to show certain parenting characteristics, often as a result of the behavioral profile associated with Down syndrome, though often families show lower levels of parenting stress than families of children with other types of developmental disabilities. Future challenges include characterizing the emergence of the Down syndrome behavioral phenotype and identifying developmental trajectories of educationally relevant areas of functioning. With a greater understanding of the nature and course of development in Down syndrome, it may be possible to develop increasingly more sophisticated interventions for children and their families.

See also: Autism Spectrum Disorders; Developmental Disabilities: Cognitive; Developmental Disabilities: Physical; Intellectual Disabilities; Learning Disabilities.

Suggested Readings

Block ME (1991) Motor development in children with Down syndrome: A review of the literature. *Adapted Physical Activity Quarterly* 8: 179–209.
Carr J (1995) *Down's Syndrome: Children Growing Up.* Cambridge: Cambridge University Press.
Dmitriev V (2001) *Early Intervention for Children with Down Syndrome: Time to Begin.* Austin: Pro-Ed.
Hodapp RM and Fidler DJ (1999) Special education and genetics: Connections for the 21st century. *Journal of Special Education* 33: 130–137.
Jarrold C, Baddeley AD, and Hewes AK (1999) Genetically dissociated components of working memory: Evidence from Down's and Williams syndrome. *Neuropsychologia* 37: 637–651.
Miller JF (1999) Profiles of language development in children with Down syndrome. In: Miller J, Leddy M, and Leavitt LA (eds.) *Improving the Communication of People with Down Syndrome*, pp. 11–40. Baltimore: Brookes Publishing Inc.
Mundy P, Sigman M, Kasari C, and Yirmiya N (1988) Nonverbal communication skills in Down syndrome children. *Child Development* 59: 235–249.
Pueschel SR and Pueschel JK (1992) *Biomedical Concerns in Persons with Down Syndrome.* Baltimore, MD: Paul H. Brookes Publishing Co.
Sigman M and Ruskin E (1999) *Monographs of the Society for Research in Child Development, 64: Continuity and Change in the Social Competence of Children with Autism, Down Syndrome, and Developmental Delays,* 114pp. Oxford: Blackwell Publishing.
Spiker D (1990) Early intervention from a developmental perspective. In: Ciccehtti D and Beeghly M (eds.) *Children with Down Syndrome: A Developmental Perspective*, pp. 424–448. New York: Cambridge University Press.

E

Endocrine System

S E Watamura, University of Denver, Denver, CO, USA

Glossary

Catecholamines – Any of a group of organic compounds (amines derived from catechol) that have important physiological effects as neurotransmitters and hormones and include epinephrine, norepinephrine, and dopamine.
Endogenous – Originating or produced within an organism, tissue, or cell.
Exogenous – Derived or developed from outside the body; originating externally.
Glucocorticoids – Any of a group of steroid hormones, such as cortisol, that are produced by the adrenal cortex; are involved in carbohydrate, protein, and fat metabolism; and have anti-inflammatory properties.
Hormone – Chemical signals secreted into the bloodstream that have effects on distant tissues.
Precursor – A biochemical substance, such as an intermediate compound in a chain of enzymatic reactions, from which a more stable or definitive product is formed.

Introduction

The endocrine system is one of two main systems in the body responsible for communication and regulation of body functions, coordinating functions such as growth, metabolism, and reproduction. The other main communication and regulation system is the nervous system. The endocrine system utilizes hormones for communication and regulation, and these are typically released into the blood. In contrast, the nervous system utilizes primarily cell-to-cell synaptic communication. While divisions are helpful for classification and specification, it is important to bear in mind the multitude of bidirectional effects between all the major systems of the body, including those between the endocrine system and the nervous system.

Hormones are chemical messengers derived from the major classes of compounds used by the body more generally, such as proteins and lipids. Endocrine coordination via the release of hormones into the blood stream presents unique problems of production, distribution, and mechanisms for action. Receptors on cell surfaces and in the nuclei of cells play a critical role in the endocrine system. Without the active participation of receptors, hormones would be incapable of executing their wide-ranging effects. Another critical aspect of the endocrine system to be discussed is regulation of hormone action via feedback loops.

Over- or under-production of hormones, autoimmune diseases, and genetic mutations can lead to a variety of endocrine disorders, some of which are life-threatening if left untreated. Diseases to be discussed below are those that are most likely to influence infant and child development, including diabetes, growth disorders, thyroid disease, adrenal insufficiency, and the rare disorder, Cushing's syndrome.

Endocrine functions also change across the lifetime, so that unique endocrine processes and profiles are found during pregnancy, in the fetus, during puberty, and in aging. Those changes that accompany pregnancy and those that are important during the fetal period will be discussed.

Endocrine System Components

Glands

A gland is a group of cells that produces and secretes chemicals. Using precursors in the blood or cell, glands create completed chemical products and release them in the body. Some glands release chemicals that act locally, for example two exocrine glands are the sweat and salivary glands that release secretions in the skin or inside the mouth. The primary glands of the endocrine system are the pituitary gland, the pineal gland, the adrenal gland, the thyroid and parathyroid glands, the pancreas, and the reproductive glands (ovaries and testes) (see **Figure 1**). Other nonendocrine organs, including the brain, heart, lungs, kidneys, liver, thymus, skin, and placenta, are also capable of producing hormones.

The hypothalamus is a region of the brain connected to the pituitary gland with short capillaries. It translates signals from the nervous system into secreted hormones that activate the pituitary to produce or inhibit specific hormones in response to the hypothalamic signal. Signals that are translated by the hypothalamus into hormones that stimulate or inhibit the pituitary are the result of both external conditions like temperature or light, and internal conditions, like fear, that have been processed by other areas of the brain and communicated to the hypothalamus by neuronal signaling. Thus, the hypothalamus serves as a critical link between the nervous system and the endocrine system.

The pituitary (also called the hypophysis) is sometimes referred to as the master gland, because it regulates the hormonal production of many other glands. It is located at the base of the brain just beneath the hypothalamus. It has two main sections, called the anterior pituitary (or adenohypophysis) and the posterior pituitary (or neurohypophysis). The anterior pituitary produces hormones that affect the thyroid, adrenal, and reproductive glands. The posterior pituitary produces antidiuretic hormone, which helps control water balance and oxytocin. The pituitary also produces endorphins, which act on the nervous system to reduce sensitivity to pain.

The two parts of the pituitary arise from very different kinds of embryonic tissue, and receive inputs from the hypothalamus in very different ways. The anterior pituitary is a classic gland in the sense that it is composed primarily of cells that secrete hormones. The anterior pituitary receives hormonal signals from the hypothalamus via a direct blood supply. The hypophyseal artery branches into a capillary bed in the lower hypothalamus, where hypothalamic hormones are secreted. This capillary bed drains into the hypothalamic-hypophyseal portal veins, which further branch into capillaries within the

anterior pituitary. Hypothalamic hormones travel the short distance from the hypothalamus to the anterior pituitary via this unique vasculature. This vasculature allows very small amounts of hypothalamic hormones to quickly and effectively signal the pituitary. In contrast, the posterior pituitary is more like an extension of the hypothalamus in that it is composed largely of the axons of hypothalamic neurons.

The pineal gland is a tiny gland located in the middle of the brain. The pineal gland produces melatonin during the dark phase of the day/night cycle. In mammals, the pineal receives signals from the suprachiasmatic nucleus (SCN) which maintains the biologic clock of the organism. The clock follows a roughly 24 h rhythm even in a continuously dark environment, however, via signals from the eye, the clock is entrained to the external day/night cycle. The pineal begins producing melatonin around 3 months after birth, and the pineal is larger in children, decreasing in size and in melatonin production after puberty.

The thyroid gland is a large gland located in the front part of the lower neck and is shaped like a bowtie or butterfly. The primary function of the thyroid is to regulate metabolism through the production of thyroid hormone. Attached to the thyroid are four glands which function together and are called the parathyroid glands. The parathyroid glands produce parathyroid hormone which, in conjunction with calcitonin released by the thyroid, regulates the level of calcium in the blood.

The adrenal glands are triangular glands, one located on top of each kidney. The adrenal glands have two anatomically and functionally distinct parts, the outer part called the adrenal cortex and the inner part called the adrenal medulla. The adrenal cortex produces glucocorticoids and mineralcorticoids. These hormones help the body regulate salt and water balance, respond to stress, participate in metabolism, regulate the immune system, and are involved in sexual development and function. The adrenal medulla produces the catecholamines epinephrine (adrenalin) and norepinephrine (noradrenalin) involved in the first line response to stress.

The pancreas produces the hormones insulin and glucagon which act together to maintain homeostasis in blood glucose levels. If blood glucose levels rise above the set-point, insulin production increases to drive glucose into cells, which decreases blood glucose, and if blood glucose levels fall below the set-point, glucagon production increases to increase blood glucose.

The reproductive glands, or gonads, are the ovaries in females and the testes in males. The ovaries are located in the pelvis and produce ova as well as release the hormones estrogen and progesterone. Both hormones are involved in healthy female sexual development, menstruation and pregnancy. The testes are located in the scrotum and produce androgens critical for healthy male sexual development, sexual behavior, and sperm production.

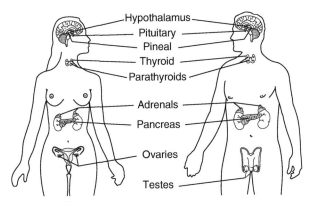

Figure 1   The endocrine system.

It is beyond the scope of this article to discuss the intricacies of each gland and the vast array of hormones produced. The focus here has been on the main glands and the best-characterized and most critical hormones. However, this necessitates leaving out the less well-characterized and more auxiliary hormones. For example, the glucocorticoid cortisol and the mineralcorticoids are mentioned; however, the adrenal cortex alone produces over 50 known steroid hormones.

Primary Endocrine Hormones

Hormones are chemical signals secreted into the blood stream that have effects on distant tissues. Hormones do not share a chemical structure and are not defined by their molecular components; rather they are defined by their actions. Hormones are produced primarily by the endocrine glands. Many hormones are produced in cascades, beginning with a signal from the hypothalamus that stimulates the pituitary to produce a hormone that then stimulates another gland (e.g., the thyroid gland, adrenal gland, or the reproductive glands) to produce a third hormone (see **Table 1** for an overview of some of the main hormones and their representative effects). Common hypothalamic hormones include corticotropin-releasing factor (CRF), gonadotropin-releasing hormone (GnRH), prolactin-releasing factor, prolactin-release inhibiting factor, growth hormone-releasing factor, somatostatin (growth hormone release inhibiting factor), and thyrotropin-releasing factor. As can be seen from their names, these hormones typically stimulate or inhibit the release of hormones by other endocrine glands.

Common pituitary hormones include oxytocin, vasopressin, adrenocorticotropin (ACTH), lipotropin (LPH), thyroid-stimulating hormone (TSH), growth hormone (GH), prolactin (PRL), luteinizing hormone (LH), and follicle-stimulating hormone (FSH). Some hormones produced by the pituitary activate tertiary hormones (e.g., ACTH activates the adrenal glands to produce cortisol), and others have primarily direct effects on target tissues, for example, oxytocin. The pineal gland produces melatonin, which is critically involved in biologic rhythms like sleep/wake behavior. The adrenal gland produces glucocorticoids and mineralcorticoids in the adrenal cortex, and epinephrine (adrenalin) and norepinephrine (noradrenalin) in the adrenal medulla. Many of these adrenal hormones are involved in the body's response to physical or psychological stress. The thyroid gland produces thyroxine (T4), which is critically involved in metabolic processes, and the parathyroid glands produce parathyroid hormone which raises blood calcium levels. The pancreas produces insulin, which works as described above to lower blood glucose levels and glucagons, which raise blood glucose levels. The reproductive glands produce estrogens, progestins, and androgens, all of which support sexual development and reproductive function.

Table 1   The major hormones of the endocrine system

Hormone	Released by	Example effects
Corticotropin-releasing factor (CRF)	Hypothalamus	Stimulates the pituitary to produce ACTH
Gonadotropin-releasing hormone (GnRH)	Hypothalamus	Stimulates the pituitary to produce FSH and LH
Growth hormone-releasing factor	Hypothalamus	Stimulates the pituitary to produce GH
Somatostatin	Hypothalamus	Stimulates the pituitary to inhibit GH and TSH
Thyrotropin-releasing factor	Hypothalamus	Stimulates the pituitary to produce TSH
Adrenocorticotropic hormone (ACTH)	Pituitary gland	Stimulates adrenal cortex to secrete glucocorticoids
Follicle-stimulating hormone (FSH)	Pituitary gland	Stimulates sex cell development (ova and sperm)
Growth hormone (GH)	Pituitary gland	Stimulates growth and metabolism
Luteinizing hormone (LH)	Pituitary gland	Stimulates ovaries and testes
Oxytocin	Pituitary gland	Stimulates uterine and mammary gland cell contractions
Prolactin (PRL)	Pituitary gland	Stimulates milk production and secretion
Thyroid-stimulating hormone (TSH)	Pituitary gland	Stimulates thyroid gland to produce thyroid hormones (T3 and T4)
Triiodothyronine (T_3) and thyroxine (T_4)	Thyroid gland	Stimulate and maintain metabolism
Parathyroid hormone (PTH)	Parathyroid glands	Raises blood calcium
Glucagon	Pancreas	Raises blood glucose
Insulin	Pancreas	Drives glucose into cells
Epinephrine and norepinephrine	Adrenal glands (medulla)	Raise blood glucose; constrict some blood vessels; increase metabolism
Glucocorticoids	Adrenal glands (cortex)	Raise blood glucose; inhibit long-term growth and restorative processes
Androgens	Testes	Support sperm formation and male secondary sex characteristics
Estrogens	Ovaries	Stimulate uterine lining growth and female secondary sex characteristics
Progesterone	Gonads	Promotes uterine lining growth
Melatonin	Pineal gland	Regulates biological rhythms

As mentioned earlier, many other organs not classified as endocrine glands also produce hormones. For example, gastrin, secretin, motilin, vasoactive intestinal peptide (VIP), somatostatin, and substance P are produced in the gastrointestinal tract; the placenta produces estrogens, progestins, and relaxin; the liver produces angiotensin II; the kidney produces calcitriol; and the heart produces atrial natriuretic peptide (ANP). While hormones are critical for health, and are capable of inducing wide-ranging effects, they are completely ineffective without appropriate receptors on target cells.

Hormone Secretion, Receptors, and Regulation

Circulating hormone levels are controlled both by the secretion pattern of glands and by binding and clearance rates. Some glands secrete hormones in short distinct pulses in response to discreet signals, for example, the secretion of insulin in response to blood glucose levels. Other hormones are secreted in rhythms coordinated by external cycles, for example, melatonin in response to day/night cycles and estrogens in response to 28-day lunar cycles. Still other hormones appear to be secreted continuously, for example, prolactin. Many hormones also have both baseline and stimulated secretion patterns, for example, cortisol is produced in basal levels following day/night cycles, and is also produced in response to stress or challenge. In the nervous system, neurons accumulate inhibitory and excitatory signals from other cells that together determine whether the particular neuron will 'fire', thus producing its own signals. Similarly, endocrine cells accumulate signals from hypothalamic hormones, peripheral hormones, nutrients, and many other mechanisms, and these accumulated signals determine the pattern and quantity of hormone secretion. This allows for subtle changes in hormone secretion in response to dynamic changes in the individual's external and internal environment.

Receptors for hormones are typically classified as either cell-surface receptors or nuclear receptors, with nuclear receptors found in the nuclei of cells. Because hormones are released into the bloodstream and are circulated all through the body, receptors are a critical mechanism of control for when, where, and how hormones exert their influence. Receptors determine which cells are affected by which hormones, the timing and degree of effect, and the nature of the effect.

Regulation occurs through at least three mechanisms: the release and binding of hormones to regulate circulating levels; the location, number, and nature of receptors; and the feedback loops elicited by hormones and their receptors that control subsequent release. Feedback loops occur when the end-stage hormonal product of a particular organ acts as an inhibitory or excitatory signal for the hypothalamic and/or pituitary hormone. For example, in the hypothalamic–pituitary–adrenal axis (HPA-axis), the hypothalamus produces CRF, which stimulates the pituitary gland to produce ACTH, which stimulates the adrenals to produce glucocorticoids (cortisol in humans). Receptors for cortisol in the hypothalamus allow cortisol levels to signal the hypothalamus to inhibit production of CRF, thus ending the cycle.

Endocrinology of Pregnancy

Preconception

Both female and male reproductive capacity is initiated and regulated by hormones. In fact, while the sex of the fetus is genetically determined by the X or Y chromosome inherited from the father (XX is female, XY is male), without the appropriate release of hormones during fetal development fetal sexual development is impaired (see the section titled The endocrinology of fetal development). In adult males, GnRH from the hypothalamus signals the pituitary to produce LH and FSH. LH stimulates the testes to produce androgens, primarily testosterone, and FSH promotes the development of sperm. Testosterone has an inhibiting effect on secretion of GnRH by the hypothalamus, completing the negative feedback loop.

In females, GnRH from the hypothalamus also stimulates the pituitary to produce LH and FSH. In females these hormones stimulate the ovaries to produce estrogens, and stimulate the follicle to mature a single oocyte (egg cell). Low levels of LH and FSH during this phase (called the follicular phase of the ovarian cycle) inhibit the pituitary in a negative feedback loop similar to that for males. However, as the follicle matures, estrogen production increases sharply. These high levels of estrogens stimulate the pituitary in a positive feedback loop, and the resulting high levels of LH supports the final maturation of the follicle and ovulation (the rupturing of the follicle and release of the oocyte). As estrogen production increases, the lining of the uterus (called the endometrium) thickens with blood and nutrients that could support an embryo. After ovulation (the luteal phase), LH stimulates the remaining follicular tissue to develop into a glandular structure called the corpus luteum. The corpus luteum responds to LH by producing progesterone and estrogen, keeping the pituitary inhibited with the negative feedback of these hormones. These hormones continue to foster development and maintenance of the endometrium, which begins secreting a nutrient fluid that could support an embryo prior to implantation. At the end of the luteal phase, if there is no implantation of a fertilized ovum, the corpus luteum disintegrates, the levels of progesterone and estrogens drop, and the pituitary hormones rise again, promoting the growth of new follicles, beginning the cycle anew. This same drop in progesterone and estrogens causes spasms of the arteries in the endometrium depriving it of blood, and the endometrium is shed in menstruation.

Conception and Gestation

After fertilization of the egg by the sperm (conception), the resulting zygote begins dividing. This process continues, leading to a ball of cells that travels to the uterus. This ball of cells becomes a fluid-filled sphere, known as a blastocyst, which will implant into the prepared endometrium. After implantation (approximately postconception day 10), the pregnancy is in the embryonic stage. The embryo begins secreting embryonic hormones that alert the mother's body to its presence and that exert control over the mother's reproductive system. For example, the embryo releases human chorionic gonadotropin (HCG), which maintains the secretion of progesterone and estrogens by the corpus luteum through the first few months of fetal development. This prevents disintegration of the corpus luteum, and thus the resulting drop in progesterone and estrogen that would initiate menstruation. HCG can be measured in the mother's urine and is used in many pregnancy tests.

The outer layer of the blastocyst and the endometrium give rise to the placenta, a unique organ that is composed of both fetal and maternal tissue. This organ allows for the exchange of nutrients and waste via the umbilical cord. The high levels of progesterone initiate changes in the mother's body, including increased mucus in the cervix which forms a protective plug, enlarged breasts, and as a result of the negative feedback loop, inhibition of the ovarian and menstrual cycles.

In the second trimester, HCG declines, the corpus luteum deteriorates, and the placenta produces the progesterone necessary to maintain the pregnancy. Interestingly, however, the placenta lacks or has reduced levels of several enzymes important for generating estrogens and progesterone and therefore requires precursors from both the mother and the fetus. This dependence has led to conceptualizing the placenta as part of a maternal–fetal–placental unit.

Estrogens have several actions during pregnancy. They help with the uptake of low-density lipoprotein (LDL) cholesterol that is important for placental steroid production; they increase utero-placental blood flow; they increase endometrial prostaglandin synthesis; and they prepare the breasts for lactation. However, conditions resulting in drastically decreased estrogen production do not result in miscarriage, thus suggesting that estrogens are not essential for maintaining pregnancy.

Parturition

Parturition (or birth) is initiated by a combination of local regulators (prostaglandins) and the hormones estrogen and oxytocin. Estrogen reaches its highest levels in the last weeks of pregnancy and promotes the development of oxytocin receptors on the uterus. Oxytocin is produced both by the fetus and by the mother, and stimulates uterine contractions and the production of prostaglandins that enhance contractions. These hormones are part of a positive feedback loop that encourages the progression of labor.

Endocrinology of Fetal Development

In addition to the role of hormones in maintaining pregnancy and initiating birth, hormones are critically involved in the development of the fetus. Hormones govern sexual development, are critical for growth, and help to prepare the fetus for birth and life outside of the womb.

Nutrients and wastes are exchanged via the placenta to support the fetus; however, the fetal hormonal environment is largely independent of the mother's. This separation is maintained in part by the impermeability of the placenta to many hormones. Hormones that cross the placenta are typically those that are lipid-soluble or smaller molecules and include cortisol, estradiol, thyroid hormones, and catecholamines. The placenta also produces many hormones, including hypothalamic, pituitary, adrenal, and gonadal hormones as well as growth factors and endorphins. The placenta has its own regulatory mechanisms. Placental hormones may modulate fetal and maternal processes, and in turn maternal and fetal hormones may regulate placental hormone production.

While many of the hormones in the fetal environment are hormones that are active later in life, some operate primarily in the fetal period. Hormones are also often present in different levels in the fetus and may be converted to inactive forms more readily than in the mother. Clearance rates also may differ. For example, in the fetus cortisol, estradiol, and thyroid hormone are quickly converted to inactive forms (cortisone, estrone, and rT3, respectively) that do not have the same effects that they would have later in life. In addition, the complexity of hypothalamic–pituitary control of hormone production requires the cortex, midbrain, hypothalamus, vasculature, and peripheral systems to have matured. While these structures and systems are maturing, circulating hormone levels may differ due to inadequate maturation. Increased conversion to inactive forms may protect the fetus from high circulating hormone levels while these regulation and clearance mechanisms mature.

As the fetus matures, changes in hormone levels support growth and development. For example, TSH and T4 increase over the fetal period and support bone and central nervous system (CNS) maturation, including neurogenesis, migration, differentiation, dendritic and axonal growth, synaptogenesis, and myelination. The fetal endocrine system is also responsive to stress, for example, in response to insufficient oxygen. Fetal catecholamines are the primary stress hormones in the fetus. Catecholamines are critical for fetal cardiovascular function and survival.

Some hormones, though present, are relatively inactive. For example, insulin and glucagon levels are both high, but secretion, clearance, and responsivity to glucose are all impaired. This may be due to the relative stability of glucose levels maintained by the placenta, because both pre-term and full-term infants quickly utilize glucagon and insulin to regulate blood glucose levels after birth. Insulin and insulin-like growth factors (IGFs) are, however, critical for normal growth in the fetal period.

In week 7 of gestation, the gonads of both male and female fetuses begin to differentiate. In males, androgens initiate the development of male primary sex organs, and later in the fetal period androgen release in the male fetus inhibits the cyclicity of the pituitary gland. In female fetuses, or in male fetuses without sufficient androgens, the female primary sex organs will develop, and the cyclicity of the pituitary will be preserved to later give rise to the menstrual cycle.

The endocrine system is also critically involved in preparing the fetus for birth and life outside of the protected uterine environment. The fetus must suddenly initiate breathing, defend against hypothermia, and prevent hypoglycemia and hypocalcemia. A cortisol surge near term supports this transition, and is achieved both by increased fetal cortisol production and decreased conversion of cortisol to cortisone. The surge supports surfactant synthesis in the lung which is critical for breathing, increases liquid reabsorption in the lung, supports duct closure, and stimulates small intestine and liver processes. Mice deficient in CRF or glucocorticoid (GC) receptors die within the first 12 h of life. Catecholamines also surge dramatically and support increased blood pressure, increased glucagon, decreased insulin, lung adaptation, and heat generation in fat tissue.

In humans and other mammals, the decreasing levels of progesterone in the mother following birth release the inhibition of the pituitary and allow the production of prolactin. Prolactin then stimulates milk production 2–3 days after birth, and oxytocin controls the release of milk from the mammary glands. Oxytocin release is regulated at least in part by the hypothalamic hormone α-melanocyte-stimulating hormone.

Endocrine System and Normal Growth

The endocrine system is critically involved in normal growth. GH, IGFs, and receptors are all involved in normal growth, and disruptions can result in abnormal growth (see the section titled Endocrine disorders relevant for infants and children).

Mean levels of GH decrease across childhood from high values in the neonatal period to lower values at early puberty. Levels then increase during mid-to-late puberty, and decrease again from late puberty across the

lifespan. Maximum GH secretion occurs at night, especially during the onset of the first slow-wave sleep. Sleep, nutrition, fasting, exercise, stress, obesity, estrogen, and testosterone all affect GH secretion.

IGFs are a family of peptides that are partially GH dependent, and that mediate many of the actions of GH. IGF-I is important for both fetal and postnatal growth and is involved in normal fertility. Levels of IGF-I are low in newborns, rise during childhood, and attain adult levels at the onset of puberty. Levels then rise to two to three times the adult levels. After 20–30 years of age, levels begin an age-associated decline. IGF-II is a major fetal growth factor and is involved in placental growth. IGF-II levels are also lower in the newborn, but adult levels are reached by 1 year and there is little-to-no decline across the lifespan. IGF-II may be involved in inhibiting excessive growth.

Androgens and estrogens do not significantly contribute to normal growth before puberty; however, during puberty they enhance GH secretion and stimulate IGF-I production. Growth during puberty is both growth in height and in bone mineral density. Thyroid hormone is also very important for postnatal growth, and untreated hypothyroidism in the infant can lead to profound growth failure and a lack of skeletal maturation (see section titled Thyroid disease). Thyroid hormone appears to influence growth by having a permissive affect on GH.

Endocrine System and Stress

Physical and psychological stress is managed in part through the efforts of the endocrine system. When a stressor is perceived by the brain, two stress systems are activated. The first is the norepinephrine sympathetic adrenal medullary system (NE-SAM), and the second is the HPA-axis. The NE-SAM system has immediate results, known as the 'flight or fight' response. This includes increased heart rate, increased pupil dilation, and increased respiration. These effects are mediated by epinephrine and norepinephrine, both produced by the adrenal glands. Epinephrine and norepinephrine are also neurotransmitters produced by nonendocrine cells in the brain where they have a number of important effects.

The first response to stress by the NE-SAM system is metabolically costly, burning through reserve glucose stores. Thus, one of the main goals of the stress systems is to generate energy. The second stress system, the HPA-axis helps to generate energy. Once activated by a stressor, the HPA-axis works to replenish the glucose stores that were quickly depleted by the NE-SAM system in preparation for a response to a second stressor or to a prolonged response to the initial stressor. All three components of the HPA-axis are part of the endocrine system; however, it is the glucocorticoid hormone released by the adrenal gland which has effects throughout the body. This hormone is cortisol in humans and corticosterone in non-human animals.

Endocrine Disorders Relevant for Infants and Children

Endocrine disorders can be the result of a variety of genetic mutations affecting the endocrine glands, hormones, and receptors. Endocrine disorders can also be the result of tumors, both malignant and benign, and can result from autoimmune destruction of endocrine glands or tissues. An important endocrine disorder is congenital hypothyroidism (also known as cretinism), resulting from iodine deficiency in the fetal, infant, or early childhood periods. Many endocrine disorders can be treated by administration of exogenous hormones, and hormones are also used to treat nonendocrine disorders, for example, steroid hormones are widely used to treat inflammation or to suppress immune response.

Diabetes

Diabetes is characterized by insufficient insulin production, insulin resistance, or both. Treatment may involve insulin replacement through intramuscular injection or oral medication to support the effective utilization of insulin by the body. Insulin-dependent diabetes (sometimes also called type 1 or juvenile diabetes) results from a genetic predisposition to the destruction of insulin-producing cells of the pancreas by the immune system. Noninsulin-dependent diabetes (also known as type 2 diabetes) results from a change in the ability of the body to utilize insulin and is often associated with obesity

Type 1

Type 1 diabetes typically does not affect infants and young children; however, it usually emerges prior to adulthood. While the genetic predisposition is present from conception, the autoimmune destruction of pancreatic insulin-producing cells occurs later in childhood. In children who develop diabetes prior to adolescence, it can be particularly difficult to maintain proper treatment as lifestyle changes may make regular meals and insulin injections difficult. However, failing to keep the glucose/insulin balance that the body intricately maintains in the absence of diabetes puts the individual at risk for a wide range of life-threatening illnesses such as cardiovascular disease and kidney failure.

Gestational

During pregnancy, the high glucose demands of the fetus are supported in part by increased insulin resistance. In gestational diabetes, the mother's body becomes unable to maintain a normal blood glucose level during pregnancy. Gestational diabetes is usually not followed by type 1 or type 2 diabetes after birth in either the infant or the mother. However, it must be treated during pregnancy and even when treated it does lead to effects on the fetus such as significantly increased birth weight.

Growth Disorders

Growth problems can be classified into four types: primary growth abnormalities as a result of genetic defects; growth problems secondary to chronic diseases or endocrine disorders; growth problems that result from prenatal or postnatal environmental factors; and those of undetermined origin. Primary growth disorders include the osteochondrodysplasias, for example, short-limbed dwarfism, which are genetically transmitted disorders of cartilage, bone, or both, and chromosomal abnormalities such as Down syndrome or Turner's syndrome. In some primary growth disorders, GH treatment can be beneficial, for example, in Turner's syndrome. Chronic diseases that delay growth include malabsorption and gastrointestinal diseases, chronic liver disease, chronic renal disease, chronic anemias, severe pulmonary disease, chronic inflammatory diseases, and HIV. In general, treatment of the primary disease is necessary to restore growth. For diseases such as severe pulmonary disease and chronic inflammation, glucocorticoids are widely used; however, minimizing exposure to glucocorticoids to the minimal dose and frequency necessary to control the underlying disease is important, as glucocorticoids used clinically can delay growth.

Endocrine disorders that involve GH as well as those that do not directly involve GH can result in delayed growth. Those that directly involve GH include central hypothalamic–pituitary dysfunction, failed or reduced pituitary GH production, and GH insensitivity. These symptoms may reflect underlying genetic abnormalities, congenital malformations, head trauma, brain inflammation due to infection, tumors, radiation therapy, or psychosocial maltreatment. Birth size may be normal or near normal, although severe early-onset GH disorder infants may be very small. Delayed growth may begin in the first few postnatal months, and by 6–12 months growth may deviate from the normal growth curve, with proportions remaining relatively normal. Weight-to-height ratios are often increased, musculature is poor, fontanel (skull bone) closure is often slow and facial bone growth may be particularly delayed. Infants with genetic GH disorder are below the 5th percentile in height, and also have documented abnormal growth velocity. As with chronic diseases, the underlying cause of the GH disorder should be treated, however, GH supplements can also be helpful and are generally regarded as safe. Prior to 1985 and the creation of recombinant DNA GH, however, GH was derived from the pituitary of cadavers, was in short supply, and has since been found to be a transmission route for Creutzfeldt–Jakob disease.

Hypothyroidism, which occurs in newborns and can develop in childhood (see section titled Thyroid disease), can retard growth. However, when treated promptly, growth and adult height are normal. Cushing's syndrome, though rare, has more severe effects, resulting in impaired skeletal growth. This impaired growth can only be partially ameliorated with exogenous GH and children may not attain target adult height. Vitamin D deficiency, which can cause rickets in infancy, can also result in delayed growth.

A number of environmental factors are very important for normal growth, the most common being malnutrition. There are two types of malnutrition, marasmus, which results from an overall deficiency in calories, and kwashiorkor, which results from mostly protein deficiency. Children with marasmus have a generally wasted appearance, while those with kwashiorkor typically have a protruding belly and very thin limbs. Stunting of growth due to malnutrition can have life-long consequences. Furthermore, protein and calories are essential for normal brain growth, thus depending on the duration and severity of malnutrition, children may have developmental delays or permanent cognitive deficits as well as an impaired immune system.

During the prenatal period, environmental agents and maternal factors can also affect normal growth. Maternal malnutrition and maternal drug use may be particularly detrimental to prenatal growth. In addition, the most common cause of infants born large for their gestational age is maternal diabetes.

Inorganic failure to thrive or psychosocial dwarfism

Infants or young children who are otherwise normal but are experiencing the extreme stress of severe maltreatment sometimes fail to grow despite a normal diet and no apparent problems with their endocrine system. When these children are relocated to a more positive environment, growth is restored, indicating that the psychosocial stress they experienced temporarily inhibited growth. Both GH and HPA-axis disruptions have been documented in this population, however GH treatment is not usually beneficial until the psychosocial situation is improved.

Precocious Puberty

The average age of puberty has decreased steadily over the last 100 years in industrialized nations and is influenced by genetic and environmental factors. Precocious puberty is premature development of body characteristics that normally occur during puberty. The declining age of the onset of puberty complicates the diagnosis of precocious puberty. Currently, in girls, precocious puberty is when any of the following develop before 8 years of age: breasts, armpit or pubic hair, mature external genitalia, or first menstruation. In boys, precocious puberty is when any of the following develop before 9 years of age: enlarged testes and penis, armpit or pubic hair, or facial hair.

The main causes of precocious puberty are structural abnormalities in the brain and hormone-secreting tumors. Medications can temporarily surpress sexual hormone secretion, however, some tumors require surgical removal. Children (of both sexes) with early sexual development are also more likely to have psychosocial problems. Their early sexual development can result in self-esteem problems, depression, acting out at school and home, and alcohol and illegal substance abuse.

Thyroid Disease

Thyroid disease is relatively common, and includes hyperthyroidism, hypothyroidism, thyroid cancer, and enlargement of the thyroid, or thyroid goiters. Hyperthyroidism results from overproduction of thyroid hormone and includes symptoms of upregulation of metabolism such as feeling hot, losing weight or increased appetite, heart palpitations, trembling hands, nervousness, insomnia, increased bowel movements, and fatigue by the end of the day. Treatment includes both temporary and long-term procedures. Short-term solutions include β-blockers, which temporarily inhibit the effects of increased thyroid hormone while not inhibiting its actual production, and antithyroid medications that temporarily block the ability of the thyroid to make thyroid hormone. More permanent treatments include oral doses of radioactive iodine and surgery. Radioactive iodine treatment is the recommended treatment as iodine is selectively absorbed by the thyroid allowing selective destruction of thyroid cells. However, with both surgical removal of the thyroid and radioactive iodine treatment, the patient must subsequently be treated for hypothyroidism as their thyroid will no longer produce sufficient quantities of thyroid hormone. 'Hypothyroidism' may affect as many as 10% of women and can result from iodine deficiency, treatment of hyperthyroidism as described previously, from temporary inflammation of the thyroid, or as the result of autoimmune destruction of thyroid hormone-producing cells. Common symptoms include weight gain, fatigue, cold intolerance, constipation, and depression. Hypothyroidism can be treated effectively with oral hormone replacement therapy.

Iodine deficiency is a serious problem, with approximately 130 countries and 29% of the world's population living in areas with insufficient iodine in the soil. This occurs most often in mountainous regions, including the Andes, Alps, and Himalayas, and in lowland regions far from oceans such as central Africa and eastern Europe. In some countries, iodine is supplemented in table salt or via the water supply. Where iodine is deficient and not supplemented, thyroid hormone synthesis is impaired. If this occurs in adults, symptoms are as described above for hypothyroidism. If this occurs in the fetus, infant, or young child, it results in the serious condition known as congenital hypothyroidism or cretinism. This condition affects CNS development and maturation and results in permanent mental retardation, neurological defects, and growth abnormalities.

Incomplete thyroid development is the most common defect, occurring in approximately 1 of every 3000 births. It is twice as common in girls as in boys. Typically few symptoms are present, as the deficiency is mild. However, infants with severe hypothyroidism have a distinctive appearance, including a puffy face, dull look, and a large and protruding tongue. Symptoms include poor muscle tone, poor feeding, choking, constipation, prolonged jaundice, and growth delays. If untreated, cognitive and growth delays are severe. However, with early diagnosis and replacement hormone therapy beginning in the first month of life normal intelligence and growth are expected. Most states routinely screen newborns for hypothyroidism to allow early diagnosis.

Thyroid disease during pregnancy

Both hypo- and hyperthyroidism can influence the regularity of a women's menstrual cycle and thus the chance that she may become pregnant. During pregnancy, women with previously undiagnosed hypo- or hyperthyroidism may assume their symptoms are related to the pregnancy. In the case of hypothyroidism, symptoms such as fatigue and weight gain are common effects of both hypothyroidism and pregnancy. Doses of exogenous thyroid hormone typically need to be increased during pregnancy to maintain appropriate blood levels. As thyroid hormone is critical for normal CNS maturation, it is important that hypothyroidism be treated. Maternal hypothyroidism has been associated with a 5–10 point IQ deficit in the child. Hyperthyroidism during pregnancy is the more serious condition, because it is associated with increased risk of birth defects and miscarriage, and this condition is difficult to treat during pregnancy without effects on the thyroid of the fetus. Women of childbearing age with hyperthyroidism may be encouraged to choose a permanent treatment of hyperthyroidism (described previously) prior to becoming pregnant.

Addison's Disease or Adrenal Insufficiency

This condition results from insufficient production of glucocorticoids by the adrenal cortex. Symptoms may include weight lost, weakness, fatigue, low blood pressure, abdominal pain, nausea, dehydration, and sometimes darkening of the skin.

Primary adrenal insufficiency, which can be acute or chronic, is most often caused by destruction of the adrenal gland as the result of an autoimmune disorder. However, destruction of the gland can also occur in other ways, including tuberculosis (TB) infection. Usually, adrenal insufficiency results when over 90% of the adrenal cortex is destroyed. Primary adrenocortical insufficiency is rare, it can occur at any age, and it is equally common in women and men.

Primary adrenal insufficiency is sometimes also one part of a more widespread endocrine disease called polyendocrine deficiency syndrome. Adrenal insufficiency may be accompanied by underactive parathyroid glands, slow sexual development, diabetes, anemia, chronic candida infections, and chronic active hepatitis. Polyendocrine deficiency syndrome is likely inherited because frequently more than one family member tends to have one or more endocrine deficiencies.

Secondary adrenal insufficiency may be caused by hypothalamic–pituitary disease, or it may result from suppression of the hypothalamic–pituitary axis by exogenous steroids or endogenous steroids (i.e., those produced by tumors). Extensive therapeutic use of steroids has greatly contributed to increased incidence.

Symptoms of adrenal insufficiency usually begin gradually. Adrenal insufficiency is most clinically problematic during times of physiologic stress. In the absence of corticosteroids, stress results in hypotension, shock, and is sometimes fatal. Adrenal insufficiency is treated with oral replacement hormones. Cortisol is replaced orally with hydrocortisone derivatives. If aldosterone is also deficient, it is replaced with oral doses of a mineralocorticoid such as fludrocortisone acetate. Patients receiving aldosterone replacement therapy are usually also advised to increase their salt intake. Because patients with secondary adrenal insufficiency normally maintain aldosterone production, they do not require aldosterone replacement therapy. Individuals with adrenal insufficiency who need surgery or who are nearing childbirth will be given additional injections of hydrocortisone and saline.

Cushing's Syndrome and Cushing's Disease

Cushing's syndrome and Cushing's disease are hormonal disorders caused by prolonged exposure of the body's tissues to high levels of the glucocorticoids. Sometimes called 'hypercortisolism', it is relatively rare and most commonly affects adults aged 20–50 years. Effects of excessive glucocorticoids can occur either as a result of endogenous glucocorticoid administration used to treat autoimmune diseases or as the result of a pituitary tumor. As with most illnesses, symptoms may vary, but most people have upper body obesity, rounded face, increased fat around the neck, and thinning arms and legs. Children tend to be obese with slowed growth rates. Other symptoms include fragile and thin skin which bruises easily and heals poorly. Purplish pink stretch marks may appear on the abdomen, thighs, buttocks, arms, and breasts. The bones are also weakened. Most people have severe fatigue, weak muscles, high blood pressure, and high blood sugar. Irritability, anxiety, and depression are common. Women usually have excess hair growth, and menstrual periods may become irregular or stop. Men have decreased fertility with diminished or absent desire for sex.

Symptoms may result from benign tumors of the pituitary, benign or malignant tumors outside the pituitary, or adrenal tumors or abnormalities of the adrenal glands. Rarely, children or young adults develop small cortisol-producing tumors of the adrenal glands.

Treatment depends on the specific reason for cortisol excess and may include surgery, radiation, or chemotherapy. If the cause is long-term use of glucocorticoid hormones to treat another disorder, the dosage will be gradually decreased to the lowest dose adequate for control of that disorder. Once control is established, the daily dose of glucocorticoid hormones may be modified to avoid symptoms.

Future Directions

Active areas of research involving the endocrine system in development include studies examining the stress systems, including their involvement in initiating labor before full term, hormonal involvement in attachment and bonding, treatment and prevention of diabetes, and the effects of treatment with exogenous glucocorticoids.

A number of investigators, including the author, are examining the development of the HPA-axis in the first few years of life as influenced by factors such as maternal stress during the prenatal period, early caregiving experiences, and temperament. Laboratories exploring HPA-axis development typically also look at factors related to individual differences in cortisol reactivity or basal cortisol levels, including attention, inhibition, and health.

Growing interest in the endocrine system's role in bonding and attachment is reflected in a number of studies of pair-bonding in monogamous species, particularly voles. Oxytocin and vasopressin appear to be critical in effective pair-bonding in this species. It may also be the case that these hormones are critically involved in bonding in humans, both in the bonding of adult mates and the bond between parents and infants.

Type 2 diabetes is becoming increasingly common in the US, at least in part because of the rising rates of obesity. A number of investigators are working to understand this disease better, including improving strategies for prevention and treatment. Type 1 diabetes is one of the diseases that may benefit from stem cell therapies, as it results from selective autoimmune destruction of insulin-producing cells in the pancreas.

Exogenous glucocorticoids are widely used in clinical practice. Particularly relevant for infants and young children are studies examining the short- and long-term effects of exogenous glucocorticoid administration to pre-term infants. This treatment is highly effective in promoting lung development to allow independent breathing. However, there may be short- and long-term effects of this treatment.

See also: Birth Complications and Outcomes; Depression; Failure to Thrive; Genetic Disorders: Sex Linked; Genetic Disorders: Single Gene; Immune System and Immunodeficiency; Obesity.

Suggested Readings

Campbell NA and Reece JB (2005) *Biology,* 7th edn. San Fransisco: Benjamin Cummings.

Greenspan FS and Gardner DG (2001) *Basic & Clinical Endocrinology,* 6th edn. New York: McGraw-Hill.

Larsen PR, Kronenberg HM, Melmed S, and Polonsky KS (2003) *Williams Textbook of Endocrinology,* 10th edn. Philadelphia: Elsevier.

National Institutes of Health. The Endocrine and Metabolic Diseases Information Service – Addison's disease. http://www.endocrine.niddk.nih.gov/pubs/addison/addison.htm (accessed on 16 July 2007).

National Institutes of Health. The Endocrine and Metabolic Diseases Information Service – Cushing's syndrome. http://endocrine.niddk.nih.gov/pubs/cushings/cushings.htm (accessed on 16 July 2007).

National Library of Medicine. National Institutes of Health – Addison's disease. http://www.nlm.nih.gov/medlineplus/endocrinesystemhormones.html (accessed on 16 July 2007).

National Library of Medicine: National Institutes of Health. Health Information – MedlinePlus, Fetal Development. http://www.nlm.nih.gov/medlineplus/ency/article/002398.htm (accessed on 16 July 2007).

Relevant Websites

http://www.diabetes.org – American Diabetes Association, Gestational Diabetes.

http://www.hgfound.org – Human Growth Foundation.

http://www.jdrf.org – Juvenile Diabetes Research Foundation International.

http://www.hormone.org – The Hormone Foundation.

F

Failure to Thrive

D R Fleisher, University of Missouri School of Medicine, Columbia, MO, USA

Glossary

Constitutional growth delay – A temporary lag in growth affecting some healthy infants and toddlers having no discernable environmental cause.

Failure to grow (FTG) – Growth deficiency, indicated by a down-shift of growth curves to lower percentile channels over time. Its causes include disease, malnutrition, psychosocial adversity and all other factors having a negative impact on a child's fulfillment of his or her genetic potential for physical growth.

Failure to thrive (FTT) – A special form of FTG caused by aberrant nurturing involving dysfunction in the parent–child relationship that impairs nutritional and developmental wellbeing.

Fundoplication – A surgical procedure that narrows the opening between the esophagus and the stomach thereby impeding gastroesophageal reflux and its resultant vomiting.

Gastroesophageal reflux (GER) – Backwash of liquid contents from the stomach up into the esophagus. It occurs normally, especially after meals, and, as such, is not pathologic.

Gastroesophageal reflux disease (GERD) – Excessive GER that causes irritation of the linings of the esophagus or airway.

Gastrojejunostomy – A surgical procedure that creates an additional opening between the stomach and the small intestine (jejunum) to facilitate emptying of the stomach.

Genetic small stature – Inherited small stature in an individual who nevertheless grows (or has grown) at normal rates, that is, near, but parallel to the lower percentile channels for height. This kind of smallness should not be mistaken for growth failure.

Hyperphagia – Overeating.

Hyperphagic psychosocial dwarfism ('deprivation dwarfism' 'pseudo-hypopituitary dwarfism') – A form of FTT associated with failure of emotional attachment between child and principal caregiver, characterized by cessation of growth resembling organic hypopituitarism along with compulsive consumption of extraordinary amounts and kinds of food. Growth resumes and eating normalizes when the child experiences nurturing.

Hypertrophic pyloric stenosis – An organic disease acquired in the first month or two of life that presents with increasing vomiting and weight loss. It is caused by thickening of the walls of the outflow tract of the stomach resulting in progressive occlusion of the channel through which stomach contents normally pass into the intestine (duodenum). It usually requires surgical intervention.

Infant anorexia syndrome – Inadequate food intake resulting from conflict between infant and caregiver around feeding and eating.

Infant rumination syndrome (IRS) – An acquired self-stimulatory habit characterized by repetitive, nearly effortless regurgitation of recently ingested food into the mouth followed by re-swallowing and/or loss to the outside. It usually has its onset between 2 and 8 months of age as a result of insufficient reciprocal interaction between infant and caregiver.

Nurturing – The process by which children's physical and emotional needs are fulfilled sufficient for normal development.

Pyloroplasty – A surgical procedure that widens the normal passageway (the pylorus) from the stomach to the intestine (duodenum) to facilitate emptying of the stomach.

Small for gestational age – A term applied to newborns whose growth *in utero* had been less than normal.
Thriving – A global concept that includes normal physical, emotional, cognitive, and motor development.
Urine-specific gravity – A measure that reflects the amount of water in urine.

Introduction

Failure to thrive (FTT) is usually defined as growth failure due to any cause. In this article, however, FTT is defined as a special kind of growth failure, namely, growth failure caused by aberrant nurturing. Although organic diseases, such as kidney failure, cystic fibrosis, or congenital heart disease, may impair growth, a large proportion of infants and children who present with growth failure have no underlying organic disease. Instead, they fail to grow because of dysfunction within their parent–child relationships, and it is this kind of growth failure to which the term FTT is specifically applied.

Philosophic Considerations

Compassionate, efficient management is based on two concepts worthy of consideration before proceeding with a discussion of FTT: (1) the distinctions between the conventional biomedical model of practice and the biopsychosocial model of practice and (2) the definitions of 'functional', as contrasted with 'organic' disorders.

The conventional, biomedical model of practice dichotomizes illness as either organic or psychogenic, the former being materialistic and the province of medicine, the latter being insubstantial or 'mental' and the province of the mental health professions. However, advances in the neurosciences have increasingly shown the unity of mind–brain–body. Sustained emotional stress, for example, has been shown to cause alterations in the anatomy and function of the brain and other organs, many of which affect behavior and influence growth and development.

The biomedical approach to diagnosis is dichotomized and biased in favor of organic disease. The process is sequential: first rule out all plausible organic causes of growth failure and only then consider psychosocial factors. Even when psychosocial pathology is evident on first encounter, the clinician adhering to the biomedical model may avoid this aspect of growth failure out of concern that an organic disease might be missed. Unfortunately, medical diagnostic procedures are not necessarily benign, especially in infants and children. They often involve pain, anguish, exposure to ionizing radiation, and other adversities. The task of the clinician is to identify the causes of growth failure in a manner that not only diagnoses them correctly, but does so in a manner that is least stressful or damaging to the patient.

The biopsychosocial approach, as described below, avoids both organic and psychogenic biases and, instead, approaches both aspects of failure to grow simultaneously, pursuing a course that is flexible, influenced by the most likely elements as they emerge during the evaluation. This lessens the likelihood of what John Apley called 'wantonness of inquiry' during which "the doctor has the notion that if he excavates long enough and deep enough the answer [i.e., the organic diagnosis] will come up."

What are the characteristics that define and distinguish organic disorders and functional disorders? Primary organic disease involves objectively demonstrable tissue damage and resultant organ malfunction. By contrast, primary functional disorders present with symptoms produced by organs that are free of organic disease. The phenomena that produce symptoms occur as part of the repertoire of responses inherent in nondiseased organs. A runner's leg cramp, for example, causes intense pain and is at least temporarily disabling, but there is no disease, no organic pathology. It is in the repertoire of healthy muscle to go into spasm when sufficiently fatigued. Recovery from this very simple example of a functional disorder is effected by a period of rest, and the expected recovery tends to confirm the diagnosis of 'normal muscle cramp' as opposed to, say, a pathologic fracture.

The central nervous system modulates the activity of the stomach. Emotional stress has long been known to cause disordered gastrointestinal motility (as exemplified by the abnormal X-ray findings of narrowing of the outflow passage of the stomach in some infants with 'nervous vomiting'). The functional nature of such vomiting, and any other presentation of FTT, can be positively differentiated from organic disease by the infant's response to a procedure referred to as a 'therapeutic trial of comfort' (analogous to the rest period that relieves a muscle cramp). This therapeutic/diagnostic procedure is described below.

This is not to say that functional and organic disorders are mutually exclusive or that functional disorders cannot have serious or even fatal organic complications. However, it would be a mistake to focus on the disease caused by a functional disorder without attending to the underlying causes of that disorder. This error is exemplified by a recommendation for surgery to prevent vomiting in an infant with FTT due to unrecognized infant rumination syndrome (IRS).

Some Misconceptions About Failure to Thrive

FTT in infants and children is characterized by lags in somatic growth often accompanied by delays in cognitive, motor, and emotional development. The complexity of FTT has lead to conceptual over-simplifications.

One over-simplification is the notion that FTT is simply equivalent to undernutrition and that the problem can be cured by getting the child to eat more. Although poor nutrition may be the most salient feature in children with FTT, nutritional deficits are merely symptomatic of their causes. Unless poor nutrition is the result of organic disease or famine, the causes of inadequate food intake in FTT almost always involve problems in the relationship between child and principle caregiver. If the nature and causes of the dysfunctional relationship are not brought to light and addressed, clinical management of FTT is not likely to achieve optimal success.

Another misconception is that FTT signifies neglect. Although neglect may be the immediate cause of FTT in some cases, FTT can also occur in children of attentive, devoted parents.

Many published series of children with FTT were reported from large city hospitals serving medically indigent populations. As a result, the impression may be gained that FTT is a manifestation of poverty. However, FTT also occurs in middle- and upper-class families.

Defining the Presence and Causes of Growth Failure

Diagnosing growth failure on the basis of one-time measurements can be very misleading. It is helpful to plot a patient's growth before eliciting the history and then, during history taking, marking on the abscissa the ages of the child at which significant events occurred. The morphology of the curve may make cause-and-effect relationships stand out. A growth curve is far superior to a single set of measurements for evaluation of growth.

Among the many growth problems that may be mistaken for FTT, three warrant special mention: children who were born small for gestational age, children with constitutional growth delay, and children with genetic short stature. Infants born small for gestational age (i.e., intrauterine growth retardation) may be proportionate in length, weight, and head circumference, or their length and head circumference may be closer to normal than their weight. Those whose measurements are abnormally small but in-proportion are likely to have sustained an insult early in gestation, such as infection, chromosomal abnormalities, or exposure to teratogens; they generally have a poorer prognosis for catch-up growth. Those whose weights are disproportionately small for their lengths and head sizes are likely to have sustained an insult later in gestation (e.g., placental insufficiency, maternal malnutrition, or hypertension) and have a generally better prognosis for catch-up growth.

Constitutional growth delay is a normal variant seen in some healthy infants. Their growth progresses normally until sometime between 4 and 12 months when height and weight gains slow causing downshifts of their curves to lower channels. Slow or arrested growth persists for several months or more with spontaneous resumption of normal growth rates by 2–3 years of age, usually along channels lower than those followed prior to the period of delayed growth.

Children with genetic short stature are healthy and typically grow at normal rates, that is, parallel to, but at or below the 5th or 3rd percentile channels. There is usually a family history of small stature.

What Constitutes Nurturing and How Can Aberrant Nurturing Cause Growth Failure?

Emotional Aspects

Nurturing is the process by which infants survive, grow, and develop. It has emotional, cognitive, and nutritional aspects. It takes place within a dyadic relationship made up of the infant and its principal caregiver. In a well-functioning dyad, mother and infant interact in a reciprocal manner so that the infant's behavior and the caregiver's behavior are mutually regulatory. Actions, responses, and reactions occur during which the infant's cues are appreciated by the mother who then reacts in a timely, sensitive, contingent manner. These interactions, over time, foster the infant's sense of existing as an individual, physically and cognitively separate from his or her mother, and able to express a need with the expectation that it will be correctly interpreted and responded to. In order for a dyadic relationship to function, the mother must have first 'fallen in love' with her infant and 'claim' her baby as her own, physically and emotionally. 'Claiming' may occur immediately in the delivery room the moment the baby is put to her breast, it may occur some time later, or may not sufficiently take place at all. Without it, however, there is insufficient motivation for devoted caring and the capacity for feeling pleasure and pride in her baby and in her achievements as a mother, all of which foster effective nurturing.

The infant's capacity to engage in dyadic interaction depends upon its ability to manage transitions of state, including those required for feeding and eating. The infant *in utero* has little experience with changes in state. Feeding is continuous; there is no experience of hunger or thirst. The fetus experiences periods of sleep and wakefulness, but, unlike sleep and wakefulness in postnatal life, it does not occur in a changing environment, neither does it have much effect upon its environment. The intrauterine environment presents comparatively few stimuli for arousal and quiescence or changes in state.

Once out of the uterus, however, the infant is inundated by an environment that changes continuously.

The ability of an infant to make transitions from one state to another (e.g., hunger/thirst, followed by feeding, followed by satiety) depends upon, for example, the infant's temperament as well as the commitment, sensitivity, and skill of the mother.

Nutritional Aspects

Nutritional adequacy is comprised of a sequence of phenomena: (1) Adequate food must be available in the environment. (2) The child must take in adequate amounts of food. If food is not offered, older children can forage, but infants and toddlers depend entirely on their caregivers' recognition of, and responses to, their hunger signals. The dyadic relationship, of which feeding and eating is a major part, must work well enough to avoid feeding disorders that impair parents' ability to feed and their infants' ability to eat in a comfortable, satisfying manner. (3) Ingested food must be retained and not regurgitated or vomited before it can be digested. (4) The food must be digested before it can be absorbed. A child with cystic fibrosis, for example, may grow poorly, even though he or she may eat more than normal amounts of food, because the pancreas fails to secrete enough enzymes to digest the food that enters her intestine. (5) The lining of the small intestine is the surface through which the products of digestion enter the bloodstream. If this absorptive surface is reduced in area, as in celiac disease, weight gain and linear growth may be severely impaired. (6) As soon as the products of digestion have been absorbed, they may be utilized for growth. The presence of sufficient nutrients in the bloodstream promotes normal growth. However, severe physical and/or emotional stress can interfere with tissue-building and promote tissue-wasting so that the nutrients available for incorporation into growing tissues are, instead, washed out in the urine along with the waste products of normal metabolism.

This sequence of phenomena essential for growth is depicted in **Table 1**.

Defective nurturing can impair growth and development at steps 1, 2, 3, and 6. Each defect has a distinctive clinical pattern.

Irene Chatoor described six feeding disorders of infancy and early childhood, three of which are often associated with FTT: 'feeding disorder of state regulation' (onset during the first 2 months); 'feeding disorder of reciprocity' (onset between 2 and 6 months); and 'infantile anorexia' (onset during the transition from bottle or breast to spoon and self-feeding). During the first 2 months, successful feeding requires the infant to achieve the state of calm alertness. Infants who have difficulty with state regulation may be difficult to calm. Even though they may feel hungry, they may be unable to reach or maintain the necessary state of calm alertness or they may

Table 1   The sequence of nutrition and its impediments

	The sequence	*The impediments*
Step 1	The availability of food	Famine or starvation
Step 2	Ingestion of food	Infant feeding disorders: • Feeding disorder of state regulation • Feeding disorder of reciprocity • Infantile anorexia
Step 3	Retention of ingested food	Nervous vomiting syndrome Infant rumination syndrome
Step 4	Digestion of food	Pancreatic insufficiency (e.g., cystic fibrosis)
Step 5	Absorption of the products of digestion	Celiac disease
Step 6	Assimilation of absorbed food (anabolism and growth)	Stress

be too sleepy, too agitated, or too easily distracted by stimuli in the environment to complete or even begin a feeding. The infant may fail to gain weight. As the mother becomes more anxious, her ability to soothe her infant may deteriorate. A vicious cycle may become established, similar to the one that perpetuates 'persistent colic'.

Feeding disorder of reciprocity has its onset beyond 2 months of age. An infant older than 2–3 months has the ability to respond to, and initiate, social interactions with its caregiver. The dyadic relationship includes communicative behaviors such as mutual smiling, cuddling with holding, and mutual vocalizations. Feeding is a major focus of mutually pleasurably engagement during which cognitive and emotional development accompanies physical satisfaction and growth. If, during this stage of development, the caregiver is unresponsive to the infant's presence or signals, the infant may withdraw, become depressed, and fail to learn behaviors that foster nurturing. Instead of the social smile, he or she may avoid eye contact. Instead of cuddling and molding into a comfortable feeding position, he or she may be either stiff or limp. A caregiver's failure to attach emotionally to her infant impairs the infant's ability to become attached to the caregiver. It may become passive, lethargic, and disinterested in food. In the absence of environmental stimulation, such infants tend to engage in self-stimulatory behaviors, such as head-rolling or rumination. Growth and development lag; malnutrition and decreased resistance to infection may result in death of the infant or, if it survives, a damaged capacity to form attachments in later life.

Infant anorexia is another feeding disorder that may impair growth. Its onset occurs between 6 months and 3 years, a period during which the infant becomes increasingly able to function more independently and willfully. The offer of food by spoon normally becomes an interaction during which any discordant desires of toddler and mother need to be negotiated. This may be especially difficult in toddlers who, by temperament, are easily distracted. Feedings take too long. The parent tries harder to get food into their child's mouth. Attempts to trick or cajole the child into taking food are met with refusal to open the mouth, refusal to swallow, turning away, throwing food or utensils, or climbing out of the highchair. Parents become increasingly worried as the child seems to never be hungry, is increasing difficult to feed, and begins to lose weight. Chatoor found that "... difficult infant temperament was associated with higher mother–infant conflict during feeding ... the most difficult infants demonstrated the highest levels of conflict and growth failure."

Case Vignette: Infant Anorexia Syndrome

A 13-month-old boy, the product of an unplanned pregnancy, was born to a 36-year-old mother of two teenage children. He was described as an 'active baby' who had colic for the first 6 weeks. At about 4 months of age, the baby refused his formula. Different formulas were tried, but taken poorly. Spoon feedings became difficult and he needed to be coaxed or forced to eat. He chewed food put into his mouth, but refused to swallow it. Weight gain continued along the 10th to 25th percentile channels until 1 month prior to being hospitalized at 13 months of age.

At the time he was hospitalized, his weight was below the 3rd percentile. He refused almost every food except apple juice. After gaining the mother's acquiescence, we tested the premise that he would not feel hunger and that he would starve if left to feed himself without being fed by a caregiver. Accordingly, the infant was placed in a crib along with several bottles of milk and an abundance of finger-foods, but no apple juice. Foods were freely available for the taking, but no feeding was attempted. His mother and other observers mostly remained out of the room. After drinking and eating nothing for almost 18 h, he reached for a grape, put it into his mouth, chewed, and swallowed it. After a minute or two, he began drinking milk and avidly eating the cookies, grapes, and other finger-foods in his crib. During the remaining 4 days of hospitalization, meals consisted of finger-foods placed on the tray of his highchair. The dramatic improvement in his intake coupled with the unequivocal appearance of a weight gain trend made it easier for the mother to comply with our recommendations that she completely abstain from feeding him and, instead, provide food for him to feed himself. During an individual diagnostic interview, the father described his wife as "overprotective...even

the older ones, if they miss lunch, she's afraid they're going to die."

The baby was brought for a follow-up visit 12 days after his release from the hospital; his weight had risen from below the 3rd percentile to just below the 10th percentile. He was feeding himself 24 oz of milk a day plus meat, pasta, rice, and other finger-foods. He was still active and distractible.

FTT can occur in infants who eat more or less adequate amounts of food, but fail to retain what they have taken in. This is exemplified by two functional vomiting disorders of infancy: 'nervous vomiting' and IRS.

Before considering these two vomiting syndromes that impair growth, it is important to recognize that about 50% or more of healthy infants vomit or regurgitate during the first 6–18 months of life. This kind of vomiting occurs in normal infants and has been termed 'innocent vomiting'. It may range from effortless regurgitation to projectile vomiting. Its main characteristics are that there is no associated pain, nausea, loss of appetite, or underlying organic disease. It does not respond to dietary, positional, or pharmacologic measures. It does not impair weight gain, presumably because, if feedings are given liberally, to satiety, the infant compensates for what has been lost by taking in more. Innocent vomiting resolves spontaneously by or before 12–18 months of age. It is an important consideration in infants who fail to thrive because innocent vomiting plus growth failure may be mistaken for organic disease (e.g., gastroesophageal reflux disease or GERD). This may result in failure to diagnose and treat existing FTT and, instead, impose stressful diagnostic tests in pursuit of nonexistent diseases.

Nervous vomiting was described by the British physician, H. C. Cameron, in 1925. It is often associated with FTT. It may mimic hypertrophic pyloric stenosis radiologically. Nervous vomiting is a visceral reaction to stress and excitement causing the stomach's motility to be functionally altered, delaying passage of food into the intestine. Food is retained in the stomach longer than normally, keeping it as a reservoir for vomiting. Infant–mother interaction becomes increasingly distressed as vomiting increases and weight lags. A vicious cycle becomes established as a result of a breakdown in the nurturing relationship which, in turn, causes irritability, vomiting, and feeding difficulties leading to FTT (see **Figure 1**).

Once suspected, the diagnosis of FTT associated with nervous vomiting can be made by a positive response to a 'therapeutic trial of comfort'. This includes simultaneous efforts to relieve both the infant's and the parent's distress. Cameron wrote that, "treatment, if it is to be successful, must aim not so much at controlling the vomiting as at allaying the nervous unrest." This begins a therapeutic process that heals the parent–infant relationship and is necessary for continued improvement beyond the period of clinical management.

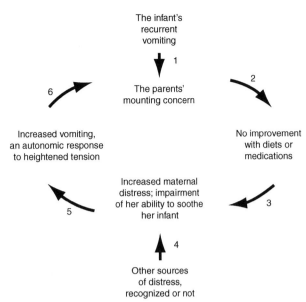

Figure 1 The vicious cycle of nervous vomiting. Modified from Fleisher D (1994) Functional vomiting disorders in infancy: Innocent vomiting, nervous vomiting, and infant rumination syndrome. *Journal of Pediatrics* 125(6) part 2: S84–S94.

Healing may be summarized schematically in terms of interrupting the vicious cycle shown in **Figure 1**. Vomiting must cease to worry the parents (step 1). To effect this attitudinal change, the parents must be shown that the infant's condition does not deteriorate when antireflux measures and dietary restrictions are dispensed with (step 2). This tests the premise that the infant is vulnerable to becoming ill when he or she is nurtured comfortably and normally, as though it were a healthy baby. This critical test may initially frighten the parents who fear that it will harm their baby. Therefore, it is best done in hospital on an infant's ward. The parents must first be assured that their child will be closely observed by a clinician who will supplement the parents' keen but unavoidably subjective observations with the objectivity of clinical practice. The infant is kept in a calm environment, comforted when fussy and fed liberally, as much as it wants whenever it wants it, vomiting notwithstanding. Burping is done during spontaneous pauses in feeding, not arbitrarily imposed in a way that interrupts a satisfying feed. Frustration and tension-producing procedures are avoided as much as possible. The baby's physical state is closely monitored by being weighed at least twice daily and by measurement of the specific gravity of spontaneously voided urine every shift. These data are charted graphically to aid in early detection of dehydration so that it can be treated without delay, in the unlikely event that it occurs.

Hospitalization also provides a supportive environment in which it might be possible for the mother to be relieved of burdensome outside responsibilities so that she can focus on the care and protection of her infant with the support of the nursing staff. Hospital personnel must not

exacerbate the parent's irrational guilt for having 'caused' their infant's illness. Diagnostic tests to screen for anatomic and metabolic causes of vomiting and/or weight lag are necessary because the infant will experience illness, like any other normal child, after the hospitalization is over. The parent's previous experience of illness may have created a sense of their child's vulnerability, predisposing them to new worries that 'something may have been missed' or that the doctor, having based his or her diagnosis on clinical impression, may have been wrong. Therefore, a prudent series of diagnostic tests based on the differential diagnosis of the infant's presenting signs and symptoms is needed. Two caveats apply, however: (1) Stressful tests (e.g., over-night fasts in preparation for X-ray studies, blood drawings) should be minimized, spread out over several days, and not done in rapid succession so as not to cause stress-induced FTT in the hospital. This also allows sufficient time for a valid therapeutic trial of comfort. (2) 'Wantonness of inquiry' should be avoided. It is counter-diagnostic and counter-therapeutic.

Time is a powerful and humane diagnostic tool provided, (1) the physician and the family are reasonably confident that no hidden, potentially serious disease has been missed and (2) they can rely on their physician's open-mindedness, accessibility, and responsiveness should they have new concerns. When these two caveats are implemented, parents, who may have initially wanted 'everything done' to find the cause of their baby's growth failure, instead become deeply appreciative of the doctor's omission of unnecessary, distressing tests.

Confirmation of the diagnosis of FTT is only possible by the resumption of thriving. This can only be ascertained during continuity of care over time. Honest mistakes are always possible. The use of time in confirming the diagnosis is safer (and more satisfying) when the relationship between the doctor and the parents is one of mutual respect, loyalty, and accessibility.

Interrupting the cycle at step 4 involves diagnostic/therapeutic interviews of the parents, together and individually, to gain insight into the conditions of their lives and the sources of stress that interfere with nurturing.

Interruption of the cycle at steps 5 and 6 occurs when the parents' optimism returns as they see their baby begin to gain weight and fuss less, and as diagnostic tests confirm the absence of organic disease.

Case Vignette: Nervous Vomiting

A 6-month-old first-born girl was hospitalized for weight loss and recurrent vomiting since 6 weeks of age. She was weaned at 3 months because her mother felt her milk was 'drying up'. Thereafter, she continued to be fussy, vomited frequently, and passed loose stools. Diagnostic studies carried out during a 10-day hospitalization, which included a therapeutic trial of comfort, showed no disease.

She rarely vomited in the hospital and passed three to six stools of varying consistency each day. She was fed the same formula as before admission, as much as she wanted, whenever she wanted it, and she gained weight. Diagnostic interviews with each parent revealed severe marital discord that worsened after the mother discovered she was pregnant. The father objected to the pregnancy and became increasingly unavailable. The mother handled her baby hesitantly during the early days of hospitalization, but became more comfortable in caring for her as the infant improved. The baby was released from the hospital with no medications and the same formula that she'd been fed before admission. During the follow-up visit 2 months later, the mother reported that her infant's fussiness had greatly improved. Although she still 'spat-up' small amounts daily, this resolved by 15 months. The mother said, "I feel a lot better now knowing that nothing is really wrong with her. She's getting to be more fun." The mother was in the process of divorcing her husband. (**Figure 2** depicts the patient's weight course.)

IRS is the second functional vomiting disorder that causes FTT and can potentially lead to an infant's death from inanition. It typically emerges between 2 and 8 months of age, during the period in which infants normally develop an increasingly strong attachment to their caregivers. The development of IRS is predisposed by failure of reciprocal interactions and, in this respect, is similar to feeding disorder of reciprocity. The caregiver is emotionally distant, unable to sense the baby's needs, and poorly responsive to his/her signals. The baby learns to regurgitate

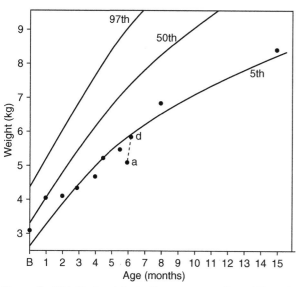

Figure 2 Weight of an infant with nervous vomiting at time of admission, a, and discharge, d, from hospital. The broken line indicates the weight gain during hospitalization (97th, 50th, and 5th percentile channels). Modified from Fleisher D (1994) Functional vomiting disorders in infancy: Innocent vomiting, nervous vomiting, and infant rumination syndrome. *Journal of Pediatrics* 125(6) part 2: S84–S94.

gastric content into its mouth for the purpose of self-stimulation and satisfaction of oral needs that would normally be supplied by the caregiver. Whereas older children and adults who habitually ruminate taste and re-swallow their regurgitated gastric content, infant ruminators are unable to contain all of it in their mouths and lose enough of it to the outside to cause progressive weight loss. Rumination is an acquired skill and is done voluntarily, without apparent nausea or distress. It ceases during sleep. It only occurs when the infant is awake, alone, quiet, and self-absorbed. It stops immediately when the baby senses the presence of another person, which might indicate the baby's intense need for social contact. The FTT does not improve with antireflux management, formula changes, arm restraints, or tube feedings. The parents' inability to nurture is one manifestation of more pervasive difficulties they have with interpersonal relationships.

The diagnosis of IRS can be confirmed by a therapeutic trial of comfort which, in this case, involves employment of a mother-substitute to hold, socially interact with, and feed the infant when it is awake. The mother-substitute should enjoy nurturing, be affectively attuned, empathic, and sufficiently observant to sense whenever the baby enters the self-absorb state of withdrawal that fosters rumination. He or she should respond to the baby with prompt engagement and interaction. A positive response consists of reversal of the weight loss trend followed by subsidence of rumination over time.

It is crucially important to foresee the likely reaction of the mother when the mother-substitute takes over the care of her baby for 1 week or more. Her feelings of guilt and resentment should be anticipated. Therefore, ask the parents' permission for this nursing procedure, the purpose of which is to help with data collection and childcare. The nurses who provide surrogate mothering should be perceived as helpers to the physician and parents, not didactic teachers of superior mothering technique. Diagnostic/therapeutic interviews with each parent alone and together strengthen rapport, provide opportunities for them to recognize their emotional pain, and explore their willingness to accept more formal psychotherapeutic help.

Case Vignette: Infant Rumination Syndrome

An 8-month-old boy began vomiting during an upper respiratory infection at 6 months of age. Respiratory symptoms cleared within a week, but frequent regurgitation persisted followed by progressive weight loss. He had been hospitalized twice for intravenous hydration and diagnostic testing. Dietary, positional, and pharmacologic measures failed to help. Finally, surgical fundoplication or gastrojejunostomy and pyloroplasty were offered, but declined by the parents. During his fourth and final hospitalization, it was noticed that his 'vomiting' ceased immediately each time he was engaged in social eye contact. The mother and maternal grandmother were enlisted in an effort to hold the patient while he was awake, watch for movements that preceded regurgitation, and immediately engage the patient. His weight stabilized, but the parents became exhausted within 2 days. The family agreed to employment of a special nurse to hold and nurture their baby. His weight increased during the next 6 days, accompanied by a decrease in urine-specific gravity indicative of improved hydration. Rumination became less frequent. He was discharged on the 20th hospital day and continued on an unlimited diet and no medication. The parents agreed to continue the special nurse at home for 10 days after his release from the hospital. On follow-up examination at 2.5 years, his weight was near the 5th percentile. He appeared well and had no further vomiting. **Figure 3** shows his weight course during hospitalization.

Table 2 compares the features of the two functional vomiting syndromes in infancy that cause FTT.

The failure of anabolism (step 6, **Table 1**) is a matter of controversy. Many accept as axiomatic that adequate nourishment automatically restores growth. The professor of social work, Dorota Iwaniec has written, "Aetiologic factors of inadequate intake of food are complex and varied, but the fact remains that all children who fail to thrive (for whatever reason) do not get sufficient calories into their systems." Nevertheless, the question remains: can emotional stress impair growth in the presence of adequate intake and retention of food? Can unhappiness stunt growth?

There are theoretical and experimental findings that would support this contention. Corticotropin-releasing factor (CRF) is a neuropeptide secreted by the hypothalamus. In nonstressed states, it regulates the cyclic secretion of adrenocorticotropic hormone (ACTH) by the pituitary gland which, in turn, controls the secretion of cortisol by the adrenal cortex. Stress increases CRF secretion, which results in activation, arousal, and anxiety. CRF is the physiologic mediator of unpleasant states associated with anger, sadness, or fear. Heightened CRF secretion has been shown in animal models to inhibit food intake and increase energy expenditure. Cortisol has catabolic effects when its secretion is increased during stress. A study of the sociologic, psychologic, and metabolic aspects of patients in the community of a metabolic ward revealed increased excretion of the products of tissue catabolism during stress, especially interpersonal difficulties between individuals having strong emotional

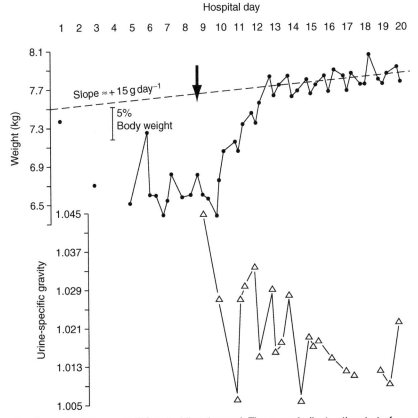

Figure 3 Response of an 8-month-old boy with IRS to 'holding therapy'. The arrow indicates the start of special nursing by a mother-substitute. There was subsequent catch-up weight gain and decreased urine specific gravity indicative of the infant's improved nutrition and hydration. Source: Fleisher DR (1979) Infant rumination syndrome: Report of a case and review of literature. *American Journal of Diseases of Children* 133(3): 266–269. © 1979 American Medical Association.

Table 2 Functional vomiting syndromes associated with FTT in infants

Features	Nervous vomiting	Infant rumination
The nature of vomiting	Involuntary Visceral Purposeless	Voluntary Behavioral Self-stimulatory
Age at onset	As early as newborn	After 2–3 months
Mothering	Attentive, but dys-synchronous; increases instead of relieves tension	Emotionally distant; little reciprocal mother–infant interaction
Typical circumstances	During the baby's response to environmental stimuli	In the absence of environmental stimuli
Prognosis if untreated	Failure to thrive	Failure to thrive and possible death
Treatment	Lessening excessive stimulation; alleviating the tension-producing quality of mother–infant interaction	Increasing environmental stimulation; satisfying the infant's needs by mothering

Modified from Fleisher DR (1994) Functional vomiting disorders in infancy: Innocent vomiting, nervous vomiting, and infant rumination syndrome. *Journal of Pediatrics* 125(6) part 2: S84–S94.

ties. Widdowson's study of 100 children 4–14 years of age in two German orphanages following World War II showed that unhappiness may be associated with impaired weight gain and that the return of happiness was associated with catch-up weight gain in children given equal amounts of food.

Whitten *et al.* disagreed with Widdowson's conclusions. In 1969, they published a study in which infants 3–24 months of age with FTT were confined for 2 weeks in a severely deprived environment consisting of a windowless room in which they were fed by personnel who were instructed to not talk to, smile at, or hold them during feedings. They were handled only for basic physical care, except during infrequent, brief visits by parents. However, the infants were fed adequate amounts of food. They did not change their abnormal behaviors (auto-eroticism, watchfulness, apathy, or developmental lags), but they did gain weight (except for two who had feeding difficulties suggestive of Chatoor's infant anorexia syndrome). The authors concluded that children with FTT, but free of organic disease, never fail to grow provided intake of food is normal.

Uncritical acceptance of this concept raises two concerns. One has to do with the effect it might have on the clinical management of FTT; the other has to do with its failure to explain a type of FTT in which supra-normal amounts of food are consumed, but growth ceases in children who failed to develop emotional attachment to their mothers.

If FTT is viewed principally as a disorder of under-nutrition that can be cured by food, the focus of management is shifted toward the immediate cause of growth failure (inadequate food intake) and away from its underlying cause (aberrant nurturing). However, the ultimate goal of treatment should be restoration of the mother's ability to love, attach, empathize, and find pleasure in her child, or if that's not possible, placement of the child with a surrogate caregiver who will provide adequate nurturing. If the child receives nutritionally and emotionally normal nurturing, the child's nutritional state and growth are likely to normalize.

The type of FTT in which anabolism and growth fail despite supra-normal intake of food has been called hyperphagic psychosocial dwarfism. It typically presents in preschool and school-aged children and is characterized by functional growth arrest resembling organic hypopituitarism. When these children are tested to determine whether their pituitary glands can secrete growth hormone or their adrenal glands can secrete cortisol, secretion fails to occur. Growth hormone injections fail to restore growth. Typical behavioral features include bizarre overeating, consumption of unusual foods and liquids, a preoccupation with food and food hoarding, social withdrawal, offensive behaviors (e.g., fecal and urinary soiling, excessive attention-seeking), and attentional deficits. Invariably, there is a failure of emotional attachment between mother and child. Surprisingly, growth resumes, aberrations of eating and drinking abate, and function of the hypothalamic–pituitary–adrenal axis returns to normal when these children are admitted to a hospital or other nurturing environment. Moreover, the abnormal behaviors and growth failure may recur when the child is returned into his or her previous environment. Although this form of FTT has been recognized for more than 60 years, it is rare and the mechanisms by which it occurs have yet to be elucidated fully. Nevertheless, this form of FTT has theoretical as well as clinical importance.

Case Vignette: Hyperphagic Psychosocial Dwarfism, That Is, 'Deprivation Dwarfism'

An 8-year-old boy, the third of four siblings, was born to a 30-year-old mother. Birth weight was 8 lb, 5 oz. He thrived during his first year. His father deserted the family when he was 18-months-old. By 2 years of age, his weight lagged and bowel movements became more frequent. He was hospitalized in a community hospital at 2 years

9 months of age with complaints of diarrhea, abdominal bloating, and listlessness after meals. Celiac disease (gluten enteropathy) was suspected, a gluten-free, milk-free diet was prescribed and he was discharged to home. One month later he was allowed to eat Christmas dinner without restrictions. His family were 'frightened at the gigantic amounts of food' he consumed. His abdomen became acutely bloated to the extent that 'he couldn't get his breath'. At 4 years of age, the patient and his siblings were abducted by their estranged father who kept them for 5 weeks. Upon his return, he had a more ravenous appetite and passed loose stools three to fives times a day. Growth continued to lag. At 6 years, he was admitted to a university hospital for evaluation. Physical examination revealed an immature boy with a 'celiac habitus' (thin limbs, distended abdomen, and flat buttocks). However, no evidence of malabsorption, cystic fibrosis, or other disease was found, except that his bones were demineralized and at a 2–3 year level of maturation.

A gluten-free diet (devoid of wheat, rye, and barley) was ordered. Nevertheless, on the first hospital day, he was found in the ward kitchen eating a sandwich. Hoarded candy was found in his bed. He surreptitiously ate cookies and saved parts of his meal for later. Painful abdominal bloating and flatulence recurred almost daily. Bowel movements were passed an average of 1.7 times a day and all but two were formed. He wet his bed every night. He gained 9.25 lb in 25 days. He was discharged after 3.5 weeks with recommendations to continue his glutin-free diet, notwithstanding how impossible it had been to impose such a restrictive diet during his hospital stay.

Six months later, worsening behavior and difficulty in keeping him from eating glutin-containing foods prompted his enrollment in a school for handicapped children. He was notorious for eating his lunch en route to school. He stole food from other children's lunches, hid food in places where he could and eat it in secret, and was often found with bread crusts and leftovers in his pockets. "We have tried all methods, short of tying him up, to avoid his getting at food that makes him ill," his teacher wrote. At home, "it was guard duty 24 h a day … he couldn't stand to let a crumb of food on anyone's plate. When he goes to the store, he just looks at the food counter, not at the toys. Food is his way of life!" his mother said. Unusual appetites appeared, for example, he might eat five packages of gum, an entire 12-oz jar of peanut butter, or a bowl of pet food at one sitting. The patient was hospitalized for the third time for 1 month at 7 year 8 months of age. He had lost weight and had hardly grown during the 18 months since his previous hospitalization. His appearance, X-ray, and laboratory findings were essentially unchanged. Growth hormone responsiveness to an insulin challenge tested on the 13th hospital day was at the lower limit of normal (Re-testing done 7.5 months later showed a more robust normal response). Psychometric testing showed intelligence quotients (IQs) between 67 and 83, but he seemed depressed and poorly motivated during testing. Receptive and expressive language was 1.5–2.5 years below expected levels for his age. The patient was offered a regular diet and free access to food. His appetite decreased somewhat and gorging and bloating lessened. He played parallel to, rather than with, his peers. He showed a striking lack of loneliness for his mother who lived 3 h away and she visited only once during his hospital stay. One day, after not seeing or speaking with her for 2 weeks, he was offered the use of a telephone and help in making a call to his mother. He declined the offer without the slightest show of emotion. Similarly, his mother showed little evidence of missing her son. The patient's mother was 38 years old, mildly obese, depressed, and emotionally continent, other than for expressions of resentment toward her son. She described herself as "a change of life baby," her next older sibling being 15 years her senior. Her father died of cancer when she was a toddler and she grew up without a step-father. She described her mother as emotionally distant. "She never went out of her way or took an interest in how I did at school". "I raised myself on my own." Her pregnancy with the patient was unwanted. She felt depressed after his delivery and attributed that to not having anyone to help her at home with the new baby. Her husband, a construction worker, was 4 years younger than she and had not been heard from in 2.5 years. The patient's three siblings were 6–14 years of age, healthy and growing normally. After 27 days, the patient was transferred to a small pediatric convalescent facility. Gorging recurred during the first week there, then subsided. He gradually began to engage in play and defend his rights with his peers. He developed a friendship with the cook and began to show spontaneous affection. He returned home after 7 months. Binging recurred the first week at home and then subsided. When seen 3.5 months after his return home, he seemed well adjusted to the second grade. Although he was still quite interested in food, gorging, bloating, stealing food, and bizarre cravings were no longer evident. (**Figure 4** depicts his growth and physical appearance before, during, and after his stays in hospital.)

Clinical Presentations of Failure to Thrive

Knowing the features of each defined syndrome does not guarantee that the clinician who encounters a child with undifferentiated growth problems will easily recognize FTT. Giulio Barbero and Eleanor Shaheen identified four presentations of FTT: (1) growth lag with no other symptoms or signs; (2) growth lag with symptoms that mimic disease, but are not pathologic and not the cause of growth failure; (3) growth lag in the presence of child abuse; and (4) children with organic diseases who have

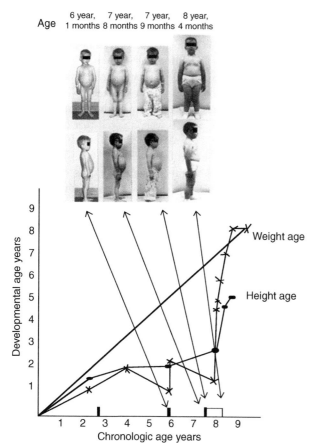

Figure 4 Changes in the appearance, height, and weight of a boy with 'hyperphagic Psychosocial dwarfism'. The ordinate indicates developmental age; the abscissa indicates chronologic age. The heavy diagonal line indicates the points at which developmental and chronological ages are equal. The solid rectangles on the abscissa indicate brief hospitalizations. The open rectangle indicates his 7-month stay at a pediatric rehabilitation facility. (All images conform to the same scale.)

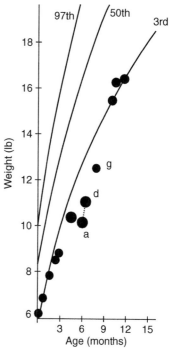

Figure 5 Type I FTT. a, weight on admission to hospital. d, weight at time of discharge. g, weight at the end of her 1-week stay in the care of her grandmother (97th, 50th, and 3rd percentile channels).

super-imposed FTT caused by distortions in the parent–child relationship resulting from the parents' knowledge or perception that their child has a life-threatening or life-altering condition. The following case vignettes illustrate each of the four patterns of presentation.

Case Vignette: Type I – Failure to Thrive Without Other Signs or Symptoms

A 6-month-old girl presented with progressive weight lag since birth. She had no illness. Her appetite was described as 'excellent'. She had no diarrhea or frequent regurgitation and she was 'always in a good mood'. She was hospitalized for 10 days. Diagnostic evaluation showed no organic disease and she remained symptom-free. Her calorie count averaged $125 \, cal \, kg^{-1} \, 24 \, h^{-1}$ which was normal for her size. Her mother was 26-years-old who grew up as a rather indulged only child, the center of an adult world. She saw herself as a 'lousy housekeeper'

and her husband, a 30-year-old computer engineer, as a 'very perfectionistic, angry man'. The parents' interaction tended to perpetuate the mother's low self-esteem, inadequate performance, and depression, which, in turn, exasperated her husband. The family home had been severely damaged by a fire the previous year. The father's job was in jeopardy, and they were financially insecure. Although they denied any effects of these stresses during interviews, they were finally able to acknowledge their emotional distress during the pre-discharge conference. The baby was seen for follow-up 3.5 weeks after discharge. She had been cranky upon their arrival home from the hospital. The parents then went on a 1-week vacation leaving her in the care of the maternal grandmother who increased the frequency of feedings. The baby gained 11 oz during the 7 days she was in her care. Catch-up weight gain continued thereafter (**Figure 5**).

Type II – Failure to Thrive Presenting with Symptoms Suggestive of Organic Disease

A 7-month-old male infant was hospitalized for vomiting and weight loss during the preceding 3 months. Two upper gastrointestinal barium studies showed narrowing of the outflow tract of the stomach, delayed gastric emptying, and gastroesophageal reflux. Although endoscopy was unrevealing, biopsy of the esophageal mucosa showed mild inflammation. Interviews with each parent revealed that the family had moved three times during the preceding 2 years, most recently a few weeks before the patient's birth. The father, a young business executive, had been transferred from another state and assigned the task of making a large, but failing business profitable. He worked long hours. The mother, a successful career woman in her own right, spent most of her time in their new home mothering her 7-year-old son and new baby. She now lived far from friends and family and had not had time to make new friends. She was self-critical, perfectionistic, and felt at fault when anything went wrong at home. The relationships in this nuclear family had become critically stressed, but the crisis had not been apparent to them, partly because of their preoccupation with their increasingly sick infant and their frustrated attempts to find the elusive food intolerance they believed caused his vomiting. The infant was hospitalized for 12 days during which he was fed on demand, shielded from commotion, and comforted whenever he fussed. Vomiting decreased. The parents became aware of their state of emotional exhaustion during reflective discussions with the attending pediatrician. Their stated fear of loosing their child subsided as a weight gain trend began to emerge on the 4th hospital day. The patient was released from the hospital on no medications or special diet. Ten weeks later, the mother wrote, "he has gone for 6 days straight without even spitting up, much less vomiting!" (**Figure 6** depicts the weight course before, during, and after his hospitalization.)

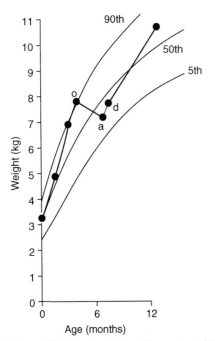

Figure 6 Type II FTT. o, onset of vomiting and weight loss. a, weight on admission to hospital. d, weight at discharge (90th, 50th, and 5th percentile channels). Adapted from Fleisher DR (1994) Functional vomiting disorders in infancy: Innocent vomiting, nervous vomiting, and infant rumination syndrome. *Journal of Pediatrics* 125(6) part 2: S84–S94.

Comment. This infant had gastroesophageal reflux and weight loss which became worse as treatments for food allergy and GERD failed and parental anxiety intensified. The possibility of nervous vomiting with FTT was considered and the approach to management was changed. The premise of organic disease was tested by omitting antireflux measures and elimination diets; this could be done provided the parents were assured that any signs of deterioration would be responded to immediately while he was closely observed in hospital. The crisis began to resolve when the parents' distress was discovered and acknowledged and when they experienced their infant's response to food and comfort as an unexpectedly welcome indication of his health rather than disease.

Type III: Failure to Thrive Accompanied by Physical Abuse

It would be wrong to assume that all children who fail to thrive are therefore abused. Such an assumption promotes judgmental attitudes that can wreck the collaborative relationship between clinicians and parents needed for successful outcomes. FTT commonly results not from abuse, but from dysfunction in the parent–child relationship, often despite the parents' sincere efforts to restore their child's health. Nevertheless, when abuse is part of the harm suffered by the child, its peril constitutes a pediatric emergency that mandates immediate hospitalization or other protective measures.

There are at least three kinds of abuse. The first kind is exemplified by the angry parent who loses control of hostile impulses and batters his or her child during a moment of frustration. The attack is not premeditated and the parents may be capable of genuine remorse afterwards. The second kind of abuse is exemplified by premeditated torture for sadistic pleasure. The third kind of abuse is also premeditated and is exemplified by the parent who creates factitious disease or suspicion of one. In the first kind of child abuse, the child must be protected from the parent, but the possibility may exist that, after treatment for anger management and/or psychotherapy, highly motivated parents may recover to the extent that it becomes safe for the child to return to their care. The second and third kinds of child abuse entail little or no possibility of safe restoration of the child to the care of its abusive parents.

Case Vignette: Type III Failure to Thrive – Factitious Disorder by Proxy (Also Known as Munchausen Syndrome by Proxy)

A 5-week-old girl born near term weighing 7 lb was said to have vomited her initial feedings and was switched to a soy-based formula. Alleged apnea spells in the newborn nursery prompted her discharge with an apnea monitor at 2 days of age. She was re-hospitalized at 4 days of age for unverified apnea and discharged 2 days later on a hypo-allergenic formula. It was reported that vomiting occurred about 12 times a day and was often projectile. At 5 weeks, she had gained only 7 oz above her birth weight and she had a severe diaper rash.

At 8 weeks, she weighed only 1 oz more, her rash was more severe, and she was scrawny, irritable, and raven-ously hungry. She was then hospitalized for 29 days. The patient consumed large amounts of formula with a calcu-lated daily caloric intake that was twice that expected of a well baby. Nevertheless, she failed to gain. On the 11th day, it was noticed that her urines were invariably dilute. A sample of leftover formula and a sample of formula from an unopened bottle were taken from her room for chemical analysis. The sodium concentration in the small amount of leftover formula was found to be about half that of the formula from the unopened bottle. Despite the mother's assurances to the contrary, the for-mula had been diluted. The patient occupied a private room and was cared for exclusively by the mother and maternal grandmother. They always declined help from the nursing staff. Observations of feeding revealed that the mother related to her 10-week-old infant as though the baby were able to obey or disobey and respond to disci-plinary measures. The mother and maternal grandmother fed the infant in an adversarial, teasing manner. In an individual interview with the father, he described his wife's medical history in terms that were typical of ongoing factitious disorder since childhood. On the 14th hospital day, the infant's malnutrition seemed life-threatening. She was transferred to the pediatric intensive care unit (ICU). The next morning, the attending, resident physicians and social worker held a conference with the family about the possibility that the patient's failure to gain weight might be caused by consumption of diluted or tainted formula. In order to test this possibility, we requested a 5-day trial during which the patient would remain in the ICU and be handled and fed only by the nursing staff. There was to be absolute physical separation of all friends and family members from the infant. They were told that, painful as the prospect of separation was, it was the only way we could explore the possibility that someone was doing something that was making their baby waste away. The parents reluc-tantly agreed to not approach the baby closer than 10 ft and a red line was taped to the floor encircling the crib which was placed directly in front of the nurses desk. The patient promptly gained weight. The diagnosis of Munchausen syndrome by proxy was confirmed and the baby was placed into high-quality foster care. When the foster-mother brought her for a follow-up visit 3.5 weeks after discharge, the patient was alert, no longer irritable, and had continued the catch-up pattern of weight gain that began in the pediatric intensive care unit (**Figure 7**).

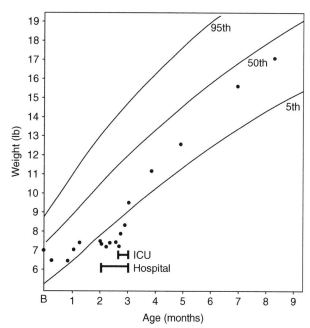

Figure 7 Type III FTT. An infant with Munchausen syndrome by proxy. The longer horizontal bar indicates the total period of hospitalization. The shorter bar indicates the part of her hospital stay during which she was closely observed in the intensive care unit, separated from her mother and maternal grandmother.

Type IV Failure to Thrive – Primary Organic Disease Complicated by Failure to Thrive

This form of FTT typically occurs in a child with an actual or perceived organic disease that may impair growth. Superimposed FTT occurs because the child's illness interferes with emotional attachment. For example, the parents may prevent themselves from attaching fully with their child because he/she might die and the antici-pated grief might be overwhelming. Therefore, without being aware of it, they avoid 'getting too close'. Or, the demands of caring for their invalid child may seem daunt-ing and even more difficult were their child unable to respond in ways that gratify and encourage his parents. The superimposed growth lag caused by aberrant nurtur-ing of this type may not be appreciated by the clinician who attributes the growth problem entirely to the child's organic disease.

Case Vignette – Type IV Failure to Thrive

Mark was born to middle-class parents weighing 4 lb, 10 oz after a pregnancy complicated by premature rupture of membranes 1 week prior to the onset of labor. Delivery was by breech extraction which caused brachial palsy and multiple cranial nerve palsies, including an absent gag reflex. A feeding gastrostomy was constructed at 2 weeks, after which he received fully adequate amounts of nourishment by tube. He was admitted to a children's hospital at 18 months for evaluation of severe lags in growth and development. Developmental evaluation showed gross motor function at the 10-month level, communication at the 9-month level and a bone age of 6–12 months. Laboratory evaluation revealed no metabolic, absorptive, or infectious diseases. There had been no vomiting, diarrhea, fever, or unusual respiratory symptoms. He passed most of his time during the 22-day hospitalization lying in a crib, receiving almost continuous infusions of food via his gastrostomy tube. Feedings consisted of 60 oz of milk plus pureed solids and vitamins in excess of twice normal requirements. Nevertheless, he gained only 4 oz in 23 days. His growth failure and retarded development were attributed to brain damage. The patient was transferred to a pediatric convalescent hospital several hours drive from his parents' home. Mark's mother remained with him for the first week, after which she returned to her husband and three children and visited on weekends. Mark remained in the convalescent hospital for 4 months during which he developed remarkable catch-up growth and accelerated development. Oral feedings were begun during the second month and he fed entirely by mouth by the end of his stay, despite an improved, but still poor gag reflex. The gastrostomy was closed several months later because his swallowing was good enough to prevent aspiration pneumonia. Follow-up at 3.25 years of age showed a happy, sociable boy with a 20–30 word vocabulary. He rode his tricycle well. He had occasional 'mild trouble chewing bulky foods', but he had not experienced aspiration pneumonia. His growth spurt in the convalescent hospital had continued at home (**Figure 8**).

In an attempt to understand what had caused the patient's remarkable improvement, the mother was asked what she had experienced the day her son entered the convalescent hospital. "I was surprised the way they handled him; they just put him in the walker, in with the other children! I felt sad and depressed when I had to feed him by the tube and the others ate at the table." When asked how she felt at the end of the first week when she decided to return home, she said, "I felt torn by having to leave Mark, but I felt a little better because he looked as though he was improving. He walked in the walker, he was happier and he had some social interest. I didn't feel so afraid for him." She indicated that the experience allowed her to overcome her fears of and for her son, as well as the feeling that he was hopelessly damaged and more than she could manage. The experience seemed to have tipped the balance in her mixed feelings and enabled her to give and receive pleasure in her relationship with her child. She felt that his outlook for normal or near-normal mental and physical function was excellent – an expectation that was confirmed when the patient was last seen at 5 years of age.

Coda

In 1980, Donald Berwick wrote an article of enduring value on FTT. In it, he summarized principles for evaluation and management of FTT in terms of eight precepts which are re-stated in **Table 3**.

The multidisciplinary tasks required for management of FTT necessitate a team led by a biopsychosocial

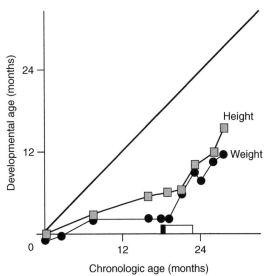

Figure 8 Type IV FTT. Growth of a prematurely born infant who sustained neurological damage during a traumatic delivery. Severe growth lag occurred during his first 18 months at home and during 22 days in hospital, despite adequate input of nutrients via feeding tube. Accelerated growth occurred during his 4-month stay in a pediatric convalescent hospital. (The ordinate indicates developmental age. The abscissa indicates chronologic age. The heavy diagonal line indicates the points at which developmental and chronologic ages are equal. The solid rectangle on the abscissa indicates the 22-day stay in hospital. The open rectangle indicates his convalescent hospitalization.)

Table 3   Principles of evaluation and management of FTT

- Involve the parents in the investigation and treatment of the child
- If the child is hospitalized, mold the physical climate of medical care to facilitate normal behavior and natural parent–child interactions
- Use laboratory investigations frugally and mainly to pursue clues from a careful history and physical examination
- Begin both evaluations and treatment with an interdisciplinary team
- Attend to interactional issues, even in the presence of organic disease
- Assure long-term follow-up
- Avoid moral judgments and threats of foster care
- Foster parental self-esteem

Adapted from Berwick (1980) Nonorganic failure to thrive. *Pediatrics in Review* 1(9): 265–270.

clinician. Otherwise, the imposition of the bias and time constraints characteristic of the biomedical model are likely to undermine the team's efforts and clinical success.

The naturalistic observations of clinicians and the data gathered by clinical investigators have created clear descriptions of FTT in its many types and presentations. However, much remains to be learned about FTT. Fortunately, contemporary neuroscience is beginning to elucidate relationships among experience, emotions, feelings, and health. The artificial designation of clinical problems as either mental or physical has outlived its usefulness. The development of a deeper, more integrated understanding of FTT shall bring us closer to its prevention and cure.

See also: Colic; Endocrine System; Feeding Development and Disorders.

Suggested Readings

Barbero GJ and Shaheen E (1967) Environmental failure to thrive: A clinical view. *Journal of Pediatrics* 71(5): 639–644.
Berwick DM (1980) Nonorganic failure to thrive. *Pediatrics in Review* 1(9): 265–270.
Chatoor I (2002) Feeding disorders in infants and toddlers: Diagnosis and treatment. *Child and Adolescent Psychiatric Clinics of North America* 11: 163–183.
Fleisher DR (1979) Infant rumination syndrome: Report of a case and review of literature. *American Journal of Diseases of Children* 133(3): 266–269.
Fleisher DR (1994) Functional vomiting disorders in infancy: Innocent vomiting, nervous vomiting, and infant rumination syndrome. *Journal of Pediatrics* 125(6) part 2: S84–S94.
Fleisher DR (1994) Integration of biomedical and psychosocial management. In: Hyman PE and DiLorenzo C (eds.) *Pediatric Gastrointestinal Motility Disorders*, pp. 13–31. New York: Academy Professional Information Services.
Heinrichs SC (2005) Behavioral consequences of altered corticotrophin-releasing factor activation in brain: A functionalist view of affective neuroscience. In: Steckler T, Kalin NH, and Reul JMHM (eds.) *Handbook of Stress and the Brain,* part 1. pp. 155–177. Amsterdam: Elsevier.
Iwaniec D (2004) *Children Who Fail to Thrive.* West Sussex: Wiley.
Powell GF, Brazel JA, and Blizzard RM (1967) Emotional deprivation and growth retardation simulating idiopathic hypopituitarism. *New England Journal of Medicine* 276(23): 1271–1278; 1279–1283.
Whitten CF, Pettit MG, and Fischoff J (1969) Evidence that growth failure from maternal deprivation is secondary to undereating. *Journal of the American Medical Association* 209(11): 1675–1682.
Widdowson EM (1951) Mental contentment and physical growth. *The Lancet.* June 16: 1316–1318.
Zeanah CH, Mammen OK, and Lieberman AF (1993) Disorders of attachment. In: Zeanah CH (ed.) *Handbook of Infant Mental Health,* 1st edn., pp. 332–349. New York: The Guilford Press.

Feeding Development and Disorders

I Chatoor and M Macaoay, Children's National Medical Center, Washington, DC, USA

Glossary

Dyadic reciprocity – Effective communication patterns between infant and caregiver during feeding or play.

External regulation – When the caregiver regulates feeding using distraction, cajoling, or force-feeding the infant regardless of the infant's hunger or satiety cues.

Failure to thrive – Infants and children who fail to gain weight or lose weight.

Infants – Birth up to 12 months.

Internal regulation – The ability of the infant/toddler to recognize his/her own inner signals of hunger and satiety.

State regulation – The ability to maintain a homeostatic mood state (e.g., calm state of alertness for feeding).

Toddlers – 12–36 months.

Transactional model – This perspective emphasizes the reciprocal, bidirectoral influence of the communication environment, between the child and his/her caregivers.

Introduction

For most infants, feeding appears to be a natural process; however, approximately 25% of otherwise normally developing infants and up to 80% of those with developmental handicaps have been reported to have feeding problems. In addition, 1–2% of infants have been found to have serious feeding difficulties associated with poor weight gain. Feeding problems may derail an infant's early development and have been linked to later deficits in cognitive development, behavioral problems, and to eating disorders during childhood, adolescence, and early adulthood.

Table 1   A classification of feeding disorders by Irene Chatoor

1. Feeding disorder of state regulation
2. Feeding disorder of caregiver–infant reciprocity
3. Infantile anorexia
4. Sensory food aversions
5. Post-traumatic feeding disorder
6. Feeding disorder associated with a concurrent medical condition

Regulation of feeding is established in the first few years of life when internal regulation of feeding by the child vs. external regulation of feeding by the parents may develop. Internal regulation is attained when the infant becomes aware of his own internal hunger and satiety cues and responds accordingly by eating or ceasing to eat. External regulation of feeding is characterized by the parent or caregiver assuming the role of regulation and feeding the infant regardless of whether the infant may be hungry or satiated.

A three-stage model of feeding development will provide a fundamental foundation of feeding behaviors, followed by a classification of feeding disorders (see **Table 1**).

Early Development and Regulation of Feeding

An important developmental process in the first years of life is the acquisition of autonomous internal regulation of feeding. The young child becomes increasingly aware of his internal hunger and satiety cues and responds accordingly by communicating his interest to eat when hungry and ceases to accept food when he recognizes fullness. Under ideal conditions, the infant is able to emit clear, unmistakable signals of hunger to his caregiver, who in turn, acknowledges these signals and responds by feeding the infant. The infant also signals when he is full by decreasing the frequency of sucking movements or by closing the mouth and not accepting any more food. When parents are attuned to their infant's hunger and satiety cues, they act as external scaffolds for the emerging abilities of the infant to self-regulate feeding. Positive reinforcement of the infant's cues during mealtimes allows the infant to trust that his basic nutritional needs will be satisfied. A nurturing and well-attuned caregiving environment establishes a solid foundation on which a secure transition from mutual regulation of feeding to the infant's own internal self-regulated feeding transpires.

The development of internally regulated autonomous feeding unfolds in three stages: (1) homeostasis, (2) dyadic reciprocity, and (3) transition of self-feeding.

Stage 1: Achieving Homeostasis

Whereas the fetus' nutritional demands were met unencumbered through the maternal umbilical cord *in utero*, upon birth, infants must actively and clearly signal hunger and satiety to caregivers. During the first few months of life, they must establish both rhythms of sleep and wakefulness, and feeding and elimination. Attaining and maintaining a calm state of wakefulness becomes a major developmental task during early feeding. Difficulties in achieving this state may result in inefficient attempts of feeding, as the infant may be too irritable or too sleepy to feed. Establishment of the infant–parent communication system is the key to establishing nutritional homeostasis – a state in which the infant's nutritional needs for growth and development are met. Appropriate perception of the infant's hunger and satiety signals by the parent and their contingent behavioral responses to the infant's signals solidifies the bonding and secure attachment between infant and caregiver.

Most infants establish a qualitatively distinct cry of hunger, in contradiction to other types of cries (e.g., pain, fear, tiredness). Ideally, these distinct cries become increasingly discernible for parents who become efficient at understanding the infant's cries during the first few weeks of life, thereby developing a communication system that allows the infant to express his needs. As the caregivers become more adept at differentiating among these cries and between infant hunger and satiety cues, they respond appropriately and thus facilitate the infant's internal regulation of feeding. However, if parents are challenged by confusing, indiscernible cues, they may respond erroneously by feeding or not feeding their infant, irrespective of their infant's state of hunger and satiety. Consequently, the infant's and the parents' distinction between hunger and satiety can become confused, which may lead to under- or overfeeding.

Stage 2: Achieving Dyadic Reciprocity

Most infants will attain state regulation (homeostatic mood state e.g., calm state of alertness for feeding) by 2–4 months of age. By that time they have become more social and infant–parent communication has become increasingly clearer. Parent and infant interactions are characterized by mutual eye contact and gazing, reciprocal vocalizations, and mutual physical closeness expressed through touch and cuddling. The adaptive infant mobilizes and engages caretakers and their interactions become increasingly reciprocal in nature. Reflexive hunger cues decrease, while intentional cues, such as vocalization for food, begin to emerge. In addition, body language that signals feeding cessation occurs with greater discern (e.g., refusing to open the mouth and turning the head). A more mature communication pattern evolves as infants begin to regulate caregivers actively and purposefully. Through receiving stronger and clearer hunger and satiety signals from the infant, caregivers are more apt to regulate the presentation and withdrawal of food accordingly. Feeding interactions become a mutually regulated process, satisfying both infant and caregiver.

The mutually regulated processes may become derailed when the infant's hunger signals are weak or inconsistent, and/or the parents lack attunement and are preoccupied with their own internal needs. These infants may be fed sporadically and inefficiently, resulting in inadequate nutrition. They may be at risk for developing a feeding disorder of failed reciprocity, as discussed later.

Stage 3: Self-Feeding Stage

The developmental stage of separation and individuation occurs between 6 months and 3 years of age. Motor and cognitive maturation processes enable the infant to become more physically and emotionally independent. Autonomy vs. dependency is negotiated daily during the feeding interactions. During each meal, mother and infant need to negotiate who is going to place the spoon in the infant's mouth. As the infant becomes more competent the parent needs to transition the infant to self-feeding. During this transition the infant not only needs to understand the difference between hunger and satiety, but also needs to differentiate the physical sensations of hunger and fullness from emotional experiences (e.g., eliciting comfort, affection, and feelings of anger or frustration).

In order for the infant to learn this differentiation, it is of paramount importance that caregivers are able to differentiate hunger and satiety cues from affective cues, and respond contingently. This includes offering food when the infant signals hunger, abstaining from offering food when the infant needs affection or calming through tactile sensations, terminating the meal when the infant appears satiated, and not insisting that the infant keeps eating until his plate is empty. This facilitative process by the caregivers ensures both the infant's awareness of hunger and satiety as well as the differentiation of physiological sensations of hunger and satiety from emotional needs.

Conversely, if the parent misinterprets the infant's emotional cues when he desires physical and emotional comfort by feeding the infant, the infant may confuse hunger with emotional experiences. He then may become conditioned to eat or refuse to eat when feeling sad, lonely, frustrated, or angry. External regulation of feeding may evolve based on the emotional experiences of the infant.

Ideally, the infant gives clear, discernible cues, and the parents interpret these signals correctly. If, however, the infant gives weak hunger cues, this may raise the parents' anxiety and cause confusion. As parents become concerned about how to deal with the nutritional needs for their infant's growth and development, they may try to override the infant's cues by feeding , even if the baby is not interested and may refuse to open its mouth. A once-envisioned happy and peaceful mealtime activity may evolve into a highly emotionally charged battleground, pitting the infant's food refusal against the parents' increasing concern about the low volume of food intake. Conversely, if an infant's weak signals of satiety or need for comfort are misinterpreted by overfeeding, parents may be unknowingly contributing to their infant's learning to eat when emotionally distressed or when seeking pleasure.

These early formative years are critical in the development of the child's internal vs. external regulation of eating. Maladaptive feeding patterns may emerge during these three developmental stages, as the infant and caregiver attempt to mutually regulate feeding behaviors. A feeding disorder may emerge if maladaptive feeding patterns become chronic, compromising the infant's growth and development. Three feeding disorders that emerge at these specific developmental stages will be discussed in the following section. In addition, other feeding disorders which can occur at various stages of development will be described.

Classification of Feeding Disorders
A Historical Perspective

Failure to thrive (FTT) was, and still is, a common term used in the medical diagnosis of feeding disorders. Clinicians initially distinguished between two forms of FTT: organic FTT, where a medical condition is considered to be the major reason for growth failure, and nonorganic FTT, where the growth failure was thought to reflect maternal deprivation or parental psychopathology. Mixed FTT and nonorganic FTT was a third category that was later added to describe growth failure that is related to a mixture of organic and environmental factors.

The diagnosis of FTT has been sharply criticized in the recent past. The main concerns are that many infants with feeding disorders do not demonstrate FTT and that it is a purely descriptive term for growth failure, rather than a diagnosis. Not until 1994, with the publication of the Diagnostic and Statistical Manual of Mental Disorders (DSM IV) by the American Psychiatric Association, was Feeding Disorder of Infancy and Early Childhood introduced as a diagnostic category to address a child's growth failure and specific feeding behaviors. Criteria include persisting failure to gain weight or significant loss of weight over at least 1 month; the disorder is not due to an associated gastrointestinal or other medical condition, another mental disorder, or by lack of available food; and onset is before 6 years of age. It is important to note that children who have feeding difficulties without weight problems or a feeding disorder associated with a medical condition are excluded from these limited criteria. Additionally, various subtypes of feeding disorders have been described by several authors that have not been addressed by this limited diagnostic definition. For example, subclassification systems of feeding disorders have been attributed to various organic and nonorganic etiologies. Other authors have used different diagnostic labels to describe the same symptomatology, or the same label to describe different symptoms. Consequently, diagnostic dilemmas have arisen as to what constitutes a feeding disorder, and how one may differentiate one feeding disorder from another or from a subclinical feeding problem. These problems in the definition of feeding disorders have also led to confusion about how to treat specific feeding problems. MaryLou Kerwin, in her literature review of empirically based treatments for severe feeding problems, noted that treatments for feeding disorders exist but the question remains for whom they are appropriate, and when, and why.

We will present a classification system of feeding disorders, developed by Irene Chatoor. Dr. Chatoor was supported in her effort to develop diagnostic criteria for these six feeding disorders by a task force of national experts in infant psychiatry. These efforts by the task force in 2004 were supported by the American Academy of Child and Adolescent Psychiatry. The criteria were further revised with the help of a work group of experts in psychopathology of infants and young children for publication in a monograph by the American Psychiatric Press Incorporated. This classification differentiates six feeding disorders that have different etiologies and require different interventions. Each feeding disorder is characterized by specific symptoms that differentiate it from other feeding disorders and healthy eating. In addition, each feeding disorder has specific criteria of impairment relating to the child's nutritional state and/or threat to the child's health and development in order to differentiate clinical feeding disorders from subclinical forms.

Feeding Disorder of State Regulation

Diagnostic criteria

1. The infant's feeding difficulties start in the first few months of life and should be present for at least 2 weeks.
2. The infant has difficulty reaching and maintaining a state of calm alertness for feeding; he/she is either too sleepy or too agitated to feed.
3. The infant fails to gain age-appropriate weight or may show loss of weight.
4. The infant's feeding difficulties cannot be explained by a physical illness.

Clinical description

Infants who have difficulty with state regulation, who are either too sleepy or too distressed and agitated, and cannot reach a state of calm alertness during feeding, are unable to suckle effectively. Consequently, their intake of milk is inadequate, which causes concern and anxiety in the mothers. As the mother becomes increasingly anxious, she is unable to help her infant in state regulation, and mother and infant become trapped in a vicious cycle of mutually distressing interactions. Newborn infants with undeveloped central nervous systems, with cardiac, pulmonary, or gastrointestinal disorders, or other medical illnesses may be at greater risk for this disorder.

Review of the literature

There is a dearth of literature regarding this subgroup of infant feeding disorder. The only study by Chatoor and colleagues posited that infants diagnosed with a feeding disorder of state regulation (homeostasis), demonstrated less positive reciprocal interactions between infants and their mothers, compared to healthy eaters and their mothers. Future studies are needed to enhance an understanding of infant and parent characteristics associated with this feeding disorder.

Treatment

Understanding infant and parent characteristics is essential in treating this feeding disorder of state regulation. The treatment may focus on assisting the mother to modulate the amount of stimulation, especially at mealtime (e.g., feeding an excitable infant in a calm and low-lighted room or massaging an infant who has difficulty waking up to feed). The intervention may target maternal factors (e.g., treating anxiety or depression in the mother to help her deal more effectively with her challenging infant). In severe cases of poor weight gain or weight loss, temporary nasogastric tube feedings may be necessary to stabilize the nutritionally compromised infant and prevent further deterioration of the infant's condition. In other cases, a combination of interventions targeting the mother and the infant may be most helpful.

Feeding Disorder of Caregiver–Infant Reciprocity

Diagnostic criteria

1. This feeding disorder is usually observed in the first year of life, when the infant presents with some acute medical problem (commonly an infection) to the primary care physician or the emergency room, and the physician notices that the infant is malnourished.
2. The infant shows lack of developmentally appropriate signs of social responsivity (e.g., visual engagement, smiling, babbling) during feeding with the primary caregiver.
3. The infant shows significant growth deficiency (acute and/or chronic malnutrition, or the child's weight deviates across two major percentiles in a 2–6-month period).

4. The primary caregiver is often unaware of the feeding and growth problems of the infant.

5. The growth deficiency and lack of relatedness are not solely due to a physical illness or a pervasive developmental disorder

Clinical description

These infants usually look ill and malnourished. They may avoid eye contact, and appear withdrawn and listless. The mothers often do not seek help for their infants, until the infants become acutely ill with an infection, and their growth and development is severely compromised. Often, the infants show poor muscle tone and impaired coordination. When held they stiffen, scissor their legs, and hold their arms up in a surrender posture to be able to hold up their heads.

Impairment in caregiver–infant interactions and communication can be observed. The mothers appear unable to engage their infants in reciprocal interactions; they often appear detached and overwhelmed by their own emotional needs. They may have been unaware of any problems, as their infants' sleeping patterns lengthened and their feeding drive lessened. They may admit to propping bottles for feeding and spending minimal time with their infant. The mothers may be guarded and distrustful, and avoid contact with medical professionals.

Review of the literature

Maternal neglect has been thought to bring on this feeding disorder, and in the early literature this feeding disorder has been referred to as Maternal Deprivation or Environmental Deprivation. In accordance with these terms, the DSM-III referred to it as 'reactive detachment disorder of infancy' and highlighted 'FTT' as the central symptom. However, in 1994, DSM-IV modified reactive attachment disorder to a selected relatedness problem without including growth failure in the diagnostic criteria. Chatoor and colleagues posited that significant issues of attachment are at the root of this feeding disorder and they called it "feeding disorder of attachment." They reported that infants with a feeding disorder of attachment and their mothers demonstrated less positive engagement and dyadic reciprocity during feedings than healthy infants and their mothers. Additionally, mothers of infants with this feeding disorder received higher maternal noncontingency ratings than mothers of healthy infants. Several studies have reported high rates of insecure attachments in the infants, and described that the mothers often suffer from psychiatric disorders (e.g., substance or alcohol abuse, mood disorders, and personality disorders). Other studies have noted that the mothers are often from a lower socioeconomic background, and may have their own history of being victims of abuse and neglect.

Treatment

Treatments, ranging from home-based interventions to hospitalization, have been proposed. The early work by Selma Frailberg, proposed an in-home approach that focused on nurturing the mother, so she could begin to nurture her infant. A study that compared three types of outpatient treatment – short-term advocacy, family-centered intervention, and parent–infant intervention – found that no treatment was superior to the other. However, outpatient treatment should be an alternative solution only in cases of mild neglect with no evidence of depriving behaviors on account of the mother, when the child is more than 1 year old, the parents have an established support system, and have a history of seeking medical care for previous illnesses and for immunizations.

More commonly, the severely malnourished and developmentally delayed infant requires hospitalization for emergency treatment. During the course of the hospitalization, treatment should address the infant's nutritional state and developmental delays while the assessment of the mother and family environment occurs. It is important that a minimum of different nursing staff are assigned to the infant and that a primary care nurse assumes responsibility for continuity of care, and for a compassionate environment for the infant. In addition, the infants may need physical therapy to address generalized hypotonia secondary to tactile understimulation in their home environment. While the rehabilitation of the infant goes on, the degree of parental awareness and cooperation with the infant's treatment needs to be assessed, as the parent's involvement with treatment is predictive of the outcome for these infants. Unfortunately, there are cases where the primary caregiver may be severely impaired or live in a chaotic environment, and may be unable to become engaged with the infant. Alternative placements have to be considered in these cases, as attention to the infant's well-being and health cannot wait.

Infantile Anorexia

Diagnostic criteria

1. This feeding disorder is characterized by the infant's or toddler's refusal to eat adequate amounts of food for at least 1 month.

2. Onset of the food refusal often occurs during the transition to spoon and self-feeding, typically between 6 months and 3 years of age.

3. The infant or toddler rarely communicates hunger, lacks interest in food and eating, but shows strong interest in play, exploration, and/or interaction with caregivers.

4. The infant or toddler shows significant growth deficiency (acute and/or chronic malnutrition; or the child's weight deviates across two major percentiles in a 2–6 month period).

5. The food refusal did not follow a traumatic event to the oropharynx.
6. The food refusal is not due to an underlying medical illness.

Clinical description

These infants characteristically have a very poor hunger drive, display minimal to no interest in food or eating, are easily distracted by other stimuli, and prefer to explore and interact with others or their environment. Caregivers report that their major concerns are the infant's intense food refusal and growth failure. Despite a variety of parental interventions to help their infants eat (e.g., coaxing, distraction techniques, feeding while playing, etc.), these measures may temporize the situation in the short term, however, over the long term, prove unsuccessful.

Some mothers report that the infants were already easily distracted while breastfeeding and would stop feeding if somebody entered the room or the phone would ring. Most commonly, by the end of the first year, these infants take only a few bites of food and then stop, refusing to eat anymore, despite the parents' attempts to feed them. The parents become increasingly worried about the infants'/toddlers' poor food intake and use great efforts to get them to eat by distracting with toys or video movies; feeding while playing, coaxing, or cajoling; feeding while the infants are sleepy; or even force-feeding them. However, in spite of all these efforts by the parents, the infants/toddlers eat inadequate amounts of food to support growth. Initially, they fail to gain appropriate weight for age, and as their feeding problems continue, they grow at a slow rate. Children at 3 years of age may look like 2 year olds, and at age 10 years, they may have the height and bone age of a 7-year-old child. However, not all children with this feeding disorder become stunted in their growth; some grow at a normal rate and become extremely thin. Interestingly, their head size tends to progress at a normal rate, and their cognitive development is age-appropriate and sometimes superior.

Review of the literature

Several studies by Chatoor and colleagues and by Massimo Ammaniti and Loredana Lucarelli have examined child and parent characteristics associated with infantile anorexia. These studies have revealed that mother–infant interactional patterns are characterized by less dyadic reciprocity, high dyadic conflict, struggle for control, and increased talk and distractions during feedings. Additional studies have found that toddlers with infantile anorexia are rated by their parents as more negative, more irregular in their feeding and sleeping patterns, more willful on the one hand and more dependent on the other than healthy eaters. In addition, toddlers with infantile anorexia exhibited more anxiety/depression, more somatic complaints, and aggressive behaviors than healthy control children. These studies also revealed that more mothers of toddlers with infantile anorexia demonstrate insecure attachment patterns to their own parents and more dysfunctional eating attitudes, anxiety, and depression than mothers of healthy control children. In addition, these studies found that toddlers with infantile anorexia exhibited a higher rate of insecure attachment relationships to their mothers than healthy eaters, although the majority of anorexic toddlers (60%) showed secure attachment patterns. However, the significant correlation between the severity of malnutrition and the degree of attachment insecurity indicated that an insecure toddler–mother relationship is associated with a more severe expression of infantile anorexia.

It is of interest that studies at both sites by Ammaniti and colleagues and by Chatoor and colleagues showed that infantile anorexia occurs with the same frequency in boys and girls, in contrast to anorexia nervosa which is seen predominantly in females.

A recent study by Chatoor and colleagues demonstrated that on average, toddlers with infantile anorexia performed within the normal range of cognitive development, although the mental developmental index (MDI) scores of the healthy eaters were significantly higher than those of the infantile anorexia group. In contrast to some of the previous reports by other authors that cognitive development is negatively affected by FTT, correlations between MDI scores and the toddlers' percent ideal body weight did not reach statistical significance, whereas the toddlers' MDI scores showed a significant correlation with the quality of mother–child interactions during feeding and play, and the socioeconomic status of the family.

In addition, a recent pilot study by Chatoor and colleagues found increased physiological arousal and decreased ability to modulate physiological reactivity in toddlers with infantile anorexia compared to a control group of healthy eaters. This study raises the question whether the difficulty of recognizing hunger, which characterizes children with infantile anorexia, may be related to a heightened physiological arousal pattern.

All of these studies were cross-sectional, and consequently, they do not allow any firm conclusions about the causality of this feeding disorder. However, the developmental histories of these children reveal that from early infancy, these children display little interest in feeding and eat only small amounts, thereby triggering anxiety and worry in the parents who try to compensate for the infant's poor food intake by falling into maladaptive feeding patterns of distracting, coaxing, and even force-feeding. These parental behaviors further interfere with the toddler's awareness of hunger and fullness and lead to increasingly conflictual interactions between mother and child, both struggling for control. As a result of these struggles, the child does not learn to regulate eating internally, but eating becomes completely dependent on the interactions of the child with the environment.

Treatment

This transactional model described above has served as a basis for an intervention to facilitate internal regulation of eating in toddlers with infantile anorexia. A treatment was developed by Chatoor and colleagues that addresses the major components of the model: (1) the parents are helped to understand the toddler's special temperament, namely the lack of awareness of hunger and fullness, and the toddler's intense interest in play and interactions with the caretakers; (2) the parents' anxiety and worry about the infant's poor growth, their difficulty in setting limits to the toddler's provocative behaviors around eating, and how these difficulties may relate to experiences with their own parents, are explored; and (3) the parents are provided with specific guidelines that detail how to structure mealtimes in order to facilitate the toddler's learning of hunger and fullness, and how to deal with the toddler's behaviors that interfere with feeding.

Sensory Food Aversions

Diagnostic criteria

1. This feeding disorder is characterized by the infant's/toddler's consistent refusal to eat specific foods with specific tastes, textures, smells, and/or appearances for at least 1 month.
2. The onset of the food refusal occurs during the introduction of a new type or taste of food (e.g., may drink one type of formula but refuse another; may eat carrots, but refuse green beans; may eat crunchy foods but refuse pureed food or baby food).
3. Eats well when offered preferred foods.
4. Does not show growth deficiency, but without supplementation, demonstrates specific dietary deficiencies (i.e., vitamins, iron, zinc, or protein), and/or displays oral motor and expressive speech delay, and/or starting during the preschool years, demonstrates anxiety and avoids social situations which involve eating.
5. The food refusal did not follow a traumatic event to the oropharynx.
6. Refusal to eat specific foods is not related to food allergies or any other medical illness.

Clinical description

This feeding disorder becomes apparent during the early years, when infants and toddlers are introduced to a variety of baby food and table food of different tastes and textures. Parents usually report that when specific foods were placed in the infants' mouths, the aversive reactions ranged from grimacing to gagging, vomiting, or spitting out the food. After an initial aversive reaction, the infants usually refuse to continue eating that particular food and become distressed if forced to do so. Some infants generalize their reluctance to eat one food to other

foods that look or smell similar (e.g., an aversion to spinach may generalize to all green vegetables). Parents frequently report that these children just look at certain foods without ever trying them and are generally reluctant to try any new foods. Some children may even refuse to eat any food that has touched another food on the plate, while others will only eat food prepared by a specific restaurant or company (e.g., French fries from McDonalds).

If infants reject foods that require significant chewing (e.g., meats, hard vegetables, or fruits), they will fall behind in their oral motor development due to lack of experience with chewing, and they may show difficulty with articulation. If children refuse many foods or whole food groups (e.g., vegetables and fruits), their limited diet may lead to specific nutritional deficiencies (e.g., vitamins, zinc, and iron). In contrast, the restricted diet of some of these children may be very unhealthy and lead to early cholesterol problems. In addition, the children's refusal to eat a variety of foods often creates conflict within their families during mealtime, and may cause social anxiety as early as in preschool, when the children are faced with eating at school, or when they get older and want to participate in events that include eating (e.g., birthday parties, sleepovers, and summer camp).

Sensory food aversions are common and occur along a spectrum of severity with some children refusing to eat only a few foods, whereas others may be limited to eating a very restrictive diet. Therefore, the diagnosis of a feeding disorder should only be made if the food aversions result in dietary deficiencies, requiring that the child needs supplementation of certain nutrients (e.g., vitamins, zinc, iron, or protein) and/or are associated with oral motor delay and speech articulation problems. In older children, social anxiety (if the child fears or avoids social situations, which involve eating with others) should be considered as a sign of impairment.

In addition to their sensitivity to certain foods; many of these children experience problems in other sensory areas as well. Parents may report that some infants with sensory food aversions do not like to touch certain foods; struggle when they need a hair cut; become distressed when asked to walk on sand or grass; or do not like to wear socks, certain types of fabric, or labels in clothing; or that they may be hypersensitive to certain odors or loud sounds.

Review of the literature

Several authors have described children's difficulty to eat certain foods, but have used a variety of names (e.g., picky eaters, choosy eaters, selective eaters, food neophobia, and food aversion). These reports are usually based on clinical case studies, they do not delineate specific diagnostic criteria, and they do not differentiate between milder or more severe forms of food selectivity. Consequently, some authors report very high numbers (25–50%) of 'picky eating' in the general population. In our own diagnostic study of feeding disorders, which was conducted in a Multidisciplinary Feeding Disorders Clinic, 'sensory food aversions' was the most commonly diagnosed feeding disorder (31% of all referrals), and 13% of the children were comorbid for sensory food aversions and infantile anorexia.

Some studies have explored whether taste sensitivities are heritable. Various models of genetic transmission have been suggested, and in 2003 Un-kyung Kim and colleagues have described that specific polymorphism of gene *Tas2r* on chromosome 7q are related to taste sensitivity in adults. A relationship between genetic taste sensitivity to propylthiouracil (PROP) and food selectivity has also been reported in preschool children. However, Lean Birch and colleagues have demonstrated that certain aspects of the eating environment can also have a strong influence on the development of food preferences, and shape selective food refusal. In summary, previous studies indicate that genetic predisposition as well as the eating environment, affect toddler's food preferences. However, further studies are needed to understand the relation between genetic and environmental influences on the development of this feeding disorder.

Treatment

Once infants or toddlers experience a food as aversive, they tend to grimace, spit out the food, or they may even gag and vomit, when they try to swallow it. After a negative experience with a particular food, they tend to refuse to accept any more of that food. Parents frequently try to coax toddlers into eating foods that they reject by promising certain privileges, for example, watching television, or getting to play with a certain toy, or they withhold a favorite food to induce the toddler to eat more healthy foods. Unfortunately, these techniques have often a significant negative effect, they make the children more anxious and lead to oppositional food refusal in general. In contrast, if parents recognize and accept that the infant/toddler experiences specific foods as aversive, and they stop offering these foods, the children can relax and consequently, they are more willing to try new foods that they may be able to tolerate. Toddlers are particularly responsive to modeling by the parents, and they are more willing to try a new food if they can observe their parents eating it. However, these clinical experiences have not been tested in any systematic research studies.

Post-Traumatic Feeding Disorder

Diagnostic criteria

1. This feeding disorder is characterized by the acute onset of severe and consistent food refusal.

2. The onset of the food refusal can occur at any age of the child from infancy to adulthood.

3. The food refusal follows a traumatic event or repeated traumatic insults to the oropharynx or gastrointestinal tract (e.g., choking, severe vomiting, insertion of nasogastric or endotracheal tubes, suctioning) that trigger intense distress in the child.

4. Consistent refusal to eat manifests in one of the following ways, depending on the feeding experience of the child in association with the traumatic event:
   - refuses to drink from the bottle, but may accept food offered by spoon (although consistently refuses to drink from the bottle when awake, may drink from the bottle when sleepy or asleep);
   - refuses solid food, but may accept the bottle; and
   - refuses all oral feedings.

5. Reminders of the traumatic events cause distress, as manifested by one or more of the following:
   - may show anticipatory distress when positioned for feeding;
   - shows intense resistance when approached with bottle or food; and/or
   - shows intense resistance to swallow food placed in the mouth.

6. Without supplementation (e.g., specific fortified formula preparations, intravenous. fluids, nasogastric or gastrostomy tube feedings, or parenteral nutrition), the food refusal poses an acute and/or long-term threat to the child's health, nutrition, and growth, and threatens the progression of age-appropriate feeding development of the child.

Clinical description

The term post-traumatic eating disorder was first coined by Chatoor, Conley, and Dickson in a paper on food refusal in five latency-age children who experienced episodes of choking or severe gagging, and later refused to eat any solid food. These children were preoccupied with the fear of choking to death, if they were to eat any solid food. Infants and toddlers with a post-traumatic feeding disorder cannot verbally communicate their fear of eating, but display fear and intense resistance to eating in their behavior. Parents may report that their infants' refusal to eat any solid foods started after an incident of choking, or after one or more episodes of severe gagging. Other parents may report that the infant's refusal to drink from the bottle started after one or more severe episodes of vomiting. After the severe vomiting, the infant would cry at the sight of the bottle and would not drink from the bottle any more. Some parents may have observed that the food refusal followed intubation, the insertion of nasogastric feeding tubes, or major surgery requiring intubation or vigorous oropharyngeal suctioning.

Reminders of the traumatic event(s) (e.g., the bottle, the bib, or the high-chair), frequently cause intense distress, and the infants become fearful when they are positioned for feedings and presented with feeding utensils and food. They resist being fed by crying, arching, and refusing to open their mouths. If food is placed in their mouths, they intensely resist swallowing. They may gag or vomit, let the food drop out, actively spit out food, or store food in their cheeks and spit it out later to avoid swallowing it. The fear of eating seems to override any awareness of hunger, and infants who refuse all food, liquids and solids, require acute intervention to prevent dehydration and starvation.

Literature review

Similar symptomatology primarily in children has been described by other authors as fear of choking or choking phobia, and as dysphagia and food aversion. However, these studies are primarily clinically descriptive and do not provide any clear diagnostic criteria. Using the diagnostic criteria listed above, Chatoor and colleagues found that toddlers with a post-traumatic feeding disorder showed intense mother–infant conflict during feeding and demonstrated the most intense resistance to swallowing food.

However, more research is needed to understand this feeding disorder better.

Treatment

This feeding disorder can be life-threatening, and many infants with this disorder may require gastric tube-feedings. Although this intervention helps infants to survive, the tube-feedings interfere with their experience of hunger and further complicate the feeding disorder. The fear of swallowing and the lack of hunger make the children very resistant to oral feedings. However, one controlled, randomized treatment study by Diane Benoit and colleagues demonstrated the effectiveness of a behavioral intervention to overcome their resistance to oral feedings and to come off tube-feedings.

A more gradual desensitization approach has been used at The Children's National Medical Center. The infants' anticipatory anxiety to the feeding situation is assessed, and through gradual exposure to the bottle, the high-chair, and the feeding utensils, the infants or toddlers are helped to overcome their fear by looking at these objects and playing with them. Food is gradually introduced, and the children are encouraged to self-feed to give them more control. This gradual desensitization process is slow and only possible if adequate food intake of the children is guaranteed through bottle-feedings or tube-feedings.

Feeding Disorder Associated with a Concurrent Medical Condition

Diagnostic criteria

1. This feeding disorder is also characterized by food refusal and inadequate food intake for at least 2 weeks.
2. The onset of the food refusal can occur at any age and may wax and wane in intensity, depending on the underlying medical condition.
3. The infant or toddler readily initiates feeding, but over the course of the feeding, shows distress, and refuses to continue feeding.
4. Has a concurrent medical condition that is believed to cause the distress (e.g., gastroesophageal reflux, cardiac, or respiratory disease).
5. Fails to gain age-appropriate weight or may even lose weight.
6. Medical management improves but may not fully alleviate the feeding problems.

Clinical description

Some medical conditions are not readily diagnosed and food refusal may be the leading symptom. For example, food allergies can be difficult to diagnose in this young age group, and silent gastroesophageal reflux may be overlooked by pediatricians because the infant does not vomit, and vomiting is usually the leading symptom of reflux. However, with silent reflux, the infant may experience regurgitations of gastric content into the esophagus, causing irritation of the esophageal mucosa without any outward signs of reflux. In addition, there is considerable individual variability in the perception of pain. Consequently, only a small percentage of infants with gastroesophageal reflux exhibit distress during feeding or after vomiting. In order to understand the individual infant's experience with gastroesophageal reflux, it is important to observe the infant during feeding. Typically, infants drink one to two ounces of milk before reflux is activated, and the infants display vomiting or show signs of discomfort (e.g., coughing, wiggling, arching, and crying) and push the bottle away. Some infants can calm themselves and resume feeding until they experience a new episode of pain. However, some others cry in distress and become increasingly agitated while their caregivers try to continue feeding.

Some infants with respiratory distress may feed for a while and take a few ounces of milk or food until they tire out and stop feeding. In general, these infants consume inadequate amounts of food, fail to gain age-appropriate weight, or even lose weight. Good medical management improves the infants' feeding difficulties. Frequently, however, the feeding problems do not remit completely, and require further psychological interventions.

Review of the literature

In the early literature, a mixed category of FTT, which is caused by a combination of various organic and nonorganic problems, has been described, and it has been generally accepted that organic conditions can be associated with psychological difficulties and lead to severe feeding problems. Some authors have reported severe feeding problems such as food refusal, and taking more than 1 hour per feeding, in infants with gastroesophageal reflux. Others have described that the food refusal associated with gastroesophageal reflux was so severe that some infants had to be tube-fed, and that even after successful surgery, the severe feeding difficulties and growth failure continued. These studies are primarily descriptive and highlight the observation that the combination of medical and psychological factors can lead to complex feeding problems, requiring combined interventions.

Treatment

Because of the interaction of organic and psychological factors in producing feeding difficulties, treatment of these infants requires close collaboration between the pediatrician or pediatric specialist and the child psychiatrist or psychologist. Direct observation of infants with their primary caregivers during feeding is most important to monitor how much distress the infant experiences during feeding and whether the medical condition is being adequately treated or requires further intervention. The observation of the feeding also reveals how parents deal with the infant's distress, whether they become anxious and inadvertently heighten the infant's distress, thus escalating the feeding problems. These observations can be used to optimize the medical treatment, and assist the parents in developing different feeding strategies to help minimize the infant's discomfort during feeding. In situations in which the medical intervention cannot control the medical illness, when infants continue to experience distress during feedings and their caloric intake is limited, supplemental nutrition through nasogastric or gastrostomy tubes must be considered. The therapist must help the parents and the medical team deal with this difficult decision and work with them to maintain the infant's interest in feeding and develop age-appropriate feeding skills, while most of the nutrition is given via tube-feedings. In general, children with this feeding disorder require individualized interventions by an experienced team.

Comorbidity between various feeding disorder subtypes

In a diagnostic study by Chatoor and colleagues, 20% of the infants and young children examined showed comorbidity of two or more feeding disorders. The most frequent comorbidity observed was between infantile anorexia and sensory food aversions, although these feeding disorders occurred more frequently in the pure form. Characteristically, children with both feeding disorders are very selective about foods which they are willing to eat, but even when given their favorite foods, the children have a poor appetite and eat little. It is important to diagnose each feeding disorder because each has a different etiology and shows different responses to treatment. Toddlers with infantile anorexia respond to the regulation of mealtimes with an increase of appetite and improved food intake, whereas toddlers with sensory food aversions will eat less or nothing if offered aversive foods, regardless of how hungry they may be. Consequently, the treatment needs to address both feeding disorders.

A problem arises when the children exhibit symptoms that appear to fit the diagnoses of three or four different feeding disorders. We recommend that the symptoms should be differentiated as much as possible to understand what the underlying diagnoses may be, because, as point out earlier, each feeding disorder requires a different therapeutic approach.

See also: Colic; Failure to Thrive.

Suggested Readings

Benoit D, Wang EE, and Zlotkin SH (2000) Discontinuation of enterostomy tube feeding by behavioral treatment in early childhood: A randomized control trial. *Journal of Pediatrics* 137: 498–503.

Birch LL (1999) Development of food preferences. *Annual Review of Nutrition* 19: 41–62.

Burklow KA, Phelps AN, Schultz JR, McConnell K, and Randolph C (1998) Classifying complex pediatric feeding disorders. *Journal of Pediatric Gastroenterology and Nutrition* 27(2): 143–147.

Chatoor I, Conley C, and Dickson L (1988) Food refusal after an incident of choking: A posttraumatic eating disorder. *Journal of American Academy of Child and Adolescent Psychiatry* 27: 105–110.

Chatoor I, Ganiban J, Surles J, and Doussard-Roosevelt J (2004) Physiological regulation and infantile anorexia: A pilot study. *Journal of American Academy of Child and Adolescent Psychiatry* 43: 1019–1025.

Chatoor I, Getson P, Menvielle E, O'Donnell, et al. (1997) A feeding scale for research and clinical practice to assess mother–infant interactions in the first three years of life. *Infant Mental Health Journal* 18: 76–91.

Chatoor I, Surles J, Ganiban J, Beker L, Paez LM, and Kerzner B (2004) Failure to thrive and cognitive development in toddlers with infantile anorexia. *Pediatrics* 113(5): e440–e447.

Frailberg S, Anderson E, and Shapiro U (1975) Ghosts in the nursery. *Journal of American Academy of Child and Adolescent Psychiatry* 14: 387–421.

Kerwin ME (1999) Empirically supported treatments in pediatric psychology: Severe feeding problems. *Journal of Pediatric Psychology* 24: 193–214.

Mahler MS, Pine F, and Berman A (1975) *The Psychological Birth of the Human Infant.* New York: Basic Books.

Fetal Alcohol Spectrum Disorders*

H Carmichael Olson, S King, and T Jirikowic, University of Washington, Seattle, WA, USA

Glossary

Active case ascertainment – 'Ascertainment' is the scheme by which individuals are selected, identified, and recruited for participation in a research study. 'Active case ascertainment' means that individuals are actively searched for so they can be identified.

Behavioral phenotype – A characteristic pattern of motor, cognitive, linguistic, and social observations that is consistently associated with a biological disorder.

Epigenetic – A factor that changes the phenotype (the observable characteristics of an individual) without changing the genotype (the entire genetic identity of an individual).

Neurobehavioral – Relating to the relation between the action of the nervous system and behavior.

Prevalence – The proportion of individuals in a population having a disease or disorder.

Teratogen – An agent capable of causing developmental malformations in the embryo or fetus when there is prenatal exposure.

Introduction

Prenatal alcohol exposure can lead to significant and lifelong developmental disabilities, now recognized under the umbrella term of 'fetal alcohol spectrum disorders' (FASDs). FASDs are a global public health problem, found worldwide and across all ethnicities. These lifelong birth defects are an especially important topic for those interested in infancy and early childhood. Not only are these birth defects preventable but, if they do occur, there is real hope that FASDs can be effectively treated. Basic animal research and human studies are building the case that diagnosis and intervention (especially early in life) can improve the developmental outcome of

individuals affected by alcohol exposure before birth. Providers working in early intervention can be among the first to grasp the real hazards of prenatal alcohol exposure for children's development, referring for diagnosis, alerting caregivers to emerging learning and behavior problems, and connecting families with needed services.

Understanding the Problem of FASDs

A Spectrum Disorder

FASDs are increasingly understood as a spectrum or continuum of effects that result from prenatal alcohol exposure. Individuals with FASDs can show adverse physical signs from prenatal alcohol exposure (such as characteristic facial anomalies or various other bodily malformations), but do not always have these physical effects. Individuals with FASDs typically do show alcohol-related deficits in many different aspects of learning, behavior, and daily function, and these are the difficulties that are the most troubling (but also the most important) to identify, diagnose, and treat. These functional difficulties vary from individual to individual, who can have very different profiles of alcohol-related deficits.

Table 1 defines diagnoses on the fetal alcohol spectrum. The range of FASDs includes the full 'fetal alcohol syndrome' (FAS), defined by growth impairment, characteristic facial features, and evidence of significant central nervous system (CNS) damage and/or dysfunction. **Figure 1** shows the 'face' of FAS. But FAS is found in only a fairly small proportion of individuals affected by prenatal alcohol exposure and, unfortunately, the effects of alcohol are not readily recognized if they do not fit the classic FAS definition. There are children born with 'partial FAS' who manifest some but not all of the characteristic physical features, and so do not meet criteria for the full syndrome. But a larger number of children, adolescents, and adults have alcohol-induced impairments without the characteristic facial features, and may or may not have growth impairment. Their functional difficulties can be just as serious, or more so, than those seen in FAS. The term 'alcohol-related neurodevelopmental disorder' (ARND) has been applied to these conditions. There are also individuals born prenatally exposed who have other alcohol-related physical abnormalities of the skeleton and certain organ systems. These anomalies are referred to as 'alcohol-related birth defects' (ARBD). Of course, a person cannot have FASDs unless there has been prenatal alcohol

*Portions of this article were previously published in: Carmichael Olson H, Jirikowic T, Kartin D, and Astley S (2007) Responding to the challenges of early intervention for fetal alcohol spectrum disorders. *Infants and Young Children* 20(2): 162–179. These sections, including Table 1, are used here with permission of © copyright owner Lippincott Williams and Wilkins, Inc.

Table 1   Criteria for diagnosing fetal alcohol spectrum disorders

Diagnosis	Diagnostic features
Fetal alcohol syndrome (FAS)	• Growth deficiency: height or weight < 10th percentile • Cluster of characteristic minor facial anomalies: small palpebral fissures (eyeslits), thin upper lip, smooth philtrum (groove above the upper lip) • Central nervous system damage (evidence of structural and/or functional brain impairment) • Reliable evidence of confirmed prenatal alcohol exposure: not necessary if the cluster of characteristic facial features is present
Partial FAS (PFAS)	• Some of the characteristic minor facial anomalies • Growth deficiency: height or weight < 10th percentile[a] • Central nervous system damage (evidence of structural and/or functional brain impairment) • Reliable evidence of confirmed prenatal alcohol exposure
Alcohol-related neurodevelopmental disorder (ARND)	• Central nervous system damage (evidence of structural and/or functional brain impairment) • Reliable evidence of confirmed prenatal alcohol exposure

[a]*The 4-Digit Code provides more detail about PFAS, as there are some cases in which growth impairment is not a necessary criterion because the expression of facial features so closely resembles the classic FAS presentation.*
Reproduced from Carmichael Olson H, Jirikowic T, Kartin D, and Astley S (2007) Responding to the challenges of early intervention for fetal alcohol spectrum disorders. *Infants and Young Children* 20(2): 162–179, with permission of Lippincott, Williams & Wilkins, Inc. Adapted from Astley SJ (2004) *Diagnostic Guide for Fetal Alcohol Spectrum Disorders: The 4-Digit Diagnostic Code*, 3rd edn. Seattle, WA: University of Washington Publication Services. (*Manual for the 4-Digit Diagnostic Code* available from the University of Washington Fetal Alcohol Syndrome Diagnostic & Prevention Network). The '4-Digit Diagnostic Code' is a system used by clinicians and researchers to evaluate the effects of prenatal alcohol exposure. While the 4-Digit Code maps onto these widely known diagnoses, the system actually uses different descriptive terms to more precisely describe how children manifest PFAS and ARND, and provides more detail. There are other diagnostic guidelines that also include a category called 'alcohol-related birth defects' (ARBDs). ARBDs exist in the presence of confirmed prenatal alcohol exposure, but children who have ARBDs do not necessarily show the characteristic facial features. ARBDs are defined as) 'Any of a number of anomalies (such as heart or kidney defects) present at birth that are associated with maternal alcohol consumption during pregnancy'. National Institute on Alcohol Abuse and Alcoholism (2000) *Tenth Special Report to the U.S. Congress on Alcohol and Health: Highlights on Current Research*. Washington, DC: US Department of Health and Human Services, Public Health Service, National Institutes of Health. Available at http://www.niaaa.nih.gov/publications/10report/chap05.pdf (Accessed February 2005).

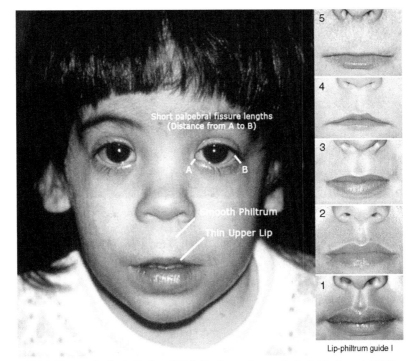

Figure 1   Based on the 4-Digit Diagnostic Code (Astley, 2004), the three diagnostic facial features of FAS are (1) palpebral fissure length (eyeslit length) of 2 or more standard deviations below the mean; (2) smooth philtrum (the vertical groove between the nose and upper lip) (Rank 4 or 5 on Lip-Philtrum Guide); (3) thin upper lip (Rank 4 or 5 on Lip-Philtrum Guide). Photo used by permission of Susan Astley, University of Washington.

exposure, although documentation or valid reports of this is not always easy to obtain.

Prevalence of FASDs and Recognition of the Risk of Prenatal Alcohol Exposure

FASDs are now known to have a higher prevalence than has been understood in the past. Reported rates vary widely and depend on the population studied and the detection and diagnostic methods used. In 2002, the number of children in the US with the full FAS was estimated by the Centers for Disease Control and Prevention (CDC) at 0.2–1.5 per 1000 live births, with much higher rates in some communities. Prevalence rates of the full range of FASDs, including FAS, ARND, and ARBD, are believed to occur about three times as often as FAS. But the full extent of the problem is still being investigated, and over the past 10 years some have estimated the rates of the full range of FASDs as high as 9 or 10 per 1000 live births in the US, approaching the latest estimated prevalence of autism spectrum disorders. There are certainly selected communities in the US with higher prevalence rates.

Prevalence rates depend on the diagnostic and detection (case ascertainment) methods used. Diagnostic issues are discussed later in this article. With FASDs, active case ascertainment is the best method for identifying the full extent of this set of developmental disabilities. Passive ascertainment methods, such as counting birth defects when a child is born and listing them in a registry, can only identify a small number of alcohol-affected individuals.

FASDs have been found worldwide. While not all countries have reliable estimates of prevalence, there are countries that have uncovered higher prevalence rates in their population or in certain communities. In Italy, for example, researcher May and colleagues have used active case ascertainment in schools and documented recent population-based estimates at 35 cases of FASDs per 1000 children. In South Africa, May and coworkers have also used active case ascertainment in schools in a selected, highly impacted community, and have shown the highest reported prevalence in any community of 68.0–89.2 per 1000 children. This is uncommonly high and alarming. In response, researchers are working together internationally because the public health problem of FASDs has become such a grave concern in some countries and communities. Around the globe, communities and governmental agencies in many locations are working on a public policy response and on efforts to build service capacity. In Canada, for example, there have been grassroots and province-wide efforts at prevention, diagnosis, and/or intervention for individuals with FASDs and their families. In the US, as another example, there have been service system interagency coordinating efforts at the federal level, momentum to build state systems, and the emergence of local and national parent support organizations – all

created in response to the public health problem of FASDs. Unfortunately, though, there are still many countries and communities, including many within the US, that have not recognized FASDs as a problem deserving a coordinated response.

While there remains great need for public and professional education worldwide, prenatal alcohol exposure is increasingly recognized as a risk factor for children's development. In the US, for example, screening for prenatal alcohol exposure is increasingly performed – especially for children in the child welfare, foster care, and adoption systems; for children born to women with chemical dependency; and for youth in the juvenile justice system. More frequently, young children with prenatal exposure to substances (including alcohol) are being recognized as at risk, referred for developmental assessment, and sent on for developmental services. Federal regulations in the US passed in 2003 and 2004 for the education, early intervention, and child welfare systems mandated that children involved in substantiated cases of child abuse and neglect be referred to early intervention systems. Educational regulations further required early intervention referral for children whose development is impacted by prenatal substance exposure. These regulations will certainly result in larger numbers of children in early intervention systems who are alcohol-exposed, who should be screened for the possibility of FASDs, and, when needed, referred for diagnosis. These children should be offered early intervention, when appropriate, either because of their at-risk status or for a diagnosed condition on the fetal alcohol spectrum.

Caregiving Burden and Costs

Families caring for individuals affected by prenatal alcohol exposure report many unmet needs for services and support, societal understanding, and modifications to existing service systems and their eligibility criteria. Parents report clinically elevated levels of stress when raising children with clearly diagnosed FASDs. Higher levels of parental stress have been clearly associated with raising a child who has complex neurobehavioral impairments, specifically executive-function deficits (that affect memory, planning, and organization), challenging problem behaviors, and poorer adaptive function.

The human costs of FASDs arise from high rates of debilitating problems in lifestyle and daily function found among affected individuals, such as mental health problems or disrupted school experiences, and the emotional and financial burdens on their families. In the US, there have been careful estimates of economic cost data for the full FAS – and these costs in care, rehabilitation, and lost productivity are striking. FAS is only one part of the larger fetal alcohol spectrum, but is actually one of the more costly birth defects. In 2004, researchers found that the median of adjusted annual cost estimates to the US economy was $3.6 billion. Little is known about costs of the wider fetal alcohol spectrum beyond FAS, but additional affected individuals can only further raise already high societal costs.

The Teratogenic Effects of Alcohol and Prevention of FASDs

A growing body of animal literature, long-term human descriptive studies, clinical studies, and neuroimaging research all come together to make clear the negative impact that alcohol use during pregnancy can have on the developing child. These teratogenic effects of alcohol continue lifelong.

Alcohol as a Neurobehavioral Teratogen

As a neurobehavioral teratogen, alcohol interferes with normal fetal growth and CNS development through multiple actions at different sites. Alcohol is a very potent teratogen, altering the developing fetal brain and CNS largely through alcohol-induced disturbance in neurogenesis and synaptogenesis (how neurons and connections between neurons are formed). But the impact of alcohol on the CNS is found at the cellular, hormonal, neurochemical, structural, and functional levels – with a further complex interplay of genetic and epigenetic factors. Researchers are now carefully and intensively studying the biochemical mechanisms underlying alcohol's effects, in part because of hope that pharmacologic treatments might eventually be used to intervene with (or prevent) alcohol-related fetal injury. Researchers are also using technology such as ultrasounds, structural and functional neuroimaging, spectroscopy, and physical measures (including electroencephalograms (EEGs)) to understand more precisely how alcohol damages the brain.

Fetal effects of alcohol exposure differ depending on the amount, timing, and pattern of maternal drinking, so deficits are highly variable from one child to another. In general, the more a pregnant woman drinks, the greater the severity of persistent CNS deficits. Episodic (or binge) drinking that creates higher maternal peak blood alcohol concentrations is associated with greater fetal damage. On an individual basis, however, any amount of drinking during pregnancy can cause harm, and alcohol use at any time during gestation is associated with a higher risk of CNS dysfunction.

Prevention of FASDs

In 2005, the US Surgeon General released an updated advisory on drinking and pregnancy. Among other information, this advisory states that no amount of alcohol consumption during pregnancy can be considered safe, that

cognitive and behavioral deficits resulting from prenatal alcohol exposure are lifelong, and that ARBDs are completely preventable. This advisory offers specific advice for women who are pregnant or considering becoming pregnant, and for their healthcare providers. But any early interventionist, educator, social service provider, or mental health provider working with families raising young children may be in a position to pass on information that will accomplish prevention of FASDs in current or future pregnancies.

Prevention of FASDs is necessary at a universal, community-wide level. Also vital are 'selective' prevention efforts targeted toward women who are pregnant or considering pregnancy and so at risk for gestational drinking, and 'indicated' prevention efforts directed toward women who are actually drinking during pregnancy and can be helped to cut down or stop.

Diagnosis of FASDs
Diagnosis in the Early Years

There have been systematic and successful research efforts aimed at how best to screen for risky drinking during pregnancy, and there is newer research focused on finding biomarkers of problematic gestational alcohol use. Research has also begun to focus on how to accomplish early detection of FASDs so that intervention can be applied. Different risk factors (such as the presence of prenatal alcohol use or small head size or a risk index based on parental characteristics) have been compared for their predictive value. Recently, ultrasound technology to image the neonatal brain has been explored as an early detection technique with suggestive but still preliminary findings. In part, this effort is prompted because of growing knowledge about the plasticity of the CNS, and because of intriguing findings in animal research on the positive developmental effects of enriched environments. Taken together, these findings strongly imply that early identification and intervention for children who are affected by prenatal alcohol exposure may be especially important, because CNS function might potentially be improved.

It is still difficult to identify children with FASDs in infancy and early childhood. This is because CNS damage or dysfunction can be hard to detect in the early years. Current FASD diagnostic guidelines require evidence of structural, neurological, and/or functional damage to the CNS. Evidence of structural/neurological damage may include such findings as microcephaly (small head size), abnormal neuroimaging, or seizure disorders. These can sometimes be found in infancy and early childhood. Evidence of CNS dysfunction includes standardized testing with scores that show significant global delays or, more commonly with FASDs, variability revealed in significant gaps in skills, atypical patterns of development, or uneven profiles of learning strengths and weaknesses. It is often hard to gather clear evidence of CNS dysfunction when children are very young. The early developmental deficits of alcohol-exposed children may be subtle and yet important precursors to later problems. Tests used with young children often cannot detect variability in learning profiles or subtle problems, so young children will less often meet diagnostic criteria for FASDs. In addition, alcohol effects may often emerge most clearly as deficits in higher-level cognitive functions or complex information processing that typically develop at age 8 years and older. As a result, the problems of children with FASDs may not even become evident until well past the window for early intervention, around second to fourth grade.

Diagnostic Guidelines

While FASDs are usually treated as developmental disabilities or behavioral concerns, these diagnoses are actually considered to be medical conditions. Current practice guidelines suggest that diagnosing physicians work with an interdisciplinary or multidisciplinary team and follow well-defined FASD diagnostic guidelines. National diagnostic guidelines have been published in the US for FAS and in Canada for the broader fetal alcohol spectrum. There is a variety of more specific diagnostic systems and techniques that are continually evolving. Currently there exist FASD diagnostic criteria developed for clinical and research use that allow diagnosis of the full range of conditions making up the fetal alcohol spectrum (e.g., see **Table 1**). There is vivid research interest in ways to improve diagnosis of FASDs (such as three-dimensional facial imaging, or defining a 'behavioral phenotype' that can be discerned through psychometric testing). Neuroimaging and neurochemistry research is being carried out to learn more about how alcohol affects the brain, which may eventually assist in diagnosis.

Co-Occurring Conditions

Diagnosed FASDs commonly co-occur with developmental delays or deficits arising from other genetic or medical causes, which are sometimes recognizable in infancy. Beginning as early as the preschool years, FASDs quite often co-occur with psychiatric disorders (such as oppositional defiant disorder or attention deficit hyperactivity disorder (ADHD)). In the school years, children with FASDs are also often found to have academic problems

or learning disabilities. For example, lowered achievement in pre-math and arithmetic skills are among the most persistent learning problems that have been identified in children across the fetal alcohol spectrum. A full understanding of an individual child's problems requires taking all co-occurring conditions into consideration.

Diagnoses on the fetal alcohol spectrum typically add an important dimension to the description of a child's problems as classified through use of medical or psychiatric diagnostic systems, or educational categories. For example, there is growing evidence that the attentional deficits caused by prenatal alcohol exposure may differ in type from those seen among children with ADHD from nonteratogenic causes. When children with prenatal alcohol exposure were directly compared with children with ADHD on measures of attention, they showed greater impairment in encoding information, while children with ADHD had more problems in focusing and sustaining attention. However, findings on the specific types of attention deficits among children affected by prenatal alcohol exposure vary depending on the sample being tested (clinical or nonclinical) and the assessment measures used. As another example, children prenatally exposed to alcohol may have associated medical complications and a complex profile of additional cognitive and learning difficulties. Therefore, knowing that a child has early-onset ADHD in the presence of FASDs can mean that commonly used interventions for ADHD (such as stimulant medication) may not have expected effects, and that a different set of treatment techniques may be needed. Learning how children affected by prenatal alcohol exposure compare to children diagnosed with other disabilities is another area of vivid research interest.

But there is a central practical benefit to understanding that a child has FASDs, which has been discussed by experienced clinicians such as Malbin. Knowing that an alcohol-exposed child's behavior problems may arise (at least in part) from that child's alcohol-induced neurological impairment can fundamentally change a parent's or provider's perception of the child's learning and behavior. This understanding can help the caregiver 'reframe' behavior problems, attributing the cause to underlying neurodevelopmental disorders rather than to willful misbehavior. For example, a 10-year-old boy with FASDs who does not cooperate when his mother asks him to 'get dressed to go to the ball game and clean your room' may actually be unable to do this because he (1) cannot mentally image what a 'clean' room looks like; (2) may not know how to organize and sequence the required behaviors; and/or (3) may not adequately process the higher-level language of his mother's multiple-step instructions. His mother will more successfully understand his behavior (and come up with effective ways to respond) if she 'reframes' her understanding of his lack of cooperation as actually arising from cognitive and language difficulties. Carmichael Olson and colleagues have made learning 'reframing' into a central treatment process in specialized behavioral consultation intervention to assist caregivers raising children with FASDs and challenging behavior problems.

Serving Children Across the Full Fetal Alcohol Spectrum

FAS is increasingly recognized as a diagnosed condition with a high probability of developmental delay, thus deserving early intervention. But there are many additional children, who do not have the full syndrome but do show diagnosable FASDs, who have a high likelihood of developmental delay and significant later psychopathology. Because of this, providing early intervention services for all children diagnosed with FASDs is vital. An even broader approach that is strongly encouraged is to classify developmentally vulnerable young children 'at-risk' because of prenatal alcohol exposure coupled with evidence of emerging learning problems and/or environmental risk. If an exposed, 'at-risk' child does not qualify for early intervention, or improves after intervention and then no longer qualifies, careful monitoring and re-evaluation at key developmental transitions is recommended. One important transition is before a child enters kindergarten; another is prior to entering second or third grade; a third is just before transitioning to middle school. One strategy that does not fit with current evidence is assuming that a young alcohol-exposed child will 'grow out of' apparently mild early delays, and therefore not providing early intervention services or developmental monitoring.

Young Children with Prenatal Alcohol Exposure and Their Families

What does current scientific evidence say about young children with prenatal alcohol exposure and their families? What are the implications for early intervention? Data come from larger clinical samples of young children referred for diagnosis, small samples of those diagnosed with FASDs, and large prospective longitudinal studies of the effects of prenatal alcohol exposure. Also referred to briefly in the following discussion are long-term studies of young children born polydrug-exposed, including alcohol, who typically have lives characterized by high levels of postnatal environmental risk.

Overview of Data from a Large Clinical Sample

There are no national data available describing FASDs, but large clinical samples are being gathered and examined.

In 2007, data from a large clinical database of children with confirmed prenatal alcohol exposure referred for diagnosis of FASDs in Washington State were reviewed by Carmichael Olson, Jirikowic, Kartin, and Astley. Highlights of their findings on nearly 800 children aged birth to 8 years are included here. The authors noted that conclusions from this database were somewhat limited by geographical context.

There was a very wide range of racial and ethnic backgrounds in this group of young children, with most no longer in the care of their birth parents and over 70% in foster/adoptive homes. The average age of identification was just over age 5 years, with only about one-third of children referred brought in during the early years before age 4 years. Surprisingly few families of these young children (<5%) were referred for diagnosis from school or early intervention settings. Instead, referrals came from medical, psychological, or social service providers. There was wide variation in prenatal alcohol exposure, ranging from reported maternal consumption during pregnancy of one single glass of wine to daily intoxication.

Of the nearly 800 children examined, only about 7% received a diagnosis of FAS or partial FAS. It is this smaller group who are most likely to be recognized and qualified for early intervention even though their CNS dysfunction is often no more severe than children with FASDs who lack the 'face' of FAS. There were 25% of this group of children aged birth to 8 years who were diagnosed with the equivalent of 'severe' ARND. This subgroup showed learning and behavior problems but were children for whom strong advocacy would likely be needed to obtain early intervention services. Importantly, there were 43% diagnosed with the equivalent of 'mild' ARND. This is a subgroup who may show more significant problems later in life but are far less likely to receive any services in infancy and early childhood, even if strong advocacy is exerted.

The authors discuss what might be early indicators suggesting a need for referral for diagnosis of FASDs. Interestingly, the presence of significant developmental delays does not seem to be a reliable early indicator, making early evaluation and identification difficult. More than 25% of these alcohol-exposed young children actually had early developmental profiles well within normal limits. Only just over half of the children referred for diagnosis showed testing evidence of marked developmental delay in the first 3 years of life – even among those with the full FAS or partial FAS.

The Developmental Impact of Prenatal Alcohol Exposure in Young Children

What are the effects of prenatal alcohol exposure on child development in the early years? In overview, it is well-established that heavy levels of prenatal alcohol exposure lead to neurobehavioral deficits, but the effects of lower levels of alcohol exposure are less clear. Neurobehavioral deficits from prenatal alcohol exposure are lifelong, but their impact on adaptive function emerges more clearly over time. These deficits can likely be improved or made worse by postnatal experiences. Gender differences in alcohol-related disabilities have rarely been examined in individuals with FASDs. Certainly, FASDs occur in both boys and girls, but the emergence of behavior problems across development may differ by gender. Limited data suggest that depressive symptoms may appear earlier for girls. It appears there are no published data available at this time about gender differences in cognition or learning. Problems in development resulting from prenatal alcohol exposure occur across multiple domains of function, as discussed below.

Problems in Early Cognitive Skills and Learning

In 2004, Kable and Coles found that infants born with higher-risk prenatal alcohol exposure had "difficulties with regulating the interactions between arousal level and the attentional system needed to provide optimal efficiency in processing environmental events" (p. 489). These infants were slow to initiate attention, and to encode visual and auditory information. They also demonstrated higher arousal levels. The authors speculated that the inability to modify arousal levels to encode information may result in slower responses to environmental events, which subsequently influences learning and later problem-solving and behavioral outcomes that depend on the interplay of these basic cognitive processes.

The enduring impact of prenatal alcohol effects on cognitive–behavioral processes and learning has been the subject of extensive research. In a 2007 literature review, Kodituwakku proposed that children with FASDs or prenatal alcohol exposure have a central, generalized deficit in complex information processing. Kodituwakku suggested that individuals with FASDs have difficulty integrating information from multiple regions of the brain and proposed this as part of the behavioral phenotype of FASDs. This overarching conclusion is drawn from synthesis of a large body of research evidence on FASDs and prenatal alcohol exposure. This evidence describes slow information processing, diminished nonverbal and verbal intellectual functioning, and difficulty with complex cognitive tasks.

In 2007, Carmichael Olson and colleagues reviewed the clinical research on infant, preschool, and older children with FASDs, which yielded consistent findings of deficits in attention, wide-ranging difficulties in higher-order cognitive processes called 'executive functions', visual–spatial processing deficits, other problems in information processing speed and efficiency, and difficulties

with mathematical problem solving and achievement. There was a wide variety in type and extent of deficits across individuals. In infancy, adverse alcohol effects were found on basic conditioned learning and other cognitive functions that reveal an impact on specific brain regions (such as the cerebellum).

Long-term prospective studies of more moderate levels of prenatal alcohol exposure find associations with cognitive and learning difficulties through adolescence and beyond, though not all longitudinal studies find effects. Prenatal alcohol has been associated in group studies with mildly decreased performance on developmental scores in infancy and with mildly lowered intelligence quotient (IQ) scores in preschoolers. Newer longitudinal research with wider ethnic diversity and somewhat more highly exposed samples (using more sensitive measures) found an association between alcohol exposure and early, specific cognitive and achievement difficulties. For example, infants prenatally exposed to alcohol have shown deficits in information processing. In response to visual stimuli under laboratory conditions, infants with prenatal alcohol exposure reacted more slowly to changing visual stimuli and gazed longer at visual stimuli, suggesting slower and less efficient information processing. These information-processing deficits, which are considered indicators of intellectual abilities in both younger and older children, appear to persist at least into the early elementary years. Additional findings among older children include decreased processing efficiency under more complex cognitive conditions and a distinctive prenatal alcohol effect on number processing. In new research, substrates in brain structure and function of many of these functional difficulties are being explored.

Deficits in Speech, Language, and Communication

A variety of problems in speech, language, and communication have been described for clinical samples of school-aged children with heavy prenatal alcohol exposure, including delays in speech acquisition, impaired receptive and expressive language, and problems in speech production. Some school-aged children with FASDs show gaps between relatively better verbal abilities (such as vocabulary or basic grammar), and reduced capacity to use these skills effectively in social communication. Social communication is an important foundation for developing social relationships and exchanging information. So far, there has been limited clinical or longitudinal study of language and communication in infants and young children with prenatal alcohol exposure. Current clinical thinking by experts such as Coggins is that young children with FASDs can often acquire basic linguistic skills in a typical manner. However, they seem to have difficulty becoming socially competent communicators later on and, as they grow older, show deficits in more complex, higher-order language skills. For instance, children with FASDs have difficulty telling coherent and cohesive narratives, which is an important communication skill used in learning situations and interpersonal relationships.

Problems in Motor Development, Neurological Soft Signs, and Sensory Processing

Alcohol-exposed individuals consistently show impairments in the development of motor control. Clinical studies of infants reveal that motor delays occur more often and/or with increased severity in the presence of heavy alcohol exposure. Among younger children with diagnosed FASDs, delays in motor skills are generally mild-to-moderate in extent, and these preschoolers show poor movement quality. In clinical samples, significant deficits in visual-motor development (but not in motor-free visual perception), and in fine motor coordination, have been described.

Some longitudinal researchers examining population-based samples have found no measurable impact of more moderate levels of social drinking on motor development in infancy or early childhood. Other long-term studies have found clinically significant effects when examining psychomotor performance on standardized tests such as the Bayley Scales of Infant Development, but only among infants at high exposure levels. However, in infants with lower exposure levels, qualitative differences in motor behaviors, such as the ability to stand, walk, and imitate have been detected and described. In early childhood, longitudinal research has found increased levels of minor neurological soft signs among alcohol-exposed preschoolers, and a positive association between greater alcohol exposure and increased deficits in fine motor steadiness and balance.

In clinical samples, parents completing questionnaires on sensory-processing behaviors documented clinically significant difficulties modulating sensory information among their young children with FASDs. Specifically, Jirikowic described behaviors that suggest fluctuating responses (i.e., both over- and under-responsivity) to sensation that include tactile, auditory, and visual sensitivity, under-responsiveness to sensory information and sensation-seeking behaviors, and poor auditory filtering.

Difficulties in Adaptive Behavior and Social–Emotional Development

Difficult behaviors and social skill deficits that persist across time are a central concern among individuals of all ages with prenatal alcohol exposure in both clinical and longitudinal prospective samples. Mental health problems have been reported for a very large majority of individuals diagnosed with FASDs in natural history research, and there are elevated rates of psychiatric disorders in childhood and beyond. Clinical studies of children with FASDs use terms such as impulsive, distractible, and 'always on the go' to describe behavior in the preschool and elementary years. In addition, while younger children with FASDs have been described as engaging, verbal, apparently alert, and bright-eyed, they likely appear more functional than they actually are. Clinicians note they seem to lack social boundaries (e.g., by showing indiscriminate affection or seeking physical proximity to strangers). There is wide variability in the level of these deficits, ranging from subtle to severe.

For school-aged children with FASDs, studies often show clinically elevated attention, social, and sometimes internalizing behavior problems and (even more frequently) problems with externalizing behavior and aggression. Adaptive behavior and social skills among preschool and young school-aged children with FASDs are reported as lower than expected for age and intellectual level. Although decreased adaptive performance has been described across most adaptive domains including daily living, social, communicative and, to a lesser extent, motor function, the development of social and interpersonal relationships appears to be especially problematic for those affected by prenatal alcohol exposure. After the age of 8 years, these deficits in adaptive function and social performance in children exposed to alcohol appear relatively greater, even than clinic-referred peers with behavior or adjustment problems. This is likely the result of the lifelong neurological impairment of children born alcohol-affected.

Longitudinal studies begun in infancy report early problems in behavioral regulation associated with prenatal alcohol exposure, including mild-to-moderate irritability, poor habituation, sleep problems, and feeding difficulties. Among preschooler children, limited longitudinal data suggest that prenatal alcohol exposure has been associated with functional compromise that includes mild-to-moderate inattention and hyperactivity, and subtle-to-moderate impulsivity, and behavior problems.

Thinking in a more complex way about developmental systems reveals how the impact of prenatal alcohol exposure (coupled with maternal drinking) on children's social–emotional development reverberates across infancy and early childhood. For example, O'Connor and colleagues described an evolving process in which alcohol-exposed infants showed increased negative affect, and their mothers had difficulty responding to these babies (perhaps because of their own depression that may be associated with a tendency to drink, and/or because of difficulties presented by the child). In this evolving developmental process, the quality of the attachment between parent and child was then compromised, and these alcohol-exposed children grew into preschooler children who showed increased levels of depression at around age 4–5 years. This process has been demonstrated among middle-income families, and shown even more clearly among low-income families who have additional risk factors that augmented the severity of this negative cycle. Additional analyses of middle-income families through age 6 years revealed this process as primarily true for girls, but there were also separate trends or significant direct effects of prenatal alcohol exposure on developmental outcome in both boys and girls. All this suggests strongly that intervention could usefully begin in infancy, and could be targeted specifically at ameliorating negative child behaviors (and providing parental support).

The Importance of Cumulative Risk

The impact of prenatal alcohol exposure is often coupled with that of other prenatal drug exposures, poor prenatal care, and life with parents who struggle with chemical dependency. Children may live in environments with health and safety concerns, relationship problems, and chaotic lifestyles. Longitudinal studies have tracked the often negative developmental outcomes of children with prenatal substance exposures in these high-risk situations. Clinical studies have examined the difficult lives of children born substance-exposed. These studies are sharp reminders that children with FASDs may often spend at least part of their early years in an environment of cumulative risk. Thinking about FASDs from a developmental systems perspective emphasizes that cumulative risk could be especially harmful for a child made biologically vulnerable by prenatal alcohol exposure.

The Potential of Treatment for FASDs

A small body of research on animal models of FAS suggests that exercise training and appropriate enrichment of the learning environment have potential to improve behavioral and learning outcomes, and to reduce alcohol-induced injury to the brain and CNS – early in life but even during the equivalent of adolescence or early adulthood. Natural history study of a large clinical sample by Streissguth and colleagues highlights 'protective factors' that are related to reduced odds that 'secondary disabilities' (negative outcomes in lifestyle and daily function) will occur among individuals with FASDs. These protective factors, which include early diagnosis, good quality of caregiving during childhood, absence of parental substance abuse and trauma, and presence of appropriate social services, can be enhanced through intervention. There may be pivotal 'turning points' in

development when intervention is most needed, with the idea of creating 'downstream effects' that push development in a positive direction. A first turning point is in early infancy, when preventive intervention may take advantage of neuronal plasticity and improve attachment quality. Secure attachment between parent and child is a powerful predictor of positive outcome in many developmental areas. A second turning point may be in preschool, a time when tailored educational techniques and focused efforts to help parents assist their children in learning behavior regulation may maintain developmental progress. Another set of turning points may occur during the time when a child grows from 5 to 11 years (and first enters kindergarten, then second or third grade, and then approaches middle school). Among children who are typically developing, these school years are a time of rapid cognitive and social development, when children master increasingly complex language and social skills, and when demands for self-reliance and self-regulation increase. For children with significant prenatal alcohol exposure or FASDs, it is during this period of time that alcohol-related deficits may start to become obvious (and troubling) to parents and teachers, and progress in the growth of adaptive behavior is likely to plateau.

A Developmental Systems Model Applied to Early Intervention for Children with FASDs and Their Families

Thinking about developmental systems can guide practice with young children with FASDs or who are at risk because of confirmed prenatal alcohol exposure. This type of thinking helps to make clear why early intervention for this population is especially important, and suggests that treatment models should be designed especially for the population served and subgroups within the population, and targeted to the individual needs of children being served. Developmental systems thinking also means that risk and protective factors specific to the population should be identified and considered.

Child and Family Characteristics in the Presence of FASDs: Risk and Protective Factors

A developmental systems model was created by Guralnick in 2001 to guide the design of early intervention with children who have special needs, and can usefully be applied to FASDs. Conceptualized from the standpoint of this model, prenatal alcohol exposure can be seen as placing a child at risk for (or creating) biological vulnerability and 'disabling child characteristics' or 'core deficits'.

Across all ages, possible disabling child characteristics for those with FASDs include sensory sensitivities and difficulty with behavioral regulation (especially in stressful or unstructured situations). In infancy, as mentioned earlier, children with FASDs may have deficits in basic cognitive processes, including the ability to regulate the interactions between arousal level and the attentional system needed to provide optimal efficiency in processing environmental events. Older children with FASDs may show a central, generalized deficit in complex information processing.

On an individual basis, the specific pattern of cognitive/behavioral deficits of a child with FASDs or significant prenatal alcohol exposure is individually variable and arises in multiple domains of development (perhaps in subtle ways). A particular child's pattern of deficits may emerge more clearly or become more debilitating over time. On an individual basis, then, a child's deficits and compensatory strengths must be comprehensively assessed.

Disabling child characteristics can disrupt existing family interaction patterns. This creates information and resource needs for parents, threats to parenting confidence, an impact on the parent–child relationship in the early years, and high levels of both caregiver and family stress. Comprehensive assessment of these 'environmental risk factors' (especially cumulative risk) is essential. One crucial family interaction risk factor identified through clinical experience centers around inappropriate caregiver reactions to deficits of the child with FASDs – deficits caregivers may not easily recognize as the result of alcohol-induced neurological impairment, but see as willful disobedience. This requires caregivers to learn 'reframing' and understanding that neurological impairment underlies problem behaviors.

Research supports the importance to developmental outcome of caregiver characteristics and quality of caregiving – in the early years and through middle childhood – for children born alcohol-exposed. In 2000, Coles and colleagues developed a cumulative risk index from data gathered during the neonatal period, based on maternal characteristics. They found this risk index was useful in predicting early growth and developmental compromise (at 6 and 12 months) in low-birthweight children exposed to alcohol before they were born. This risk index had more predictive power than when using other early indicators such as the presence of heavy alcohol exposure or small head size. Other pivotal family risk factors have been documented in natural history research on FASDs by Streissguth and workers. For this population, past or current parental substance use, exposure to violence, and poor quality of the childhood caregiving environment, are all significantly associated with the occurrence of poor outcomes later in life.

The developmental disabilities and early intervention literatures stress that protective factors, such as family strengths and coping skills, are also important and should be assessed. There are specific protective factors hypothesized by Carmichael Olson and colleagues as important for the population of children born with FASDs. In infancy, these include the quality of attachment security and treatment for parental alcohol abuse or dependency (a protective factor for a child of any age). Starting in the preschool years, protective factors include the parent's level of optimism and sense of parenting efficacy, use of specialized parenting practices, advocacy skill, knowledge of FASDs, use of respite and beneficial social support, and appropriate linkage to community resources and social services.

Developing Interventions Based on a Developmental Systems Model

Early intervention should aim to reduce both the impact of disabling child characteristics and cumulative environmental risk, while at the same time enhancing protective factors. For 'at-risk' young children with prenatal alcohol exposure who may or may not yet show clinically concerning behaviors, preventive interventions are needed. This could include careful and ongoing developmental monitoring, providing anticipatory guidance to parents, daycare providers, and school staff, general environmental enrichment, and very early substance abuse education.

For the diagnosed child, a comprehensive intervention program can first provide thorough and tailored assessment, so that all caregivers understand the child's 'disabling characteristics' and can 'reframe' their understanding of the child's behavior in light of neurological impairment. Then intervention can provide resource, social, and information supports, and direct treatment to enhance family interaction patterns, adjusted to the family's unique needs and targeted to the disability.

If the caregiving relationship is strongly affected, early in life it may be vital to provide ongoing infant mental health interventions that help caregivers behave in ways that foster attachment security, even in the face of negative affect or unresponsiveness from the infants born prenatally exposed. This may have to be adjusted depending on whether the caregiver is from a birth, foster, or adoptive home. Intervention will likely become 'multimodal' as a child with FASDs grows older. For example, if a preschooler with FASDs has sensory sensitivities and deficits in information processing arising from prenatal alcohol exposure, then environmental modification and supportive occupational therapy services, caregiver education about the child's cognitive processing, and advocacy for later special education, all might be necessary. Home visiting or clinic-based services to help caregivers understand alcohol-related brain damage, modify attitudes, learn specialized parenting skills, and learn effective advocacy to access existing community supports may be required when preschool-aged and school-aged children with FASDs have especially difficult behavior problems. Intervention models for such services have been developed by researcher Carmichael Olson and colleagues.

An Emerging Body of Evidence on Intervention for FASDs

General intervention approaches to FASDs have been developed based on expert opinion and research on related disorders, and are reviewed in a set of guidelines published by the National Center on Birth Defects and Developmental Disabilities and discussed by other authors. Carefully designed FASD intervention studies are beginning to show positive effects for children and families. The broader child treatment literature also suggests strong potential for positive change if early intervention is designed based on scientific data now available about child development and early psychopathology.

Examining the efficacy of relationship-based infant mental health treatments, which have been useful for families raising children with polydrug exposure, is an important next step in research on early intervention for children with FASDs and their families. New research by several investigators, funded by the CDC, including Carmichael Olson, Chasnoff, Coles, Gurwitch, and O'Connor, suggests that treatment for children with FASDs in the preschool and school years can (among other outcomes) improve social skills and/or reduce disruptive behavior, and improve self-reported parenting attitudes and knowledge. There are many field-initiated research projects underway examining a wide variety of interventions for FASDs, although mostly for older children and youth. Intervention for youth in juvenile justice, coordinated state service responding to FASDs, and intervention for high-risk chemically dependent women and their young children (who are likely drug- and alcohol-exposed) are only some of the interventions being actively explored. Successful intervention may prevent or reduce secondary disabilities and debilitating family strife – and intervention earlier in life has the potential for powerful positive change. Although only family and expert clinical experience support the idea – even as late as adolescence and adulthood, diagnosis and intervention for individuals with an FASD are deemed crucial (especially holistic treatment and management of associated mental disorders). Even later in life, intervention can likely reduce suffering and cost to affected individuals and those who care for them.

Acknowledgments

The authors gratefully acknowledge the Centers on Disease Control and Prevention (Grant No. U01-DD000038-02, awarded to Heather Carmichael Olson) and the National Institute on Drug Abuse (Grant No. 5 T32 DAO 7257-14) for postdoctoral support of Dr. Jirikowic for support and facilitation during preparation of this manuscript.

See also: ADHD: Genetic Influences; Birth Defects; Depression; Developmental Disabilities: Cognitive; Intellectual Disabilities; Sensory Processing Disorder; Teratology.

Suggested Readings

Carmichael Olson H, Jirikowic T, Kartin D, and Astley S (2007) Responding to the challenges of early intervention for fetal alcohol spectrum disorders. *Infants and Young Children* 20(2): 162–179.

Families Moving Forward Program (2007) Families moving forward. http://depts.washington.edu/fmffasd/index.html (accessed 13 July 2007).

Fryer SL, McGee CL, Matt GE, Riley EP, and Mattson SN (2007) Evaluation of psychopathological conditions in children with heavy prenatal alcohol exposure. *Pediatrics* 119(3): 733–741.

Kable JA and Coles CD (2004) The impact of prenatal alcohol exposure on neurophysiological encoding of environmental events at six months. *Alcoholism: Clinical and Experimental Research* 28(3): 489–496.

Kalberg WO and Buckley D (2006) FASD: What types of intervention and rehabilitation are useful? *Neuroscience and Biobehavioral Reviews* 31: 278–285.

Kodituwakku PW (2007) Defining the behavioral phenotype in children with fetal alcohol spectrum disorders: A review. *Neuroscience and Biobehavioral Reviews* 31: 192–201.

National Center on Birth Defects and Developmental Disabilities (NCBDD) (2004) *Fetal Alcohol Syndrome: Guidelines for referral and diagnosis.* Washington, DC: Centers for Disease Control and Prevention. Available in hard copy from CDC or at http://www.cdc.gov/ncbddd/fas/documents/FAS_guidelines_accessible.pdf.

O'Connor MJ, Frankel F, Paley B, *et al.* (2006) Controlled social skills training for children with fetal alcohol spectrum disorders. *Journal of Consulting and Clinical Psychology* 74(4): 639–648.

Spadoni AD, McGee C, Fryer SL, and Riley EP (2007) Neuroimaging and fetal alcohol spectrum disorders. *Neuroscience and Biobehavioral Reviews* 31: 239–245.

Spohr HL, Willms J, and Steinhausen HC (2007) Fetal alcohol spectrum disorders in young adulthood. *Journal of Pediatrics* 150(2): 175–179.

Streissguth A (1997) *Fetal Alcohol Syndrome: A Guide for Families and Communities.* Baltimore, MD: Paul H. Brookes.

Streissguth AP, Bookstein FL, Barr HM, *et al.* (2004) Risk factors for adverse life outcomes for fetal alcohol syndrome and fetal alcohol effects. *Journal of Developmental and Behavioral Pediatrics* 25(4): 228–238.

Substance Abuse and Mental Health Services Administration (SAMHSA) (2007) *FASD Center for Excellence.* Multiple fact sheets available at http://fascenter.samhsa.gov (accessed 13 July 2007).

Surgeon General's Advisory on Drinking and Pregnancy (2005, February). United States Department of Health & Human Services. Available at http://www.hhs.gov/surgeongeneral/pressreleases/sg02222005.html (accessed 13 July 2007).

Tenth Special Report to the US Congress on Alcohol and Health: Highlights on Current Research. Available at http://www.niaaa.nih.gov.

Fragile X Syndrome

M Y Ono, University of California, Davis, Medical Center, Sacramento, CA, USA
F Farzin, University of California, Davis, Davis, CA, USA
R J Hagerman, University of California, Davis, Medical Center, Sacramento, CA, USA

Glossary

Autism spectrum disorder – The category that includes PDDNOS and autism.

Cortisol – The glucocorticoid produced by the adrenal cortex upon stimulation by adrenocorticotropic hormone (ACTH) that mediates various metabolic processes, has anti-inflammatory and immunosupressive properties, and whose levels in the blood may become elevated in response to physical or psychological stress.

Dyspraxia – The impairment of the ability to perform coordinated movements.

Echolalia – The pathological repetition of what is said by other people, echoing.

Hyperarousal – The state of having excessive arousal.

Hypotonia – The state of having deficient tone or tension.

Macroorchidism – The condition of having large testicles.

Otitis media – The acute or chronic inflammation of the middle ear.

Strabismus – The inability of one eye to attain binocular vision with the other because of imbalance of the muscles of the eyeball, also known as lazy eye.

Introduction

Fragile X syndrome (FXS) is a heritable form of mental retardation that affects approximately 1 in 4000 individuals. Not only is it the most common cause of mental retardation, but it is also a common cause of developmental delay, that is, learning disabilities, in addition to psychological and behavioral problems among children.

Genotype

FXS is caused by a mutation on the fragile X mental retardation 1 (*FMR1*) gene, which was discovered in 1991 to be located on the lower end of the X chromosome of Xq27.3. This mutation involves an expansion of the CGG trinucleotide repeat within the promoter region of the *FMR1* gene. Depending on the size of the expansion, the gene can become silenced, resulting in a diminished or complete lack of transcription into messenger RNA (mRNA) and subsequent lack of translation into FMR1 protein (FMRP). The lack of FMRP leads to the classic phenotype of FXS.

In general, the degree of affectedness is determined by the size of the CGG repeat expansion. In normal individuals, the CGG repeat size is 5–44. The gray zone category is 45–54 repeats and the allele can become unstable when transmitted to the next generation. Individuals with 55–200 repeats are categorized as premutation carriers and they typically are more mildly affected by FXS compared to the individuals who have the full mutation. The full mutation is defined by having more than 200 repeats and usually involves the gene being completely methylated and thus silenced. Males with the full mutation and complete methylation do not produce FMRP and therefore display the most severe symptoms of FXS. In contrast, females with the full mutation are less affected because of their second X chromosome. Depending on their X activation ratio, that is, the proportion of cells that express the allele without the mutation, the amount and severity of symptoms will vary. There are also individuals who are mosaic, meaning they have some cells with the premutation and some cells with the full mutation or they have the full mutation but they are partially unmethylated, which allows them to produce some FMRP.

Physical and Medical Phenotype

During infancy, the physical features of a child with FXS commonly appear to be normal. Most individuals with FXS are not diagnosed until 3 years of age or older because there is a lack of awareness of this disorder among clinicians and the fact that the physical features are somewhat common among the general population. The classic features include prominent ears, long face, high-arched palate, hyperextensible finger joints, soft or velvet-like skin, and flat feet (**Figures 1** and **2**). However, approximately 30% of children and adults with FXS do not have obvious physical features.

Retrospective studies have found that many males with FXS also have various medical conditions. For example, approximately, 85% have otitis media (middle-ear

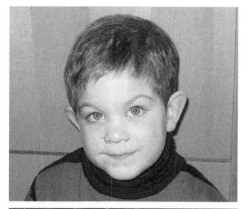

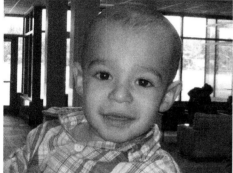

Figure 1 Young boys with fragile X syndrome.

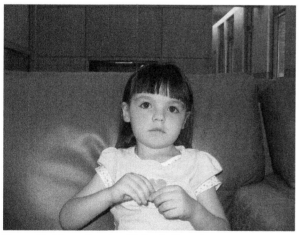

Figure 2 Young female with fragile X syndrome.

infection), 36% have strabismus, 31% have emesis, 23% have a history of sinusitis, 22% have seizures, and 15% have failure to thrive in infancy. Loose connective tissue is thought to lead to some of these features, including hyperextensible finger joints, soft or velvet-like skin, flat feet, and otitis media.

One study, conducted by Jean-Pierre Fryns in 1988, found an unexpectedly high rate of sudden infant death syndrome (SIDS) in babies with FXS. Eight per cent (17/219) of males and 4% (6/169) of females died of

SIDS before the age of 18 months. Although SIDS had not been thoroughly studied in FXS, there were various hypotheses of why it occurred, that is, central nervous system (CNS) disturbances, hypotonia leading to obstructed airway, seizures, mitral valve prolapse (MVP), or cardiac arrhythmias. SIDS also occasionally occurs in older individuals with FXS and these cases are thought to relate to cardiac arrhythmias.

Neurobiology and Brain Development

FMRP is a regulator of translation that binds to approximately 4% of all mRNAs in the neuron. It typically suppresses translation such that the absence of FMRP leads to enhanced translation of many messages in the CNS. One pathway that is remarkably enhanced is the metabotropic glutamate receptor 5 (mGluR5), which leads to enhanced long-term depression (LTD). LTD is the weakening of a neuronal synapse thought to result from changes in postsynaptic receptor density, and subsequently results in weak and immature synaptic connections, particularly in the hippocampus and cerebellum and this is thought to be a significant cause of the mental retardation in FXS. Synaptic connections are weak and immature in the fragile X knockout (KO) mouse model and there is a lack of synaptic plasticity and pruning. The identification of enhanced mGluR5 activity in KO mice and humans with FXS suggests that mGluR5 antagonists might be a specific treatment for FXS. Studies in the KO mouse and Drosophila models of FXS have demonstrated benefits of the mGluR5 antagonist, 2-methyl-6-phenylethynyl-pyridine (MPEP). In addition, lithium, which downregulates the mGluR5 system, has been shown to be helpful for the KO mouse in decreasing seizures and improving cognition and for the Drosophila in enhancing cognition and lifespan. In humans with FXS, lithium improves behavior, but improvements in cognition have not yet been demonstrated, although studies are currently being conducted.

There is limited information regarding the brain development of infants and toddlers with FXS, primarily due to the late diagnoses. One study, by Hill Karrer *et al.* in 2000, used event-related potentials (ERPs) to measure electrical brain activity through the scalps of infants with FXS, Down syndrome (DS), and typical development when they viewed visual images. Results indicated exaggerated early visual processing, possibly related to the deficit in dendritic pruning, in infants with FXS.

Children with FXS typically have large heads and prominent foreheads in early childhood. Neuroimaging studies have shown overall larger brains with significant enlargement of the caudate and a smaller size of the cerebellar vermis. Those with FXS and autism also have larger heads than individuals with FXS without autism.

Learning, Cognition, and Perception

Learning and Cognition

Research to-date on infants and young children with FXS has been restricted by the ages included and methodologies used. In 1998, Don Bailey *et al.* published a study describing a prospective examination of the development of infants with FXS. This study administered three developmental screening tests (Denver-II, Battelle Developmental Inventory Screening Test, and Early Language Milestone Scale-2) and two comprehensive assessment measures (The Mullen Scales of Early Learning and the Receptive-Expressive Emergent Language Scales) to 18 infants and toddlers with FXS (13 boys and 5 girls). One of the main objectives of the study was to assess the predictive validity of individual screening measures that might be useful in picking up delay in children with FXS at early ages. It was found that all of the screening tests and both comprehensive assessment measures were successful at detecting developmental delays in most children with FXS.

Another set of findings by Don Bailey's group examined the early developmental trajectories of males with FXS by employing a longitudinal design. Children in this study varied in age from 24 to 72 months and were evaluated on overall development in the domains of cognition, communication, adaptive, motor and personal–social, using the Battelle Developmental Inventory. The application of hierarchical linear model analysis revealed that the overall rate of development in the boys with FXS was approximately half of that expected for typically developing children. Also, although stable patterns of development were observed within individual subjects, development was not uniform across the sample. Significant variability was reported among subjects in both the levels of performance at each age, and in the rate of developmental change over time. Communication and cognitive skills were typically lower than social, adaptive, and motor skills.

In early childhood, intelligence quotients (IQs) are in the borderline to mildly mentally retarded range in 80–90% of males with FXS. In contrast, 30–35% of females with FXS test in the mild mental retardation range and 20–30% are in the borderline normal range. IQs in the normal range are seen in 40–50% of females with FXS; however, approximately half of those testing in the normal range have learning disabilities. In males with FXS, the level of FMRP correlates with the overall IQ.

IQs typically decline in most males and in many females with age. By adulthood, most males with FXS have IQs in the 40s. However, approximately 15% of males have an IQ greater than 70 and are called high-functioning males. They usually have FMRP levels greater than 50% and their DNA pattern is unmethylated or mosaic. IQ decline is not seen in individuals with FMRP levels greater than 50%.

One of the common cognitive weaknesses in children with FXS is sequential learning. For example, processing of verbal directions that require keeping both the instructions and their sequence in mind is difficult for children with FXS. Also, learning how to read using the phonics system, and performing the steps involved in math functions can be a struggle. Executive function is another common weakness in individuals with fragile X since it is difficult for them to store information in their short-term working memory as they attempt to complete a task, such as putting pictures in a specific order. Lastly, children with FXS often think in concrete terms and have difficulty with concepts that they cannot see, hear, or touch. As a result, their abilities to solve problems and think abstractly are compromised.

Perceptual Development

Much of the evidence about perceptual development in FXS comes from the field of visual processing. A number of studies have suggested that FXS is not associated with a global deficit in visual processing, but rather, that deficits in this group are specific. In particular, a finding that emerges consistently across studies is that affected individuals perform worse on tasks that require coordinated visual–spatial activity. It has been shown that individuals with FXS are worse than those with DS on block construction and drawing completion tests. Similarly, Kim Cornish's group conducted a comprehensive study that compared males with FXS to chronological age (CA) and mental age (MA)-matched and (DS) controls on a series of visual–motor (e.g., the block design and object assembly subtests of the Wechsler Intelligence Scales for Children, the triangles subtest of the Kaufman-ABC test, and the Annett pegboard) vs. a visual–perceptual task (the gestalt closure task). Males affected with FXS performed worse than both the CA-matched and DS control groups on all visual–motor tasks, but performed relatively and significantly better than the DS group on the visual–perception task. Together, these findings converge on a picture of visual information processing in FXS in which performance deficits are consistently reported for tasks that require visual–motor but not visual–perceptual processing.

Most recently, two studies by Cary Kogan *et al.* provided both molecular and behavioral evidence for the claim that the visual–motor deficits evident in FXS are attributable to a selective M pathway and dorsal stream deficit. First, they conducted immunohistochemical staining of the lateral geniculate nucleus (LGN) of a normal human male, and showed high FMRP basal expression selectively within the magnocellular (M) layers, suggesting an increased susceptibility of these neurons to the lack of FMRP as occurs in FXS. They also performed staining of the LGN of a male FXS patient, which revealed, unlike the normal male, a population of small-sized neurons within the M layer, providing anatomical and morphological support for the idea that M pathway pathology exists in FXS. For the behavioral evidence, they tested male patients with FXS on tasks that probed either the M pathway or the P pathway and found that they had reduced contrast sensitivity only for those stimuli probing the M pathway. Lastly, they demonstrated that male patients with FXS performed poorly on a global motion task, but not on a form perception task, again suggesting a selective deficit of M pathway (dorsal stream) functioning in FXS.

Auditory processing is another domain that has been found to be impaired in FXS. One study by Maija Castrén assessed auditory processing using ERPs by comparing N1 responses (the occurrence of a negative peak in response to repeated presentations) to tones in school-aged children with FXS to the responses of CA-matched controls. N1 amplitude to standard tones was significantly larger in FXS than in controls. Perhaps most interestingly, children with FXS exhibited no habituation of N1, indicating increased sensory sensitivity for auditory stimuli in FXS. These results are in line with previously reported findings in adults with FXS.

Motor and Language Development

Motor

Clinically, young males with FXS often present with hypotonia, or low muscle tone, which can affect joint stability, fine and gross motor coordination, and sensory integration. For example, hypotonia can lead to a delay in sitting up on one's own and crawling or walking. Children with FXS also have difficulty with sensory integration, particularly integrating and processing touch, sound, sight, and movement. Children with FXS may also experience dyspraxia, trouble with planning a sequence of movements. Often they will toe walk. Approximately 60–90% of boys with FXS are tactile defensive, meaning they do not like people to touch them, the feeling of their clothing, and/or the texture of the food.

Language

While FXS is considered to be a common genetic disorder associated with a varying array of developmental delays, language impairment has been recognized as a characteristic hallmark associated with FXS. Still little is known about the very early developmental course of language in FXS, and its link to atypical sensory information processing that may affect subsequent language outcomes in social communication contexts. But, recent studies on the emergence of deviance in language in FXS have documented word-retrieval deficits, linguistic and cognitive profiles, and deficits in conversational skills. In addition,

a study prospectively examined the developmental trajectories of receptive and expressive communication in 39 young males with FXS (aged 20–86 months) who were given a standardized language test. Results revealed marked delays in language development, but substantial individual variability. In general, it was found that expressive language skills were acquired more slowly over time than were receptive skills. Gain of receptive language progressed at about half the rate expected for typically developing children and expressive language progressed at about one-third the rate.

In general, boys with FXS will develop single words approximately at the age of 3 years and two-word phrases around 4 years. In contrast, girls with FXS usually have single words at the age of 2 years and full sentences at the age of 4 years. Once these children acquire the skill to speak, they tend to perseverate and have echolalia, characteristics often seen in autism. Eventually, the majority of children with FXS will develop functional speech; however, approximately 10–15% of males do not have useful speech, which may be related to dyspraxia.

Social and Emotional Development

An important aspect to understanding the early social development of infants and young children with FXS is to determine how these features are changed with the comorbid diagnosis of autism spectrum disorders (ASD). Rates of ASD comorbidity range from 25% to 40% in males and 3% to 17% in females, and while a considerable amount is known about the overlap between FXS and ASD, much remains unanswered about the factors that predispose an infant with FXS to develop an ASD. Given that FXS can be diagnosed accurately in late infancy, the determination of ASD risk factors in FXS will also inform our understanding of the emergence of the symptoms of ASD in other more heterogeneous groups for which the etiology is unknown.

The behavioral phenotype of infants and young children with FXS includes a relatively pervasive pattern of anxiety symptoms and social problems that reach prominence and clinical attention by perhaps 3–5 years of age. It is critical to study this phenomenon early in development for several reasons. First, there is an overlap in anxiety-related social deficits in FXS (e.g., gaze avoidance and social withdrawal), raising questions about whether social anxiety, early in development, contributes to or predisposes an infant with FXS to more significant social problems or perhaps even autism in later childhood. Anxiety may be manifested by gaze aversion in novel social situations, withdrawn behavior and social isolation, distress with changes in routine and desire for sameness, obsessive compulsive behavior, and repetitive and tangential speech. Some stereotypic behaviors associated with autism, such as hand-flapping and hand-biting, seem to occur more often during periods of increased anxiety, stress, or excitement.

Eye gaze provides a link to social competency in infancy, in addition to being one of the earliest regulators of perceptual input, visual attention, visual processing, and integration. There are several published studies documenting abnormal eye gaze in children with FXS, and recently, it has also been suggested that deviant processing of gaze in FXS may be indicative of dysfunction of underlying neural systems serving these functions. In studies examining attention shifts in typically developing children vs. children with autism, the latter group demonstrated a lack of attention to social stimuli. This has obvious implications for the development of an infant's social system whereby dyadic interactions are not experienced the same. Studies on eye gaze in children with FXS found that the children with FXS are more avoidant of direct eye contact when someone looks at them, suggesting a reactive avoidance, as opposed to children with autism who avoid direct eye gaze whether people are looking at them or not.

Autism Spectrum Disorders

The characteristics of autism in FXS, including the hand-flapping, hand-biting, perseveration in speech, shyness, and poor eye contact, are often present, but some researchers believe the core social deficits typical of autism present less commonly. Usually, individuals with FXS tend to be interested in social interactions and they typically are aware of facial emotional cues from others. In contrast, a study by Sally Rogers et al. in 2001 involving 24 children with FXS, 27 children with autism, and 23 children with developmental delay (DD) ages 21–48 months, demonstrated that the FXS and autism group had a similar profile on the autism measures to the autism only group, but performed lower on the developmental measures, specifically the fine and gross motor domains. This study also found two distinct groups in the FXS sample, one group had autism and the other did not. The FXS group alone was identical to the DD group on the autism measures and the developmental instrument. The two distinct FXS groups may imply possible additional genetic contributions acting synergistically with the *FMR1* mutation, thus leading to the presence of autism.

There are not many studies that have evaluated the role of molecular outcomes, such as FMRP, in the presence of autism in FXS. In addition to the limited number of studies, the measures used to evaluate ASD or symptoms of ASD are not always the same, which also contributes to inconsistencies in the findings. For example, a study by David Hessl et al. in 2001 found that FMRP, after controlling for IQ, predicted symptoms of autism on the Autism Behavior Checklist (ABC) in girls with FXS; but not in boys. In contrast, Deborah Hatton et al. in 2006 found levels of FMRP were negatively correlated to scores on the Childhood Autism Rating Scale (CARS) in males and females. Specifically, low levels of FMRP were related to higher scores on the CARS, indicating more autistic behavior. A small study by Beth Goodlin-Jones et al. in 2004 found that individuals with the premutation and ASD had lower FMRP levels compared to individuals with the premutation alone using the CARS, autism diagnostic observation schedule (ADOS), and autism diagnostic interview-revised (ADI-R) or social communication questionnaire (SCQ).

In females with FXS, ASD is not as well studied, primarily due to the low incidence in females compared to males. The few studies on ASD prevalence in females with FXS have found rates of 3–17%. One study by Michele Mazzocco et al. in 1997 found that females with lower activation ration (percentage of cells expressing the normal allele) had more repetitive behaviors, a characteristic of autism. When autism is present in females with FXS, it indicates the most severe end of the spectrum of social anxiety and withdrawal.

Hyperarousal, Anxiety, and Attention Deficit Hyperactivity Disorder

Studies have looked at physiological indices of enhanced reactions to sensations. For example, the electrodermal responses (EDRs) in FXS, as compared to controls, to olfactory, visual, auditory, tactile, and vestibular sensations which were presented in a 'sensory challenge protocol'. They reported that the FXS group differed significantly from the controls demonstrating greater magnitude, more responses per stimulation, responses on a greater proportion of trials, and lower rates of habituation to these stimuli. In addition, within the group of FXS subjects, the EDR patterns were related to their FMRP expression. Because EDR activity indexes the sympathetic nervous system, and because of the link between FMRP and development in the limbic system, researchers have suggested that the overarousal to sensation often reported in FXS may be due to a sympathetic nervous system dysfunction, possibly caused by a deficiency or absence of FMRP.

Based on early studies documenting hypothalamic and endocrine abnormalities in individuals with FXS, a comprehensive in-home study of anxiety was conducted to examine salivary cortisol (a hormone related to levels of stress) levels in 109 children with FXS (ages 6–17 years) in comparison to their unaffected biological siblings. The results of the study documented that the children with FXS, especially males, had elevated baseline cortisol during the day and before bedtime, and they had a greater cortisol response to the diverse challenges of the home visit (meeting the examiners, undergoing neuropsychological testing, and engaging in tasks designed to elicit social anxiety), in comparison to their unaffected biological siblings. Salivary cortisol levels were positively associated with severity of behavior problems, predominantly withdrawn behavior, social problems, and attention problems. The association in FXS was present after accounting for several other factors shown to predict behavior in these children, including IQ, FMRP, parental psychopathology, and the quality of the home environment, indicating a unique association between anxiety and behavior in children with FXS. Approximately 70% of young males and 60% of young females with FXS have anxiety. In some females with FXS, the anxiety is so severe that they can become selectively mute, where they are silent in some situations, usually at school, but are able to talk in other situations, usually at home.

Research by Maria Boccia and Jane Roberts in 2000 found autonomic dysregulation and hyperarousal in FXS by comparing heart rate variability in young males with FXS compared to CA-matched normal controls. Results showed those with FXS had a faster heart rate and lower parasympathetic activity, but similar sympathetic activity compared to the normal controls. The lowered levels of parasympathetic activity indicate autonomic dysfunction and another mechanism of hyperarousal. Hyperarousal and anxiety in children with FXS can often lead to aggression and tantrums. Studies have shown as high as 42% of young males and 28% of young females with FXS have aggression.

Research evaluating the prevalence of attention deficit hyperactivity disorder (ADHD) in young males with FXS has documented 70–80% meet criteria for ADHD, but studies have also indicated that with age, hyperactivity decreases. For example, 80% of young males with FXS compared to 54% of older school-aged males with FXS had ADHD. In females with FXS, ADHD is seen less frequently with studies showing approximately 35% meeting criteria, which is not significantly different from CA and IQ-matched female controls. The young females with FXS and ADHD typically have less hyperactivity compared to their male counterparts; however, other symptoms, that is, impulsivity and short attention span, can be a significant issue.

In summary, the socioemotional presentation of children with FXS involves symptoms of ADHD and autism with behaviors, such as hand-flapping, hand-biting, poor eye contact, hyperactivity, perseveration, anxiety, and tantrums. Two factors, low FMRP expression and a high degree of autistic behavior, are linked with poorer cognitive outcomes in young children with FXS. In particular, social and communication skills are typically lower for children who have both FXS and autism.

Involvement in Premutation Carriers

As stated earlier, individuals with the premutation have between 55 and 200 CGG repeats. Although carriers were initially thought to be completely unaffected, advances in our understanding of their clinical phenotype and the molecular abnormalities which occur in the premutation have changed this opinion.

Some children with the premutation present with clinical problems including cognitive deficits, mental retardation, autism, ADHD, or emotional difficulties. For children who are in the upper premutation range, a CGG repeat greater than 130, there is often a deficit of FMRP production which lead to features of FXS, including prominent ears and hand-flapping. The majority of individuals with the premutation do not exhibit the clinical features of FXS, although ADHD, shyness, and even social avoidance, can be common. A recent study by Farzin et al. compared boys with the premutation who presented clinically (probands) to boys with the premutation who were identified in families after cascade DNA testing (non-probands) and to brothers who do no have the fragile X mutation. The probands demonstrated ADHD in 93%, whereas the nonprobands had ADHD in 38% and the typical controls had ADHD in 13%. Most striking was the symptoms of ASD which occurred in 71% of the probands, 8% of the nonprobands, and 0% in the typical controls. The probands were significantly different in the number of autistic features from the typical controls; but the nonprobands also demonstrated a significant increase in autistic features compared to the typical controls. Shyness and social aloofness were common in the nonprobands even when they did not meet criteria for ASD. The importance of these findings is that a clinician should not ignore the finding of the premutation allele in a child who presents with developmental delay or behavioral problems.

As previously mentioned, some children with the premutation have lowered FMRP levels which lead to their fragile X involvement. However, we also see an increase of mRNA in premutation carriers. The *FMR1* mRNA levels are increased from two to 10 times the normal. Once the CGG repeat is higher than 200 and into the full mutation range, the level of mRNA drops to zero, particularly if the full mutation is completely methylated. Some individuals with the full mutation will have a lack of methylation or they may have mosaic status, which is a mixture of the premutation and full mutation alleles in the cells. In these cases, the level of mRNA may be elevated or below normal, but it is usually detectable. The elevated mRNA also includes the expanded CGG repeat and this forms a hairpin structure which is 'sticky' and will bind to other proteins in the neuron, leading to a dysregulation of other protein function. Some of the proteins bind to the elevated mRNA, myelin basic protein, αB-crystallin, and lamin A/C.

Research has shown that in individuals who are aging with the premutation, the elevated mRNA combined with the bound protein will form inclusions in the neurons and it is more likely for the neurons to die, leading to brain atrophy. These neuropathological changes lead to the development of the fragile X-associated tremor/ataxia syndrome (FXTAS) in approximately 40% of older adult male carriers and in a subgroup of older adult female carriers. The prevalence of FXTAS in aging male carriers includes 17% in individuals in their 50s, 38% in individuals in their 60s, 47% in individuals in their 70s, and 75% in individuals in their 80s. These numbers were seen in male carriers and the prevalence of FXTAS is significantly decreased in female carriers, most likely related to the protective effects of the second X chromosome. The effect of the elevated mRNA in aging carriers is an RNA toxicity problem, which is similar to what occurs in myotonic dystrophy. We do not yet know if the problems that are seen in some children with the premutation relate to a developmental RNA toxicity effect. This will require further studies of children with the premutation.

The premutation is also the most common single gene associated with premature ovarian failure (POF). In population studies of POF, anywhere from 6% to 14% of women, will have the premutation with the higher rates related to studies of women who have familial POF. Overall, 20% of women with the premutation will have POF, menopause before age 40 years, although a higher percentage will have some degree of ovarian dysfunction including irregular periods or elevation of their FSH. Sometimes POF can occur in the 20s and so genetic counseling is important, particularly if a woman wants to have children.

The premutation can also be associated with psychiatric problems in adults and children. Anxiety and social phobia is a frequent problem, in addition to depression. Depression is more common in the adults, particularly when they have children affected by FXS. The emotional problems related to the premutation may also be related to an RNA toxicity effect in the CNS. The level of psychiatric problems in adult carriers is significantly different from controls and correlates with the degree of mRNA levels.

Newborn Screening

The technology now exists for screening blood spots in newborns for the *FMR1* mutation. Early identification will facilitate genetic counseling, which is critical for this disorder. Once a child is identified, the entire family tree should be reviewed. If the patient has a full mutation, then the mother is the carrier. If the mother's father is the carrier then all of the mother's sisters are carriers and are at risk of having children with FXS. Often extended family members will not have been identified and cascade testing in the family will reveal others who are involved with fragile X, either with premutation or full mutation involvement. Families should be referred to a genetic counselor for further counseling. Reproductive options are reviewed, including prenatal diagnosis, *in vitro* fertilization, egg donation, and adoption. Newborn screening also facilitates early and intensive interventions which can be molded to the needs of infants with FXS.

Treatment and Intervention

Early intervention and specialized services are known to improve outcomes for children with developmental disorders such as FXS, but no study has ever measured the progress of individual children before and after receiving early intervention. In light of this, and given the current discussions about the possible initiation of newborn screening procedures for FXS, there is a need to describe the early developmental profiles, which can be utilized to better understand the benefit of early interventions using behavioral, medical, and education-based treatments.

To reach full potential, a child with FXS may need speech and language therapy, occupational therapy, and physical therapy to help with the many physical, behavioral, and cognitive impacts of the disorder. For young children with FXS, or any type of developmental disability, the Individuals with Disabilities Education Act mandates the early intervention services, special education, speech and language, occupational, and physical therapies be provided for qualified individuals. To gain access to these services, the first step is to have the child assessed for specific strengths and needs. Pediatricians routinely refer children for developmental evaluations, although a developmental evaluation can also be scheduled by calling the local health department.

For very young children with FXS, early intervention services may include family counseling, home visits to help families with nursing, parent/infant programs to encourage language, play, and sensory development. During the preschool years (ages 3–5 years), the local public school system can provide information on the services that are available. Therapies are specialized interventions that can be accessed either through the public systems or privately through the healthcare system. Health insurance coverage of therapeutic interventions varies widely. Therapies may be offered as individual sessions where the child is pulled out of the classroom or integrated into the class routine. Special education programs should be created to fit a child's individual needs to modify classes and assignments. A special educator will often use a variety of tools to meet the needs of each child, such as special equipment, strategic room arrangement, behavior management system, visual communication techniques, and shortened assignments. It is important for parents to be involved in the various steps of their child's educational plan and to implement the recommended practices at home as well.

The association between FXS and autism makes it especially important to identify the children with FXS who also meet criteria for a diagnosis of autism. Several intervention strategies have been shown to be beneficial for individuals with autism, which may also benefit children with FXS and autism. For example, the applied behavior analysis (ABA) technique involves the application of basic behavioral practices (positive reinforcement, repetition, and prompting) to reach a desired outcome. Discrete trial teaching (DTT) is a primary methodology, but not the only instructional method used in ABA programs for individuals with autism. DTT involves breaking down skills into small sub-skills and teaching each subskill, intensely, one at a time. It involves repeated practices with prompting to insure the child's success. DTT also uses reinforcement to help shape and maintain positive behaviors and skills. Also, the Denver model, created by psychologist Sally Rogers, has been a successful treatment program for children with autism. The model is a developmental approach which has two foci, one on intensive teaching and the other on developing the social-communicative skills. The model advocates that social-communicative development originates from emotional relatedness, and so, emphasizes affective connection, relationship building, and understanding communication and emotional exchange between people. Overall, intensive behavioral interventions are helpful in young children with autism and may also benefit young children with FXS and autism combined.

Medication

If the social–emotional dysfunction is detectible in the young children with FXS, there is a great potential for early psychopharmacological intervention, in addition to behavioral therapies as discussed above, to address the antecedent difficulties before well-established maladaptive social, emotional, and behavioral patterns are established.

Early use of psychopharmacological agents, such as selective serotonin reuptake inhibitors (SSRIs), which increase serotonin levels at the synapse, can be helpful for autism and anecdotally in children with FXS who are 3 years or older. Folic acid therapy has also been used in infants and toddlers with FXS, but the results are not consistent. Benefits in behavior are seen in about 50%, but controlled studies are mixed regarding outcome. The advent of mGluR5 antagonists, that is, MPEP and lithium, may have a targeted effect in children with FXS, but studies on these medications have not yet been initiated.

Conclusion

FXS can affect the entire lifespan of an individual, often beginning with motor and language delays in infancy and toddlerhood; cognitive, socioemotional, and behavioral deficits in early childhood; and continued intellectual, behavioral, and emotional problems in adults. Thus far, there has been limited research on FXS in infancy and early childhood; however, research in this younger age range is growing as methods for earlier detection advance and a greater awareness develops in medical settings, schools, and communities overall. The earlier an individual is diagnosed, the sooner the symptoms can be treated, leading to better prognosis. This article reviewed the existing research on FXS in infancy and early childhood, in addition to involvement in older children and adults and intervention strategies.

Acknowledgments

This work was supported by NICHD (grants HD36071, HD02274), NINDS (grant NS044299), a collaborative agreement with the Center for Disease Control and Prevention (grant U10/CCU925123), and the M.I.N.D. Institute at the University of California at Davis. We also thank the families who have supported our research.

See also: ADHD: Genetic Influences; Autism Spectrum Disorders; Developmental Disabilities: Cognitive; Genetic Disorders: Sex Linked; Genetic Disorders: Single Gene; Intellectual Disabilities; Learning Disabilities; Obesity; Sensory Processing Disorder; SIDS.

Suggested Readings

Bailey DB, Jr. (2004) Newborn screening for fragile X syndrome. *Mental Retardation and Developmental Disabilities Research Reviews* 10: 3–10.

Bailey DB, Jr., Hatton DD, Tassone F, Skinner M, and Taylor AK (2001) Variability in FMRP and early development in males with fragile X syndrome. *American Journal on Mental Retardation* 106: 16–27.

Bailey DB, Warren SF, Hatton DD, and Brady N (2007) *Intervention Strategies for Young Children with Fragile X Syndrome.* Baltimore, MD: Brookes Publishing Company.

Berry-Kravis E and Potanos K (2004) Psychopharmacology in fragile X syndrome – present and future. *Mental Retardation and Developmental Disabilities Research Reviews* 10: 42–48.

Cornish KM, Sudhalter V, and Turk J (2004) Attention and language in fragile X. *Mental Retardation and Developmental Disabilities Research Reviews* 10: 11–16.

Hagerman RJ and Hagerman PJ (2002) *Fragile X Syndrome: Diagnosis, Treatment, and Research,* 3rd edn. Baltimore, MD: The Johns Hopkins University Press.

Mirrett PL, Bailey DB, Jr., Roberts JE, and Hatton DD (2004) Developmental screening and detection of developmental delays in infants and toddlers with fragile X syndrome. *Journal of Developmental and Behavioral Pediatrics* 25: 21–27.

Rogers SJ, Wehner EA, and Hagerman RJ (2001) The behavioral phenotype in fragile X: Symptoms of autism in very young children with fragile X syndrome, idiopathic autism, and other developmental disorders. *Journal of Developmental and Behavioral Pediatrics* 22: 409–417.

Scerif G, Cornish K, Wilding J, Driver J, and Karmiloff-Smith A (2004) Visual search in typically developing toddlers and toddlers with fragile X or Williams syndrome. *Developmental Science* 7: 116–130.

Relevant Websites

http://www.fpg.unc.edu – FPG Child Development Institute, The University of North Carolina at Chapel Hill.

http://www.fraxa.org – FRAXA Fragile X Research Foundation.

http://www.cdc.gov/ncbddd – National Center on Birth Defects and Developmental Disabilities, Centers for Disease Control and Prevention.

http://www.fragilex.org – The National Fragile X Foundation.

Genetic Disorders: Sex-Linked

J Isen and L A Baker, University of Southern California, Los Angeles, CA, USA

Glossary

Autosome – Any chromosome other than the sex Chromosomes (X and Y). Humans have 22 pairs of homologous autosomes.

Diploid – Cells containing two sets of chromosomes, usually one from the mother and one from the father. Somatic cells in humans are diploid.

Haploid – Cells containing only one chromosome from a homologous pair, as in the case of human gametes. Males are also haploid with respect to the X chromosome, while females are diploid.

Heterozygotic – The presence of two different alleles on homologous chromosomes at a given locus. This is contrasted with the homozygotic state of possessing two identical alleles at a given locus.

Imprinting – A phenomenon in which the expression of a given allele depends on whether the allele was inherited from the mother or father.

Proband – An individual affected with a disorder under investigation, and from whom other family members are identified for study. Also called 'index case'.

Sex-influenced – A trait influenced by different processes in males and females, usually as a function of different hormonal exposure in the two sexes.

Sex-limited – Different sets of genes influence a trait in males and females.

Sex-linked – A trait controlled by one or more genes on the X or Y chromosome.

X-inactivation – The process in females whereby one X chromosome is randomly inactivated in each cell line, resulting in genetic mosaicism.

Introduction

Many heritable disorders affect one particular sex much more frequently. This sex difference in prevalence may suggest that the genetic mechanisms are either 'sex-linked' (influenced by one or more genes on the X or Y chromosome) or 'sex-limited' (different genes affecting males and females). A skewed sex ratio is especially salient for developmental disorders such as autism and language/speech disabilities, as well as childhood aggression. The prevalence is invariably higher in males, indicating that a sex-linked, sex-influenced, or sex-limited process may account for the etiology of these complex disorders.

Sex-linkage occurs when a trait is controlled by genetic loci on either the X or Y chromosome. However, there are few traits or disorders known to be directly influenced by Y-linked genes, so these will not be discussed here. The expressive effect of a given allele can span anywhere from recessive (an allelic effect is completely masked in the presence of another allele on the homologous X chromosome) to dominant (one allele is always expressed independently of the homologous allele). Some alleles can also act in a semi-dominant (additive) manner, such that a heterozygous combination of two different alleles leads to a quantitatively intermediate phenotypic expression (e.g., medium height) compared to the phenotypes produced by the two homozygous combinations (short or tall). The dominant–recessive nature of X-linked gene action determines whether males or females are more affected at the phenotypic level. For X-linked traits that are recessive or semi-dominant, males will typically show a higher prevalence. Since most single-gene disorders (sex-linked or otherwise) are recessive, the bulk of affected cases will be male.

A gross disparity in prevalence indicates the possibility that a genetic disorder may be sex-linked, although there are alternative interpretations. Sex-limiting or sex-influencing factors, such as testosterone exposure, may instead explain sex differences in prevalence. Autosomal genes may account for some disorders, although these alleles may function differently in males and females due to interactions with other X-linked genes. In general, the mere existence of sex differences in prevalence or mean trait levels does not necessarily imply sex-linkage. Nor does the fact that sex chromosomes are implicated for a disorder guarantee that the disorder is sex-linked.

Sex-linkage, sex-limitation, and sex-influenced models are described in detail here, followed by a review of several known sex-linked disorders as well as syndromes caused by sex chromosome abnormalities. Finally, we turn to autism as an example demonstrating how one can evaluate evidence for sex-linkage and sex-limitation.

Theoretical Background

In general, males suffer a poorer developmental outcome than females. There are higher rates of prenatal disturbances, birth complications, and childhood disorders in males. This phenomenon is mirrored by a male–female sex ratio that progressively declines from conception to adulthood. Male embryos greatly outnumber females at conception. Not surprisingly, the male–female ratio of fetal deaths is immense, reportedly reaching 2:1 within some populations. Nonetheless, the male–female ratio among live births lingers around 1.05, which is small but still significantly greater than 1. It is only with further male attrition during childhood that gender parity is finally reached by adulthood; males who survive gestation and infancy manifest much higher levels of developmental disorders than females. These skewed sex ratios support the argument that males, due to genetic disadvantages, are more sensitive to environmental perturbation than females. That is, they experience greater difficulty overcoming early developmental challenges.

What accounts for this increased male frailty? While the ultimate source of this phenomenon is linked to Darwinian sexual selection, the actual genetic mechanism is poorly understood. There are at least two competing explanations: sex-linkage and hormonal sex-limitation. Briefly stated, both mechanisms will result in a sexually divergent prevalence for a disorder. However, sex-linkage models assume that the genetic etiology of a disorder is the same across sex, whereas sex-limitation asserts that the causes are essentially different between the sexes.

Sex-Linked vs. Sex-Limited Traits

Sex-linkage exists when traits are influenced by alleles located on the X chromosome. The phenotypic prevalence for a sex-linked trait differs between the sexes as a

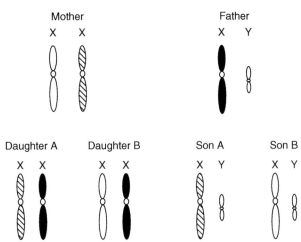

Figure 1   Diagram representing the transmission of sex chromosomes from parents to offspring (via the gametes). Mothers transmit one of their two X chromosomes to each child. Fathers can pass either an X chromosome or a Y chromosome to their offspring. In the former case, the product would be XX (female). In the latter case, the child would be XY (male). Note that daughters receive an identical copy of the X chromosome from their father. (Maternal transmission is more complicated, however, since sections of the mother's two X chromosomes recombine during gamete formation, so that the maternal X chromosome received by each offspring is effectively different than what is received by any other sibling.)

result of the unique karyotype (46, XY) of males, and, less perceptibly, due to the mosaicism of the female cell line (i.e., different X-chromosomes being expressed in different cells). For females who carry two X chromosomes (see **Figure 1**), full phenotypic expression of a trait only occurs in the homozygous condition (in which both alleles are present). If females are heterozygous for an X-linked gene, the process of X-inactivation guarantees that a given allele will be expressed in only a proportion of developing cells. (One X chromosome is randomly inactivated during development, ensuring that females do not possess twice as many gene products as males.) For males, genes on the sex chromosomes generally operate in a haploid (single chromosome) state. Alleles on their single X chromosome will have a higher likelihood of being expressed (i.e., higher penetrance) due to their hemizygotic (XY) status. Moreover, the expressivity of an allele will be especially enhanced in males if traits are X-linked recessive.

All sex-linked traits stem from genetic variation on the X chromosome. Interestingly, sex-linked traits are not confined to reproductive-related processes, but instead exert influences on a wide array of domains. This contrasts with the Y chromosome, which is solely involved with sex determination and male fertility. Although a condition known as hairy ears syndrome was thought to be Y-linked, more recent evidence has cast doubt on that speculation. The most significant gene on the Y chromosome is the

SRY gene, which determines testes formation and appears to be structurally invariant in humans.

Sex-limitation occurs when genes are only expressed in one sex or the other (e.g., breast development in females; beard growth in males). Genes may also be sex-influenced, where the same genes are expressed differently in males and females. Although many genetics textbooks typically distinguish between sex-limited and sex-influenced traits, many studies in practice refer to both of these effects as sex-limited, indicating that the underpinnings of a disorder are fundamentally different between the sexes. These effects may result from different hormonal environments, socialization processes, or other environmental factors which may lead to different relative effects of (autosomal) genes in the two sexes. For example, a disorder might be heritable in males but more environmentally caused in females. Furthermore, sex-limitation occurs if different sets of genes are operating between the sexes. This contrasts with sex-linkage, in which the etiology is the same for males and females. For example, if color blindness is a recessive sex-linked condition, then color-blind females should possess a double dose of the same allele that colorblind males possess. However, if color blindness were a sex-limited trait, we would find that males are generally colorblind for different and perhaps nongenetic reasons (e.g., greater frequency of head injury).

The distinction between sex-linked, sex-limited, and sex-influenced mechanisms is a recurring theme, and will be discussed with regard to a potentially sex-linked developmental disorder. For theoretical purposes here, we place these mechanisms in the context of the broad developmental process.

The higher male morbidity in early childhood is often thought to reflect a sex-linked genetic mechanism. Since females have a second ('backup') copy of the X chromosome, the risk associated with a deleterious mutation is considerably lower. The diploid state of females leads to greater stability during development. It is true that some X-linked mutations can severely disrupt development in females, as in the case of Rett syndrome. However, for most conditions, the effect of a deleterious mutation is more debilitating in males (and, in the case of Rett syndrome, spontaneously aborts the male fetus with few exceptions).

An alternative to the sex-linkage model is that the hormonal milieu differs between the sexes. This often takes a sex-limited form, since testosterone exposure in early infancy overlaps little between males and females. Such theories claim that testosterone suppresses immune functions and stifles language-related abilities. Norman Geschwind, for example, hypothesized that prenatal testosterone is tied to a constellation of quirks and disorders that are more often observed in boys: immune diseases, left-handedness, and reading disabilities. Although this hypothesis has not been well supported, a similar and more compelling theory has been applied to autism. The

presence of a Y chromosome should dramatically increase susceptibility to the disorder, since the fetus' testes are a major source of testosterone in the uterus.

These two mechanisms, sex-linkage and sex-limitation, do not necessarily have to be mutually exclusive. However, the former is more directly genetic, while the latter may operate through hormonally mediated channels. Additionally, sex-linkage is not generally concerned with the domain of sexual development and differentiation, whereas sex-limitation is tied to sexually dimorphic processes. They each entail unique predictions, which can be compared when information about the biological relatives of affected individuals is available. It is difficult to distinguish these two mechanisms in the absence of genetically informative data, as both may lead to a similar level of sexual divergence in prevalence.

Known Sex-Linked Disorders

It is considerably easier to determine the genetic mechanism when a disorder is controlled by allelic variation at a single genetic locus. There are several well-known disorders that are inherited in a Mendelian fashion, meaning that they are transmitted by a single allele, which can behave as recessive or dominant. This type of transmission can be contrasted to a multifactorial polygenic process, in which the effects of multiple genetic loci additively increase vulnerability to a disorder.

Most alleles are not completely dominant or recessive, but rather possess an intermediate level of expressivity. However, it is convenient to describe sex-linked traits using the classic Mendelian approach. Some sex-linked disorders are indeed purely recessive (e.g., color blindness), while other disorders such as fragile X syndrome are less so. When the inheritance of a recessive sex-linked gene is involved, prevalence will be much higher in males. Conversely, for genes that are best described as dominant, prevalence may be higher in females. This is because females can receive a mutation from either their mother or father, and therefore the chance of inheriting a disorder may be twice that of males (who can only inherit an X-linked mutation from their mother); note that this is more of a technical possibility than an actual phenomenon.

Consistent with most autosomal-linked diseases, sex-linked Mendelian disorders are typically recessive. As mentioned before, X-linked disorders are not necessarily tied to sexual development, but affect domains as wide-scoping as color vision, blood clotting, and neuronal growth. The sex-linked nature of these disorders was demonstrated prior to the availability of molecular genetic tools. This is because sex-linked recessive traits have specific inheritance patterns. At the pedigree level, transmission of the disorder must pass from mother to son. Furthermore, a female carrier will transmit the disorder to half of her male offspring.

At the population level, one should observe that the prevalence of affected females is the square of the proportion of males who are affected. (The odds are squared to reflect the fact that females require a homozygous combination of mutations to manifest the disorder.) This prediction assumes that affected males have equal mating success relative to female carriers. If the condition is lethal in childhood or renders affected males sick and undesirable, such males will be less likely to produce children compared to female carriers. Girls would therefore be less likely to inherit the allele from their father, and the proportion of females affected will be less than the square of males. This caveat does not apply to sex-linked color blindness since it does not affect mating success or mortality, but would be relevant to developmental disorders.

Color vision deficiency, or color blindness, is a relatively common disorder that interferes with perception of red and green hues. It reportedly occurs in about 8% of white males and in about 0.7% of white females. This pattern in prevalence remarkably coincides with quantitative predictions of a recessive condition; the proportion of affected females is the square of the proportion of affected males. Another notable X-linked recessive disorder is androgen insensitivity syndrome. It is unique among the sex-linked disorders in that it has powerful implications for our understanding of sexual development. A single genetic mutation renders the androgen receptor severely compromised or missing. Although an affected fetus might produce normal amounts of testosterone, the lack of binding sites for androgen prevents masculine sexual differentiation. Affected individuals are almost always genotypic males who appear phenotypically indistinguishable from females. Other recessive conditions include Lesch–Nyhan syndrome and hemophilia, but these are extremely rare.

A few sex-linked disorders are influenced by genes that are not recessive. Fragile X syndrome is the most prominent to fall under this category. Due to the semi-dominant nature of the alleles leading to this disorder (i.e., variations in the *FMR1* gene), female carriers often exhibit less severe symptoms. The deleterious forms of the *FMR1* gene frequently cause mental retardation in males but milder learning difficulties in females. Fragile X syndrome is the most common form of inherited mental retardation. (Down syndrome, which is more prevalent, is not hereditary.) It is thought that the prevalence is twice as high in males, although ascertainment in females is less straightforward. The detection rate in females is probably lower, since they are usually able to live independently.

Fragile X syndrome has a very complex inheritance that defies simple Mendelian descriptions. A mutation of the *FMR1* gene leads to a variety of physical anomalies and cognitive defects. Moreover, the defective gene itself (an expansion in a repeating triplet nucleotide sequence) becomes more deleterious across generations, since the expansion increases in each transmission. Production of the FMR1 protein is severely curtailed in individuals with fragile X syndrome, and the effect worsens across generations. Since the FMR1 protein is necessary for normal brain function, affected individuals will present with intellectual disabilities. Such individuals often exhibit social impairment and autistic behavior. Thus, fragile X syndrome is interesting in that it contains features that closely parallel pervasive developmental disorders.

Rett syndrome is a pervasive developmental disorder which is transmitted in a dominant X-linked fashion. Unlike fragile X syndrome, the mutation is highly penetrant. In other words, the mutation is extremely potent and will invariably be expressed if present. Rett syndrome is caused by a mutation of the *MECP2* gene. Due to its dominant and debilitating nature, most cases of Rett syndrome are sporadic in which the *MECP2* mutation spontaneously arises in a parent's gonad.

Nearly all cases of Rett syndrome are female, although a few male cases have been reported. The sex difference in prevalence can be interpreted as reflecting a much higher lethality in male fetuses. This is supported by observations that affected females have fewer male siblings than would be expected. The male lethality of this disorder portends the debilitating consequences experienced by its female survivors. In general, development appears to follow a normal trajectory until 1–2 years of age. At that point, intellectual growth is suddenly stunted and psychomotor abilities begin declining. Affected individuals are relegated to a life of profound mental retardation.

At least one X-linked gene has also been shown to affect impulsive and aggressive behavior in humans. Specifically, monoamine oxidase A (MAO-A) is an enzyme (found in the human brain) controlled by a single gene on the X chromosome, and is involved in the metabolism of neurotransmitters serotonin (5-HT), norephinephrine (NE), and dopamine (DA). In a large Dutch pedigree, Han Brunner's group found a point mutation in the *MAO-A* gene that was associated with abnormal aggressiveness in adult males. Further support for the role of MAO-A on aggression comes from Jean Shih's studies of knockout mice (i.e., an inbred strain bred to be missing the normal MAO-A allele), which exhibit elevated levels of aggressive and violent behavior. In children, MAO-A mutations have been shown to confer a greater risk of aggression and violence, but only in those who experienced elevated levels of physical maltreatment by their parents. Adverse environments, therefore, may enhance the effects of some X-linked genes.

Sex Chromosome Abnormalities

Some genetic disorders are not caused by mutations, but rather stem from the failure of sex chromosomes to properly separate during gamete formation – a process called nondysjunction. This will lead to numerical abnormalities, in which individuals have more than two sex chromosomes (either X or Y) or lack one copy. In addition, a chromosome may be present but functionally faulty. Unlike those with autosomal abnormalities (i.e., Down syndrome), affected individuals usually do not suffer global mental retardation. Instead, sex chromosome abnormalities often lead to learning disabilities and difficulty in specific cognitive domains. The most common types of cases are XYY syndrome, Klinefelter syndrome, and Turner syndrome (TS).

XYY males possess a trisomy of the sex chromosomes instead of the normal two. Most XYY males appear physically normal (aside from taller stature) and do not experience unusual deficits. However, there may be an increased risk of learning disorders and language problems. Additionally, there was early speculation that XYY males are more prone to aggression and criminal behavior, but this view was made obsolete in 1976. A study by Herman Witkin and colleagues showed that higher rates of XYY males in prison populations could be explained by lower intelligence rather than higher aggression or violence.

Some males possess an extra copy of the X chromosome. These XXY males exhibit Klinefelter syndrome. Unlike males with the XYY karyotype, Klinefelter males are usually sterile and often possess a variety of physical anomalies. Klinefelter boys tend to exhibit selective deficits in reading and language skills. Arithmetic skills may also be compromised, but visuospatial skills are remarkably intact. This often results in a large discrepancy between verbal intelligence quotients (IQ) and performance IQ.

One conclusion is that boys with sex chromosome abnormalities manifest a cognitive profile exaggerative of typical males. That is, delayed language skills tend to be coupled with normal visuospatial abilities. This observation is useful because it may shed light on disorders that are genetically more elusive (i.e., dyslexia, autism, stuttering). Interestingly, TS girls exhibit the opposite profile.

Girls with TS have only one intact X chromosome. Their second copy is a nonfunctional stub or is altogether missing. In over two-thirds of cases, it is the X-chromosome of paternal origin that is missing. The girls possess extremely short stature and a variety of medical problems. However, their condition often goes unnoticed until adolescence, when it is found that they are not developing secondary sexual characteristics. In terms of academic performance, they generally have verbal skills in the normal range but show deficits in spatial skills and mathematical problem solving.

This cognitive profile has attracted interest because it refutes hypotheses that superior visuospatial skills are X-linked recessive. However, females with TS also experience gonadal dysgenesis, which causes the ovaries to degenerate and thwart all secretion of hormones. Perhaps optimal spatial intelligence results from the interaction of sex steroids with genetic loci on the X chromosome. In 2003, a group led by Judith Ross evaluated that possibility by experimentally treating TS girls with androgen replacement. Surprisingly, girls who received androgen did not show increases in spatial cognition, but did show improvement in working memory.

Finally, some investigators have drawn a link between autism and TS, noting that the risk of autism is 200-fold in females with TS. Autism is present only among TS girls who inherited an intact X chromosome from their mother; no cases of autism are observed among those who possess a paternally derived X chromosome. David Skuse and colleagues have argued that genetic imprinting (i.e., different gene expression depending on which parent transmitted it) might explain the male vulnerability to autism, insomuch that superior social–emotional processing is associated with an X chromosome of paternal origin.

Blueprint for Evaluating Potential Sex-Linked Disorders

When a disorder is controlled by a single mutation, it is rather straightforward to determine whether sex-linkage is at work, based on patterns of transmission across generations and associations with measured polymorphisms on the X-chromosome. For complex polygenic disorders, however, it is necessary to carefully weigh evidence of sex-linkage and sex-limitation in order to discover the underlying biological process. For example, if family pedigree data supports evidence for sex-linkage, then an intensive hunt for relevant loci on the X chromosome will be warranted. However, if sex-limitation is demonstrated, then hormonal and/or environmental influences should be explored. This is because there are two major routes by which genetic differences between the sexes are manifested at the phenotypic level: (1) an X-linked route and (2) an 'indirect' hormonal route.

The second route is described as 'indirect' because the disorder is influenced by an epigenetic mechanism in which sex steroids alter transcription of genes. For example, substances produced by the gonads (androgen and estrogen) might interact with genes carried on the autosomes. If liability for the disorder can be shown to correlate with androgen levels (prenatal or otherwise), then sex-linkage is unlikely a source of the gender skew in prevalence. A sex-influenced steroid pathway is essentially different from a sex-linked genetic mechanism.

These two models can be tested at the molecular level (i.e., genetic linkage studies) as well as at the latent or phenotypic level (i.e., family transmission studies). Evidence for sex-linkage occurs when a disorder is associated with specific polymorphisms on chromosome X. The genetic signature of affected individuals is compared to that of unaffected individuals. Sex-linkage is demonstrated if a specific marker on the X chromosome can successfully discriminate the two groups. Sometimes, however, when stratifying a sample by gender, it is found that the genetic loci associated with the disorder in males are different from the trait loci in females. This would be an example of sex-limitation, since the genes contributing to the disorder in males would be different from those influencing females.

When working with pedigree data, sex-linkage can be demonstrated if transmission of risk tends to run from mother to son but not from father to son. Also, since daughters inherit the same X chromosome from their father, sisters will share on average 75% of their alleles identical by descent. Therefore, symptoms of a sex-linked disorder should be most similar among sister–sister and father–daughter pairs. Sibling resemblance should weaken among brother–brother and opposite-sex pairs. Finally, the genetic loading of risk should be higher in families with affected females than in those with male-only cases. Since females require a higher genetic dosage to manifest a sex-linked disorder, a higher prevalence of the disorder should be observed in the biological (particularly paternal) relatives of female probands.

Autism: An Illustrative Example

These predictions can be used to evaluate the sex-linked status of candidate disorders. Autism serves as a good example to illustrate the methods for detecting sex-linked effects, as the male–female ratio is 4:1. This has led investigators to propose that X-linked mutations may increase vulnerability, although testosterone-related individual differences have also been endorsed as a potential source of the sex difference in prevalence. It should be noted, however, that autism is considered a complex disorder with genetic heterogeneity, such that several different genes (including several autosomal ones) may account for different forms of autism. Still, the sex difference in prevalence has led investigators to consider sex-linkage as one potential etiological source of autism.

Sex differences in prevalence are not necessarily the product of genotypic differences between the sexes. However, autism appears a strong candidate as a sex-linked genetic disorder because it is unlikely that environmental influences would lead to systematic gender bias. Autism emerges too early in life to be caused by gender-specific socialization patterns. Indeed it would seem bizarre that

parents could treat infant boys in such a fundamentally different way that would cause them to develop severe impairments in communication and social skills.

Evidence for sex-linkage is based on autistic features in boys with fragile X syndrome. A substantial proportion of fragile X boys suffer social anxiety, repetitive/stereotyped behaviors, and language disturbances such as echolalia. However, the deficits observed in these boys may qualitatively differ from those with pure autism. Also, the amount of FMR1 protein is not related to the degree of autistic behavior in fragile X boys. This suggests that X-linked mutations affecting the *FMR1* gene are not directly responsible for the high prevalence of autism.

The absence of gender effects on familial risk also runs contrary to sex-linkage. In 2000, Andrew Pickles and colleagues reported that the prevalence of broadly defined autism is no higher in the biological relatives of female probands than in the relatives of male probands. This indicates that the genetic threshold necessary for manifestation of autism is not higher in females, thereby undermining a key argument for sex-linkage. Furthermore, among parents of male probands, the rate of autism is actually lower in mothers than in fathers. This result departs from the sex-linked expectation that risk is primarily transmitted from mother to son.

Molecular studies, however, have met with more success. In a genetic linkage study, a group led by Hugh Gurling explored a region of the X chromosome involved in the encoding of MeCP2 and FMRP. (Mutations of the *MECP2* and *FMR1* gene cause Rett syndrome and fragile X syndrome, respectively.) Genetic markers in this region produced a likelihood ratio of approximately 100:1 that autism is X-linked. Similarly, Merlin Butler and colleagues observed a highly skewed X-inactivation pattern in a significant portion of autistic females. The control group was composed of unaffected sisters, who showed a much more random (and typical) pattern of X-inactivation. (Skewed X-inactivation is comparable to the male [haploid] disadvantage of 'putting all your eggs in one basket'.) The interpretation, then, is that random inactivation buffers females from the deleterious effect of any single allele.

It should be noted that molecular evidence in favor of sex-linkage for some forms of autism has emerged quite recently. Previous genome-wide searches had consistently pointed to autosomal linkage. In fact, even sex-limited expression of autosomal genes had been implicated. A group led by Stan Nelson, for example, discovered a linkage site on chromosome 17 among families possessing at least two children with broadly defined autism. However, linkage was specific to families possessing male-only cases of autism. No significant linkage sites were found for the remaining families who possessed female cases. This suggests that the genes influencing autism may differ between the sexes, although it does not imply that the overall magnitude of genetic influence is different. Indeed, twin studies demonstrate that the heritability is equally high for males and females.

Equal heritability in the face of a marked sexual divergence in prevalence may occur in the presence of sex-specific hormonal thresholds. For example, the 'extreme male brain' theory of Simon Baron-Cohen describes a neurodevelopmental trajectory that is typified by high androgen levels. Elevated exposure to testosterone should lead to enhanced growth of the brain's right hemisphere at the expense of left hemisphere development. As a result of these mean differences in prenatal testosterone, males will normally develop an asymmetry favoring the right hemisphere. This bias is reflected in males' superior functioning in right hemisphere-specialized tasks, such as mental rotation. The drawback is that language skills are delayed. As a result, female infants begin verbally interacting at a younger age and are more effective at gesture-based communication, two skills that autistic children generally lack.

According to this theory, the traits that contribute to autism are an extreme magnification of the same characteristics that typical males possess to a greater degree than typical females (e.g., fiddling with objects instead of chatting on the telephone, systematizing instead of empathizing). One extension of this argument is that intellectual impairment in autistic males should follow a more normal distribution within a more typical range. Autistic females, in contrast, should adhere to a more deviant IQ distribution. Cognitive development in autistic females should be more qualitatively deviant because autism is essentially the unfolding of a masculine developmental process.

There is a general consensus that autistic females possess lower IQs than their male counterparts. In fact, the sex ratio in autism is least distorted among those with the lowest levels of intellectual functioning. As one approaches the higher-functioning end of the spectrum, the sex ratio climbs to 9:1. This contrasts with the pattern observed for fragile X syndrome, in which mental retardation is proportionately more common among males than among females. This suggests that a sex-linked model is inferior to a sex-limited or sex-influenced interpretation.

Evidence for a sex-influenced hormonal mechanism comes from females who possess an autosomal-recessive condition known as congenital adrenal hyperplasia. Females with this disease are often exposed to abnormally high levels of testosterone during early development. Consistent with the 'extreme male brain' theory, they score as high as male controls (and significantly higher than female controls) on a self-report autism questionnaire. Furthermore, the digit length ratio of autistic children tends to cluster at the very masculine end of the spectrum. (The length of the index finger in relation to

the ring finger is sexually dimorphic; low ratios serve as a putative index of increased fetal testosterone.) Interestingly, the digit length ratio is similarly low in the fathers of autistic children, indicating that genetic risk may be transmitted from father to son.

Concluding Remarks

The sex distribution of a disorder may provide important clues concerning its genetic origins. Indeed, understanding the source of the disparity in prevalence is tantamount to identifying the etiological roots of the disorder. Therefore, it is important to discern the various genetic mechanisms that might lead to a systematically higher prevalence in one gender. Sex-linkage is one of several processes that might account for the greater male vulnerability to developmental disorders.

The evidence regarding autism as a sex-linked disorder, however, is mixed. The gender skew in prevalence may stem from a combination of sex-influenced, sex-limited, and sex-linked processes. This ambiguity reflects the fact that the genetic and environmental factors contributing to autism are diverse. As with any polygenic disorder, each predisposing gene (X-linked or otherwise) probably exerts only a small effect on overall risk. Heterogeneity further complicates matters, since it is unlikely that the same mechanisms account for the entire spectrum (i.e., Asperger syndrome, autism with speech, autism without speech).

All sex-linked disorders that have hitherto been established involve mutations at a single genetic locus. However, as clinicians continue to refine the diagnostic categories, it is likely that X-linked alleles will emerge as significant risk factors for polygenic disorders. Single-gene disorders and sex chromosomal abnormalities provide an ideal starting base from which to search for genetic loci involved in the pathology of more complex disorders.

See also: Autism Spectrum Disorders; Endocrine System; Fragile X Syndrome; Genetic Disorders: Single Gene; Intellectual Disabilities.

Suggested Readings

Baron-Cohen S and Hammer J (1997) Is autism an extreme form of the 'male brain'? *Advances in Infancy Research* 11: 193–217.
Brunner HG, Nelen MR, van Zandvoort P, et al. (1993) X-linked borderline mental retardation with prominent behavioral disturbance: phenotype, genetic localization, and evidence for disturbed monoamine metabolism. *American Journal of Human Genetics* 52: 1032–1039.
Pickles A, Starr E, Kazak S, et al. (2000) Variable expression of the autism broader phenotype: Findings from extended pedigrees. *Journal of Child Psychology and Psychiatry* 41: 491–502.

Ross J, Roeltgen D, Stefanatos G, *et al.* (2003) Androgen-responsive aspects of cognition in girls with Turner syndrome. *Journal of Clinical Endocrinology and Metabolism* 88: 292–296.

Skuse DH (2005) X-linked genes and mental functioning. *Human Molecular Genetics* 14: R27–R32.

Stone JL, Merriman B, Cantor RM, *et al.* (2004) Evidence for sex-specific risk alleles in autism spectrum disorder. *American Journal of Human Genetics* 75: 1117–1123.

Talebizadeh Z, Bittel D, Veatch O, Kibiryeva N, and Butler M (2005) Brief report: Non-random X chromosome inactivation in females with autism. *Journal of Autism and Developmental Disorders* 35: 675–681.

Vincent JB, Melmer G, Bolton PF, *et al.* (2005) Genetic linkage analysis of the X chromosome in autism, with emphasis on the fragile X region. *Psychiatric Genetics* 15: 83–90.

Witkin H, Mednick S, and Schulsinger F (1976) Criminality in XYY and XXY men. *Science* 193: 547–555.

Relevant Website

http://www.ncbi.nlm.nih.gov – Online Mendelian Inheritance in Man (OMIM).

Genetic Disorders: Single Gene

E L Grigorenko, Yale University, New Haven, CT, USA

Glossary

Developmental science – Studies of complex systemic changes in human occurring over life-span.

Epigenetics – Studies of changes in gene functioning (silencing and transcription initiation) that occur without changes in the genes themselves.

Genetics – Studies of heredity investigating how genes are transmitted from generation to generation.

Genomics – Studies of the whole genome and how it functions as a complex system of interacting genes in an environment.

Proteomics – Studies of proteins and their functions.

Introduction

We refer to development as a complex process of realization of biological mechanisms uniquely defining a human being. These biological mechanisms cannot unfold in a vacuum; they unfurl in the environments defined by 'humanness', that is, in the human habitat. The idea that both internal forces hidden in an individual, as well as the external characteristics of the habitat, guide the development of a human being has been central to social and behavioral sciences since their very emergence. Relevant challenges and debates have not really been about whether either matters, but rather about what constitutes internal and external forces of development and how their various elements interact with each other. One of the charges of developmental sciences is to define these internal and external 'black boxes' and to understand, as much as possible, direct, indirect, and interactive mechanisms of their functioning.

The objective of this article is to sample from the modern body of knowledge on the content and function of one of the many internal forces guiding development – the human genome. With amazingly rapid developments in genetics and genomics, the genetic 'draw' of the internal forces black box is gradually being filled by a summary of the roughly 24 500 genes carried by individuals from the moment of conception. Genetics and genomics are on their way to characterizing every individual in terms of his or her genetic 'script', but scientists today understand that it is environments, in their infinite variability, that guide the interpretation of the genetic script by its carrier into the actual performance, which is always a unique realization of the inherited genetic script. Yet, understanding what these genes do and whether or not their functions are modifiable by environment is a very important task that is greatly relevant to both developmental and health sciences.

The article is structured into three parts. First, a number of concepts that capture the vocabulary used throughout the article are introduced. Second, a general description of single-gene disorders (SGDs), depicting their common and specific features, and introduces a number of examples of such disorders are provided. Third, comments on selected common characteristics of SGDs that might be of interest to developmentalists in the context of understanding genetic forces of development are made.

Concepts and Definitions

Broadly defined, genes are sources of information that define growth patterns and functions of human cells; genes are units of inheritance forming the bases of heredity. Genes are contained in a complex chemical known as deoxyribonucleic acid (DNA). This complex polymer is made of simpler chemicals referred to as nucleotides. Nucleotides are basic constituents of DNA; they are organic molecules that consist of a nitrogenous base (adenine (A), guanine (G), thymine (T), or cytosine (C)), a phosphate molecule, and a sugar molecule. Thousands of nucleotides link together in a long chain forming DNA in such a way that C matches with G and A matches with T to establish a base pair (bp). Because of this selective pairing of nucleotides, although DNA is usually double-stranded, it is enough to know the sequence of nucleotides on one DNA strand to reproduce a complementary sequence on the other DNA strand. Each human has ∼3 billion bp of DNA, which together form the human genome. Within an organism, DNA is contained in cell nuclei and organized into chromosomes. Chromosomes enfold both genes and intergenetic DNA. Genetic DNA (i.e., DNA that forms genes) is presented by segments that contain the information necessary to manufacture a functional ribonucleic acid (RNA) needed for subsequent synthesis of proteins. Genes themselves are complex structures that contain, chiefly:

1. regions determining specifics of the RNA product to be produced (so-called promoter regions);
2. transcribed regions establishing the content of the RNA product (so-called exons);
3. noncoding intra-exonic pieces of DNA that are not transcribed (so-called introns); and
4. other functional sequence regions (e.g., 3′ UTR). Functionally, genes can be 'working' (i.e., expressed) or 'not working' (i.e., silent, not expressed). Expressed genes can produce different gene products, which result in protein synthesis or in regulation of other genes.

The human genome is characterized by the presence of 46 chromosomes – 22 pairs of autosomal (nonsex) chromosomes and two sex chromosomes. Chromosomes 1–22 are identical for males and females, whereas sex chromosomes differ. Sex chromosomes are defined as X and Y; males are '46, XY' and females are '46, XX'. Each pair of autosomal chromosomes is formed by a maternal and a paternal chromosome; thus, each individual has two copies of the same gene – one inherited from the mother and one from the father. Paternal and maternal chromosomes essentially carry the same information: each chromosome contains the same set of genes, but their nucleotide sequences can vary slightly (by less than 1%). The pairwise relationships between the two chromosomes and genes harbored by chromosomes determine various patterns of genetic transmission.

Decoding DNA for the sake of revealing its bp constitution is referred to as 'sequencing'. The first draft of the human genome became available with the completion of the Human Genome Project in 2003. Now various gaps in this draft have been closed and pieces of the genomes of many individuals from different ethnic backgrounds have been sequenced. From the rapidly accumulated mass of human DNA sequences completed to date, it is evident that two unrelated individuals have, on average, one different nucleotide per 1000 bp. Although when considered across the whole human genome these differences amount to 3 million per person, when two people are compared with each other, the differences amount to only ∼0.1%. The places in the genome where these differences occur are referred to as polymorphic sites (or loci) and the differences themselves are referred to as polymorphisms (or variants). When people differ at particular sites, they are said to have different alleles at those sites. There are two main types of polymorphisms: (1) those for which only two types of different alleles can be observed, called di-allelic polymorphisms; and (2) those for which multiple different alleles can be observed in the population, called multi-allelic polymorphisms. The chief examples of di-allelic polymorphisms are single nucleotide changes called SNPs (pronounced 'snips', or single nucleotide polymorphisms). An illustration of an SNP is when, at a particular site, a certain percentage (e.g., 60%) of the population will have a T nucleotide and the remaining percentage (e.g., 40%) will have a C nucleotide. The chief examples of multi-allelic polymorphisms are DNA variants involving multiple nucleotides, so-called STRPs (pronounced 'es-ti-ar-piz', or short tandem repeat polymorphisms). For this type of polymorphism, multiple alternative alleles exist in the general population in which each allele is characterized by a particular frequency. To establish what particular allele an individual carries at a particular polymorphic site, this individual's DNA needs to be genotyped or sequenced. Both genotyping and sequencing, among other techniques, are widely used in studies of the genetic bases of human disorders. If a person has the same alleles at a given site, this person is referred to as homozygous for that allele; if the alleles differ, the person is referred to as heterozygous.

DNA polymorphisms arise as a result of mutations. Mutations change a so-called wild (i.e., original) type of allele into a mutant type. Generally, mutations are subdivided into functional (i.e., resulting in some kind of a change) and nonfunctional (i.e., not leading to any registrable change) types. Functional mutations, in turn, can be advantageous (e.g., leading to particular advantages such as the human ability to speak) or detrimental. The focus of this article is on detrimental mutations that form the genetic bases for SGDs. Mutations are either newly acquired (i.e., happening in a given individual *de novo* or anew) or heritable. Yet, the presence of a mutation in an individual (i.e., the mutation is structurally present in the DNA sequence) does not guarantee this mutation will play a role in development because of internal, so-called epigenetic processes that regulate the function of the genome in a human being. Thus, genetic does not mean deterministic; it means probabilistic. Mutant genes might code for an abnormal protein; these abnormalities can be either structural (i.e., an abnormal protein will be synthesized) or functional (i.e., more or less of a particular protein than needed will be synthesized).

Genetics refers to studies of heredity (i.e., how genes are transmitted from generation to generation), whereas genomics refers to studies of the whole genome and how it functions as a system in an environment (i.e., how the inherited genes are expressed within a particular individual). Proteomics is the study of proteins and their functions. Collectively, all three disciplines contribute to understanding the genetic bases of human disorders in general and SGDs in particular.

Single-Gene Genetic Disorders

The Centers for Disease Control and Prevention (CDC) of the Department of Health and Human Services (DHHS) defines SGDs as a group of conditions caused by a deleterious change (mutation) in one specific gene. The CDC recognizes more than 6000 SGDs. Each specific SGD tends to be rare (i.e., its prevalence in the general population is typically <0.01–0.001%). Examples of very rare SGDs are severe hydroxylase deficiencies, inborn conditions caused by genetic alterations in the *CYP11B* gene on chromosome 8, which are characterized by dehydration, occasional vomiting, poor feeding, failure to gain weight, and intermittent fever. These deficiencies are seen in fewer than 200 000 individuals in the US (i.e., less than 0.001% of the population). The incidence of hyperphenylalaninemia, an inborn metabolic disorder (see below) is higher, affecting 1 in 15 000 newborns, with a wide range of prevalence in different populations around the world (e.g., 0.001% in the US, 0.003% in Ireland, and 0.0001% in Finland). When considered as a group, however, SGDs may be seen in 1 in 300 individual births. Thus, collectively, although rare individually, these conditions constitute a substantial number of pediatric illnesses.

SGDs can be subdivided into three types: (1) Mendelian disorders; (2) repeat expansion disorders; and (3) disorders involving epigenetic mechanisms. In the literature at large, SGDs are also referred to as monogenetic disorders; these terms can be used interchangeably.

Mendelian Single-Gene Disorders

A large number of SGDs conform, in their patterns of inheritance, to laws discovered by Gregor Mendel and are thus referred to as Mendelian. Mendelian SGDs are transmitted in families. These families are typically ascertained

through an individual with a disorder, who is referred to as a 'proband'. The family of a disordered individual is referred to as a nuclear family if it includes only first-degree relatives (i.e., parents and siblings) or extended family (or kindred) if it includes other types of relatives. Families are typically represented graphically by pedigrees; these representations use conventional symbols to illustrate males and females, disordered or nondisordered individuals, types of relationships among relatives, and probands.

There are five basic patterns of single-gene inheritance, two of which describe modes of transmission of mutant genes located on autosomal chromosomes 1–22 (autosomal dominant and recessive patterns of inheritance) and three of which describe modes of transmission of mutant genes located on sex chromosomes (two for X chromosome, X-linked dominant and X-linked recessive, and one for Y chromosome, Y-linked).

Under an autosomal-dominant pattern of inheritance, the disorder usually appears in every generation. In such families, every affected child has an affected parent and each child has a 50% chance of inheriting the disease from the affected parent and, if affected themselves, passing the mutant gene to their children. In this pattern of inheritance, only one copy of the mutant gene is needed for the manifestation of the disorder. It is important to mention that autosomal-dominant conditions are also characterized by incomplete penetrance (i.e., the probability of expressing a phenotype given a genotype); penetrance of autosomal dominant SGDs is low compared with other types of inheritance. Correspondingly, although only one mutated gene (either maternal or paternal) is required for the disorder, a substantially smaller proportion of the individuals compared with the carriers of the mutant allele will develop the disease. An example of a SGD transmitted in the autosomal dominant fashion is Marfan syndrome (MFS), a disorder of the connective tissue. This disorder was first described by French pediatrician Antoine Marfan in the late nineteenth century in a 5-year-old girl named Gabrielle. MFS is characterized by less than normal stiffness of tendons, ligaments, blood vessel walls, cartilage, heart valves, and many other structures supported by connective tissue because of abnormal biochemistry. Data from research studies indicate that the estimated prevalence of MFS is 1 in 5000 with no predilection for either sex. Although the penetrance of MFS is high, its degree of severity varies dramatically, so that the presentation ranges from few (if any) symptoms to life-threatening heart problems. The syndrome cannot be diagnosed by a single test and requires a sophisticated scoring system. Phenotypically, people with MFS present with disproportionately long limbs and fingers, a relatively tall stature, and predisposition to cardiovascular abnormalities. The chief mechanism for the development of MFS is a mutation in the gene *FBN1* (located on the long arm (q) of chromosome

15, 15q21.1) encoding the production of the protein fibrillin, one of the components of microfibrils, constituting connective tissue. Today, scientists have identified more than 600 different mutations associated with MFS. The overwhelming majority of these mutations ($\sim$75%) are familial, that is, transmitted in families, but there are also cases in which the syndrome is cased by *de-novo* mutations in *FBN1*. Also, $\sim$10% of individuals with MFS do not have any detectable mutations in *FBN1*; thus, it is possible that the syndrome can be caused by some other genetic mechanism, likely involving two other genes whose proteins interact with the protein encoded by *FBN1*, *TGFBR1*, and *TGFBR2*, which code for receptors of the transforming growth factor-beta (TGFβ). To manage MFS, doctors might encourage patients to restrict physical activity, reduce emotional stress, monitor cardiovascular functioning, and take possible preventive measures such as β-blocker medication for aortic protection and prophylactic surgery (e.g., replacement of the aortic root). Correspondingly, children diagnosed with MFS are recommended to avoid highly demanding isometric exercise and competitive or contact sports, but to remain active by engaging in specific aerobic exercise and eating healthy diets to prevent obesity.

For a disorder to be inherited in the autosomal recessive mode of inheritance, a person needs to have two copies of the mutated gene. Often a proband with a recessive disorder has unaffected parents, each of which has a copy of the mutant. If both parents are carriers (i.e., they have one copy of the mutated gene, but not the phenotype), they have a 25% chance of having a child affected by the disorder. This distinctive pedigree pattern, in which there are mutant genes for recessive disorders, is 'horizontal', meaning that the disorder is observed more often within a generation (i.e., within a sibship) than across generations (i.e., between parents and offspring). A well-known example of an autosomal recessive disorder is hyperphenylalaninemia (HPA), also referred to as phenylketonuria (PKU). The first systematic description of a case of HPA was done by Norwegian physician Ivar Følling in the 1930s. HPA is a genetic disorder of metabolism caused chiefly by the lack of or malfunctioning of the enzyme phenylalanine hydroxylase (PAH); this enzyme converts dietary phenylalanine, which is present in dairy products, into tyrosine. The production of the PAH enzyme is controlled by the gene *PAH*, situated on the long arm of chromosome 12 (12q23.2). Scientists have reported somewhere in the neighborhood of 450 mutations in the gene that vary in origin and create a range of severity in the manifestation of HPA. HPA presents an example of a disorder whose molecular basis is well understood and can be interfered with therapeutically to prevent associated mental retardation. In its untreated form, HPA can result in severe neurological and functional disability. Studies have shown that dietary restrictions aimed at

maintaining the plasma concentration of phenylalanine (and, consequently, the cerebral tissue) within safe limits of nontoxic concentration (120–360 mmol/L) have made remarkable improvements in the lives of people carrying two copies of the mutant gene. Although if diagnosed early (prenatally) and treated attentively for life, the presentation of mental retardation can be avoided, HPA has been associated with other outcomes, including structural and functional changes in the brain, abnormalities of visual function, and emotional and behavioral difficulties, which require professional attention.

If a mutant gene of which only one copy is required for manifestation of the disorder is located on X chromosome, the mode of transmission is referred to as X-linked dominant. In pedigrees with this pattern of inheritance, males are affected more often than females. The chance of transmitting the mutant allele also differs for men and women; because all sons of an affected male will receive his Y chromosome, all of them will be unaffected, and because all daughters of an affected male will received his mutant X chromosome, all daughters will be affected. In turn, because she has two X chromosomes, a woman with an X-linked dominant condition has only a 50% chance of transmitting her mutant X chromosome. Thus, half of her sons and half of her daughters, on average, are expected to be affected. As an example of this pattern of transmission, consider Aicardi syndrome, named for the French neurologist who systematically described the syndrome in the 1960s. This syndrome is lethal for males and thus is observed only in females. Its frequency is very low and is estimated at 300–500 cases worldwide. Phenotypically, this syndrome is characterized by the partial or complete absence of the corpus callosum, the structure that links the two hemispheres of the brain. The onset of the syndrome unfolds at the age of 3–5 months and presents through infantile spasms (a form of seizures), brain microcephaly and deviant structure, lesions of the retina of the eye, and mental retardation. There is a substantial amount of variation in the severity of the syndrome, both anatomically (i.e., the number and severity of abnormalities) and behaviorally (i.e., the extent of mental retardation). The genetic causes of Aicardi syndrome are unknown.

The X-linked recessive mode of transmission requires two copies of the mutant gene on X chromosome. Similar to the X-linked dominant mode, males are affected more often than females and risk of transmission is different for males and females. Because males have only one copy of X chromosome, they cannot transmit the disorder to their sons, but they can transmit the disorder to their daughters. Affected women will transmit the mutant X chromosome to all their children. In addition, women can be carriers of these disorders – even if they have no phenotypic manifestation, they have a 50% chance of transmitting the mutant X chromosome to their children. If this happens, all their sons will be affected and some of their daughters might be affected as well, provided they receive the second copy of the mutant chromosome from their fathers. An example of this type of disorder is muscular dystrophy of Duchenne type (MDD), named after the French neurologist Guillaume Duchenne, who first described a case of MDD. The estimated prevalence of MDD is 1 in 3500 male births. It is a disorder that presents with rapidly worsening muscle weakness and a loss of muscle mass (wasting) that starts in the lower limbs (legs and pelvis) and spreads to the whole body. MDD usually onsets before the age of 6 years and can manifest its first symptoms as early as infancy. By mid-childhood (age 10 years or so), walking might require braces, and by late childhood (age 12 years or so) confinement to a wheelchair might be necessary. MDD can also present through many other symptoms (e.g., breathing and bone disorders). The disorder is caused by mutant versions of the *DMD* gene (located in the short arm (p) of chromosome X, Xp21), which codes for the protein dystrophin, an essential cell membrane protein in muscle cells. A distinct feature of the *DMD* gene is that it is the largest and most complex known gene in the human genome. Studies show that this gene is characterized by large numbers of mutations, deletions, and duplications of genetic material. There is no known cure for MDD, but there is a significant ongoing effort to develop state-of-the-art pharmacological treatments as well as attempts at gene therapy.

Finally, the last type of Mendelian transmission is exemplified by Y-linked disorders caused by mutations on Y chromosome. Although Y chromosome is very small and home to relatively few genes (compared with other chromosomes), it is far from being the genetic 'badlands' it was once considered. Clearly, this type of inheritance is relevant to males only; females do not have Y chromosome and, thus, cannot transmit or manifest a disorder. Y-linked disorders are rare and there are few examples of them. One such example is a late-onset sensorineural deafness. In addition, Y chromosome contains a number of genes involved in spermatogenesis; mutations in these genes have been reported to lead to genetic disorders of infertility.

Repeat Expansions Single-Gene Disorders

The 24 500 genes and DNA between them form ~3 billion DNA bp. Of note is that a large portion of these bp are composed of recurring motifs of repetitive DNA (e.g., STRPs, see above; repetitive DNA sequences in specific parts of the human chromosomes, the telomeres and centromeres, and heterogeneous DNA regions). These recurring motifs can occur both within and outside genes. When inside genes, they can disrupt the function of these genes. These repetitive motifs are heritable and transmitted from generation to generation. They form another, non-Mendelian type of mechanism for SGD. Fragile X syndrome is an example of one such non-Mendelian SGD.

Fragile X syndrome is a genetic condition associated with a variety of developmental problems ranging from learning difficulties to mental retardation. The symptoms are variable and can include anxiety, hyperactive behavior (e.g., fidgeting and excessive physical movements), impulsivity, problems with social interactions and communication, and seizures. The syndrome's incidence is ~1 in 4000 boys and 1 in 8000 girls, with greater severity of symptoms in males. Many males also have characteristic physical features of fragile X syndrome that strengthen with age (long and narrow face, high-arched palate, high-pitched speech, large ears, prominent jaw and forehead, unusually flexible fingers, enlarged testicles). The heritable nature of the syndrome and its connection with sex was first noted in the 1940s, but the nature of the disorder was established only in the late 1970s. The syndrome is caused by mutation in the gene known as *FMR1* (located on the long arm of chromosome X, at Xq27.3), which codes for production of a protein called fragile X mental retardation 1, or FMRP. FMRP is ubiquitous in the human body and observed in higher amounts in the brain and testes; it is hypothesized that in the brain FMRP is involved in the regulation of synaptic plasticity by binding and transporting a number of essential neuronal RNAs. The *FMR1* gene has a region containing a repetitive motif composed of repeated sequences of three nucleotides, CGG. In most people, the number of repeats varies from a low of six to a high of 54 and the repeats appear are interrupted by a different three-base motif, AGG. In people with fragile X syndrome, the repeat is observed from 200 to more than 1000 times. The result of this expansion is that it results in the disruption of the $3'$ region ($3'$ UTR) of the gene, which inactivates its proper translation or silences it. This alteration, in turn, results in the disruption of production, so that FMRP protein is deficient, not sufficiently present, or absent. Malfunction, shortage, or loss of the FMRP protein is what leads to the development and manifestation of fragile X syndrome. If the repeat is observed 55 to 200 times, the situation is referred to as a permutation expansion. Carriers of such a variant of the *FMR1* gene do not demonstrate typical fragile X features or behaviors. However, they are at risk for the development of a disorder called fragile X associated tremor/ataxia (FXTAS). FXTAS is a progressive disorder of movement (ataxia), tremors, memory loss, reduced sensation in the lower extremities, and mental and behavioral changes. Women who carry 35–200 copies of the repeat are also at risk for premature ovarian failure, which can result in infertility. The repeat is inherited with an X-linked dominant pattern. However, inheriting the permutation does not necessarily lead to inheriting the disorder. What is characteristic of fragile X syndrome is that a mother who carries a permutation and does not present any symptoms of the syndrome might have a child with fragile X syndrome. This is possible because the permutation in the *FMR1* gene can expand to more than 200 CGG repeats in cells that develop into eggs. All the mothers of males with fragile X syndrome have been reported to be carriers, thus it is possible that new mutations are very rare or only occur in males. The permutation appears to be passing through the maternal germline, gradually expanding until a critical level has been reached and the expanded repeat has been inherited by the male child manifesting the syndrome.

Since the identification of the molecular mechanism of fragile X, scientists have associated various DNA repeated sequences with a number of disorders. In fact, today there are more than 40 neurological, common neurodegenerative, or neuromuscular disorders associated with DNA repeat (especially trinucleotide repeat) instability. The signature characteristic of these disorders is in the instability of the number of DNA repeated motifs, which might result in the expansion of the number of the repeats over a threshold that, in turn, might trigger molecular pathological effects leading to manifestation of a disorder.

Single-Gene Disorders Involving Epigenetic Mechanisms

The last category of SGDs briefly described in this article includes disorders involving so-called epigenetic mechanisms (i.e., mechanisms that produce genetic changes without changes in genotype). To illustrate this category of SGDs, consider Rett syndrome.

Rett syndrome is a postnatal developmental disorder presented in initially normally developing children through loss of acquired motor and language skills, slowed brain and head growth, gait abnormalities, and seizures. The disorder was initially described in the late 1960s by Austrian pediatrician Andres Rett. The syndrome occurs almost exclusively in women, with estimated prevalence of 1 in 10 000–15 000 newborns. The overwhelming majority (more than 99%) of cases of Rett syndrome appear to occur in individuals with no family background for the disorder, although the literature contains descriptions of a few families with more than one affected individual. Based on the patterns of genetic transmission in these families, it was incorrectly suggested that Rett syndrome demonstrated an X-linked dominant pattern of inheritance that caused prenatal lethality in males. Yet, the investigation of these families and sporadic cases of Rett syndrome led to the identification of the gene, located on the long arm of chromosome X (Xq28) and known as *MECP2*. This gene codes for a protein called methyl cytosine binding protein 2 (MeCP2), which regulates other genes through use of biochemical switches that can either silence or activate a gene (i.e., trigger or shut down production of specific proteins). Various mutations (more than 2000 known today) in *MECP2* explain ~95% of cases of classic Rett syndrome. Mutations in another gene located on chromosome X, *CDKL5* (Xp22.13), have also been reported to be associated

with phenotypes similar to that of Rett syndrome and usually referred to as atypical cases of Rett syndrome. Of interest is that proteins produced by *MECP2* and *CDKL5* have been shown to interact. The identification of both genes as the foundation of Rett syndrome has led to a series of investigations of molecular functions of these genes. There is now a substantial body of research indicating that MeCP2 epigenetically regulates genes that are involved in neuronal maturation. It appears that its regulation is not global, but specific, that is, targeted at certain genes. Among such targets of MeCP2 is, for example, the gene that encodes brain-derived neurotrophic factor (BDNF). Levels of BDNF were found to be differentially informative in postmortem studies of brains from patients with Rett syndrome. It is the targets regulated by MeCP2 that are thought to contribute to Rett syndrome pathogenesis. The disruption of regulation by MeCP2 might set off a chain of molecular events controlled by the proteins produced by gene-targets of MeCP2 that leads to the manifestation of Rett syndrome.

Single-Gene Disorders and Developmental Sciences

Several comments can be made.

The first set of comments pertains to the realization that rare SGDs are, actually, quite common when considered collectively. Specifically, although the general population risk for a newborn to have a SGD has been estimated at 1%, family history drastically changes risks for children of individuals from such families (for up to 25% for recessive and 50% for dominant conditions). Thus, conditions that can be very infrequent in the general population might be quite frequent in particular families. Correspondingly, knowledge of SGDs is very important for developmentalists working with families at higher risk for rare developmental disorders. Besides, as stated earlier, although each individual condition can be rare or very rare, collectively, SGDs form a large group of children with special needs. This group of children requires professionals working with them to have knowledge of their conditions and to use special developmental and pedagogical practices.

Second, understandably, families with a child with a SGD and practitioners who work with individuals with SGDs often ask what the future holds. The answer to this question varies, of course, depending on a particular SGD. However, the general thought here is related to the status of research linking genes and phenotypes (disorders). One of the fundamental realizations since the 1980s pertains to the rarity (if not absence) of absolutely deterministic outcomes involving the human genome. Whereas genetics typically leads to an identification of a particular gene controlling the manifestation of a particular disorder, genomics provides knowledge on how this gene interacts with other genes, which it might regulate or cowork with within a pathway or which can be regulated by it, and proteomics unravels complex patterns of associations between proteins produced by this gene. Consider the illustration from the studies of MFS. As indicated earlier, selected manifestations of MFS appear to be caused by mutations in *TGFBR1* and/or *TGFBR2*, the genes coding for receptors of the TGFβ. Mouse models of MFS have indicated the presence of increased TGFβ-signaling in aortic aneurysm; this rise in signaling can be prevented by TGFβ-antagonists [e.g., TGFβ-neutralizing antibody or an angiotensin II type 1 receptor (AT1) blocker]. For example, researchers have shown that the administration of losartan, an AT1 antagonist, to a mouse model of MFS prevents aortic aneurysm in this mouse. This basic work has direct implications for clinical outcomes, creating new hope of reversing cardiac symptomatology for MFS patients. Thus, the initial identification of the *FBN1* gene as the basis for the majority of cases of MFS (a genetics finding) leads to understanding the pathways in which this gene is involved and identification of other 'players' in this pathway (a genomics finding), which, in turn, leads to understanding proteins interactive within these pathways (a proteomics finding). And the hope is that all this knowledge can lead to clinical discoveries essential to remediation and treatment of both symptomatology and syndromatology of SGDs. Thus, the message communicated through research studies of SGDs is that the more the field understands about SGDs, the more it departs from the initial simplistic notion of deterministic deleterious mutations that initially dominated the field. Rapidly developing molecular medicine presents individuals with SGDs and their families with high levels of hope.

Third, as is evident from the discussion earlier, genetic heterogeneity of SGD is rather impressive. The presentation of genetic heterogeneity is twofold. First, although the majority of cases of a particular disorder are typically explained by a single gene, often there are other genes in the pathway in which the protein synthesized by the gene in question operates and the disorder might be caused by mutations in these other pathway-related genes (consider the example of MFS). Second, within a single gene there are often multiple mutations that can result in the manifestation of a disorder. Consider an example of cystic fibrosis (CF) – a recessive disorder of progressive damage to the respiratory and digestive systems. In the US, the incidence of CF is 1 in 3200 in Caucasian American newborns, 1 in 15 000 African American newborns, and 1 in 31 000 Asian American newborns, but the estimated carrier frequency is much higher across all groups. CF is caused by mutations in the *CFTR* gene (located on the long arm of chromosome 7 at 7q31.2) coding for a protein called the cystic fibrosis transmembrane conductance regulator, whose function is to form channels across the membranes of cells that produce mucus, sweat, saliva, tears, and digestive enzymes for the transport of charged particles in and out of such cells. These mutations either change the coding sequence or delete a small amount of DNA, thus altering the coding instruction for the CFTR protein. As a result, the production, structure, or stability of the membrane channels can be altered, preventing them from functioning properly and leading to symptoms of CF. As of today, more than 1000 mutations in the *CFTR* gene are known. Among these mutations, 23 are common and account for more than 90% of detectable mutations. In other words, heterogeneity of mutations is remarkable and this heterogeneity is associated with the presentation and severity of CF. Thus, it is important to consider a range of variability in ways the same disorder can be manifested in different children.

Fourth, frequencies of deleterious disorder-related mutations differ substantially in individuals from various ethnic backgrounds. For example, Tay-Sachs disease (TSD) is an autosomal-recessive disorder of lysosomal storage caused by a deficiency of hexosaminidase A and characterized by developmental delay followed by substantial worsening of conditions (paralysis, seizures, blindness) and subsequent death in early childhood; this disorder is caused by mutations in *HEXA* gene, situated on the long arm of chromosome 15, 15q24.1. The carrier frequency of TSD is 1 in 300, but it ranges substantially for different ethnic subgroups (e.g., 1 in 30 in the Ashkenazi Jewish population and 1 in 52–92 in individuals of Irish background).

These first four remarks lead to the fifth comment, which considers the issue of genetic screening for SGDs. As we rapidly expand our knowledge of how the human genome operates, we come across a number of ethically charged issues, one of which is genetic screening, which is characterized by both remarkable benefits and frightening downfalls. For example, as a result of prenatal screening of Ashkenazi Jews for TSD begun in the 1970s, today the incidence of TSD has decreased by more than 90% in this population. Obviously, this is a tremendous success on par with the success of immunization. Yet, there are examples of failed screening policies. At the same time TSD screening was launched, 12 US states and the District of Columbia instituted mandatory sickle cell screening programs for African Americans because of high rates of disease-related mutations in this population (in the general US population, 1 in 3700 Americans but 1 in 500 African Americans have some form of sickle-cell diseases). Today, 44 US states, the District of Columbia, Puerto Rico, and the US Virgin Islands test all newborns for sickle-cell anemia (sickle-cell disease is the generic name for a group of disorders affecting hemoglobin, red blood cell molecules delivering oxygen to body cells, with common features of anemia, repeated infections, and periodic episodes of pain. This is a recessive disorder caused by the *HBB* gene, located on the short arm of chromosome 11 (11p15.4); in the remaining six states the tests are available but not mandatory. The result was stigmatization of carriers, denial of health and life insurance and employment opportunities, and a variety of other limitations (e.g., denial of acceptance into the US Air Force Academy).

Although this happened 30 years ago, this history emphasizes the importance of public education, privacy protection policies, autonomy of any screening institution, and laws against discrimination based on genetic disorders. In addition to these issues, characteristics of SGDs raised in the earlier comments are directly linked to questions such as:

1. Who do we screen? Do we screen all fetuses or newborns or only those whose families have histories of SGDs?
2. Do we screen families and babies of all ethnic backgrounds or only of those backgrounds where frequencies of particular SGDs are elevated? Does that mean that there should be different, ethnicity-specific screening tools?
3. Given genetic heterogeneity of SGDs, do we screen only for the dominant gene or for all genes associated with particular SGDs? And how many mutations in each gene should screening include?
4. Finally, what are the purposes of genetic screening in the context of SGDs? These and many other questions are at the heart of discussions of SGDs.

The final remark pertains to the fact that the role of the environment in the development and manifestation of various SGDs has been neglected. Little is known about phenotypic variation in presentation of specific SGDs in patients with the same mutations living in different physical and cultural environments. Accumulation of data on the variability in manifestation of the same genetic syndrome (especially when attributed to the same mutations) in different environmental conditions may be of considerable importance for understanding the pathogenesis and prognosis of monogenetic disorders. And these environmental conditions should be defined broadly, ranging from climatic conditions, to cultural and religious practices, to specific dietary and leisure/stress-avoidance and remediation practices.

In summary, the term SGD might be misleading in that it is associated, at least superficially, with an image of a straightforward, deterministic chain linking 'the' mutation in 'the' gene to 'the' disorder. It turns out that there is a considerable amount of clinical variability in the disorder (often there are many disorders under a collective umbrella of a particular SGD). It also turns out that the disorder in question is characterized by a considerable amount of genetic heterogeneity, both from the point of view of what gene causes that disorder and what particular mutant allele within the gene is responsible for that disorder. In fact, if anything, the chain linking the human genome and disorders is not deterministic, but probabilistic. And this means that this chain can be broken by interventions, both biochemical (pharmaceutical) and environmental (developmental and pedagogical). Developmentalists just have to find ways of breaking these chains.

Acknowledgments

Preparation of this article was supported by Grants R21 TW006764 (PI: Grigorenko) from the Fogarty Program as administered by the National Institutes of Health, Department of Health and Human Services, and R01 DC007665 as administered by the National Institute of Deafness and Communication Disorders (PI: Grigorenko).

See also: ADHD: Genetic Influences; Endocrine System; Fragile X Syndrome; Genetic Disorders: Sex Linked.

Relevant Websites

http://www.cdc.gov – Centers for Disease Control and Prevention, Single Gene Disorders and Disability (SGDD).
http://ghr.nlm.nih.gov – Genetics Home Reference, Cystic fibrosis.
http://ghr.nlm.nih.gov – Genetics Home Reference, Sickle cell disease.
http://www.ornl.gov – Oak Ridge National Laboratory, Human Genome Project Information.

Immune System and Immunodeficiency

A Ahuja, National Jewish Hospital, Denver, CO, USA

Glossary

Adaptive immune system – Comprised of specialized T cells, B cells, and plasma cells that protect the host from infection in a highly specific manner; the immune response adapts antibody formation and cell-mediated immunity (CMI) to the specific antigen it encounters, and with subsequent attacks from the same antigen it is able to eliminate it more quickly and efficiently.

Anaphylaxis – A severe immediate allergic reaction to an antigen resulting in a constellation of symptoms including shortness of breath, wheezing, vomiting, diarrhea, urticaria, swelling, hypotension, and even death.

Antibody – A molecule produced by B lymphocytes and plasma cells in response to an antigen.

Antigen – Any substance that elicits an immune response.

Apoptosis – Also known as programmed cell death; a series of enzyme reactions that leads to cell death without disruption of the cell.

Cytokines – Proteins released by cells of the immune and hematopoietic systems that act as intercellular mediators of the immune response and inflammation.

Degranulation – Release of the contents of cytoplasmic granules.

Hematopoiesis – The generation and development of blood cells.

Hypoplasia – Incomplete or underdevelopment of an organ or tissue.

Immunoglobulins (Ig) – The classes (isotypes) of proteins secreted by plasma cells that contain antibodies; the five immunoglobulin isotypes are Igs G, A, M, D, and E.

Innate immune system – Comprised of cells and mechanisms that protect the host from infection in a nonspecific manner and without conferring specific immunologic memory.

Interleukins – A subgroup of approximately 30 cytokines, abbreviated IL.

Isotype – One of five types of immunoglobulins (Igs G, A, M, D, and E) that differ in structure and function.

Isotype switching – The process by which the cell switches from secreting one isotype of immunoglobulin to another.

Lymphadenitis – Infection of a lymph node.

Mannose – A sugar residue expressed on the surface of many microbes.

Microbes – Another term for microorganisms – bacteria, viruses, protozoa, mycoplasma, and chlamydia.

Opsonin – An antibody or complement component that coats an antigen and makes it more susceptible to phagocytosis.

Osteomyelitis – Infection of the bone.

Otitis media – Infection of the middle ear.

Passive immunity – Transfer of humoral immunity in the form of antibodies from one individual to another.

Pathogen – A microorganism that causes disease.

Phagocytosis – The act of engulfment of a microorganism by a phagocyte (neutrophil, monocyte, or macrophage), which normally results in microbial killing.

Phagosome – A membrane-bound vesicle in a phagocyte containing a microbe engulfed during phagocytosis.

Introduction

The immune system is the body's primary defense against infectious agents. The term immunity refers to protection from adverse events, such as infections and malignancies.

This system includes numerous cells, enzymes, and proteins that together function to maintain the integrity of the human body. However, if essential parts of the immune system become dysfunctional, increased susceptibility to infections and malignancies can result. Additionally, dysregulation of the immune system can lead to various autoimmune disorders such as systemic lupus erythematosus and rheumatoid arthritis, which will not be discussed in this article. The human immune system can be divided into two parts, the innate immune response and the adaptive immune response. The innate response is the first component of the immune system to respond to foreign pathogens. The second arm of human immunity is the adaptive immune response, which consists of humoral and cell-mediated immunity (CMI). These components work integrally in a sophisticated manner to optimize the host's defense against invasion of infectious agents such as bacteria, viruses, and fungi.

Development

The development of the human immune system begins during fetal gestation. Hematopoiesis (the generation and development of blood cells) appears in the yolk sac at 3 weeks, and by 6-weeks, gestation, these hematopoietic stem cells are detected in the fetal liver. During gestation weeks 8–12, the stem cells migrate to primary lymphoid organs, the bone marrow, and thymus. Secondary lymphoid organs (spleen, lymph nodes, tonsils, gastrointestinal lymphoid tissue) develop soon thereafter and serve as sites for further cell maturation and differentiation. Lymphoid stem cells differentiate into T, B, or natural killer (NK) cells. From the bone marrow, T cells migrate to the thymus where they undergo further maturation and gain characteristic cell markers. Once T cells mature, they can travel to secondary lymphoid organs, where they may perform their effector functions. B lymphocytes undergo their maturation and differentiation in the bone marrow. Once mature, B cells can differentiate into plasma cells, which secrete antibodies for use in the humoral immune response. NK cells develop from bone marrow precursors, just as B and T lymphocytes do, and can be found in the thymus, spleen, and lymph nodes.

Innate Immunity

The innate immune system is the first defense mechanism the body has against pathogens. This component of the immune system recognizes patterns and structures common to microbes but unlike those on host cells. Different types of microbes can share similar structures and constituents that are common to microbes and foreign to the host. Structures or components such as RNA or DNA sequences that are inherent to many pathogens can elicit an immune response. Cells of the innate system have receptors that recognize lipopolysaccharide (LPS), which is a component of the cell walls of Gram-negative bacteria (bacteria that do not retain crystal violet dye with standard Gram staining technique). The innate immune system relies on pattern recognition of pathogens through a limited repertoire of receptors. Because of this it has limited diversity and lacks specificity for microbial killing, unlike the adaptive immune system. However due to effective recognition of microbial specific patterns, the innate immune system is quite efficient at discriminating self (host) from foreign (microbial) molecules.

Components of the innate immune system include host physical barriers, effector cells, and certain proteins, particularly those of the complement system, which will be described (**Table 1**). Physical barriers include epithelial layers such as the skin, respiratory mucosal surfaces, and intestinal mucosal surfaces. These are the first line of defense against environmental pathogen entry. The epithelia also produce peptides, including defensins that have natural antibiotic function.

The effector cells of innate immunity function to combat pathogens that actually make it through the physical epithelial barriers. These cells are phagocytes (neutrophils, monocytes, and macrophages) and NK cells. All of these arise from hematopoietic stem cells in the bone marrow during fetal development. When a microbe evades the host's physical barriers and enters the body, it is recognized as being foreign and elicits an immune response. Monocytes, which mature into tissue macrophages, and neutrophils (together with lymphocytes, termed 'leukocytes') represent the initial influx of inflammatory cells. Their primary functions are to identify, phagocytose, and kill microbes.

Table 1   Major components of the immune system

Components	Innate immunity	Adaptive immunity
Physical and chemical barriers	Skin, mucosa antimicrobial chemicals	Ephithelial lymphocytes and antibodies
Blood proteins	Complement	Immunoglobulins (IgG, IgA, IgM, IgE, IgD) complement
Cells	Phagocytes (neutrophils, monocytes, macrophages), NK cells	T lymphocytes (helper and cytolytic), B lymphocytes

Neutrophils and macrophages have receptors for particular structures that are expressed only by microbes. These structures as well as substances released by microbes elicit an immune response. This includes a release of inflammatory proteins, known as cytokines at sites of infection. The cytokines attract phagocytes to sites of microbial invasion by increasing their adherence to the endothelium. Through a sophisticated mechanism, neutrophils roll along the endothelium encountering proteins that enhance adhesion and eventual migration to the site of infection. Once on site, neutrophils and macrophages are able to phagocytose the microbes that have been coated with opsonins (antibody and complement). During phagocytosis, the cells release numerous enzymes and reactive oxygen and nitrogen radicals that kill the ingested microbe.

Neutrophils are the first cells to respond to a microbe. They migrate to the site of an infection within a few hours and can remain viable for up to 12 h. Monocytes are immature forms of macrophages derived from a different lineage of stem cells in the bone marrow than neutrophils. These cells respond to infection almost as quickly as neutrophils, but are able to survive longer.

Macrophages have numerous functions other than phagocytosis and are an integral part of both the innate and adaptive immune systems. They release numerous cytokines that promote inflammation and activate other inflammatory cells to sites of infection in both types of immune responses. Macrophages have a distinct ability to facilitate tissue repair by removing debris and enhancing wound healing. Macrophages also assist in antibody formation and CMI, which will be discussed later in this article.

NK cells are a subset of lymphocytes found mostly in the blood and spleen. Their primary function is to kill host cells infected with viruses and intracellular bacteria. NK cells are normally in an inhibited state but can be activated and recruited to sites of infection by various cytokines released by other inflammatory cells such as activated macrophages and T and B lymphocytes. NK cells kill infected cells by degranulating and thereby releasing their enzyme products. These enzymes enter the infected cells and induce apoptosis. Another significant function of NK cells is to promote further macrophage activation. When macrophages become activated due to a microbial infection, they secrete the cytokine interleukin-12 (IL-12), which promotes activation of NK cells. Activated NK cells kill cells infected with viruses and intracellular bacteria and also secrete a cytokine known as interferon-gamma (IFN-γ), which further promotes macrophage killing of microbes.

Adaptive Immunity

The adaptive immune system is the second arm of the human immune response. Similar to the innate system, adaptive immunity is able to recognize the difference between foreign substances and host cells and so has the ability to not react against itself. However, some pathogens are able to evade killing mechanisms of the innate immune response and thus challenge the killing tactics of the adaptive system. Recall that the innate immune response lacks specificity and kills microbes based on pattern and structural recognition. The adaptive system is highly sophisticated in that its immune response is specific to individual antigens that characterize specific microbes. Because of this specificity, adaptive immunity is able to respond to a much larger variety of microbes and other molecules. This specific immunity can distinguish even very closely related pathogens. Also it has memory, thereby facilitating a heightened and more effective immune response when an antigen is encountered for a second time.

The two types of adaptive immune responses are humoral and CMI. Lymphocytes are the key cellular components and immunoglobulins (Igs) are the key humoral proteins of these systems. T and B lymphocytes are derived from lymphoid stem cells in the bone marrow. B lymphocytes undergo maturation and differentiation in the bone marrow and T lymphocytes mature in the thymus and migrate to peripheral organs. Both humoral and CMI mechanisms use these cells in an integrated fashion to fight infection. Cells and cytokines of the innate immune system are also used along with cells and proteins of the adaptive system for microbial killing.

Humoral Immunity

Humoral immunity is the main adaptive defense mechanism against extracellular microbes and toxins. The principal mediators of this function are the antibodies secreted by plasma cells. Once extracellular microbes or toxins are encountered by the host, B lymphocytes are stimulated to mature into plasma cells, which secrete antibodies that bind these antigens to neutralize or eliminate them.

B Lymphocytes

As noted earlier lymphocytes originate from stem cells in the bone marrow. B lymphocytes continue to mature in the bone marrow, whereas T lymphocytes migrate to the thymus for further maturation. As lymphocytes mature, they acquire specific cell-identifying markers. These cell-surface markers, known as cluster of differentiation (CD) markers, denote a particular cell lineage and/or particular stage of lymphocyte maturation. By using CD markers, a T or B lymphocyte can be identified and its stage of development can be elucidated. B lymphocytes begin as pre-B cells and progress through stages of immature, mature, and activated B lymphocytes, and finally antibody-secreting plasma cells. Most mature B cells express CD19 and CD20 cell markers. B cells will lack these markers if full B-cell maturation does not occur, which can be detected with laboratory testing.

Immunoglobulins

Plasma cells are able to secrete the Ig isotypes that contain antibody function. There are five isotypes IgG, IgA, IgM, IgE, and IgD. The basic structure of these molecules is similar; however, each can be stimulated to respond to distinct types of antigens. They can all function to kill microbes in conjunction with complement proteins and phagocytes, and to neutralize microbial toxins. They also have the ability to present antigens to T lymphocytes in order to facilitate microbial killing through other mechanisms that will be discussed later in this article.

The core structure of an antibody is made up of two heavy chains and two light chains of amino acids bonded together. Each Ig is made of a constant region and two variable regions (see **Figure 1**). The variable regions are on one end of the molecule and are comprised of heavy and light chains, and the constant region consists of two heavy chains on the other end of the molecule. The variable regions can bind a wide variety of antigens with tremendous specificity. The high specificity and variability of antigens that can be bound is partially due to sophisticated recombination of the amino acids of the variable regions. The different classes of antibodies are determined by the structural difference of their constant regions. The constant region (Fc) of the various Ig is recognized by a variety of circulating cells and proteins, for example, complement components.

IgG is the most abundant antibody in human serum followed by IgA, IgM, IgE, and IgD. It is the only Ig

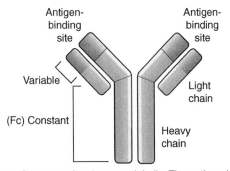

Figure 1 Structure of an immunoglobulin. The antigen-binding site is the site where the antigen binds to the molecule and is located on the variable region. There are two variable regions, each made up of a light chain and a heavy chain. The constant region (Fc portion) is made up of two heavy chains. The isotype and function of the immunoglobulin is determined by the constant region.

transferred from the mother to the baby via the placenta during fetal development. IgM and IgD are present on B cells during their later stages of maturation. The function of IgD is not well defined. IgM is the largest Ig and is the first to respond to foreign antigens during an immune response, followed by IgG. IgA is mostly present in mucosal surfaces such as those of the gastrointestinal and lung. It helps to eliminate pathogens from these sites. Also IgA is the only maternal antibody that can be passively transferred to the baby via breast milk. Secretion of IgE increases in response to antigens such as parasites and helminths. IgE is also the predominant antibody involved in the inflammatory process of severe allergic reactions such as anaphylaxis and to airways inflammation in asthma.

Plasma cells can produce different forms of antibodies based on the particular immune response. Antibodies can be made in membrane-bound and secreted forms. They also have the capability of isotype switching in response to antigen. The variable regions do not change, but to facilitate elimination of invading organisms, the constant regions switch to the appropriate isotype for the particular antigen encountered. For instance, the IgM isotype switches to the IgG isotype, which is more efficient and lives longer in the circulation. Also, the constant region of an IgG molecule may switch to that of an IgE antibody in response to a parasitic antigen.

Passive Immunity

Lymphocytes begin formation and maturation during fetal development, as discussed previously. Antibodies are not secreted into fetal circulation until the second trimester. The newborn immune system relies on maternal IgG antibodies passively transferred via the placenta and maternal IgA antibodies transferred via breast milk during the first few months of life. This constitutes passive immunity. Breastfeeding is commonly encouraged for this reason.

Memory

One of the hallmark features of the adaptive immune response is the ability to maintain memory. When a foreign antigen is encountered by the host, the appropriate antibody response occurs and works to eliminate the infection. This is the primary immune response, in which there is proliferation of B lymphocytes and antibodies specific for that antigen. After the infection subsides, a reservoir of memory antibody-producing cells migrates from peripheral lymphoid organs to the bone marrow, where they remain for months to years. When that same antigen or infection is encountered again, the long-lived memory cells are recruited from the bone marrow into the circulation and lymphoid organs where they secrete antibodies to eliminate the antigen quickly and effectively. This phenomenon of more rapid antibody response is known as the secondary immune response. This principle is behind the protective humoral immunity provided by vaccinations.

Complement System

The complement system is made up of several proteins that interact in a series of sequential steps leading to the killing of microbes. It plays a role in both innate and adaptive immune responses. The complement system consists of the classical, alternative, and lectin pathways. The central event in complement activation is the cleavage of the complement protein C3 which yields C3b, the active protein that binds the microbe or antibody. Each of these pathways is triggered by different stimuli; however, they all lead to a common killing mechanism, referred to as the membrane attack complex (MAC).

Microbes can activate the alternative pathway directly. The complement fragment C3b has the capability to bind to microbial surfaces, thereby initiating activation of this cascade. Through a series of steps, as shown in **Figure 2**, the C3 cleaving enzyme is generated, which splits C3 into two fragments. The major fragment, C3b, makes up part

of the C5 cleaving enzyme, which cleaves C5 and initiates the next steps leading to the formation of the MAC. C3b is an important protein fragment because not only does it help form the MAC for microbial killing, but it binds microbes and serves as an opsonin and also initiates the alternative complement cascade, as schematized in **Figure 2**.

The classical pathway requires an antibody that is bound to a microbial antigen for activation. IgM and IgG can activate C1q (a component of the complement protein C1), and thereby the rest of the complement system after binding microbial antigen. Antibody and C3b then opsonize the microorganism. Opsonization prepares the microbe for phagocytosis, leading to microbial killing. This is another way in which the innate and adaptive immune systems work together to eliminate foreign antigens from the host. Different complement proteins are needed for the classical pathway and the alternative pathway to generate the C3 and C5 cleaving enzymes, but the end result, formation of the MAC, is the same.

As described earlier, a common feature in the innate immune system is recognizing common molecular patterns on microbes to target for killing. This pattern recognition is used in the lectin pathway. Serving as the initiating step, a circulating plasma lectin, mannose-binding lectin (MBL), binds mannose residues on microbial cell walls. MBL acts as C1 does in the classical pathway, but the remaining steps are

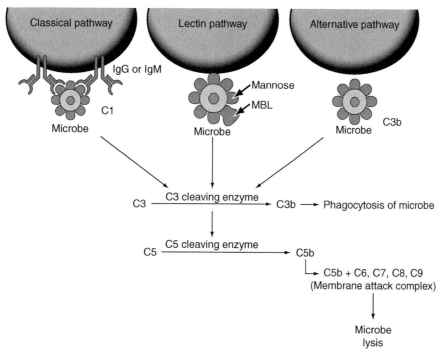

Figure 2   The complement cascade denoting the classical, lectin, and alternative pathways. The classical pathway is activated by a microbe bound to IgG or IgM, plus the complement protein C1. The alternative pathway is activated by a microbe coated with the C3b complement protein. Mannose-binding lectin (MBL) binds to a mannose residue on the microbe for initiation of the lectin pathway. After the initial activation of each pathway, they all commonly cleave C3 to generate C3b which promotes phagocytosis and killing of the microbe. C5 is also cleaved to generate C5b, which in conjunction with C6–9 forms the membrane attack complex (MAC) for microbial lysis.

identical to those in the classical pathway and lead to formation of the MAC.

The MAC complement proteins form a circular complex that kills the microbe by forming pores in the microbial cell membrane, thereby allowing water and salt ions into the cell. The water and salt ions cause cellular swelling and eventual rupture of erythrocytes and death by apoptosis in nucleated cells.

There are several regulatory proteins that help to control complement system activation. Regulation is needed to ensure that the system is active for the killing of microbes and not for normal host cells. If the complement system is not tightly regulated, it can become overly activated, which can cause unwarranted harm to host cells.

Cellular Immunity

The second branch of the adaptive immune system is CMI. This is the host's principal defense mechanism against intracellular microbes and viruses. T lymphocytes are the primary mediators of CMI. In CMI, T lymphocytes must contact specialized cells known as antigen-presenting cells (APCs), which present antigens to T cells for recognition and subsequent elimination (see **Figure 3**).

CMI can enhance the microbial killing mediated by innate and humoral immune responses in numerous ways. Recall that B cells undergo isotype switching from IgM to the more versatile IgG; however, T cells must release specific cytokines that mediate this switch. Isotype switching of humoral immunity would be impaired without the presence of T CMI. Some microbes may escape the innate killing mechanisms of phagocytes and survive in phagosomes. When this occurs T cells can release cytokines such as IFN-γ to enhance intraphagocytic killing and elimination of these intracellular microbes. Macrophages mediate many of the effector functions of CMI, and thus they serve

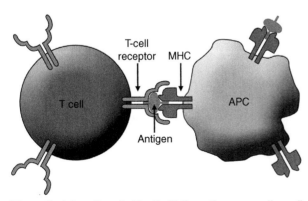

Figure 3   Interaction of a T cell with the antigen-presenting cell (APC)-antigen-major histocompatiblity complex (MHC) complex. An antigen must be bound to the MHC in order for an APC to present it to the T lymphocyte. The T-cell receptor then is able to bind the antigen that is presented by the APC.

as a continuous link between adaptive and innate immune responses.

Professional APCs are mainly macrophages, dendritic cells, and B lymphocytes. These cells first recognize and bind foreign antigens for presentation to T cells. Antigens on the APCs must also be bound to the major histocompatibility complex (MHC) in order for T cells to become fully activated (**Figure 3**). The MHC is a group of proteins encoded together on a gene locus that varies from individual to individual. The task of displaying the APC-associated antigen to T cells is the function of the MHC. MHC proteins can be divided into two groups, MHC class I molecules and MHC class II molecules.

T lymphocytes, like B lymphocytes, have cell surface (CD) markers that distinguish various T-cell subsets functionally. Mature T cells are CD3+ cells. Also, like B cells, T cells have the capability of memory. Memory T cells have different cell-surface protein markers that distinguish them from naive or unstimulated T lymphocytes. T lymphocytes that are not antigen stimulated are known as naïve T cells and are CD45RA+ cells. Memory T cells that develop after antigen stimulation are CD45RO+ cells. These memory cells, like B lymphocyte-derived memory cells, survive for up to years without the need for antigen exposure. Once T cells are activated after antigen recognition, they differentiate into either helper T cells or cytolytic T cells. Helper T cells are CD3+CD4+ and cytolytic T cells are CD3+CD8+. There is a 2:1 ratio of helper T cells to cytolytic T cells in circulation under normal circumstances. APCs that display antigens bound to MHC class I molecules preferentially bind to CD4+ T helper cells. MHC class II molecules preferentially bind CD8+ cytolytic T cells.

CD4+ T helper cells have different effector functions from cytolytic CD8+ cells. Through the release of various cytokines, helper T cells can have numerous effector functions such as to activate macrophages; enhance T and B lymphocyte proliferation; stimulate cytolytic T-cell differentiation; and upregulate release of inflammatory mediators, such as ILs. CD4+ T helper cells can be divided into the two subsets Th1 and Th2. Each of these releases different cytokines that mediate functions specific for that subset. The cytokines from one subset can inhibit functional responses from the other subset.

Whether the immune response gravitates toward the Th1 response vs. the Th2 response depends on the type of stimuli or antigen encountered. Bacteria and viruses that involve innate immune components such as macrophages and NK cells cause stimulation of the Th1 pathway of inflammation and microbial killing. Antigens, such as parasites, that do not significantly challenge innate immunity or macrophages stimulate the Th2 pathway. This is the inflammatory pathway that predominates in allergic disorders. Cytokines released from the Th2 pathway upregulate production of IgE and numbers of circulating eosinophils, which can contribute to IgE-mediated disorders such as asthma, atopic dermatitis, food allergy, allergic rhinitis, and anaphylaxis.

Cytolytic T cells become activated after recognition and binding of intracellular microbes or viruses. Cytolytic killing can occur through release of enzymes and other proteins that enter and kill the infected cell. A second mode of killing is through induction of apoptosis of the infected cells.

Immunodeficiency Diseases

The human immune system consists of several sophisticated and complex mechanisms to fight infection. Dysfunction or deficiency of any of various proteins or cells among these defense mechanisms can lead to an increased susceptibility to recurrent or severe infections. It is estimated that approximately 1 in 500 individuals in the US have some type of defect in their immune system. There are numerous immunodeficiency syndromes that have been described as a result of these defects. When there is a genetic abnormality of the immune system leading to disease, the condition is termed a 'primary or genetic immunodeficiency'. When an immunodeficiency develops as a consequence of an underlying condition such as cancer, drugs, or infection, the immunodeficiency is said to be 'secondary or acquired'. The immune system can also lose the ability to distinguish self from nonself so that immune cells attack the host, leading to autoimmune diseases such as thyroiditis, lupus, or juvenile diabetes. Individuals with an immunodeficiency have a greater tendency to develop autoimmune diseases as well as frequent infections.

Cells or proteins of the innate immune system or those of the adaptive immune system may be adversely affected and lead to an immune disorder in which the individual becomes more susceptible to recurrent infections. Infections may be very invasive leading to severe symptoms, and at times death. Depending on the nature of the defect, the types of infections and the organisms causing them can be predicted.

In innate immunity, interruption of physical barriers or phagocyte dysfunction can lead to recurrent bacterial infections. A deficiency of a type of phagocyte or a defect in the steps required to perform phagocytosis and microbial killing can lead to recurrent infections with bacteria such as *Staphylococcus* species, enteric bacteria such as *Escherichia coli*, and other pyogenic organisms, which refers to bacteria that make pus or form abscesses. These infections commonly occur in the respiratory tract or on the skin.

Essential complement protein deficiencies are rare. Since the complement system acts as a cascade of reactions, one reaction leading to the next, one protein or enzyme deficiency can affect the development of others downstream in the cascade. Proteins such as C3 are needed for opsonization and phagocytosis; and a deficiency of this component can result in serious infections with pyogenic bacteria. Deficiencies of components of the MAC can result in recurrent infections with *Neisseria* bacteria, such as meningitis due to *Neisseria meningitides* or infection with *N. gonorrheae* at multiple body sites.

In humoral immunity deficiencies there can be B lymphocyte abnormalities or defects in the antibodies they generate. This can result in recurrent bacterial infections of varying severity. Also since IgG or IgM are needed for activation of the classical complement cascade, oposonization and phagocytosis can also be impaired due to Ig defects.

Those that suffer from T-cell, or CMI, dysfunction will often have an increased susceptibility to viral, intracellular microbial, and fungal infections. T-cell function plays a vital and integral role in humoral and innate immunity. For instance, recall that macrophages are activated by proteins (cytokines) released by T cells, which increases macrophage phagocytic killing and antigen presentation. Also isotype switching of Igs require T-cell function. Those unfortunate individuals who have combined humoral and cell-mediated immunodeficiencies are prone to suffering from all types of infections including invasive bacterial, viral, and fungal infections.

The following section will discuss examples of primary immunodeficiencies that should be recognized by healthcare providers despite their rare occurrence. Additionally, HIV-AIDS, the most common acquired immunodeficiency, will be briefly discussed.

Immunodeficiencies of the Innate Immune System

Chronic granulomatous disease (CGD) is an immunodeficiency syndrome resulting from a defect in the phagocyte oxidase enzyme system necessary for killing of ingested bacteria and fungi by neutrophils and macrophages. Without this enzyme phagocytes do not generate the reactive oxygen intermediates that kill microbes. This rare disorder has an incidence of 1 per 200 000 individuals. Clinical presentation can occur as early as the newborn period and as late as young adulthood. Patients suffering from this disease are plagued with recurrent bacterial and fungal infections. The most common infections are pneumonia, skin abscesses, lymphadenitis, and osteomyelitis. Bacteria that do not produce hydrogen peroxide such as *Staphylococcus aureus*, intestinal bacteria and fungi are the most common pathogens. Defective phagocyte production of microbicidal oxidants can be detected through laboratory testing. These patients are best treated aggressively with antibiotic and antifungal therapies aimed at cultured organisms and with surgical drainage of abscesses. Patients are placed on antibiotics prophylactically to help prevent bacterial infections.

An immunomodulating agent, IFN-γ, is a more recent treatment option shown to enhance other phagocytic enzymes and therefore microbial killing. The only cure for CGD to date is bone marrow transplantation.

Leukocyte adhesion defect (LAD) is characterized by an inability of neutrophils and monocytes to adhere normally to blood vessels around the site of an infection. Defective cells do not express certain outer membrane proteins termed integrins that allow leukocytes to adhere to endothelial cells. Since the leukocytes are not able to adhere to the vessel wall, they cannot penetrate the endothelial lining to enter the underlying area of infection. This defect also inhibits phagocytosis of complement-opsonized organisms.

The incidence of the major form of LAD is approximately 1 in 1 000 000. Patients suffer recurrent bacterial and fungal infections, as well as impaired wound healing. The defect varies in severity. Children with severe defects present early in life with recurrent bacterial infections, including skin infections, skin ulcers, and gingivitis. Infants can present with delayed separation of the umbilical cord (beyond 3 weeks after birth). Infections are present without signs of pus since pus formation requires leukocyte adhesion and migration to sites of inflammation. Clinical laboratories can test for the presence of the integrin proteins. Bone marrow transplantation is the best treatment option for severe LAD. Other treatment modalities include prophylactic antibiotics and supportive care such as aggressive treatment of infections with appropriate antibiotic therapy.

Immunodeficiency of the Humoral Immune System

Hypogammaglobulinemia is a condition in which one or more of the different Ig isotypes is very low or absent. The most common of these Ig deficiencies is 'selective' IgA deficiency, with an incidence of approximately 1 in 700 Caucasian individuals. Patients with this condition may actually be asymptomatic, but others will have an increased incidence of bacterial infections such as otitis media, chronic bronchitis, and sinusitis. Laboratory values will show absent or very low IgA levels in the serum. There is no treatment for IgA deficiency other than prevention and aggressive treatment of the bacterial infections.

Bruton's agammaglobulinemia, or X-linked agammaglobulinemia (XLA) is a disorder characterized by very low or no Igs of all isotypes. This condition affects males with an incidence of 1 in 100 000–200 000 individuals. The defective protein, Bruton's tyrosine kinase (Btk), is essential for mediating early B-cell maturation. Individuals have low or no B cells in their circulation or lymphoid organs and are antibody deficient, so that they have an increased susceptibility to severe bacterial infections, such as abscesses,

pneumonia, and meningitis. Most patients with XLA present during their first year of life with invasive bacterial infections. However, some may have milder symptoms and may not be diagnosed until later in childhood. Genetic testing for the *Btk* gene is available for diagnosis. Ig levels as well as the B-cell markers CD19+ and/or CD20+ will be low or absent. There is no cure for this disease, but treatment with monthly intravenous infusions of gamma globulin (IVIG) minimizes symptoms and allows patients to live a near normal life. Some patients may also need maintenance prophylactic antibiotics.

All infants are relatively hypogammaglobulinemic and rely during their first 6 months of life on IgG antibodies transferred from the mother during pregnancy. However, in transient hypogammaglobulinemia of infancy, patients have low levels of Igs that extend beyond 6 months of age. These patients may have an increased susceptibility to bacterial infections while their antibody levels are low. Their antibody response to vaccines will be normal, although their circulating Ig levels will be low. Patients suspected to have transient hypogammaglobulinemia of infancy should be monitored closely and have regular testing of Ig levels. This developmental delay in Ig synthesis is transient and usually resolves by 2 years of age. Intravenous gamma globulin is sometimes needed for these patients.

Hyper-IgM syndrome is a rare disorder which can be caused by several genetic defects. Males are most commonly affected, but females can be affected as well. Both IgM and IgD are expressed on the cell surface of B cells during maturation. The IgM isotype must undergo isotype switching to other Ig classes. When there is a defect in the genes involved in isotype switching or if T CMI is impaired, isotype switching may not occur normally, and super-normal synthesis of IgM can develop. Individuals with this condition suffer from recurrent bacterial infections and invasive, opportunistic infections such as *Pneumocystis carinii* pneumonia. Patients will often present during childhood. Upon testing, IgM levels will be high, but IgG and IgA levels will be low. There is no cure for this disease, but treatment is similar to that for hypogammaglobulinemia, and monthly IVIG infusions are protective.

Common variable immunodeficiency (CVID) refers to a group of immunodeficiency disorders with common features but with variable presentations and severity. Patients may present during infancy, although presentation is usually later in life in the form of recurrent infections. These individuals also have an increased susceptibility to autoimmune disorders and malignancies. Patients often suffer more from symptoms resulting from these autoimmune disorders and malignancies than from the CVID. Ig levels are low and there is decreased antibody responsiveness to vaccines or infection. B cells and CMI may be normal or decreased. Treatment for these patients involves monthly IVIG as well as aggressive treatment of secondary disorders that may be present.

Disorders of Cell-Mediated Immunity

A malformation in fetal life leading to defective development of the thymus can adversely affect T-cell maturation. Thymic hypoplasia is a hallmark feature of DiGeorge syndrome, along with other anatomical abnormalities, including cardiac anomalies and unusual facies. Parathyroid glands are usually also hypoplastic, and patients may present with symptoms related to decreased circulating calcium levels. Most patients present early during infancy. DiGeorge syndrome is the result of a deletion of the genes on the 22q11 chromosome. Because T cells are not able to mature in the thymus, they lack cell-mediated defense mechanisms. Also some humoral and innate responses that rely on T lymphocyte help are impaired. Patients are susceptible to intracellular microbial and opportunistic infections. Genetic testing for the chromosomal deletion is available. Total T lymphocytes and CD4+ and CD8+ T-cell subsets may be low, and T-cell function may be impaired. Many patients with DiGeorge syndrome have small amounts of thymic tissue which may be enough to maintain at least partial T-cell maturation and activation. These patients may have normal T-cell function in laboratory tests and no significant immunodeficiency. However, they should undergo regular testing of T-cell numbers and function and review of infection history during the first few years of life to be certain that they are not predisposed to serious infections.

Combined Immunodeficiencies

Severe combined immunodeficiency (SCID) refers to disorders of humoral and CMI responses because of underlying T-cell and B-cell abnormalities. SCID can be caused by a variety of gene defects. The resulting clinical disorder, however, is relatively the same, with an increased incidence of recurrent bacterial, viral, and fungal infections. Because of the severe immunodeficiencies that are typical in SCID patients, they present early in life, usually with recurrent invasive infections. T- and B-cell function and levels are usually low. Diagnostic genetic testing for particular mutations is available. Treatment includes monthly infusions of IVIG. Depending on the etiology, enzyme replacement therapy may be warranted as well. Bone marrow transplantation can be curative, with the best prognosis being transplantation with a related matched donor.

AIDS

As opposed to the immunodeficiencies that result from a primary defect in the immune system, AIDS is the most common of all immunodeficiencies. AIDS is caused by infection of HIV. This epidemic has infected millions of people across the world and has caused millions of deaths of adults and children. The disease may be contracted through infected bodily secretions such as semen or vaginal fluid or via intravenous routes such as with transfusions or infected drug needles. Helper CD4+ T cells are the main cells targeted by HIV. Numerous other cells such as macrophages and dendritic cells are affected as well.

When the HIV viral load increases and the CD4+ T cells decrease, AIDS develops. Patients with AIDS suffer from invasive opportunistic infections, severe immunosuppression, malignancies, and central nervous system degeneration. Research in this field has made remarkable strides in treatment for this deadly disease. While there is no cure for the disease currently, patients with HIV can now live over 20 years without the development of AIDS because of antiviral therapy.

HIV-AIDS is a devastating disease for the patients and their families. All racial and socioeconomic groups are affected worldwide. Although HIV was once considered to infect mainly homosexual males, the incidence of HIV is highest in the heterosexual population. Unprotected sexual intercourse with someone who has the virus is the leading means of transmission. In the US, one of the fastest rising prevalence of HIV is among heterosexual African-American females. Children born to mothers with HIV require early identification and intervention. Transmission of HIV to the fetus can be prevented by early detection and treatment of HIV infection in the pregnant woman.

Conclusion

Certain immunodeficiencies are X-linked and occur only in males, but most immunodeficiencies can affect all races and both genders in all socioeconomic groups. These diseases are not only physically strenuous, but also emotionally and mentally challenging for the patients and their families. Treatment should be focused on these aspects as well. In addition to physicians and nurses taking care of the recurrent infections, particular attention should be addressed to other facets of the illness and its impact on the patients and their families.

Commonly, a multispecialty approach is beneficial to the well-being of these individuals and the family unit. Nutritionists can concentrate on helping the patient avoid malnutrition. Psychologists, psychiatrists, counselors, and social workers can play vital roles in treating depression, anxiety, and daily stress on quality of life. Social workers can identify available resources to address various economic and financial stressors. Child life specialists can be particularly a great source of support for children with these diseases. Finally, because of the genetic basis of the immunodeficiencies, genetic counseling can be important for family planning.

See also: AIDS and HIV; Allergies; Asthma.

Suggested Readings

Abbas AK and Lichtman AH (2005) *Cellular and Molecular Immunology,* 5th edn. Philadelphia: Elsevier Saunders.

Behrman R, Kliegman R, and Jenson H (2000) *Nelson Textbook of Pediatrics,* 16th edn. Philadelphia: W.B. Saunders Company.

Leung D, Sampson HA, Geha RS, and Szefler SJ (2003) *Pediatric Allergy Principles and Practice.* St. Louis: Mosby.

Rich R, Fleisher TA, Shearer WT, Kotzin BL, and Schroder HW (2001) *Clinical Immunology Principles and Practice,* 2nd edn. Philadelphia: Mosby.

Stiehm R, Ochs H, and Winkelstein J (2004) *Immunologic Disorders in Infants and Children,* 5th edn. Philadelphia: Elsevier Saunders.

Relevant Website

http://www.primaryimmune.org – Immune Deficiency Foundation. The National Organization dedicated to research, education and advocacy for the primary immune deficiency diseases.

Intellectual Disabilities

D J Fidler and J S Jameson, Colorado State University, Fort Collins, CO, USA

Glossary

Adaptive behavior – The ability of an individual to perform behaviors that evidence age-appropriate and culturally appropriate levels of personal independence and social responsibility.

Behavioral phenotype – The observable expression of behavioral traits; in this case a profile of behaviors associated with a specific genetic disorder.

Diagnostic overshadowing – The tendency of a clinician to attribute co-morbid psychiatric symptoms to the presence of mental retardation/intellectual disability or a syndrome associated with mental retardation/ intellectual disability.

Dual diagnosis – The diagnosis of comorbid psychiatric disorders in addition to intellectual disability.

Early intervention – A comprehensive set of services that are provided to children from birth to age three and their families to enhance a child's developmental potential.

Familial mental retardation – According to Zigler, mental retardation that results from the interaction between inherited and environmental factors, leading to a designation.

Indirect effects – The impact that behavioral characteristics associated with specific genetic disorders impact family members, educators, and other members of the community.

Individualized education plan – A plan that describes the educational program that has been designed to meet the unique needs of a child receiving US special education services (ages 3–18 years); it outlines the needs, goals, strategies, and methods of assessment that will guide instruction and intervention strategies.

Individualized family service plan – In the US, contains information about the services necessary to facilitate a child's development (ages 0–3 years) and enhance the family's capacity to facilitate the child's development; family members and service providers work as a team to plan, implement, and evaluate services tailored to the family's unique concerns, priorities, and resources.

Mental retardation/intellectual disability – According to the 2002 definition from the American Association of Mental Retardation, "a disability characterized by significant limitations both in intellectual functioning and in adaptive behavior as expressed in conceptual, social, and practical adaptive skills" that originates before the age of 18 years.

Organic mental retardation – According to Zigler, mental retardation that results from a biological insult on the genetic, neurodevelopmental, or pre/perinatal level.

Special education – Specially designed educational instruction, including supplementary aids and related services that allow a child with a disability to benefit meaningfully from his or her educational program.

Undifferentiated mental retardation – According to Zigler, mental retardation that cannot be reliably attributed to either organic or familial causes.

Introduction

According to the most current definition put forth in 2002 by the American Association on Mental Retardation (AAMR), the term mental retardation refers to "a disability characterized by significant limitations both in intellectual functioning and in adaptive behavior as expressed in conceptual, social, and practical adaptive skills." To highlight the developmental nature of mental retardation, this definition specified that cognitive limitations and adaptive behavior deficits must originate before the age of 18 years. The AAMR also stipulated that there are additional assumptions that should be made when applying the current definition of intellectual disability/mental retardation. First, functioning difficulties must be understood within the context of the community and environments that are appropriate for an individual's chronological age and cultural background. Second, appropriate assessment techniques that lead to a diagnosis of mental retardation must take both cultural/linguistic background and issues related to motor, sensory, and communicative functioning into account. The third assumption relates to the recognition that challenges in functioning often occur simultaneously with areas of strength in functioning. Fourth, one of the main purposes of identifying an individual's challenges relates to developing a profile of supports to address the individual's needs. And the final assumption of the AAMR definition relates to the idea that well-planned support systems implemented over time should lead to improvement in the functioning of the individual with intellectual disability/mental retardation.

While this definition of the construct 'mental retardation' is widely used in clinical and educational settings, it is the product of many decades of change. The most recent changes relate to the use of the term 'mental retardation' itself, which has increasingly fallen out of favor in both the advocacy and practice communities. In 2006, the majority of members of the AAMR voted to change the name of their organization to the American Association on Intellectual and Developmental Disabilities. This is the culmination of a larger movement worldwide to discontinue the use of the term mental retardation, in favor of terms such as intellectual disability, cognitive disabilities, and the more global term developmental disabilities. Thus, while the term mental retardation is still currently used in clinical and some educational settings, the term is becoming increasingly obsolete as organizations formally adopt other, more socially acceptable, terms. For the purposes of this article, the term mental retardation will be used to discuss any historic issues involving the definition of the phenomenon, but the term intellectual disability will be used for all current issues and topics. In addition, to illustrate the complex nature of this construct, in the following sections we will focus on the history of mental retardation/intellectual disability in the US, though additional cross-national information will be included in the discussion of service delivery.

Definition and Categorization

Definition History

In addition to changes in terminology, throughout much of the twentieth century, the behavioral sciences have struggled to operationalize a definition of mental retardation that defines accurately and humanely the specific characteristics that are common among individuals in this category. The many changes in terminology and the definition of mental retardation/intellectual disability reflect a century-long history of challenge regarding the science and study of individuals with impaired or delayed cognitive development. These struggles have led to many definitions, technical terms, and clinical criteria that often changed in accordance with broader political and societal movements. Regardless of the variations, the definition of mental retardation has had importance beyond the scientific community as throughout much of its recent history, the definition has had a direct impact on eligibility for services from government agencies.

The earliest definitions of mental retardation focused mainly on intellectual functioning exclusively, with the use of IQ tests serving as the main diagnostic criterion. In the 1920s, the AAMR introduced a classification scheme that categorized individuals according to the severity of their impairments, dividing the IQ ranges by 25 point ranges, with the cut-off IQ score for mental retardation designated at 75. With the introduction of the first edition of the Diagnostic and Statistical Manual in the 1950s, the term mental deficiency was introduced by the American Psychiatric Association (APA), with severity of impairment denoted by the terms mild deficiency (IQ range 70–85), moderate deficiency (IQ range 50–69), and severe deficiency (IQ of 49 and below). In one of the many controversial turns in the definition's history, this competing definition put forth by the APA designated the cut-off for mental deficiency at 10 IQ points higher than the earlier AAMR definition. This is the first of several differences between the APA and AAMR definitions to come in the latter part of the twentieth century. While these early definitions focused exclusively on intellectual functioning and IQ scores, during the first half of the twentieth century various opinions were expressed that IQ-only definitions were insufficient to characterize the true nature of mental retardation. By the 1930s and 1940s, the discussion of the definition of mental retardation widened to include competence in one's own environment. This led to an updated AAMR definition in the 1960s, that included impairments in a construct titled 'adaptive behavior', in addition to subaverage intellectual functioning that originates in the developmental period. This 1960s definition also raised the IQ score cut-off to 85, in line with the APA definition at the time, and established five categories of severity of impairment: borderline, mild, moderate, severe, and profound mental retardation.

Those who have analyzed the history of the definition of mental retardation often note that this change mirrored the 1960s movement to be more inclusive in providing services to individuals in need. However, it is also noted that changes in the IQ cut-off raised the number of individuals who met at least the borderline definition of mental retardation to 16% of the general population, with concerns raised that there was an over-representation of minorities included in this range.

In addition, the introduction of the adaptive-behavior aspect of the definition proved controversial, with difficulties relating to reliability of assessments of this dimension, and the practicality of its use in actual diagnostic situations. The 1970s definition of mental retardation put forth by the AAMR made some minor changes in wording, specifying that subaverage general intellectual functioning must be 'significant', and that it must 'exist concurrently' with adaptive-behavior deficits. But one change had a strong impact, as the IQ cut-off was lowered to 70, lowering the percentage of individuals meeting the criteria to roughly 2% of the general population. Minor wording changes were also made to the AAMR definition in the 1980s, with specifications that the onset of mental retardation should occur before the age of 18, rather than the more general wording regarding manifestation during the developmental period as mentioned earlier. Perhaps the most controversial changes to the AAMR definition of mental retardation were introduced in the 1990s. Substantial changes were made to the AAMR definition of mental retardation, with specification that an individual must show impairment in two of 10 specific adaptive behavior skill areas. In addition, another major change related to the categorization scheme, that shifted from an IQ-based 'severity of impairment' approach to categorization of 'intensities of needed supports' (intermittent, limited, extensive, and pervasive), though the use of this system was challenged by the lack of readily available instruments for measuring these levels of need. Finally, this definition imprecisely identified the IQ cut-off as '70 to 75 or below', leaving the range of individuals meeting the criteria ranging from 2% to 5% of the general population. These changes proved to be so controversial that many organizations and agencies rejected the categorization scheme, and some voiced the need to develop their own definition for mental retardation. Others, like the APA, opted to adopt the new categorization scheme, but maintained clarity regarding an IQ cut-off with their prior designation of 70 (rather than 70–75). The 2002 definition of mental retardation, however, has reverted back to a severity of impairment categorization scheme and more general notions of adaptive behavior.

Adaptive Behavior

The term adaptive behavior refers to the ability of an individual to perform behaviors that evidence age-appropriate and culturally appropriate levels of personal independence and social responsibility. The inclusion of the adaptive behavior construct in the formal definition of mental retardation in the latter half of the twentieth century reflected awareness that intellectual functioning was not the sole predictor of one's ability to function in society. In addition, the inclusion of this construct was meant to encourage clinicians and educators to focus on remediation of disabilities, rather than simply categorizing children according to specific groups.

Adaptive behavior assessment became an important means of identifying behaviors that facilitated deinstitutionalization in the 1960s and brought about an increased awareness of the need for rehabilitation for individuals with disabilities in their communities. With the shift in focus from treatment and service delivery in the 1960s to normalization and legal rights in the 1970s, legislation was passed in some states that designated adaptive behavior assessment as a crucial measure of functioning. This reflected a concern that without adaptive behavior assessment and consideration of performance outside of academic contexts, there would be an over-representation of minorities in special education settings. By the 1980s, adaptive behavior assessment was seen as foundational for developing instructional approaches that would prepare individuals for living in their communities. The 1980s also brought about increased research attention into the construct of adaptive behavior in individuals with intellectual disability, leading to some specific criticism of the construct from researchers' perspectives. Some researchers argued that problematic aspects of the adaptive behavior construct – including lack of cohesive factor structure, lack of consensus regarding the best method for assessment, differing opinions regarding the relationship between intelligence and adaptive functioning – limited its utility.

Over the last few decades, the notion of adaptive behavior shifted from a broad concept to a more specific delineation of competence in specific areas. In the 1992 definition of mental retardation, adaptive behavior was redefined as adaptive skills comprising the following areas: communication, self-care, home living, social skills, community use, self-direction, health and safety, functional academics, leisure, and work. While these skill areas were thought to be related to the need for supports, and thus improved the characterization of individuals with mental retardation, these changes did not silent the debate regarding the utility of the adaptive behavior construct. Among the main criticisms of the construct was the argument that, practically speaking, most clinicians did not use the construct when making a diagnosis. The 2002 definition of mental retardation has reverted back to the term adaptive behavior (instead delineating adaptive skill areas), with a renewed focus on adaptation in conceptual, social, and practical areas; however, the debate over the use of the construct in clinical and educational settings continues.

Two-Group Approach

Amidst these definitional issues, an additional view for categorizing individuals with mental retardation became prominent in the latter half of the twentieth century. This new categorization approach arose when researchers began to note that there are more cases of children with IQ scores lower than 50 than would be expected, based on a normal statistical distribution. Various theorists began to speculate that there were various pathways leading to mental retardation, culminating in Edward Zigler's argument that there are two distinct groups of individuals with mental retardation. The first pathway is through the interaction between inherited and environmental factors, leading to a designation of familial or cultural mental retardation. The second pathway is through a biological insult that could happen on the genetic, neurodevelopmental, or pre/perinatal level, leading to a designation of organic mental retardation. Zigler argued that the distinction between familial and organic mental retardation is so important that it should be included alongside intellectual functioning for the classification of individuals with mental retardation. Included in this scheme was also a group of individuals with 'undifferentiated' mental retardation, for whom a reliable assignment to a group was not possible. This undifferentiated group has historically received very little research attention, and thus, Zigler's approach has been called the 'two-group' approach for its primary distinction between mental retardation due to organic versus nonorganic causes.

Within this two-group approach to categorization, additional designations were made by Zigler and his colleagues. Within the familial group, they included children who had at least one parent with mental retardation; isolated cases of children who had parents of normal intelligence and from appropriate home environment, but inherited low intelligence; and children who experienced sociocultural deprivation. Within the organic group, Zigler included children with chromosomal disorders, metabolic disorders, neurological impairments, congenital birth defects, and perinatal complications. He theorized that children in the familial mental retardation group would show 'similar sequences' of development, and thus would pass through the stages of typical development in the same sequence as typically developing children, albeit at a slower pace. He also argued that children in the familial mental retardation group would show 'similar structures' of development, thus showing the same organization of developmental constructs as typically developing children. It is important to note that Zigler did not argue that the similar sequence and similar structure hypotheses would apply to children in the organic mental retardation group. Subsequent researchers argued for a more 'liberal' application of Zigler's developmental theories, suggesting that children with organic etiologies of mental retardation, such as Down syndrome, may conform to the similar sequence and similar structure hypotheses as well.

Etiology-Specific Approach

As an extension of Zigler's two-group approach to classifying individuals with mental retardation, Robert Hodapp, Jake Burack, and other researchers in the developmental approach argued that greater differentiation was needed within the organic mental retardation group. Specifically, they argued that it would advance both science and practice in mental retardation to distinguish among children with different organic syndromes, particularly among children with different genetic disorders. There are currently over 1000 known genetic disorders associated with intellectual disability that have been identified to date. Research on a small subset of these disorders suggests that there are identifiable patterns of outcome associated with these disorders, which may inform both the basic science of gene–brain–behavior pathways, as well as the delivery of educational and intervention services for individuals with intellectual disability.

In the past few decades, many research endeavors have been aimed at characterizing behavioral phenotypes, or the various patterns of behavioral outcomes associated with specific genetic disorders. Though there have been debates over what constitutes a behavioral phenotype, especially with respect to the issues of specificity and pervasiveness of specific symptoms, there is some emerging consensus regarding a middle ground. Elisabeth Dykens' definition of a behavioral phenotype includes the probabilistic notion that children with a given genetic disorder may have a heightened probability of showing a specific outcome or set of outcomes relative to children without the syndrome. Implicit in her definition is the notion that not every child with a specific genetic disorder will show the phenotypic outcomes associated with the disorder, and that an outcome need not be totally unique to a specific group.

In further discussion on the uniqueness of the effects of genetic disorders, Robert Hodapp has noted that some outcomes are partially specific, or shared characteristics among a handful of disorders, and some characteristics are totally specific, or unique to a specific syndrome. Amidst these debates, research on behavioral phenotypes has become increasingly advanced in recent years, involving the use of more sophisticated developmental protocols, brain-imaging techniques, and genetic sequencing. These studies have made it possible to characterize the impact of genetic disorders such as Down syndrome, fragile X syndrome, Williams syndrome, Prader–Willi syndrome, Smith–Magenis syndrome, and 5p-syndrome on development in the areas of cognition, language, social and emotional functioning, motoric functioning, and outcomes related to psychopathology.

Dual Diagnosis

While the term 'intellectual disability' has referred to individuals with cognitive impairments and difficulties with day-to-day adaptation, individuals with intellectual disability are often at risk for showing other behavior problems beyond those captured in this definition. As a result, many individuals have been dually diagnosed with both intellectual disability and other co-morbid conditions, such as psychiatric disorders. The reported prevalence of individuals with dual diagnoses varies from study to study, with some reports as high as 40–50% of children with intellectual disability in middle childhood showing some degree of psychiatric symptomatology.

In addition, children with specific causes of their intellectual disabilities may be vulnerable to some psychiatric conditions, but not others. For example, individuals with Prader–Willi syndrome show increased rates of obsessive-compulsive behavior, including hoarding behavior, as well as well-documented obsessive food ideation symptoms. Children with Williams syndrome are at increased risk of showing difficulties in the area of anxiety and heightened fear responses. While children with Down syndrome tend to show lower levels of psychopathology than other children with intellectual disability, there is evidence to suggest that these individuals are at increased risk for autism and autism spectrum disorders, relative to the prevalence rates observed in the typically developing population.

Diagnosis of a comorbid psychiatric condition along with intellectual disability may pose many challenges to clinicians and therapists. Researchers in this area have noted that many clinicians are prone to attribute the behavior problems associated with psychiatric conditions to the diagnosis that a child already has, leading to the phenomenon called diagnostic overshadowing. In other words, the diagnosis that a child already has – for example, Down syndrome – becomes the explanation for poor communication and impairments in social interaction, rather than exploring the alternative possibility that the child might meet criteria for autism as well. This is notable in that impairments in social interaction are unusual in most children with Down syndrome, who tend to show competence in achieving early intersubjective milestones in infancy and toddlerhood. Thus, understanding the relative contributions of the intellectual disability and

a possible comorbid disorder may make it possible to improve the precision with which decisions are made regarding appropriate services and intervention strategies.

Yet, making dual diagnoses of this nature can be challenging for a number of reasons. First, the manifestation of a psychiatric disorder may be modified in an individual with intellectual disability. For example, an anxiety disorder may manifest itself differently in a child who has pronounced expressive language delays versus a child who has an age-appropriate ability to express his/herself. In addition, when a child has pronounced intellectual disability that are in the severe or profound IQ score range, additional difficulties present themselves with regard to accurate dual diagnosis. If a low-functioning child with Down syndrome shows many of the behavioral hallmarks of autism, including poor joint attentions skills, poor initiation, language delays, or a lack of pretend play, it is possible that the child simply has not yet reached an overall developmental level wherein a clinician would expect to observe those behaviors. As a result, an autism diagnosis may not be appropriate in this situation, especially if these deficits are observed in the context of some other, more basic behaviors that evidence impairment in social interaction (e.g., sharing enjoyment or interest).

Identification, Intervention, and Education

Identifying Young Children with Intellectual Disability

Evaluation of young children during the first 2 years of life involves identifying children who already show pronounced developmental delays, as well as identifying children who are at high risk of showing later developmental delays. Newborn assessment begins in the earliest moments of life with Apgar scoring. Lower Apgar scores indicate an increased risk of neurological impairment, and newborns with low scores generally require close observation during the first weeks of life. Additional screening during the first few months of life includes assessment of reflexes and screening for genetic abnormalities via blood testing, if needed.

The pathways into the referral process vary internationally. For example, in Spain and many other countries, children are monitored by pediatricians or pediatric nurses, who use protocols that detect warning signs for developmental delays during regular visits. The Israeli early intervention system stresses both the importance of parent-initiated referrals, as well as referrals through the public well-baby care centers that are found throughout the country. In addition, infants determined to be at greater risk because of low birth weight or other factors, are referred to a child development center for closer monitoring. In Sweden, referrals can come from parents or Child Health Services, but often children who do not have established disabilities are referred by preschool professionals because of the general system of preschool services provided to all children in that country.

Though systems for identifying children with or at risk for intellectual disability vary greatly internationally, there are some features that are commonly found. In general, the first line in detecting developmental delays involves those professionals who have the greatest interaction with infants, including pediatricians and other healthcare workers. If delays are suspected, additional professionals are recruited into the clinical team, including developmental specialists, social workers, and other interventionists. Subsequent to the newborn-screening process, additional evaluation of development can take place throughout infancy, with measures such as the Bayley Scales of Infant Development and the Mullen Scales of Early Learning.

Specific assessment of the development of areas such as language, social–emotional functioning, and adaptive behavior can also be conducted with standardized measures that have become the norm for typically developing infants and other infants with delays. Because of their psychometric properties, in the US, commonly used measures in infancy include the Preschool Language Scales IV, the Reynell Developmental Language Scales, the Battelle Developmental Inventory, the Brazelton's Neonatal Behavioral Assessment Scale, and the MacArthur Communication Development Inventories (Infant and Toddler form). For preschool-aged children, assessment of various aspects of development continues. To assess cognitive development, commonly used measures include the Wechsler Preschool and Primary Scale of Intelligence – Revised and the Stanford Binet. Language assessment is often assessed using the *Peabody Picture Vocabulary Test* (3rd edn.) and the *Preschool Language Scales* (4th edn.). Social and adaptive behavior development is often measured using the Vineland Adaptive Behavior Scales and the AAMR Adaptive Behavior Scales.

In general, children with lower IQ scores tend to be identified earlier in development than children with more mild impairments. Thus, the prevalence of children with IQ scores below 50 or so remains somewhat steady throughout development. In contrast, children with milder intellectual disability tend to be identified later in development, often upon beginning formal schooling. As a result, the prevalence of children with mental retardation tends to increase for children once they reach school years.

Early Intervention

Beyond identification of intellectual disability in young children, a primary goal of early assessment is to enable children with identified intellectual disability to receive appropriate early intervention services. Early intervention is a comprehensive set of services that are provided to children from birth through the early childhood years (generally lasting through to ages 3–6 years, depending on the country) and their families to enhance a child's developmental potential. The family-focused approach to early intervention is found in many different countries, including the US, Austria, Canada, the UK, Israel, Spain, and Sweden, among others. The structure and implementation of early intervention services internationally varies greatly. In this section, we explore the model implemented in the US, though references for additional information are given ahead about early intervention in other countries.

In the US, federal law Individuals with Disabilities Education Act (IDEA), with the 1997 Amendment (Public Law 105–17), specifies that children under the age of three years are eligible for early-intervention services should they show delays in one or more areas of development or if they have a diagnosis of a condition that is generally associated with developmental delays. Named 'Part C', early-intervention services include a few over-riding principles: families are at the center of the early-intervention process; and services should be provided to young children within natural contexts (typically the child's home). A service coordinator is assigned to each child to act as the family's main point of contact for the provision of these services. In many cases, early intervention involves a teacher (or an early-intervention specialist), various therapists, the family, and the child, working together to minimize the effects of the child's disability on his or her development. Specialists in the area of family training, counseling, respite care, home visits, physical therapy, occupational therapy, speech-language therapy, audiological services, and many other areas may be included in this team according to each individual child's and family's needs.

In the US early intervention involves the development of an individual family service plan (IFSP), which is created by a team in order to identify both short- and long-term goals and strategies for early intervention. The IFSP contains information about the services necessary to facilitate a child's development and enhance the family's capacity to facilitate the child's development. Through the IFSP process, family members and service providers work as a team to plan, implement, and evaluate services tailored to the family's unique concerns, priorities, and resources. According to IDEA, included in the IFSP are the following elements: (1) Current level of functioning – this section includes a detailed description of the child's present levels of development in all areas (cognitive, communication, social or emotional, and adaptive development). (2) Resources – this area outlines the family's resources and concerns relating to enhancing the development of their child. (3) Desired goals and outcomes – this section lists the major outcomes to be achieved for the child and the family. It includes the criteria, procedures, and timelines used to determine progress; and whether modifications or revisions of the outcomes or services are necessary. (4) Access to early intervention services – specific early-intervention services are identified that are necessary to meet the unique needs of the child and the family. This section also indicates the frequency, intensity, and the method of delivery for recommended services. (5) Integration into environments with typically developing peers – this section describes the natural environments in which services will be provided, including reasoning as to the extent, if any, to which the services will not be provided in a natural environment. (6) Timeline – the timeline documents the projected starting and ending dates for delivery of services. (7) Identification of service provider – this section, unique to the IFSP, identifies the specific service provider who will be responsible for implementing the plan and coordinating with other agencies and persons. (8) Plans for transition into the formal educational environment – this final section identifies the steps to support the child's transition to preschool or other appropriate services upon reaching the age of three.

Special Education

Special education services refer to specially designed educational instruction, including supplementary aids and related services, that allow a child with a disability to benefit meaningfully from his or her educational program. These strategies include both instructional accommodations and developmentally designed learning environments inside the classroom and outside intervention programs with specialists. The changes in attitudes toward educating children with intellectual disability are reflected in the twentieth century history of disability law in the US. Prior to the passage of IDEA, in the US, the standards for educating children with disabilities varied tremendously among states. When it was first enacted in 1975, IDEA introduced the notion of guaranteed 'free, appropriate public education' to children with disabilities and mandated that, to the 'maximum extent appropriate', they be educated with their nondisabled peers in the 'least restrictive environment'. In addition to creating standards for the education of children with intellectual disability and other conditions, IDEA brought into the public schools slightly more than 1 million children with disabilities who had previously received only limited educational services.

Beyond guaranteeing children an education that was free and appropriate, an important shift in education for children with intellectual disability in the US came in the stipulation that children should be educated in the 'least restrictive environment'. Prior to this landmark legislation, children with disabilities who were permitted into public schooling environments were often assigned to self-contained classrooms. The implementation of IDEA in educational settings was not without controversy. Teachers and administrators cited issues related to a lack of preparation and training to accommodate the needs of children with developmental delays, and parents of typically developing children expressed concerns over the issues of equity and access to quality. In particular, some parents were concerned that the quality of the education that their child would receive might be in some way compromised by the presence of a child with intellectual disability in the classroom.

The concept of full inclusion calls for teaching students with disabilities in regular classrooms, rather than in special classes or pull-out sessions, and is now adopted in many countries, including the UK and Australia. In the US, federal special education law states that, to the 'maximum extent appropriate', children with disabilities should be educated with nondisabled peers in the 'least restrictive environment possible'. While inclusion has grown more common, most severely disabled students are still typically included in regular education classes for only a few subjects a day, such as art or physical education. The inclusion of children with disabilities in the general education classroom and access to a developmentally appropriate curriculum has improved in recent years with increased training for teachers in all classrooms and a better understanding of intervention strategies and assessments.

Individualized Education Plan

Education planning for older children with intellectual disability

From age 3 to 21 years, children with intellectual disability in the US may qualify for special education services through the public educational system. Criteria state that the child must have a disability that interferes with their ability to benefit from a regular educational program. Within an educational environment, specialists, educators, and parents work together to identify common goals and strategies to assist the child with developmental disabilities in achieving critical developmental milestones. Once a child reaches the age of 3, they no longer receive an IFSP through Part C services. Rather, children over the age of three are given an individualized education plan (IEP) to guide their development and learning both in and out of the classroom. Each child's IEP describes, among other things, the educational program that has been designed to meet that child's unique needs. It is created in collaboration and reviewed at least once per year, possibly more often, if requested by a parent or teacher.

The IEP includes pertinent information outlining the needs, goals, strategies, and methods of assessment that will guide instruction and intervention strategies. Included in the IEP are the following elements: (1) Current performance – the IEP must describe the child's current performance (known as present levels of educational performance). The statement about current performance includes how the child's disability affects his or her involvement and progress in the general curriculum. (2) Annual goals – these are goals that the child can reasonably accomplish in 1 year. Goals are broken down into short-term objectives or benchmarks. Goals may be academic, address social or behavioral needs, relate to physical needs, or address other educational needs. The goals must be measurable; it must be possible to quantify whether or not the student has achieved the goals. (3) Special education and related services – this section outlines the particular intervention strategies and how they will be implemented during the child's time at school. (4) Participation with nondisabled children – addresses the amount of time spent in a classroom with typically developing peers and the amount of time in pull-out intervention programs. (5) Dates and places – the IEP must state when services will begin, how often they will be provided, where they will be provided, and how long they will last. (6) Measuring progress – the IEP must state how the child's progress will be measured and how parents will be informed of that progress.

The IEP differs from the IFSP in several ways. First, the IFSP revolves around the family, as opposed to the educational environment where older children spend the majority of their day. The IFSP includes outcomes targeted for the family, while the IEP focuses primarily on the eligible child. The IFSP includes the notion of natural environments that encompass home or community settings such as parks, childcare, and gym classes. This community-oriented focus allows for learning interventions in everyday routines and activities, rather than limiting the implementation to formal educational settings. Finally, it names a service coordinator who will assist the family during the development, implementation, and evaluation of the plan.

Etiology and Education Planning

With a new wealth of knowledge regarding the impact of specific genetic syndromes on behavioral outcomes, there is a growing awareness that this information might be used to inform intervention and educational planning for children with intellectual disability. Given that children with different genetic disorders can be predisposed to very different profiles of strength and weakness in areas such as cognition, language, social–emotional functioning, and other important areas of development, it may be possible to incorporate these profiles into the educational planning process for children with different disorders. This approach can be incorporated into educational programming for children in primary and elementary education settings, as well as early intervention programs for infants, toddlers, and preschool-aged children.

In terms of instruction in educational settings, it has been recommended that aspects of a child's syndrome-specific predispositions be used to modify the presentation of materials and to inform the selection of instructional techniques. For example, children with Williams syndrome are predisposed to deficits in various aspects of visuospatial processing, but they show relative strengths in the area of verbal processing. Children with Down syndrome show the opposite profile, evidencing pronounced deficits in verbal processing and strengths in visual processing. Thus, in coordinating instructional techniques for a child with Down syndrome and a child with Williams syndrome – even if they show similar overall severity of impairment – it would be advantageous to take into account these diverging profiles with subtle modifications. A simple example might be to support verbal instruction with visual scaffolds for a child with Down syndrome, and to support visually based instruction with verbal scaffolds for a child with Williams syndrome. A teacher who is informed regarding these information-processing profiles might make such decisions seamlessly, without needing to disrupt his/her instruction in a larger class setting, with great impact. Other etiology-linked aspects of learning may be taken into account in this type of instructional modification, including executive function, simultaneous/sequential processing, and motivation.

In terms of early-intervention planning, it may be possible to use information regarding etiology-specific predispositions to identify potential areas of vulnerability during the earliest stages of development. Interventionists may take into account, for example, that the majority of middle childhood-aged children with Down syndrome show strengths in receptive language and pronounced delays in expressive language. When treating a toddler with Down syndrome, rather than waiting for a distinct split between receptive and expressive language to emerge in order to begin to address the issue with intervention, an interventionist could use knowledge about this predisposition to target a potential split from very early stages of development. They may choose to monitor early precursors of expressive language to identify an evidence of a disrupted pathway, and make effective intervention-planning decisions from the beginning. Thus, using an etiology-specific approach it may be possible to monitor areas of later strength and weakness from the earliest stages of development in order to detect and target subtle manifestations of a later, more pronounced, profile.

Critics argue that such an approach might not be cost-effective in that not all children with a given syndrome show a given outcome. In addition, there are concerns regarding defining groups too narrowly in the educational system such that it becomes both costly and cumbersome to address the needs of each identified group. These issues will doubtlessly be explored in debates regarding special education policy in upcoming years. Yet, as scientific research in the area of behavioral phenotypes continues to become more sophisticated, it may be inevitable that families and educators work together to connect phenotypic learning profiles in various syndromes with educational pedagogy.

Families of Children with Intellectual Disability

Though a great deal of attention was placed on the definition of mental retardation during the first half of the twentieth century, little attention was placed on families of individuals with mental retardation. In the 1960s, however, families became a focus of research attention as a greater emphasis was placed on improving child outcomes. It was theorized that families can have a direct influence on a child's achievement and their adaptation to their environment, and targeting home environments might be an important way to improve outcomes for children with mental retardation.

The main focus of initial research on families of children with mental retardation was on negative outcomes in the family, with an emphasis on issues such as social isolation, divorce, sibling identity, and parental depression. Case reports focused largely on parental experiences of mourning and the responses of parents to the loss of the 'ideal' typically developing child they had expected. More current research continues to focus on negative outcomes to some degree, though the focus of such work has been updated to include issues such as work–family balance and quality of the spousal relationship. In addition, more recent work has focused on the notion of stress in families of children with intellectual disability, where such a child is viewed as one stressor in the larger family environment. The notion of stress in this line of research refers to a perceived disparity between the situational demands and one's ability to respond to them. Thus, in families of children with intellectual disability, stress may result from a mismatch between the demands of caring for a child with cognitive impairments and the resources available to the family to address those needs.

Recent research on outcomes in families of children with intellectual disability has also begun to focus on positive aspects of the parenting experience, such as feelings of satisfaction and enjoyment. Parents in these studies have reported feelings of reward in watching their child make small achievements, enjoying the various aspects of everyday life, enjoying when demands were decreased, or the child's prognosis was good. Other positive outcomes in research on families of children with intellectual disability are parents reporting that their child with intellectual disability may provide challenges but also makes them feel needed, and even provides a sense of purpose in life. Research on families of children with intellectual disability has also focused on coping style and family supports. Factors impacting parental coping involve demographic factors such as Socioeconomic status, and also cognitive factors such as being problem-focused versus emotion-focused. Social support networks can influence outcomes like maternal stress and family adjustment, though some characteristics of support networks, such as increased density (many members of the support network are known to one another), may be less helpful than others.

Specific child characteristics may also have an impact on family outcomes as well. Some studies show that the child's age is positively correlated with family stress. These findings may support a 'wear-and-tear hypothesis', where the stress associated with parenting a child with a disability builds up over time. Other studies do not show this positive association between child age and stress, and some suggest that there is a lack of linearity in the relationship between the two. A nonlinear model of stress in families of children with intellectual disability suggests that specific periods in the child's development may increase a family's vulnerability to stress, while other periods of time may place families at lower risk for stress. For example, certain age milestones throughout development may lead parents to make normative comparisons to typically developing children, leading to 'wistful' thoughts about what their child may have been experiencing if they did not have intellectual disability.

Another child characteristic that has been shown to impact family outcomes is maladaptive behavior. Problem-behavior, associated with outcomes such as parental depression, pessimism, time demands, dependency and management, lifespan care, and maladaptive behavior, is a stronger predictor of parenting stress than some other possible factors, such as severity of cognitive impairment. Family outcomes may also be influenced by the specific etiology of the child's intellectual disability. It has been hypothesized that genetic disorders predispose children to specific outcomes, and that these outcomes may indirectly affect family stress, coping, and other outcomes. Robert Hodapp termed this phenomenon the indirect effects of genetic syndromes associated with intellectual disability, and has shown that different genetic disorders indirectly affect families in various ways. For example, families of children with Down syndrome report lower levels of overall family stress than families of children with other genetic disorders, such as Williams syndrome, and Smith–Magenis syndrome. These findings have been replicated in several studies, and possible reasons for the disparity may be related to child-personality characteristics, lower levels of maladaptive behavior, perceived immaturity, and parent-demographic characteristics.

Summary

In the past century, important advances have been made in both science and practice in intellectual disability. The needs of children with intellectual disability and their families have moved to the center of education service delivery in many countries, and early-intervention practices have become standard in many countries for children who are at risk or identified as having intellectual and developmental disabilities. However, the historical struggle to define and treat intellectual disability in the most humane and appropriate ways will likely continue into the next century. As attitudes continue to shift, it is likely that the political, economic, and social environments will continue to intersect and influence the ways in which children with intellectual disability are identified and educated.

See also: Autism Spectrum Disorders; Down Syndrome; Genetic Disorders: Sex Linked; Genetic Disorders: Single Gene; Learning Disabilities; Mental Health, Infant.

Suggested Readings

Borthwick-Duffy SA, Palmer DS, and Lane KL (1996) One size doesn't fit all: Full inclusion and individual differences. *Journal of Behavioral Education* 6: 311–329.

Dykens EM (1995) Measuring behavioral phenotypes: Provocations from the 'new genetics'. *American Journal on Mental Retardation* 99(5): 522–532.

Guralnick MJ (1997) Second-generation research in the field of early intervention. In: Guralnick MJ (ed.) *The Effectiveness of Early Intervention*, pp. 3–20. Baltimore, MD: Paul H. Brookes Publishing.

Guralnick MJ (2005) *The Developmental Systems Approach to Early Intervention*. Baltimore, MD: Paul H. Brookes Publishing.

Hodapp RM (1997) Direct and indirect behavioral effects of different genetic disorders of mental retardation. *American Journal on Mental Retardation* 102: 67–79.

Hodapp RM (2004) Behavioral phenotypes: Beyond the two group approach. *International Review of Research in Mental Retardation and Developmental Disabilities* 29: 1–30.

Hodapp RM and Fidler DJ (1999) Special education and genetics: Connections for the 21st century. *Journal of Special Education* 33: 130–137.

Lipsky DK and Gartner A (1998) Factors for successful inclusion: Learning from the past, looking toward the future. In: Vitello SJ and Mithaug DE (eds.) *Inclusive Schooling: National and International Perspectives*, pp. 98–112. Mahurah, NJ: Lawrence Erlbaum Associates.

MacMillan DL and Reschly DJ (1997) Issues of definition and classification. In: MacLean WE, Jr. (ed.) *Ellis' Handbook of Mental Deficiency, Psychological Theory and Research*, 3rd edn., pp. 47–74. Mahwah, NJ: Lawrence Erlbaum Associates.

Relevant Websites

http://www.aamr.org – AAIDD, The American Association on Intellectual and Developmental Disabilities.

http://www.assid.org.au – Australasian Society for the Study of Intellectual Disability.

http://www.dh.gov.uk – British Department of Health, Providing Health and Social Care Policy, Guidance and Publications.

http://www.iassid.org – International Association for the Scientific Study of Intellectual Disabilities.

http://www.mencap.org.uk – MENCAP, Understanding Learning Disability.

http://www.psych.org – The American Psychiatric Association.

http://www.thearc.org – The Arc.

http://www.cec.sped.org – The Council for Exceptional Children, The Voice and Vision of Special Education.

http://idea.ed.gov – U.S. Department of Education, Promoting Educational Excellence for all Americans.

L

Lead Poisoning

R L Canfield, Cornell University, Ithaca, NY, USA
T A Jusko, University of Washington, Seattle, WA, USA

Glossary

Anthropogenic – Arising from human activity.

Biokinetics – The ways substances behave after they enter the body, how are they distributed to various organs, and how long they persist in the body.

Brain death – A total and irreversible cessation of brain function as manifested by the absence of consciousness and absence of all brainstem functions, including spontaneous movement and respiration.

Cellular proliferation – An increase in the number of cells through cell division and in the size of cells through growth.

Computed tomography (CT) scan – A diagnostic imaging procedure that uses a combination of X-rays and computer technology to produce detailed cross-sectional images of the body.

DMSA (dimercaptosuccinic acid) – Also known as succimer (Chemet) is an orally active chelating agent often used to treat lead poisoning in children with blood lead concentrations $>45\,g\,dl^{-1}$.

Encephalopathy – A general term describing degeneration or dysfunction of the brain, which can be defined more specifically by reference to a set of symptoms.

Erythrocyte – A red blood cell, containing hemoglobin, which is responsible for transporting oxygen throughout the body.

Executive functions – Cognitive operations that control and manage lower-level cognitive processes, such as those involved in planning, the selection of relevant and filtering of irrelevant sensory information, attentional flexibility, abstract thinking, rule acquisition, and inhibiting inappropriate actions.

Glial cell – Any of the cells making up the network of branched cells and fibers that support and nourish the tissue of the central nervous system.

Half-life – The time required for a biological system to eliminate by natural processes half the amount of a substance, such as toxin, that has entered it.

Hippocampus – A brain structure involved in forming, storing, and processing memory.

K-XRF (bone scan) – X-ray fluorescence method used to estimate lead-exposure in bone.

Meta-analytic study – A collection of statistical methods for analyzing the results of multiple independent studies for the purpose of integrating the findings.

Migration – The movement of nerve cells from where they were originally generated in the neural crest to their eventual location in the mature brain.

Myelination – The process of forming a fatty sheath (myelin) around axons and dendrites, thus enabling neural impulses to travel faster.

Neural plasticity – The malleability of brain structure and function as a result of experience.

Osteoporotic – A condition that affects especially older women, characterized by a decrease in bone mass with decreased bone density and enlargement of bone spaces producing porosity and brittleness.

Protein kinase C – An enzyme found throughout the body's tissues and organs that is capable of modulating many cellular functions, including neuronal growth, ion channel function, and gene expression.

Socioeconomic status (SES) – A measure of an individual or family's relative economic and social ranking.
Synaptogenesis – The formation of nerve synapses.

Introduction

A simple axiom of human development is that growth and change result from a confluence of genetic and environmental forces that shape individual life trajectories. Environmental toxins can be among the most influential forces for permanently altering the course of development. Although recognized as a serious health threat for more than two millennia, more children are known to be adversely affected by lead (Pb^{2+}) than by any other environmental pollutant. In the US today, as many as 1 in 10 children will be exposed to a potentially dangerous amount of lead at some time during infancy or early childhood. Largely as a result of human activity, this confirmed neurotoxin has been distributed throughout the environment in a manner that makes infants and young children likely targets of exposure, making it especially regrettable that infants and children are also the most vulnerable to lead's potentially devastating effects. It has long been known that at very high levels of lead exposure children suffer encephalopathy (acute brain swelling), resulting in extensive permanent brain damage and even death. Only since the 1970s has it become widely appreciated that children with low-level lead exposure and who show no clinically observable symptoms nevertheless have impaired iron, calcium, and vitamin D metabolism, and also lasting cognitive and behavioral deficits – the primary focus of this article.

Childhood lead poisoning is a problem as multifaceted as the study of child development itself. To understand this toxin's personal and societal impact requires the collective efforts of researchers in the physical and biological sciences, the social and behavioral sciences, medicine, public health, and policy studies. These efforts focus on addressing several questions, including (1) what are the sources of lead in the environment and how do children become exposed; (2) what happens to lead after it enters the body and what are the mechanisms of toxicity; (3) what are the harmful effects of lead and how do they relate to the amount of exposure, the age of exposure, and other characteristics of the individual; and (4) are the adverse effects of lead permanent, or can they be reversed or reduced in severity by removing lead from children's bodies? Answers to these questions are used to guide the medical treatment of lead-exposed children, to inform regulatory agencies about appropriate standards of environmental management of lead contaminated homes and

industrial sites, and for setting permissible lead content in consumer products. The knowledge also provides guidance to parents whose children might be at risk, and motivates the broader society to ensure that no child's developmental potential is limited by exposure to lead. This article will review these four questions in detail, providing information on exposure to lead, its mechanisms and effects, and whether and how those effects can be mitigated.

Human Exposure to Lead

Lead is a naturally occurring element that has been part of human culture for millennia. Its malleability and durability make it useful for creating products that meet a broad range of practical and esthetic human needs. Examples of these include decorative lead beads discovered in Turkey, dating to about 6500 BC, and a small lead statue discovered in Upper Egypt dating to approximately 3800 BC. Use of lead bowls and jugs for oil and wine is evident from 3000 to 2500 BC, and lead's use as a pigment for pottery glazes, paints, and cosmetics are similarly ancient.

The more extreme symptoms of acute lead poisoning, such as severe abdominal pain and paralysis of the extremities, were described by Nikander (185–135 BC), a Greek physician writing about poisons and their antidotes. We now know the progression of symptoms to include colic, muscular weakness and clumsiness, disorientation and confusion, encephalopathy, paralysis, and death. The Romans used lead to build an elaborate system of pipes to convey freshwater into their city, and some attributed the poor health among pipe fitters to lead exposure. A modern English word for pipe fitter, plumber, is derived from the Latin word for lead, plumbum, which gives us a term for lead poisoning, plumbism. Medical concern with lead poisoning lagged behind concerns about many other poisons that are more obviously linked to their consequences. Symptoms of arsenic poisoning occur about 30 min after it is ingested, whereas lead poisoning generally progresses more slowly, obscuring the temporal relation between cause and effect. Also, lead poisoning has always tended to be a malady of the poor, such as slaves who worked in lead mines, potters, and laborers. Even today, lead disproportionately affects those of lower socioeconomic status (SES).

In modern times, exposure to lead extends well beyond those who mine, smelt, or otherwise work directly with the metal. Lead's value as a pigment in paint, as an additive to increase octane in gasoline, and in many industrial processes has resulted in its widespread distribution throughout the environment. Consequently, many children in the industrialized world, and increasingly in some developing countries, are exposed to 20–100 times as much lead as was common during prehistoric or preindustrial times.

Although historically high, the average exposure of children in the US today is less than one-seventh of what it was only 30 years ago.

Especially when exposures are low, the symptoms of lead poisoning can be very subtle. Also, the delay between the exposure and the adverse outcome can be very long, which directly affects the sense of urgency needed to adequately address the problem. The need to establish a cause–effect link between lead exposure and children's health, and the need to know the minimum exposure required to produce a meaningful adverse effect are the overarching motivations for the study of childhood lead poisoning.

Sources of Environmental Lead, Exposure Mechanisms, and Biokinetics

Although a naturally occurring element, the primary sources of environmental lead are anthropogenic. Prior to the banning of leaded gasoline in the US, Europe, and many other countries, most of the lead released into the environment was from automobile emissions. The gradual removal of leaded gasoline was one of the most important environmental health successes of the twentieth century, and children's blood lead levels (BLLs) declined in concert with the gradual removal of lead from gasoline. Although the lead content of gasoline was greatly reduced beginning in 1986, it was not completely banned until 1996. **Figure 1** shows two time series, spanning the years 1970–2000, illustrating the relation between the total

amount of lead used for transportation in the US and the average BLL in children. During this 30-year span of time the average BLLs of young children declined from about 15 to about 2 $\mu g\,dl^{-1}$. The similar rate of decline in the two time series suggests that leaded gasoline was the primary source of children's exposure. In countries where gasoline still contains lead, children's BLLs are similar to those in the US prior to its ban.

The major sources of environmental lead, the pathways of exposure, and biological fate of lead after it enters the body are illustrated in **Figure 2**. Currently, industrial activity is the largest contributor of lead released into the environment, which includes lead released from smelters, from the manufacture of lead-acid batteries for automobiles and computer backup systems, and from chemical production. The current source of greatest exposure to children living in the US is from lead-based paint. In 1990, the US Food and Drug Administration estimated that 75% of the total lead exposure for a typical 2-year-old child originates from household dust contaminated with small particles of lead, with only 16% coming from food, 7% from water, and 2% from soil and other sources.

In part because paint is the primary source of exposure, the age and quality of housing is an important predictor of the amount of lead found in a child's body. Children living in houses built prior to 1940 (when lead content in paint was highest) are more than twice as likely as other children to have elevated blood lead. The correlation between lead-based paint and housing quality means that lead exposure is not equally distributed

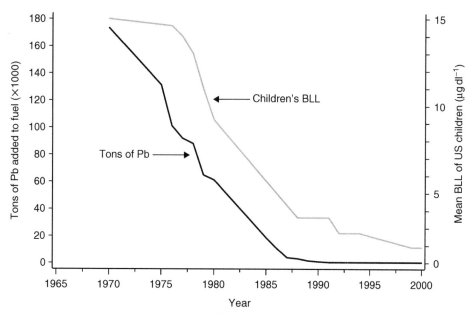

Figure 1 Declining use of lead in transportation fuel and declines in children's blood lead levels (BLLs) in the US: 1970–2000. The black line corresponds to the left axis, showing the yearly use of lead (in thousands of tons) for all transportation purposes in the US. The gray line corresponds to the right axis, showing the change over time in the mean BLL of children during the same historical period. The similar rates of decline of the two time series suggests the importance of leaded gasoline as source of children's exposure. Lead was completely banned as an additive for commercial gasoline in 1996.

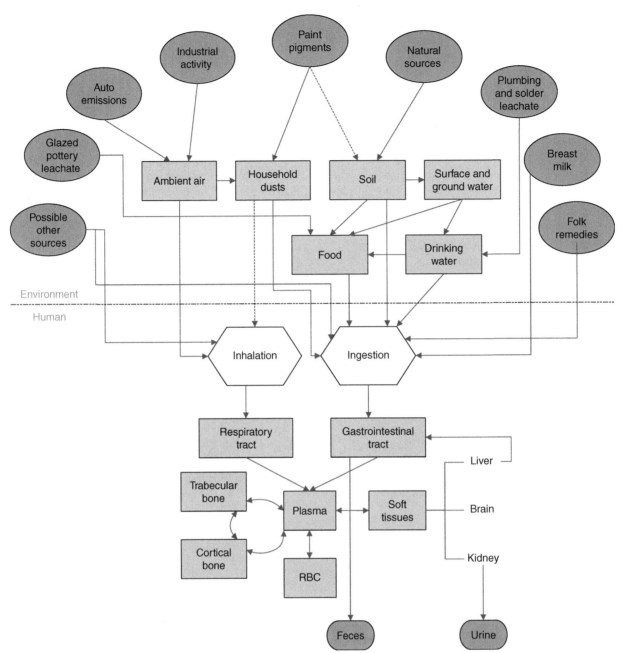

Figure 2 Sources of environmental lead, routes of exposure, and biologic fate. The figure shows the flow of lead from the environmental sources through the human body. The most common source of exposure in children is lead-based paint, although some children are poisoned by more idiosyncratic sources, such as inexpensive metallic jewellery items and toy soldiers; plastic lunch boxes; Tamarindo jellied fruit candy from Mexico; calcium supplements; canned foods; imported vinyl miniblinds and some plastics; crystal decanters and glasses; cosmetics; hair dyes; tobacco; Lozeena, an orange powdered food coloring from Iraq; metal urns and kettles, and curtain weights. RBC, red blood cells.

across groups defined by income and ethnicity. Children from low-income families, who are more likely to live in older buildings that are in poor condition, have been found to be eight times more likely than are children from high-income families to have dangerously elevated BLLs. For similar reasons, non-Hispanic black children are nearly 2.5 times more likely to have dangerous levels of lead in their blood than are non-Hispanic white children (see **Figure 3**).

Other aspects of a child's environment can also influence their exposure to lead. For example, soil lead levels can be high in some urban areas near roadways that were heavily traveled when leaded gasoline was in use. Children living near smelters or other past or present

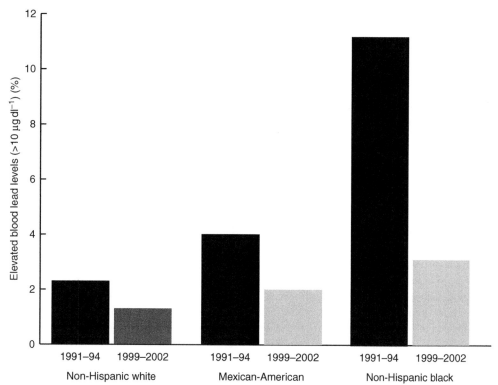

Figure 3 Racial and ethnic group differences in the percentage of children the US with blood lead levels greater than 10 μg dl^{-1} in 1991–94 and 1999–2002.

industrial sites are also at greater risk of harmful exposure. Less frequently, children are exposed to dangerous amounts of lead from toy jewelry and other metal trinkets, from lead-pigmented plastic consumer products (e.g., lunch boxes, window blinds), and from imported foods (e.g., candy stored in lead-glazed pottery).

Lead Exposure in Early Childhood

Lead enters the body mostly through inhalation or ingestion (see **Figure 2**). As noted above, the primary route of exposure for infants and children, at least in the US, is ingestion of contaminated household dust. Leaded paint applied to friction areas such as door frames and double-hung window frames gradually wears away, releasing lead particles that collect on the floor, sills, and other flat surfaces. Cracking and peeling paint on ceilings and walls can also release lead particles. Contaminated soil can be tracked into the house, and lead from the parent's workplace or lead used in hobbies can increase their children's exposure. Very dangerous amounts of lead can be released when lead-based paint is disturbed during home remodeling.

Infants explore the world and learn about the properties of objects and about their own bodies by sucking on their fingers and mouthing toys, blankets, and other objects. In a house contaminated by lead, these objects, especially when

wet with saliva, will accumulate lead particles that can be readily ingested. When infants begin crawling and walking, they cover much more territory and are at risk of greater exposure than pre-locomotor infants; consequently, it is during toddlerhood, from about age 18–36 months, that children's BLLs tend to reach their maximum. Declining hand-to-mouth behavior and improving personal hygiene usually result in less exposure and declining BLLs throughout childhood and adolescence.

In addition to ingesting more lead during infancy than later in life, infants absorb lead more efficiently than adults. Up to 70% of the lead ingested by children and pregnant women can be absorbed into the body, compared to 20% for adults. Also, whereas adults excrete approximately 99% of the lead they absorb, children excrete only about two-thirds of absorbed lead.

In the body, lead is distributed and redistributed among three compartments: blood, soft tissues, bones, and teeth (see **Figure 2**). Lead is initially taken up into blood plasma and then distributed to erythrocytes (where 99% of blood lead is found), soft tissues, and bone. Soft-tissue lead is found mostly in the liver, kidney, lungs, and brain, and eventually 90% or more of an adult's total body lead burden is stored in the bones and teeth.

The half-life of lead in adult bone can be several years to several decades. However, during skeletal growth, pregnancy and lactation, osteoporotic bone loss and other periods of bone remodeling and calcium stress, lead is released from the bones to circulate in the blood and accumulate in tissue and other body compartments. Recirculating pre-pregnancy bone lead can account for one-third or more of lead in the blood of pregnant women and, because the placenta does not protect the fetus from lead in maternal blood, maternal pre-pregnancy lead exposure can enter fetal tissue. Maternal body lead can also be transmitted to the infant through breast milk.

Lead Neurotoxicity

Measuring Exposure

Identifying lead poisoning and linking it to a health outcome depends on knowing how much lead has been absorbed into the body. Although lead damages the brain, it is not possible in humans to measure brain lead levels. Thus, methods have been developed for measuring lead concentration in the other body compartments – blood, bones, and teeth. The concentration of lead in whole blood is the most common measure of exposure. Blood lead reflects primarily current and recent exposure and is the most widely used measure in both clinical and research settings.

Possible Biological Mechanisms of Lead Neurotoxicity

The overt symptoms and potentially lethal sequelae of acute lead poisoning in children were clearly described in the medical literature more than a century ago, and are briefly reviewed below. However, only since the 1970s has it become widely accepted that lead poisoning can cause subtle deficits in the cognitive and behavioral performance of children who show no overt symptoms of poisoning – children for whom their exposure would go unnoticed without a biological indicator such as BLL. The specific biological mechanisms responsible for these subtle neurobehavioral deficits are not well understood, but it is established that lead affects fundamental inter- and intracellular biochemical processes. Using animals and *in vitro* preparations it has been possible to manipulate directly the amount of lead exposure and then examine the damaged tissues and cells thought to be the basis of functional behavioral deficits in the whole organism. This research has shown that lead does not act through a single biochemical mechanism. As a divalent cation (Pb^{2+}), lead shares properties with calcium (Ca^{2+}), iron (Fe^{2+}), and zinc (Zn^{2+}), all essential micronutrients. And although it has no nutritional value, lead can mimic the actions of these other minerals, allowing it to participate in and potentially disrupt a wide range of critically important cellular processes.

Lead's similarity to calcium may be responsible for many of its adverse effects at low exposure levels. For example, lead has been implicated as a cause of abnormal programmed cell death (apoptosis) by activating a cascade of intracellular processes normally regulated by calcium. Even very low concentrations of lead can alter calcium homeostasis in ways that produce an abnormal buildup of intracellular calcium. This excess calcium can trigger a sequence of events that will induce otherwise healthy cells to activate the enzymes involved in normal apoptosis.

Other calcium-related processes are also highly sensitive to lead. For example calmodulin, a binding protein involved in intracellular calcium homeostasis, is activated by lead at nanomolar concentrations. Protein kinase C (PKC), normally a calcium-activated enzyme, can be activated by lead in picomolar concentrations, much lower than it can be activated by calcium. PKC is involved in a broad range of cellular functions including neuronal growth and differentiation, and in specific biochemical processes fundamental to learning and memory, including long-term potentiation (LTP) in the hippocampus.

Altered calcium homeostasis can also affect neural function by disrupting both the spontaneous and the evoked release of neurotransmitters such as dopamine (DA) and alter dopamine D1 and D2 receptor protein expression in nucleus accumbens, hippocampus, and frontal cortex. Some studies indicate that the mesocorticolimbic DA system is especially sensitive to lead exposure. Other mechanisms of lead toxicity include the inhibition of N-methyl-D-aspartate (NMDA) receptors, delayed differentiation of glial cell progenitors, and reduced growth and abnormal branching of dendrites.

Frank Lead Poisoning

Individuals differ greatly in their sensitivity to lead. Some infants begin to exhibit overt symptoms of lead poisoning at blood concentrations as low as 40–50 $\mu g\,dl^{-1}$, and at about 60 $\mu g\,dl^{-1}$ in young children. These levels are sometimes seen in children who have ingested household dust contaminated with particles of high lead-content paint, or in children who frequently eat food stored in lead-glazed pottery. At these BLLs, highly sensitive children show abdominal cramping and become irritable. This can progress to increased intracranial pressure, edema, and other forms of encephalopathy. Children who experience encephalopathy nearly always suffer permanent deficits in cognitive and behavioral functioning.

Extremely high BLLs can result from ingesting paint chips or other objects with high lead content. In two recently described cases, BLLs greater than 100 $\mu g\,dl^{-1}$ were observed in children who swallowed pieces of low-cost jewellery. In one case, a 4-year-old boy swallowed a charm from a metal bracelet that had been provided as a free gift for purchasing a pair of athletic shoes. Approximately 2 days after seeing a physician for unexplained abdominal complaints, the child was admitted to the hospital with severe gastric pain, persistent vomiting, and listlessness. Ten hours after admission the boy became agitated and aggressive and shortly thereafter suffered seizure and respiratory arrest. After being resuscitated, a computed tomography (CT) scan revealed cerebral edema. Subsequent studies on the following day revealed that the boy had suffered brain death; his BLL was 180 μg dl^{-1}. Upon autopsy, the metal charm was found in the boy's stomach. Chemical analysis showed the charm to contain 99.1% lead.

A very different outcome was seen in another 4-year-old boy who swallowed a medallion from a toy necklace purchased at a vending machine. After 3–4 weeks the medallion was discovered and the boy was diagnosed with lead poisoning; at that time his BLL was 123 μg dl^{-1}. The child was immediately treated with several courses of chelation therapy using succimer (dimercaptosuccinic acid; DMSA). Chelation therapy is a means of removing circulating lead ions; the chelator tightly binds to lead and forms a water-soluble compound that is excreted through urine. After chelation, the child's BLL had declined to approximately 25 μg dl^{-1}. Surprisingly, extensive psychometric, neuropsychological, and electrophysiological evaluation revealed no obvious cognitive impairment. Repeated cognitive testing over a period of more than 1 year revealed no immediate evidence of adverse effects in this child.

These two cases illustrate that children vary greatly in their sensitivity to lead. Indeed, cases of fatal poisonings have been reported in children with BLLs of only 80 μg dl^{-1}, but there also are reports of children who are asymptomatic with lead levels as high as 300 μg dl^{-1}. The reasons for these individual differences are unclear, but it is possible that children who appear especially sensitive have had one or more previous poisonings that went unreported. Genetic differences, nutritional status, and previous or concurrent exposure to other toxins might be involved also.

Neurobehavioral Correlates of Low Blood Lead Levels

Medical experience with lead-exposed children established that BLLs as low as 60 μg dl^{-1} – exposure sufficient to cause gastric symptoms in most infants and young children – were strongly associated with subsequent cognitive and behavioral deficits and were, therefore, recognized to be unsafe as early as the 1930s. However, after it was discovered that BLLs as low as 40 μg dl^{-1} interfered with heme biosynthesis in otherwise asymptomatic children, the notion of insidious lead poisoning was proposed. Insidious poisoning refers to the idea that when severe damage is caused by acute high-level exposure to a toxin, lower-level chronic exposure will produce more subtle adverse effects. The possibility of insidious lead poisoning was identified as a top research priority in a 1972 National Academy of Sciences report

to the US Environmental Protection Agency (EPA). As a result, the primary focus of research during the past 35 years has been to establish what amount of exposure, if any, can be considered safe for the health and long-term development of infants and young children.

Methods for detecting insidious lead poisoning

Case reports and descriptions of the long-term developmental outcomes of lead-poisoned infants and children were an inadequate basis for detecting possible subtle neurobehavioral effects of BLLs less than about 40 μg dl^{-1}. Thus, researchers began formal studies that involved large numbers of children and more sophisticated research designs. These studies also used sensitive measures of cognitive and behavioral functioning that allow for making fine distinctions between levels of performance. The primary outcome measure used in these early studies, and in nearly all subsequent studies of pediatric lead exposure, was some form of a standardized psychometric intelligence test. These tests yield a global index score to represent the quality of general intellectual functioning. Although the terminology for the global index scores differs, for ease of presentation we use the term 'intelligence quotient' (IQ) to refer to the omnibus score from any such test.

In addition to examining the possible effects of lead on IQ scores, several studies have assessed the relationship between lead exposure and more specific areas of cognitive function. These studies employ neuropsychological tests originally developed for the diagnosis and evaluation of patients with psychiatric problems or probable brain damage. Also, several studies have investigated the possible effects of lead exposure on children's social, emotional, and psychological function – focusing primarily on a link between early exposure and later externalizing behaviors (e.g., conduct problems, aggressiveness, and delinquency).

Lead exposure and intelligence test performance

Early formal studies of what, at that time, was considered low-level lead exposure employed cross-sectional research designs for which the exposure measure (typically BLL) and the outcome (typically IQ) were measured at a single time point. Importantly, these studies were designed with the recognition that exposure to lead is only one of many factors that can influence a child's performance on an IQ test. As a result, information was obtained about possible prenatal and birth complications, postnatal health, family structure, SES, and parental education, among other possible influences. This information was then used in statistical analyses to estimate the independent contribution of lead exposure on IQ. Although the findings of individual studies were not fully consistent, when the results of 24 cross-sectional studies were systematically analyzed, a broad consensus emerged among most researchers studying lead exposure: that BLLs as low as 25 μg dl^{-1}, and possibly as low as 10 μg dl^{-1}, adversely affect children's intellectual functioning. Taking a precautionary approach, in 1991 the Center for Disease Control and Prevention (CDC) lowered the definition of an elevated BLL from 25 to $10 \, \mu g \, dl^{-1}$.

Although the cross-sectional studies were highly influential in shaping public policies, research using that methodology cannot rule out critically important alternative explanations. For example, suppose that brain damage was caused by an undetected prenatal event not related to lead exposure. It is possible that neurologically compromised infants engage in more hand-to-mouth behavior, which causes them to ingest more lead. In this case, one would observe an inverse association of BLL and IQ but the conclusion that lead causes lower IQ scores would be unwarranted.

Criticisms of the early studies also revolved around the issue of confounding. Confounding occurs when a variable (measured or unmeasured) is associated with the exposure and the outcome of interest. Maternal IQ would be a potential confounder because it reflects the mother's genetic contribution to her child's IQ, but also because it can contribute to economic disadvantage and poor housing quality, and therefore to the child's exposure to lead. In this way, maternal IQ is associated with children's BLLs (exposure) and also with children's IQ (outcome). If confounding is present and not adequately addressed, the estimated association between blood lead and IQ could be either spuriously strong or weak. Although the cross-sectional studies did attempt to identify possible confounders and adjust for them, they often lacked measurement of key confounding variables such as maternal IQ and the quality of stimulation in the home environment. Based on these and other challenges to the validity of these early studies, the scientific basis for the CDC action was vigorously questioned by some.

Prospective, or longitudinal, cohort studies address many of the limitations of the cross-sectional design, and in the late 1970s and 1980s prospective studies were initiated in Boston and Cincinnati, in the US, Kosovo in the former Yugoslavia, Mexico City, and Port Pirie and Sydney in Australia. Although originally designed to examine the effects of prenatal substance abuse, a prospective study conducted in Cleveland also examined childhood lead exposure in relation to intellectual development. These studies followed children, typically from birth, to ascertain BLLs and measure neurobehavioral performance on multiple occasions during infancy and childhood. Again, the primary outcome was the child's score on an IQ test, but other outcomes were examined in one or more individual studies.

These longitudinal studies also focused more intensely than earlier studies on the problem of possible confounding by parental IQ, SES, and the quality of the childrearing environment (e.g., maternal warmth and responsivity, encouragement of learning, and provision of competence-building toys). Pregnancy and birth complications and many other indicators of child health were also considered.

The Boston study was unique in that the average BLL of the children who participated was consistently below $10 \, \mu g \, dl^{-1}$, which contrasted with the higher lead levels found in Cincinnati, Cleveland, Sydney, and Port Pirie. In the Yugoslavia study, approximately one-half of the subjects resided near a lead smelter, refinery, and battery plant, whereas a comparison town had much less environmental exposure and thus BLLs ranged considerably, from 1 to $70 \, \mu g \, dl^{-1}$, in that study cohort. Five of the seven prospective studies (Boston, Cincinnati, Cleveland, Mexico, Port Pirie, Sydney, Yugoslavia) reported that higher BLL, measured either as cumulative exposure or exposure at a particular age during infancy or early childhood, was associated with lower IQ scores – after statistical control for many possible confounders. Moreover, for each study that reported adverse effects, the lead–IQ association was replicated at two or more ages. Reports from the Cleveland and Sydney studies indicated no association between BLL and IQ. No studies have reported significant positive associations between BLL and children's intelligence test performance. When the results from all the prospective cohort studies were subjected to meta-analysis, the effect of an increase in BLL from 10 to $20 \, \mu g \, dl^{-1}$ was estimated to be a 1–4-point decrease in children's IQ scores.

Specific cognitive and neuropsychological functions

Intelligence test scores reflect a sort of average of a person's performance on multiple individual subtests, each assessing competence in a general domain of cognitive functioning. Although IQ scores are reliably associated with children's BLLs, they reveal little about the specific types of cognitive functions that are affected. If, as is found with many toxins, lead selectively affects some biochemical or neurophysiological processes but spares others, then the cognitive functions most dependent on those more vulnerable processes would be disproportionately damaged. Consequently, a better understanding of the types of cognitive processes affected by lead could uncover more sensitive measures for indicating the presence of adverse effects of lead, and it might also open avenues to possible behavioral or neuropharmacological interventions for lead-exposed children.

Researchers have used two main methods to identify what some have called a behavioral signature of lead toxicity. One method has been to examine patterns of performance across the individual subtests used to derive an overall IQ score. A potentially stronger methodology has been to use clinical neuropsychological tests initially developed to characterize the pattern of behavioral deficits associated with localized brain damage. Studies using these methods are suggestive of several broad areas of cognitive function that are especially vulnerable to lead exposure – visual–motor integration, attention, and executive functions.

Visual–motor integration involves the ability to coordinate fine motor skills with visual–spatial perception in order to draw and copy geometric forms, assemble puzzles, and arrange blocks to create a specified configuration. Reviewing patterns of subtest performance across studies suggests that lead-related deficits in the overall IQ score are influenced by a particularly strong inverse association between BLL and performance on block-design tasks. The block-design subtest is also the most consistent among all subtests in showing a statistically significant association with BLL. Studies using neuropsychological tasks designed specifically to assess visual–spatial abilities and visual–motor integration and have produced a consistent set of findings; namely, that BLL is inversely related to fine motor skills, eye–hand coordination, and standardized testing of the ability to copy geometric forms. Although these results are mostly consistent, in one longitudinal study visual–spatial abilities were most impaired at age 5 years, whereas extensive neuropsychological testing conducted at age 10 years revealed no clear deficit in visual–spatial skills.

Attention, a second area of possible special vulnerability, involves cognitive functions for sustaining performance over time, and for selecting particular stimuli for intensive cognitive processing. Some studies have used index scores based on combinations of IQ subtests and neuropsychological tests thought to reflect sustained and focused attention. Although sustained attention is generally unrelated to lead exposure, more highly exposed subjects in these studies showed poorer performance on tasks requiring focused attention.

Executive functions enable planning and goal-oriented cognition based largely on the ability to coordinate the activities of more specialized cognitive functions, such as memory, attention, and visual–spatial processing, and to flexibly apply these cognitive functions to meet changing task demands. Importantly, the line between certain aspects of attention and executive functioning is not clearly drawn. For example, focused attention involves the controlled use of attention and therefore is sometimes included as a component of executive functioning. Attentional flexibility is more generally considered to reflect executive functioning and involves the ability to shift the focus of attention between different sources of information or to consider alternative problem-solving strategies.

Two prospective studies have examined children's performance on classical measures of executive functioning, arriving at similar but not identical conclusions. In one study of 10-year-old children, BLL during childhood was associated with an increase in several measures of perseverative behavior. For example, although childhood BLL was unrelated to how quickly children learned a simple rule, children with higher BLLs appeared to be less cognitively flexible – after the rule changed they were

more likely to continue making the previous, but now incorrect, response. Cognitive rigidity was also seen in a study in which 5-year-old children completed a computerized test battery. Lead exposure was unrelated to the ability to sustain attention on a simple task, but children with higher BLLs made more errors when they were required to shift to a new rule. These children also showed planning deficits when solving multistep problems. Children with higher BLLs made impulsive choices on the first step of the problem, which made subsequent steps more difficult, thereby causing them to make more errors. Finally, a study of young adults given a large battery of neuropsychological tests showed that tooth lead levels were inversely related to performance on groups of tasks that assessed focused attention and attentional flexibility (although not sustained attention).

Externalizing behaviors and juvenile delinquency

A curious symptom during a period of acute lead poisoning is a high level of aggressiveness and combativeness, even in young children. Lasting effects of lead on behavior problems were described in an early case study of the long-term outcomes of boys treated for acute lead poisoning. As adolescents, many years after being treated, these boys were found to have extremely high rates of delinquency. This report was one motivation for studies investigating whether lead exposure at subacute levels is associated with problems of behavioral and emotional self-regulation. Based on parent and teacher ratings on child behavior checklists, children with higher lead exposure early in life were found to have more conduct problems and were more defiant, withdrawn, and destructive than children with lower lead levels. Studies of behavior problems in older children focus on antisocial, delinquent, and pre-delinquent behaviors. For example, in one study of 300 boys, the frequency of their antisocial and delinquent behaviors at ages 7 and 11 years was rated by their parents and teachers using the Child Behavior Checklist (CBCL). One major scale of the CBCL assesses behaviors such as disobedience at home and school, destructiveness, cruelty, and truthfulness. The boys rated their own behaviors using the Self-Reported Antisocial Behavior (SRAB) and Self-Reported Delinquency (SRD) scales. SRAB measures nonviolent and violent antisocial behavior in terms of frequency, whereas SRD defines delinquent behavior operationally as activities that violate legal statues and often involve some risk of arrest. Childhood cumulative lead exposure was measured using K-XRF at age 12 years. Evidence for lead-related influences on delinquency was inconsistent. When the boys were rated at age 11 years, CBCL ratings of problem behaviors were positively associated with bone lead. However, there was no association between bone lead and self-reported behaviors, or between bone lead and parent and teacher ratings at age 7 years. Because many children might under report their socially undesirable activities, and because eventual levels of delinquency and problem behaviors might not have developed by age 7 years, these findings provide some, albeit limited, support for the hypothesis that exposure to lead increases the risk of problem behaviors among boys during late childhood.

A subsequent study addressed the age issue by selecting adolescents, and the reporting bias issue by selecting children who already had been arrested and adjudicated. In this case-control study design, cases were those adjudicated as delinquent and controls were nondelinquent age-mates selected from high schools in the same county as the cases. Results from this study indicated that, compared to nondelinquent controls, adjudicated delinquent adolescents were four times more likely to have a bone lead concentration greater than 25 parts per million (ppm).

Whereas the previously described studies lacked detailed information about subjects' history of lead exposure during childhood, one study measured blood lead more than 20 times between birth and 6.5 years. When they were 19–20 years old, the young men and women reported on their delinquent and predelinquent behaviors and their parents provided independent reports. After controlling for a range of other factors that might predict both lead exposure and delinquent behavior, this study revealed that children with higher BLLs as neonates engaged in more problem behaviors later in life; average childhood lead concentrations were also positively associated with self-reports and parent reports of delinquency.

The consistency of findings from studies using different measures of problem behaviors and different measures of lead exposure (bone, blood, and dentin) suggests the possibility of a causal relation between early lead exposure and later delinquency. Although the BLLs among the children in the studies just described were substantially greater than what is common in the US today, these findings cannot be dismissed as irrelevant. Still today, thousands of children living in substandard housing in many inner cities of the East and Midwest are likely to experience similar amounts of lead exposure as the children in these studies. Also, the relation of lead and delinquency has been little explored in samples of children with very low exposure and so it remains unknown whether behavior problems are significantly increased in such children, or whether there is a threshold exposure below which lead and delinquency are unrelated.

Susceptibility

Is There a Safe Level of Exposure?

In 1991, the CDC issued its fourth statement on preventing lead poisoning in young children. The main outcome of

this report was a change in the definition of an elevated blood lead from $25 \, \mu g \, dl^{-1}$ to its present level of $10 \, \mu g \, dl^{-1}$. In this report it was explicitly acknowledged that some studies indicated harmful effects at levels at least as low as $10 \, \mu g \, dl^{-1}$, and that no threshold had been identified. Partly in consideration of the inadequate base of evidence, $10 \, \mu g \, dl^{-1}$ was described as a level of concern. The CDC also established recommended courses of action for treating lead-exposed children. For example, for a 1-year-old infant with a BLL of $10 \, \mu g \, dl^{-1}$ or less, it is recommended that the lead test be repeated at age 2 years. If the result is again of $10 \, \mu g \, dl^{-1}$ or less, then no additional testing is recommended. Implicit in this approach is that BLLs of $10 \, \mu g \, dl^{-1}$ are safe. However, because no safety threshold had been indicated by research carried out prior to the 1991 statement, some researchers and policymakers were concerned that using $10 \, \mu g \, dl^{-1}$ as a cutoff lacked a strong scientific justification. Of particular concern was that nearly all the research findings available in 1991 were based on populations of children with BLLs greater than $10 \, \mu g \, dl^{-1}$.

Concerns about using $10 \, \mu g \, dl^{-1}$ as an implicit safety threshold were heightened by findings from a prospective study initiated in the late 1990s to track the development of children in Rochester, New York. Reflecting secular trends in lead exposure (see **Figure 1**), the children who participated in this study had very low BLLs throughout infancy and early childhood. Indeed, most children had BLLs less than $10 \, \mu g \, dl^{-1}$ at every assessment (i.e., at 6, 12, 18, 24, 36, 48, and 60 months). The results of intelligence tests administered when the children were 3 and 5 years of age showed an inverse association between IQ scores and average BLL during infancy and childhood. More specifically, after controlling for nine pre-specified covariates, it was estimated that as lifetime average BLLs increased from 1 to $10 \, \mu g \, dl^{-1}$, children's intelligence test scores declined by an estimated 7.4 points. These results suggested that subtle adverse effects on children's cognitive functioning occurred at BLLs well below $10 \, \mu g \, dl^{-1}$. Statistical modeling revealed the dose–response curve shown in **Figure 4**. The shape of this curve did not indicate a safety threshold at around $10 \, \mu g \, dl^{-1}$. Indeed, rather than there being no change in IQ as BLL increased from 0 to $10 \, \mu g \, dl^{-1}$, the results indicated a substantial decline in IQ across that range of exposures. Indeed, the shape of the nonlinear function suggests that at lower levels of exposure a one unit increment in blood lead is associated with more than a one unit decrement in performance. However, at higher exposure levels (approximately $10-15 \, \mu g \, dl^{-1}$), the function appears approximately linear (see **Figure 4**). The linear slope in this region of the curve is consistent with previous research based on children with BLLs greater than $10 \, \mu g \, dl^{-1}$.

Using the Rochester data it was possible to address a more focused question of central importance to public

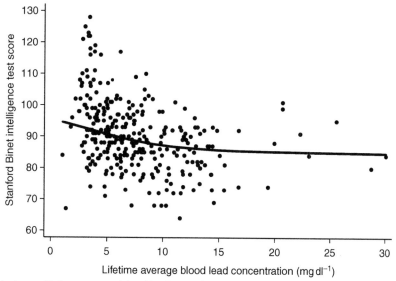

Figure 4 The relation between lifetime average blood lead levels (BLL) and children's Stanford Binet intelligence test score when tested at both 3 and 5 years of age. The points represent the IQ–BLL values for individual children and the smoothed curve is the empirically derived dose–response function estimated by a nonlinear regression model. The function shows that the rate of decline in IQ scores is greater at BLLs below 10 μg dl^{-1} than above 10 μg dl^{-1}. As estimated by the function, as children's blood lead concentration increases from 0 to 10 μg dl^{-1}, IQ decreases by 7.4 points. By contrast, the estimated decline in IQ across the range from 10 to 30 μg dl^{-1} is only 2.5 points. The biological interpretation of a faster-than-linear decline in IQ at very low BLLs remains unclear. Adapted from Canfield, RL, Henderson, CR, Cory-Slechta, DA, *et al.* (2003) Intellectual impairment in children with blood lead concentration below 10 μg per deciliter. *The New England Journal of Medicine* 348: 1517–1526.

health; namely, for children who, throughout infancy and early childhood, have BLLs consistently below the CDC definition of an elevated BLL, do they nevertheless show detectable adverse effects of lead? The answer to this question pertained in particular to the performance of the more than 100 children in the Rochester study whose BLLs were less than 10 μg dl^{-1} at each of the seven blood draws. This group would be comparable to many children in the general population whose blood lead tests are considered normal throughout early childhood. Results of this analysis indicated that even in this group of children, higher lead exposure was associated with significantly lower IQ scores.

These surprising and potentially troubling results motivated two reanalyses of previous studies to test the generality of the findings. The first reanalysis involved data from the 48 children in the Boston cohort that had BLLs less than 10 μg dl^{-1} through age 10 years, and the results were consistent with findings from the Rochester study. Remarkably, the two studies generated nearly identical statistical estimates for the size of the lead effect on IQ.

The close correspondence of results from the Rochester and Boston studies is especially notable because the subject samples differed in many ways. Children from Rochester were 70% non-white and largely from low-income families in which 70% of the mothers had 12 or fewer years of education. In the Boston cohort children were 80% white, and approximately 50% of the parents had some

postcollege education. In addition, the average child IQ in the Rochester study was approximately 90, whereas the average child IQ was approximately 115 in the Boston study. Obtaining such similar results from samples at opposite ends of the SES is inconsistent with a leading alternative explanation of the magnitude of the low-level lead effects estimated from the Rochester study, that is, that children suffering from multiple risk factors in addition to lead exposure will be more severely affected by lead. Instead, the effects appear consistent across samples with very different risk profiles.

Because both studies were limited by a small sample size, a second reanalysis was carried out using the combined data from nearly all the previous longitudinal cohort studies of pediatric lead exposure. The study included 1333 children, 244 of whom had peak BLLs less than 10 μg dl^{-1}. Consistent with the Boston and Rochester studies, the dose–response function indicated that an increase in BLL from 2.4 to 10 μg dl^{-1} was associated with a decline in IQ of almost 4 points.

The effects of very low BLLs estimated by these studies suggest that the IQs of children with BLLs of 10 μg dl^{-1}, the current CDC definition of an elevated BLL, will be approximately 5 points lower than for children with BLLs of only 1–2 μg dl^{-1}. These results have been used to support arguments favoring primary prevention of lead exposure in children, as opposed to waiting to find that a child has an elevated BLL (currently defined as 10 μg dl^{-1}) and only taking action after the test results are confirmed.

Timing of exposure

As noted above, the developmental timing of exposure to a toxin is likely to affect the nature and severity of its effects on the developing organism. Environmental influences typically are most influential when neural plasticity is greatest, during the period of gestation and, especially in humans, during infancy and childhood. During this time the brain is rapidly developing the basic structural organization, connectivity, and functional capacities that are the foundation for learning, cognition, and behavioral self-regulation. Timing of exposure to lead is indisputably an important factor in determining the magnitude of the adverse outcomes. The time of greatest vulnerability, in both humans and non-human animals, is during gestation, infancy, and early childhood. However, it is unclear whether there are specific times during this period of vulnerability when exposure is most damaging. It is also poorly understood which neurodevelopmental processes, for example, cellular proliferation, migration, synaptogenesis, myelination, or apoptosis, are most disrupted by lead.

The biokinetics of lead, the chronic nature of childhood exposure, and the lack of infant tests that are good predictors of later neurobehavioral functioning all limit our ability to identify critical periods of vulnerability. Unlike some toxins, absorbed lead remains in the body for weeks, months, or years so that even a single exposure event can cause elevated lead for a prolonged period. Studying age-specific effects in children is further complicated because in most cases exposure is chronic for a period of years. As a result, BLLs in children are highly correlated from one age to the next, making it conceptually and statistically problematic to determine whether exposure at any specific age is the most important cause of later deficits.

Although not fully surmounting the methodological difficulties, several of the prospective longitudinal studies described above have examined the relative predictive capacity of prenatal vs. postnatal lead exposure, with varying results. Across studies, prenatal maternal BLL is inconsistently associated with cognitive and behavioral outcomes in the child. However, few data are available for exploring the possible special importance of exposure during a particular stage of prenatal development. Studies of postnatal exposure are somewhat more consistent, typically finding that BLLs measured during the first year of life are poor predictors of concurrent or later behaviors. Instead, BLL during the second and third years of life, the period when BLLs are generally highest, tend to be most strongly related to neurobehavioral outcomes. However, some studies report that IQ scores at ages 5–7 years are most highly correlated with BLL when the two are measured concurrently. Together with studies suggesting that prenatal and postnatal lead exposure have independent effects on cognitive outcomes, these findings are difficult to reconcile with the view that

vulnerability to lead is when the brain is developing most rapidly or when particular structures and functions are emerging. These varied results likely reflect the complex interactions between lead and brain development, which are further veiled by differences among studies in terms of the amount and timing of exposure, characteristics of the study sample, age when lead exposure is assessed, age when outcomes are assessed, types of outcomes measured, covariates considered, and approaches to statistical analysis. At this time, however, the combined evidence does not justify the singling out of any particular age or developmental stage as a window of special vulnerability.

Are the effects of early lead exposure transient or permanent?

Evidence from long-term follow-up testing of children who participated in the prospective cohort studies suggests that early deficits endure into the later teenage years. Follow-up testing has been completed through age 10 years in the Boston and Mexico cohorts, age 11 years in the Yugoslavia cohort, age 13 years in the Port Pirie cohort, and age 16 years in the Cincinnati cohort. In every case, even though children's lead levels had declined greatly, prenatal or early postnatal BLLs were inversely associated with the cognitive outcomes. These results suggest that lead effects are enduring.

If exposure to lead during infancy and early childhood results in lasting cognitive deficits, then it was hoped that by reducing BLLs in highly exposed infants and children that lead's detrimental effects on cognition could be reduced or avoided altogether. To test this hypothesis, the treatment of lead-exposed children (TLC) study enrolled children with elevated BLLs and randomized them to placebo or succimer. The TLC study was carried out simultaneously at several research sites, enrolling 780 children between 1 and 3 years of age who had a confirmed BLL between 20 and 44 $\mu g\,dl^{-1}$. A main objective of this study was to determine whether neurobehavioral deficits can be prevented or lessened by administering succimer – presumably by reducing lead concentrations in blood and tissue, including brain.

At baseline, children in the TLC trial were given tests of intelligence, behavior, and neuropsychological function, and then randomly assigned to treatment or placebo. Treatment consisted of up to three 26-day courses of succimer, administered orally. After 3 years of follow-up, children's cognitive function was reassessed. Although BLLs were, at least initially significantly lower in the treated group, scores on cognitive, behavioral, and neuropsychological tests did not differ between the groups. A second round of assessments was conducted when children were 7 years old, but again no benefits of succimer therapy were observed.

The implications of the TLC trial are clear: according to this protocol, chelation therapy with succimer has no affect on subsequent cognitive function for young children with

BLLs in the range studied. One interpretation of these results is that the children were permanently damaged by their lead exposure prior to the age when they began chelation. Another possible reason for the lack of a beneficial effect of chelation is suggested by the findings from research with children having very low BLLs; namely, that the benefits of chelation might be evident only after children's BLLs are reduced to much less than $10\,\mu\mathrm{g\,dl^{-1}}$. Whether a more aggressive regimen would be deemed safe and whether it would produce measurable long-term benefits to children's cognitive functioning remain open questions. In agreement with other evidence, the results from the TLC trial emphasize the importance of taking effective environmental action to prevent children from being exposed to lead.

A Perspective on Lead Exposure during Infancy and Early Childhood: The Importance of Small Effects

Research into pediatric lead exposure reveals a consistent pattern of findings showing that early lead exposure, at levels that produce no overt symptoms, is associated with decrements in later IQ scores, and that these deficits persist into later adolescence. Emerging evidence also suggests that early exposure might cause an increase in antisocial and delinquent behaviors. It must be emphasized, however, that all of these effects are small relative to other factors that shape a child's life. For example, nearly all studies of low-level lead exposure find that parental education, and the quality of the childrearing environment are more important than low-level lead exposure for shaping children's intellectual development and social adjustment. Specifically, whereas lead generally

accounts for less than 5% of the variability in intelligence test scores, measures of the childrearing environment typically account for between 10% and 20% of the variance – independent of what is explained by lead. Nevertheless, small effects can have important ramifications for the affected individuals and for society as a whole.

Over the past several decades IQ test scores have been viewed with an increasingly skeptical eye. Concerns are commonly expressed about cultural bias, about the narrow range of abilities tested, and about the value of these tests for predicting success in both academic and nonacademic settings. Nevertheless, scores on IQ-like tests can have profound practical significance for an individual person. Most affected would be individuals with an ability test score that is, merely by chance, near one of the mostly arbitrary cutoff values routinely used to inform decisions about school placement, aptitude for college work, or opportunities for training and advancement in the workplace. For example, inevitably each year some proportion of high school students is denied access to college because of poor admission test scores. In some of those cases, an increase of only a few points on an IQ-like aptitude test would have allowed an otherwise qualified student the opportunity to obtain higher education. It is sobering to realize that early lead exposure, even at blood lead concentrations below the current level of concern, could be very costly to such a person.

The importance of a small adverse effect of lead also can be gauged by taking a societal or population perspective. **Figure 5** depicts the normal distributions of IQ scores for two groups of children. One distribution represents children drawn from a population not exposed to lead. The mean IQ of this unexposed group is 100. The second distribution represents the predicted IQ scores for a population of children who experienced average BLLs

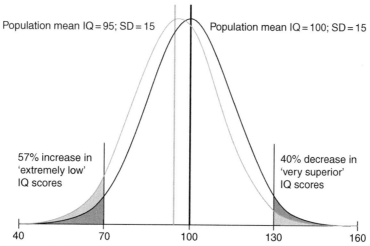

Figure 5 Population-level effects of lead exposure. Hypothetical distributions of IQ scores in two populations of children. The distribution shown by the black line represents children who are unaffected by lead exposure, and the distribution shown by the gray line represents children with a 5-point lead-induced decrease in IQ test scores. Note that a 5% difference in the population mean IQ is associated with a disproportionate difference at the tails of the distributions.

of about $10\,\mu g\,dl^{-1}$ during infancy and early childhood. The estimated mean IQ for that group, based on the combined evidence from the longitudinal cohort studies, is approximately 95. As illustrated in **Figure 5**, one consequence of this 5-point (5%) downward shift in IQ for the exposed group is a disproportionate (57%) increase in the number of children with IQ scores in the extremely low range (<70). An IQ test score less than 70 is consistent with the need to place a child in a special education program – an unfortunate necessity for the child and an approximate doubling of the cost for his or her education. Similarly, this 5% downward shift in the average IQ of a population would cause a disproportionate 40% reduction in the number of children who score in the very superior range (IQ > 130). An IQ score of 130 is often a requirement for access to accelerated courses in high school. Thus, a small effect of lead can be very costly for individuals and for society as a whole.

Summary

Despite the long and cheerless history of lead's detrimental effects on human health, the efforts of public health advocates over the past half-century have resulted in an impressive reduction in childhood exposure throughout most of the industrialized world. However, although lead exposure is almost entirely preventable, millions of children throughout the world continue to suffer the adverse effects of excessive exposure to this potent neurotoxin. The neurobehavioral effects of lead are subtle, but they can be detected in children with blood concentrations below the CDC definition of an elevated BLL, and they appear to be lasting. Moreover, efforts to restore cognitive function in lead-exposed children through medical treatment suggest little reason for optimism. The shared perspective of developmental psychologists and medical and public health specialists is that only through primary

prevention of lead exposure during gestation, infancy, and childhood is it possible to protect children from this ancient threat to human health.

See also: Developmental Disabilities: Cognitive; Neurological Development.

Suggested Readings

Agency for Toxic Substances and Disease Registry: ATSDR Toxicological Profile on Lead. http://www.atsdr.cdc.gov – (accessed on 14 July 2007).

Canfield RL, Henderson CR, Cory-Slechta DA, *et al.* (2003) Intellectual impairment in children with blood lead concentrations below 10 μg per deciliter. *The New England Journal of Medicine* 348: 1517–1526.

Centers for Disease Control and Prevention: Prevention of Lead Poisoning in Young Children. http://www.cdc.gov – (accessed on 14 July 2007).

Dietrich KN, Ware JH, Salganik M, *et al.* (2004) Treatment of Lead-Exposed Children Clinical Trial Group. Effect of chelation therapy on the neuropsychological and behavioral development of lead-exposed children after school entry. *Pediatrics* 114(1): 19–26.

Koller K, Brown T, Spurgeon A, and Levy L (2004) Recent developments in low-level lead exposure and intellectual impairment in children. *Environmental Health Perspectives* 112(9): 987–994.

Markowitz G and Rosner D (2000) Cater to the children: The role of the lead industry in a public health tragedy, 1900–1955. *American Journal of Public Health* 90: 36–46.

Relevant Websites

http://www.asmalldoseof.org – A Small Dose of Toxicology by Steven Gilbert, A Small Dose of Lead.

http://www.atsdr.cdc.gov – Agency for Toxic Substances and Disease Registry: ToxFAQs for Lead.

http://www.cdc.gov – US Center for Disease Control and Prevention (CDC). CDC Childhood Lead Poisoning Prevention Program.

http://www.hud.gov – US Department of Housing and Urban Development (HUD), Office of Healthy Homes and Lead Hazard Control.

http://sis.nlm.nih.gov – US National Library of Medicine Enviro-Health Links: Lead and Environmental Health.

Learning Disabilities

H Liang and E Simonoff, King's College London, London, UK

Glossary

Autosomal dominant – A form of genetic (Mendelian) inheritance in which a single copy of a mutant gene will cause the disorder. Autosomal dominant disorders affect both sexes equally and are passed from parent to child, on average in 50% of cases.

Autosomal recessive – A form of genetic (Mendelian) inheritance in which two copes of a mutant gene, one from each parent, are required to cause the disorder. Autosomal recessive disorders affect both sexes equally. Parents are usually unaffected carriers and each child has, on average, a 25% chance of developing the disorder.

Global learning disabilities – Learning disabilities that affect all domains of thinking or intellectual functioning. Sometimes referred to as mental retardation or intellectual disability.

Macrocephaly – An abnormally large head, compared to body size. This may indicate an underlying disorder that can be associated with learning disability.

Microcephaly – An abnormally small head compared to body size. This may indicate an underlying disorder that can be associated with learning disability.

Non-disjunction – A failure of the two chromosomes in a pair to split during cell division. This can lead to an abnormal complement of chromosomes in the offspring, causing disorders such as Trisomy 21, where there are three copies rather than the normal two of chromosome 21, causing Down syndrome.

Specific learning disabilities – Learning disabilities where overall intellectual functioning is within the normal range but where specific abilities, most commonly reading, spelling, and mathematics are operating at a level well below that predicted by overall ability.

Trisomy – Having three rather than the normal two chromosomes, one from each parent. The most common is Trisomy 21 or Down syndrome.

Twin concordance – The percentage of cases where, if one twin is affected with a disorder, the other twin is also affected. Differences in twin concordance rates between identical (monozygotic)) and non-identical (dizygotic) twins provide an index of how important genetic factors are in causing the disorder (heritability).

Variable expression – Some single gene (Mendelian) disorders show a range of expression among individuals with the same mutation, from few and mild signs to a very severe presentation. Mild cases may not be identified until another family member presents with a more severe condition.

X-inactivation – The X chromosome is present in two copies in females and only one in males (who also have a much smaller Y chromosome). During fetal development, one of the two X chromosomes becomes inactivated in females, ensuring that they have the same dose of gene products as males. This process occurs in each cell separately and is a random phenomenon.

X-linked – A form of genetic (Mendelian) inheritance in which the X chromosome carries the mutant gene. Because males have one X chromosome and females two, the disorder is usually apparent only in males while females are generally carriers passing on the mutant copy to their offspring.

Introduction

The field of learning disabilities is confused by a range of terminology, used in various ways. In this article, we are referring to 'global learning disabilities', which are also called 'mental retardation' or 'intellectual disability' and affect all domains of thinking or intellectual functioning. Global learning disability needs to be distinguished from 'specific learning disabilities', also referred to as (specific) 'learning difficulties', where overall intellectual functioning is within the normal range but where specific abilities, most commonly reading, spelling, and mathematics, are operating at a level well below that predicted by overall ability. In this article, we shall use the terms mental retardation and learning disability interchangeably. There are three major classification systems for mental retardation: the American Association of Mental Retardation (AAMR), the Diagnostic and Statistical Manual (DSM), and the International Classification of Diseases (ICD) (**Table 1**). All three systems require the presence of not only globally reduced intellectual functioning but also significant impairment in adaptive functioning, that is, the ability to function in an age-appropriate way in areas of everyday life including learning, working, enjoying relationships, caring for oneself, and living independently.

Intellectual functioning is usually assessed by tests of cognitive functioning that produce a measure called the intelligence quotient (IQ). The IQ is measured by tests that examine thinking and knowledge in a range of areas. These areas usually include both verbal skills such as vocabulary knowledge, the ability to understand conceptual similarities between words and short-term (working) memory for verbal material, and nonverbal skills, such as completing puzzles, identifying missing parts of pictures and completing pictorial sequences. Because ability to complete such tasks changes with age, IQ tests are standardized across a range of ages. The IQ is the mental age divided by chronological age multiplied by 100, where mental age refers to the average score achieved by children of a certain chronological age. Therefore, an IQ of 100 is average. The scores on IQ tests are usually standardized to produce normally distributed scores with not only a mean of 100 but also a standard deviation of 15. People with mental retardation are expected to have IQs at the extreme low end of the normal distribution of IQ.

Table 1   Classification of mental retardation

Classification of mental retardation International Classification of Diseases (World Health Organization, 1992)			Diagnostic and Statistical Manual-IV			American Academy of Mental Retardation (2002)	
General: Arrested or incomplete development of the mind, characterized by impairment of skills which contribute to the overall level of intelligence			General: Subaverage intellectual functioning that is accompanied by significant limitations in adaptive functioning in several (at least two) skill areas			General: Mental retardation is a disability characterized by significant limitations both in intellectual functioning and adaptive behavior, originating before age 18 years	
Term		Definition	Term		Definition	Statement	Component
Mild	F70	IQ 50–69	Mild	317.0	IQ 50/55–69		Mental retardation is a disability
Moderate	F71	IQ 35–49	Moderate	318.0	IQ 35/40–50/55	First requirement	Significant limitations in intellectual functioning
Severe	F72	IQ 20–34	Severe	318.1	IQ 20/25–35/40	Second requirement	Significant limitations in adaptive behavior as expressed in conceptual, social and practical adaptive skills
Profound	F73	IQ <20	Profound	318.2	IQ <20/25		
Other	F78		Unspecified	319.0			
Unspecified	F79						

Subheadings relating to behavioral impairment
.0   No or minimal behavioral impairment
.1   Significant behavioral impairment requiring attention or treatment
.8   Other behavioral impairment
.9   Without mention of behavioral impairment

IQ, intelligence quotient.

Degree or severity of mental retardation is largely classified by the IQ or an equivalent measure of intellectual ability. Mild mental retardation is defined in the ICD-10 and DSM-IV as IQ 50–69, moderate retardation as IQ 35–49, severe retardation as IQ 20–34, and profound retardation an IQ less than 20 (**Table 1**). IQ estimates are approximate and particularly difficult to measure precisely in more severely affected individuals. While the classification systems state that a criterion of impairment should also be met, none specify how this should be determined. Much of the epidemiological and biological research on mental retardation has collapsed the categories of moderate, severe, and profound retardation and referred to this group as having severe mental retardation.

Epidemiology

Using an IQ of less than 70 (2 standard deviations below the mean) as the criterion for learning disability or mental retardation should result in prevalence rates of 2.3% based on the properties of the normal distribution. Studies of mild mental retardation have produced widely varying prevalence estimates, however, from less than 0.5% to over 8%. There are at least several reasons for this variation. First, identification, or ascertainment, of the 'at risk' population affects the rate, with studies that survey the entire population producing higher rates than those relying on cases formally identified because of health or educational problems, as many people with IQs between 50 and 70 may not be formally registered. Second, the test administered may affect the rates identified. Because performance on IQ tests has improved over the years (a phenomenon called the Flynn effect), the use of older and 'easier' tests may produce a lower rate of learning disability. There may also be real differences in the rate of mental retardation across different populations, with more advantaged populations having lower rates of learning disability. Some of this population difference may be due to bias in test content, so that children from developed countries who attend school from an early age may be more familiar with the type of items on conventional IQ tests. However, use of the supposedly culture-fair test does not eliminate the differences in rates of learning disabilities.

For severe mental retardation, however, the reported prevalence rates have been more consistent and average around 0.4–0.5%, which is about 10 times greater than expected where the normal distribution maintained. This extra 'hump' at the bottom of the normal IQ distribution is likely to represent the children whose learning disabilities have a clear 'organic' origin whether caused prenatally, perinatally, or postnatally.

These findings have led to a suggestion of a 'two-group' approach to learning disability. The first group represents the lower end of a normally distributed population, for which no organic cause can be ascertained and encompasses the majority of children with mild learning disability. Environmental deprivation has classically been cited as the cause of cognitive delay in this group, although this is now criticized for being too simplistic. The second group consists of those children with defined organic or biological cause for their cognitive impairment, which may be more severe. Again, this is likely to be an oversimplification of the heterogeneity of learning disability, and as advances are made in molecular genetics, increasing numbers of children with mild learning disability are likely to be found to have genetic disorders. However, the division of learning disability into these two broad etiological groups has been a useful starting point for researchers in this field.

There is also criticism of the use of IQ as sole discriminator of learning disability for both epidemiological studies and administrative purposes. In terms of judging prevalence rates based on IQ, problems arise due to the fact that IQ may not remain stable throughout development and IQ scores in infancy typically have only low correlations with scores in later childhood. Further, researchers found that although once formal schooling begins IQ scores tend to be more robust, individual cases can still show major gains or losses in cognitive ability. Up to now, however, there has been no agreement on the way in which adaptive behavior should be measured and impairment defined to meet this additional criterion for diagnosis.

The term 'administrative prevalence' has been used to mean the numbers for whom services would be required in a community which made provision for all who needed them. Here again, using IQ alone as discriminator is inadequate as IQ scores do not correlate with social adaptation in all instances. Indeed, researchers found that although 2.5% of children in the study could be classified as having learning disability based on their IQ scores, only half of these children were sufficiently impaired in their daily lives to require the additional provision of services. Functional impairment is dependent not only on the child's developmental level, but on wider social issues of available family and community resources. Thus, it is unsurprising that administrative prevalence is somewhat higher in lower socioeconomic groups.

Gender differences are also apparent in the rates of learning disability with a male to female ratio of 1.5:1, which may reflect the male preponderance in certain genetically mediated disorders affecting cognitive ability. These differences are more clear-cut for those with severe learning disability.

Etiology

As suggested in the two-group approach, learning disability is heterogeneous and it is likely that multiple factors and their interaction contribute to its etiology. These factors can largely be divided into environmental and genetic factors.

Environmental Factors

Social factors

Learning disability is associated with adverse social conditions: low socioeconomic status, poverty, poor housing, and an unstable family environment. To establish whether this is a cause or consequence of learning disability, researchers endeavored to manipulate the outcomes for at risk children. A group of deprived children in residential care were given a special education provision and these children were found to have higher IQ scores compared to a control group 20 years later. Indeed, positive social environmental influences may increase IQ scores by as much as 20 points. However, other studies indicate that environmental enrichment may not 'normalize' IQ, so that deprived children receiving enrichment do better on IQ tests and measures of educational attainment than deprived children without enrichment but less well than advantaged children. Large-scale projects aimed at early environmental enrichment, such as Head start, have suggested that the improvements in IQ may be short term only, although there may be wider benefits of such programs for overall development.

Obstetric factors

Pregnancy and birth factors have traditionally been thought of as important causes of learning disability. Indeed fetal alcohol syndrome, associated with maternal alcohol consumption in pregnancy, can cause up to 10% of mild learning disability. Intrauterine infections (including rubella, toxoplasmosis, cytomegalovirus, and herpes) are recognized causes of learning disability in the offspring. Maternal malnutrition and irradiation during pregnancy may increase the risk of learning disability, particularly during vulnerable periods of fetal brain development. Prematurity and low birth weight have been associated with learning disability, but earlier studies estimating that clinically recognizable birth injuries accounted for about 10% of learning disability have fallen out of favor. The relationship to severe prematurity, for example, 32 weeks' gestation or less, birth weight less than 2500 g, and significant anoxia during delivery remains clear, and is often associated with abnormalities observed on brain scans. However, the relationship to more subtle obstetric adversity is less certain. Studies finding a link between milder obstetric adversity and later developmental delay have not adequately addressed whether there is a direct link or whether minor obstetric adversity is indexing other factors that are responsible for the association. Babies born with genetic disorders associated with learning disability, such as Down syndrome and

Prader–Willi syndrome, have increased rates of mild obstetric adversity, presumably due to fetal abnormalities. Thus, it cannot be differentiated whether the adversity resulted in learning disability, or that existing fetal brain abnormalities led to complications at birth. Current thinking supports the latter explanation. Furthermore, some of the milder obstetric adversity is more common in mothers from socially disadvantaged backgrounds, who may themselves have lower cognitive ability, raising the possibility that obstetric adversity is a confounder.

Other environmental factors

Postnatally, important environmental factors include lead poisoning, meningitis, malnutrition, and hypothyroidism (e.g., due to iodine deficiency). Severe or prolonged seizures, head injury, brain tumors and their treatment, and brain irradiation are all causes of acquired learning disability. While these factors are less significant causes of learning disability in developed countries compared to genetic, social, and perinatal factors, these environmental factors are the main causes of learning disability in developing countries and malnutrition in the first 2 years of life is probably the most common cause of learning disability worldwide.

Genetic Factors

Genetic factors can cause or contribute to learning disability in different ways. Some specific genes are recognized to cause particular syndromes which present with cognitive impairment. More complex genetic influences involving the operation of multiple genes or the interaction of genetic vulnerability with the environment may also play a part.

As advances in medical genetics have been made, over 100 genetic disorders that present with learning disability as a symptom have been identified. Most of these are extremely rare, but some such as Down syndrome and fragile X syndrome are relatively common. They also provide good examples of chromosomal and single-gene abnormalities that can lead to learning disability.

Chromosomal abnormalities

Chromosomal abnormalities can cause learning disability. Down syndrome is the most common single cause of severe learning disability, accounting for up to a third of all cases and occurring in 1 in 600 live births. A trisomy (having three rather than two copies) of chromosome 21 due to nondisjunction is the cause of 95% of Down syndrome, with the remaining 5% due to translocations and mosiaicism. Nondysjunction is associated with increasing maternal age, and hence, the incidence of Down syndrome in older mothers is increased. Children with Down syndrome have distinct physical features (e.g., short stature, small head, round face, and epicanthic folds)

in association with cognitive impairment and frequently cardiac and gut abnormalities.

Having too many sex chromosomes (XXY males, XYY males, and XXX females), or too few (XO females) may also cause learning disability to varying extents. More subtle deletions and rearrangements of chromosomal material, invisible under the microscope but identifiable with DNA probes, called microdeletions, have been demonstrated in several conditions, including William's syndrome, Smith–Magenis syndrome, and velo-cardio-facial syndrome. These can now be diagnosed reliably using a laboratory technique called fluorescent *in situ* hybridization (FISH). In addition to being implicated in causing distinct syndromes, researchers found that subtle chromosomal abnormalities were present in 7% of children with moderate to severe learning disability compared to 0.5% of children with only mild mental impairment. These as yet unidentified abnormalities may be an important cause of learning disability.

Single gene effects

After Down syndrome, fragile X syndrome is probably the next most common cause of learning disability and occurs in 1 in 2000 males and 1 in 4000 females, and is the most common to be inherited (because Down syndrome is usually not inherited). Fragile X syndrome is caused by an expanded triplet repeat of DNA sequence (CGG) on the X-chromosome (Xq27.3). X-inactivation of one of the two X syndrome chromosomes in girls explains the reduced prevalence in females. It is thought that the expanded triplet repeat interferes with the transcription of the gene *FMR1*, whose protein product familial mental retardation protein (FMRP) is thought to be important in regulating proteins important in brain signaling pathways. Fragile X syndrome largely causes moderate learning disability, but can present with mild learning disability or normal intelligence. Its associated physical features in males include large protruding ears, long face, prominent jaw, and enlarged testicles. Because the expansion of the triplet repeat DNA sequence occurs over the course of generations (but only in female germ cells), it is common for the phenotype, or outward characteristics, to appear *de novo*.

Rett syndrome is another X-linked disorder that only occurs in females because the presence of the Rett mutation in the *MECP2* gene is lethal in males. However, other mutations have been identified in the *MECP2* gene causing a range of syndromes associated with mild to moderate learning disability and frequently also spasticity. It is uncertain how prevalent these mutations are but it has been suggested that they may be as common as fragile X in causing learning disability. There are a large number of other X-linked mutations associated with learning disability and, as single gene causes of learning disability, they appear to be disproportionately represented.

Autosomal recessive disorders causing learning disability include phenylketonuria and a range of other metabolic disorders. Many of the autosomal dominant disorders show either high rates of spontaneous new mutations, such as in tuberose sclerosis, or variable expression, as in neurofibromatosis, consistent with the reduced reproduction rates in people with significant learning disability.

Imprinting effects
Some genetic abnormalities vary in the features depending upon whether the mutation is maternally or paternally derived. Prader–Willi and Angelman syndromes are two genetic disorders with distinct characteristics. Prader–Willi syndrome is associated with mild learning disability (and nonverbal ability may be in the normal range), early hypotonia, small hands, and feet. Characteristic features include compulsive overeating, skin-picking, and emotional lability. Angelman syndrome, on the other hand, is associated with severe to profound learning disability, epilepsy, an abnormal gait, and jerky movements. Both disorders are caused by abnormalities in the same region of chromosome 15, and may occur where this area is deleted in one of the chromosomes. However, Prader–Willi syndrome occurs where the deletion is from the chromosome of paternal origin and Angelman syndrome where it is of maternal origin.

Multiple gene effects
Many family, twin, and adoption studies have consistently shown that polygenic inheritance (such as that involved in other attributes such as height) is important in determining IQ within the normal range. In comparison, surprisingly few studies have investigated polygenic inheritance in learning disability. Available evidence, however, points toward a moderate role for genetic factors.

One study of siblings of learning disability children found that siblings of mildly impaired children also tended to have lower than average IQ scores. The familial component of mild learning disability is further supported by a study of the families of people with mild learning disability. This showed that if one parent has mild learning disability, the risk of a similar diagnosis in their offspring was 20%. If both parents were affected, almost half their children would also suffer from mild learning disability. These findings show that mild learning disability runs in families and suggests genetic factors may have a role.

In the first major twin study of mild learning disability, including a sample of 3886 twins, twin concordances were 74% for monozygotic (identical) twins, 45% for same-sex disygotic twins, and 36% for opposite-sex dizygotic (fraternal) twins, indicating substantial genetic influence. Group heritability (the amount of variance in the phenotype, learning disability that is explained by genetic

factors) was about 50%. These results suggest that mild learning disability is genetically influenced and is therefore a good target for research on global brain function and dysfunction.

In contrast to findings for mild learning disability, in the same sibling study mentioned above, siblings of moderately and severely impaired children were found to have average intelligence. New gene mutations and chromosomal abnormalities or environmental insults (such as those described above) could explain the nonfamilial nature of moderate and severe learning disability. This lends support to the two-group approach suggesting that mild learning disability is familial, possibly representing the lower tail of intelligence which is determined by polygenic inheritance, while moderate and severe learning disability is nonfamilial and could represent the 'hump' of learning disability caused by biological factors.

Gene–Environment Interplay

Interplay between genes and environment in learning difficulties is likely to be very common but it is difficult to detect until individual susceptibility genes are identified. However, the role of family stress on behavioral problems in boys with fragile X syndrome has been documented, highlighting that even disorders caused by a single gene are influenced by environmental factors.

Clinical Features of Learning Disability

Typically, learning disability affects all aspects of cognitive ability (learning, memory, problem-solving, language) uniformly; however, it is not uncommon for some children to have a more varied profile of ability. Identifying particular weaknesses can help predict areas where the child may struggle and require extra assistance in order to prevent frustration and the consequent behavioral problems which may result.

Of children with learning disability, the vast majority (85%) will have mild disorder. Moderate learning difficulty children account for 10%, with severely and profoundly affected children accounting for 3–4% and 1–2%, respectively. Children with mild learning disability are often unremarkable in appearance and with only slight motor or sensory deficits if any. Their language and social behavior develop close to normally and they are able to manage activities of daily living independently. They are often undiagnosed and attend mainstream schools without extra educational provision, albeit many may feel that they have to struggle to keep up at school. Of the moderately learning disabled, receptive language skills are often superior to expressive language, which is often easier for carers to understand than strangers. Use of simplified signing systems, such as Makaton or picture exchange, may be useful in this group to allay the frustrations of being misunderstood. Activities of daily living can usually be mastered with rehearsal and time in these children. In contrast, children with severe and profound learning disability will usually require close supervision at all times. Severely learning disabled children may be able to learn simple activities of daily living with supervision and may be able to communicate basic needs. In the profound group, support and supervision are generally required for all activities of daily living, and function in all domains is equivalent to that of a 1-year-old child.

Behavioral Phenotypes

On studying children with particular syndromes associated with learning disability, certain nonadaptive behaviors have been commonly identified in affected children. Such behaviors include hand-wringing in Rett syndrome, voracious eating in Prader–Willi syndrome, bouts of inappropriate laughter in Angelman syndrome, self-injury in Lesch–Nyhan and Cornelia de Lange syndrome, self-hugging in Smith–Magenis syndrome and a shrill cat-like cry in Cri-du-chat syndrome. For these and other syndromes, there appears to be a strong correlation between the behavior and the syndrome. As the genetic basis of these syndromes is known, research is now focused on identifying the links between the genetic basis and the phenotypic behavior shown. Not only will elucidation of the pathway from gene to abnormal behavior gain greater understanding of the syndrome and brain function in general, but offer potential avenues for treatment.

Further study has shown that other behaviors appear to span a variety of syndromes. Inattention and hyperactivity are frequent in fragile X syndrome, William's syndrome; sequential processing deficits are common in fragile X and Prader–Willi syndromes. Individuals with velo-cardio-facial syndrome have a markedly increased rate of psychosis. Thus, a number of syndromes have distinctive but not necessarily unique behavioral features. Dykens suggests that such behavioral phenotypes involve an increased probability or likelihood that people with a given syndrome will show certain behavioral features relative to those without the syndrome. Researchers are now also beginning to study such 'between-syndrome' behavioral phenotypes: examining genetic, environmental, and psychosocial correlates which may predispose to the observed behaviors. The identification of behavioral phenotypes and its study is a move forward from the broad two-group approach and has allowed finer dissection and closer examination of the etiology of learning disability in particular syndromes.

Common Comorbities

Associated problems, or comorbid conditions, are common in learning disability. The cause of the learning disability may have a range of effects on the brain and other organ systems. Other central nervous system disorders are frequent. Cerebral palsy is frequently associated with learning disability. Epilepsy is much increased occurring in some 20–30% of children with learning disability compared to 1% of the general population. The seizures often begin in the first few years of life in those with learning disability as opposed to a later onset in other people.

Children with learning disability are more likely to have motor, hearing, and vision problems. Some of these may be immediately apparent, such as severe cerebral palsy, blindness, and deafness. Although individuals with some syndromes and/or more severe learning disability are particularly likely to have such impairments (so that about 50% of those with Down syndrome have hearing problems), the rates of such problems are also increased in those with mild learning disability (with hearing problems occurring in about 20% and visual impairment in about 4%). However, many deficits are more subtle and are unlikely to be detected unless routine screening is undertaken. Children with learning disabilities are also more likely to have chronic physical health problems requiring increased medical treatment, and are more likely to miss school because of such problems. This may add to poor educational attainments.

Almost all child psychiatric problems are substantially increased in children with learning disabilities but Emerson showed that autism and attention deficit hyperactivity disorder (ADHD) are those most strongly associated with lower IQ. Between 50% and 75% of people with autism also have an IQ less than 70 and the mean IQ among children with ADHD is about 7–12 points below the general population. Other emotional problems, such as anxiety, depression and obsessive-compulsive disorder, and conduct problems, such as oppositional defiant disorder, are more frequently seen in children with learning disability. While delinquent problems and conduct disorder are more common in those with borderline low and mild learning disabilities, those with moderate and severe learning disabilities are relatively protected from such problems at least in part become they are more socially isolated. However, less organized aggression is common in children with moderate to severe learning disability. In addition, as learning disability becomes more severe, it is increasingly difficult to identify psychiatric disorders as they are expressed in typically developing children. This is partly because children with significant learning disability may lack the communication skills to describe their emotional state. Behavior may seem odd or unpredictable because parents and carers are unaware of the child's experiences and internal mental state. In addition, there are also some behavioral problems that are almost exclusive to the learning disability population; these include certain forms of self-injury (biting, chewing skin-picking, eye-poking) and pica (eating nonfood material).

Children with global learning disabilities are not exempted from having specific learning disabilities such as reading and spelling problems (dyslexia) but such problems are often less likely to be identified. A diagnosis of a specific learning disability requires that the problems in that area exceed what is expected based on overall intellectual functioning. Children are not generally expected to have achieved many reading milestones before the age of 7 years, so that children with a mental age of less than this age will not be recognized as having dyslexia. However, with children and young adults functioning at a higher mental age, the possibility of specific learning disabilities exists, especially if they are struggling with basic numeracy and literacy despite an appropriate educational placement.

Assessment

Assessment starts from the point of referral. From here it is important to establish why the referral has been made and who has raised concern. Parents and teachers are usually good judges of a child's ability level and can often give a good estimate as to the child's developmental level. Even so, sometimes a child's ability can be misjudged; in particular, where the cognitive profile is varied, strengths in one area may allow the child to hide weaknesses in others. Teacher and parental expectations may differ and, again, lead to differences in their judgments of developmental level. It is also useful to consider the timing of the referral. Children with mild learning disability often only present when they are older and are referred for emotional or behavioral problems (somewhat

often consequent to their learning disability) rather than for developmental delay. Any pre-existing family beliefs and expectations should also be evaluated.

Assessment of learning disability is largely directed at three areas: (1) establishing etiology of the learning disability; (2) establishing level of cognitive function, adaptive behavior and social skills; and (3) assessing for the presence of any comorbid psychiatric and physical difficulties (**Table 2**).

Assessment of Etiology

Establishing any underlying etiology for learning disability is dependent on a thorough history and physical examination. The history should pay particular attention to any family history of inherited disorders and abnormalities in the pregnancy or birth of the child, including maternal alcohol consumption. A full developmental history including milestones should be taken as well as documentation of any associated medical conditions such as congenital defects, epilepsy, and cerebral palsy. The physical examination should include observation for dysmorphic features and neurocutaneous skin signs. Relevant dysmorphic features include the round face and up-slanting eyes of Down syndrome and the long face and prominent ears of fragile X syndrome. Relevant skin signs include the neurofibromata of neurofibromatosis, adenoma sebaceum of tuberose sclerosis and port-wine stain of Sturge-Weber. Examination under Wood's lamp for typical ash-leaf like skin patterns may be required if tuberose sclerosis is suspected. Head circumference, height, and weight should be documented against standardized gender-specific norms, certain conditions being associated

Table 2   Features of the assessment of learning disability that aid identification of etiology, developmental level, and associated comorbidity

	History	*Examination and investigations*
Etiology	<ul><li>Family history of inherited disorders</li><li>Pregnancy and birth abnormalities</li><li>Developmental history including milestones</li><li>Medical history</li></ul>	<ul><li>Examination of dysmorphic features and neurocutaneous skin signs</li><li>Measurement of head circumference, height, and weight</li><li>Neurological examination</li><li>Neuroimaging, electroencephalogram, and genetic testing may be indicated</li></ul>
Developmental level	<ul><li>School reports and previous psychological reports should be sought</li><li>Parental estimate of developmental level is often an accurate predictor</li></ul>	<ul><li>General standardized psychometric testing (e.g., Wechsler Intelligence Scales for Children, Mullen Scales, Vineland Adaptive Behavior Scales)</li><li>Additional specific tests may be indicated (e.g., Autism Diagnostic Interview)</li></ul>
Associated comorbidity	<ul><li>Systematic review of symptoms (e.g. inattention, overactivity, impulsivity, eating, sleeping, emotional and behavioral difficulties)</li><li>Structured instruments (e.g., Strengths and Difficulties Questionnaire, Conners' Rating Scales) may be helpful</li><li>Good behavioral examples should be sought</li></ul>	<ul><li>Behavioral observation in clinic setting</li><li>Behavioral observation in school setting</li></ul>

with macrocephaly (autism), microcephely (cri-du-chat, fetal alcohol syndrome), short stature (Down syndrome), and tall stature (Soto syndrome). A neurological examination is also important, and should include assessment of vision, hearing, coordination, and gait. Asymmetry in motor skill, tone, reflexes, or limb size may suggest hemisphere dysfunction or other pathology. Specialist assessment of hearing and vision should be undertaken if there is any suspicion that these are abnormal.

Investigations may need to be undertaken to supplement history and examination findings. This may include neuroimaging, electroencephalogram, and genetic testing for chromosomal abnormalities, fragile X syndrome or metabolic diseases. The likelihood of finding a medical condition is greatest in children with severe and profound learning disabilities.

Assessment of Developmental Level

Cognitive assessment by an educational or clinical psychologist using standardized psychometric tests is invaluable in assessing learning disability. Ingenuity and patience are required to allow a child to maintain interest and perform at their best. Tests should be selected to suit the expected developmental level of the child and start with tasks well within the child's capabilities to avoid early frustration. A variety of psychometric tests have been developed, among the most popular being the Wechsler Intelligence Scales for Children and the Stanford-Binet. Whenever possible both nonverbal and verbal aspects of ability should be assessed as these may vary and building on a child's strengths can promote their development. In some cases, a test that has not been standardized for the child's developmental age is the most appropriate; this will produce age equivalents, which can be used to give a ratio IQ [(age equivalent ÷ chronological age) × 100]. Although the latter may be less accurate, it nevertheless gives a broad estimate of the child's level of functioning. On occasion, it is not possible to gain a child's cooperation in testing; in such instances an assessment based on parent/carer report of skills, such as the Vineland Adaptive Behavior Scales, will give an estimate of a child's functional level. The results of such testing should always be evaluated in the light of all other available information. Further standardized tests are also available for specific developmental problems and neuropsychological deficits, such as reading, language, problem solving, or social development.

Assessment of Comorbidity

A systematic approach should be taken to the assessment of possible comorbid problems, including physical disorders, psychiatric problems, and additional cognitive impairments. Close liaison with pediatricians caring for the child is essential as many physical problems may present in unusual ways, including as an exacerbation of or new behavioral difficulties. Children with learning disability are at increased risk of a range of psychiatric disorders as well as emotional and behavioral difficulties. It is more difficult to identify comorbid conditions in children with learning disabilities as they may not be able to express difficulties as well as other children. Further, comorbid psychiatric diagnoses are often underdiagnosed in this group of children as it is often assumed that their difficulties are due to the underlying learning disability. A systematic review of symptoms in the history, including symptoms such as inattention, overactivity, impulsivity, and eating, sleeping, emotional, and behavioral difficulties should be conducted. Structured instruments such as the Children's Behavior Checklist (CBC-L), the Strengths and Difficulties Questionnaire, and the Conners' Rating Scales may be administered to parents as an aid to identifying and assessing difficulties. Scales particularly designed for children with learning disability include the Developmental Behavior Checklist and the Aberrant Behavior Checklist. Behavioral observation is an important tool and parents should be asked for specific behavioral examples in the history. Careful observational assessment of the child in clinic or school setting may also be beneficial.

Treatment

Treatment should focus on two areas: learning disability and comorbid conditions. As treatment options for learning disability are limited, identification of comorbid disorders, which play a key role in overall morbidity, becomes a priority.

Treatment of Learning Disability

Prevention is one of the most important aspects of learning disability and treatment. In relation to prenatal care, healthy pregnancy and delivery can significantly reduce the rate of mental retardation due to obstetric factors and is likely to be one reason why there are lower rates of mental retardation in developed countries with national health systems. The identification of potential genetic disorders either prior to conception or during early pregnancy allows prospective parents greater choice in their family choices. However, many genetic disorders are impractical to identify prenatally. Where prenatal testing is possible, it is unclear that additional active population-based screening, for example for fragile X syndrome, would lead to a significant reduction in the number of cases. However, genetic testing for high risk groups, such as Ashkenazi Jews at risk of Tay-Sachs disease, or cascade screening of at-risk relatives of affected people, as in fragile X syndrome, can reduce genetic disorders causing mental retardation in targeted groups. Population-based postnatal screening is practical where the test is automated and straightforward to interpret, and most importantly where early detection has treatment implications. Hence, population screening for phenyl-ketonuria and hypothyroidism has been implemented in many countries. Malnutrition is rare in developed countries and most likely to occur in the context of other medical problems but routine infant healthcare is important in its identification.

The underpinnings of any treatment for learning disability include clear identification of the overall level of functioning, along with areas of strength and weakness, as these will aid in appropriate educational placement and psychoeducation for the family and other carers. Policies regarding education in mainstream vs. special schools/units have varied across time and countries. There is almost certainly a place for both alternatives. In either instance, the objective is to provide an individual educational plan that builds on the student's areas of strength. Education should also ensures the student achieves his potential both scholastically and in life skills. Very often those with milder degrees of learning disabilities will benefit from at least some attendance in mainstream classes to allow participation in less academic subjects and to mix with peers, to extend their social skills. However those with severe learning disability, particularly at secondary levels of education, may require a differentiated curriculum and may also have different social needs, so that mainstream education is unlikely to meet their needs. Educational goals and placement should be reviewed regularly.

Providing parents and other carers with as much information as possible will help them to set realistic goals. Many parents have difficulty in coming to terms with their child's mental retardation and may need considerable support in understanding and accepting the situation. As the child gets older, the gap in comparison to typically developing children widens (a 4-year-old child with an IQ of 50 roughly behaves like a child of 2 years of age while a 16-year-old child with an IQ of 50 behaves like a child of 8 years of age), so the developmental abnormalities often become more apparent with age. In addition, parents frequently require additional support at certain points in development. Children with learning disability (and especially those with autism) have difficulty coping with their emerging sexual feelings during puberty. At a time when increased privacy and independence is the norm for typically developing children, those with learning disability may not have attained sufficient awareness for parents to allow this.

Parents often find it helpful to know the cause of mental retardation, where it has been identified. Often societies exist for particular disorders to provide information and support to families and are usually perceived as extremely helpful. Where a cause has not been identified

or no such group exists, the voluntary organizations focusing on families affected by mental retardation and disability can offer a similar role. There is also an important role for social services in providing family assistance, including respite care. The family should be supported in engaging in the full range of family activities, including time alone for the adults and also with their other children. While siblings may benefit from taking a caring role in relation to a child with learning disability, they are also likely to get less attention and nurturing from their parents.

Treatment of Associated Problems

As mental problems are increased in children with learning disability, professionals should be alert for early signs. The evidence for prevention, for example, by behavioral advice and support to parents, is limited. Although it is unlikely to be harmful, it is uncertain whether prevention and early intervention services are effective or efficient. However, in certain instances, alerting parents to common problems and how to prevent them may reduce their incidence. For example, in disorders such as Cornelia de Lange syndrome where self-injury is common, informing parents about the early signs and describing appropriate management strategies may help to avoid serious problems.

When they present, emotional and behavioral problems should always be systematically assessed, looking for comorbidities as well as identifying the main problem. In most instances, there is limited evidence for treatment efficacy specifically for children with learning disability and treatment choices will be similar to those without learning disability. Where behavioral treatments are to be used, appropriate modification should be made for the child's cognitive level, including simple explanations to the child, use of visual as well as verbal prompts, and immediate and frequent reinforcement of behavior. Generalization of treatment is often more difficult for children with learning disability so consistency across home, school and other situations is especially important. Cognitive-behavioral approaches can sometimes be successfully simplified to work directly with children, but parallel intervention with parents so they can reinforce the treatment between sessions is usually necessary. Pharmacotherapy has a place but the increased sensitivity of the brains of children with learning disability to both beneficial and adverse effects should be borne in mind. Initial low doses, cautious increases and frequent monitoring for adverse effects should be the rule.

As physical health problems are more common in children with mental retardation, regular reviews should be undertaken by a pediatrician with expertise in their examination and treatment. Dental care also requires personnel with expertise and patience in achieving compliance. A frequent cause of new or exacerbations in behavior problems, where no environmental precipitant can be identified, is a physical problem causing pain.

Prognosis

Parents frequently want information about their child's longer-term prospects, particularly about the ability to live independently, work, and have intimate relationships in adult life. Prediction about adult outcome can be difficult in early childhood as developmental trajectories may vary. Some conditions, such as Down syndrome and fragile X syndrome, may show a plateau in development in late adolescence or early adult life. In part, this may reflect that the type of new cognitive abilities acquired by typically developing adolescents involve a higher level of abstraction that is not achievable with certain forms of learning disability. About one-third of people with Down syndrome will develop early onset Alzheimer's disease, usually in their 40s. In other instances, people may continue to develop new skills and cognitive abilities well into adult life. Often by late childhood or early adolescence it is possible to make more specific predictions about the degree of adult independent living anticipated and this is very helpful for families in longer-term planning.

Physical health remains poorer amongst those with learning disability. In part, this is due to the physical problems associated with the underlying causes of mental retardation but also aspects of the life style of people with learning disability increase their risk of poor health; opportunities for exercise are reduced and obesity is common. However, tobacco, alcohol and substance use/misuse are less common, especially amongst those with severe retardation. The health needs of those with learning disability are more likely to go untreated and in many countries transfer from pediatric to adult healthcare is associated with the cessation of regular health reviews and screening.

Research Directions

Research into the molecular basis of learning and cognition is likely to make significant advances in the next decade. Alongside animal models of genetic defects that affect cognition, these should have important implications for human learning disability. However, previous experience with nonbrain-based disorders has shown that applications of such knowledge, for example, through gene and stem cell therapy, present a new and different set of challenges. While it is likely that such interventions will have a role in treatment and prevention, of learning disability the extent of their applicability is uncertain. For this reason, research should continue to focus on

prevention, both through pre-pregnancy and prenatal identification of single gene mutations and also the reduction in environmental factors causing learning disability. The latter involves higher-quality universal healthcare in both Western and developing countries and also better public education in relation to the effects on the fetus and child of maternal alcohol and substance use and the importance of regular prenatal care. In developing countries, adequate nutrition and protection from infectious disease can play an important role in prevention.

For those with learning disability, future research needs to focus on better prevention and treatment of associated physical and mental health problems. Such research needs to include both basic science components aimed at exploring the underlying causes of associated disorders and also applications that focus on effective treatment strategies. The latter approaches should consider the challenges of improving identification of comorbid conditions. Finally, there is a strong need for research involving people affected with learning disability to discover their priorities for health, education and social services. Frequently the extra effort required to communicate effectively with people with learning disability interferes with the process of discovering their own service priorities and identifying the factors that impair their quality of life. While each of these research areas presents many challenges, the rewards of meeting these to reduce the burden of learning disability are great.

See also: ADHD: Genetic Influences; Autism Spectrum Disorders; Cerebral Palsy; Developmental Disabilities: Cognitive; Down Syndrome; Fetal Alcohol Spectrum Disorders; Fragile X Syndrome; Genetic Disorders: Sex Linked; Genetic Disorders: Single Gene; Intellectual Disabilities; Mental Health, Infant; Teratology.

Suggested Readings

Dykens EM (2000) Psychopathology in children with intellectual disability. *Journal of Child Psychology and Psychiatry* 41: 407–418.

Knight SJ, Regan R, Nicod A, Horsley SW, Kearney L, and Homfray T (1999) Subtle chromosomal rearrangements in children with unexplained mental retardation. *Lancet* 354(9191): 1676–1681.

O'Connor TG (2003) Early experiences and psychological development: Conceptual questions, empirical illustrations, and implications for intervention. *Development & Psychopathology* 15(3): 671–690.

Rutter M, Graham P, and Yule W (1970) *A Neuropsychiatric Study in Childhood.* London: Spastics International Medical Publications.

Simonoff E, Bolton P, and Rutter M (1996) Mental retardation: genetic findings, clinical implications and research agenda. *Journal of Child Psychology and Psychiatry* 37: 259–280.

Sternberg RJ (2004) Culture and intelligence. *American Psychologist* 59 (5): 325–338.

Tizard JP (1975) Etiology of mental retardation. *Proceedings of the Royal Society of Medicine* 68(9): 561.

Zigler E, Balla D, and Hodapp R (1984) On the definition and classification of mental retardation. *American Journal of Mental Deficiency* 89: 215–230.

Mental Health, Infant

P D Zeanah, M M Gleason, and C H Zeanah, Tulane University Health Sciences Center, New Orleans, LA, USA

Glossary

DC:0–3R – The revised edition of the *Diagnostic Classification of Mental Health and Developmental Disorders of Infancy and Early Childhood*, published by Zero to Three in 2005. This document was developed by an advocacy and professional development organization to specify criteria for disorders of early childhood because of the belief that DSM-IV-TR did not adequately describe the problems seen in young children.

DSM-IV-TR – The fourth edition (text revision) of the *Diagnostic and Statistical Manual of Mental Disorders*, published by the American Psychiatric Association in 2000. This document specifies criteria used in the diagnosis of psychiatric disorders. The criteria are developed by expert committees who review relevant research and use it to inform the criteria.

Neuronal synapses – The connections between the axon of one neuron (nerve cell) and the dendrite of another in which neurotransmitters are released and taken up as electrical impulses are discharged.

RDC-PA – This document, the 'Research diagnostic criteria – preschool age', was published in the *Journal of the American Academy of Child and Adolescent Psychiatry* in 2003 and describes criteria for early childhood disorders. The purpose was to modify existing DSM-IV-TR criteria so that they could be applied to young children with a degree of specificity that would help investigators achieve uniformity in studies of early childhood disorders.

Strange situation procedure – A laboratory paradigm involving a young child, a caregiver (parent), and an adult who is unfamiliar to the child (the stranger). The procedure involves a series of episodes in which the child's behavior with the caregiver (parent) is compared with the child's behavior with the stranger. Based on the child's behavior, the child's attachment to the caregiver (parent) is classified as secure, avoidant, resistant, or disorganized. Each of these types or patterns of attachment is preceded by certain patterns of interaction and predictive of subsequent outcomes in the child. The attachment classification may vary with different caregivers (parents) and is thought to reflect a characteristic of the relationship rather than a characteristic of the child.

Strengths perspective – In clinical work, the conscious attempt to discover strengths in individuals, families, and situations that may be used as the clinician attempts to reduce or eliminate problems or risks. This does not mean overlooking problems, vulnerabilities, or weaknesses, but rather, not focusing on them exclusively.

Introduction

There is more interest at present in infant mental health than ever before. In part this is because enhanced infant survival in the developed world has shifted focus to quality of life issues. This interest has been bolstered by unprecedented gains in scientific advances in our understanding of early life experiences and the impact of these early experiences on later social, emotional, and cognitive development. Neuroscientific advances have begun to address how experiences affect brain development (and vice versa), increasing interest in the kinds of experiences that lead to adaptive and maladaptive outcomes.

Definitions

Although there are a number of ways to think about infant mental health, it is usually considered to be essentially synonymous with healthy social and emotional development. It has been defined as the developing capacities to experience, regulate, and express emotions; to form close interpersonal relationships; to explore the environment; and to learn in the first 3 years. In this definition, infant mental health must be considered in the context of family, community, and cultural expectations for young children. This definition incorporates a broad range of risk and protective factors that impact current and future functioning and development.

In addition, infant mental health is relationship-focused; that is, the infant's dependence on the caregiver means that any interventions undertaken to either enhance development or address problems must consider the caregiver's capacity to care for the infant, as well as the psychological 'fit' between the infant and caregiver. Infant mental health is also intergenerational in approach. In addition to attending to both parent and infant, the parents own sense of their childhood relationships, as well as ongoing interactions with their family of origin are often central to work with infants and their families. Clinical efforts are likely to be aimed at parents or extended family members in addition to the infant. Further, infant mental health is culturally bound, with different values defined by different cultures about childrearing.

Infant mental health is also prevention-oriented; activities are aimed at enhancing normal development and preventing problems from getting worse or from disrupting normal developmental trajectories. In this sense, it may be considered health promoting as well as distress alleviating.

Infant mental health has traditionally been transdisciplinary – enriched by the frameworks and perspectives of numerous professional disciplines that contribute to our understanding of the early experience of children. As an integrative discipline, infant mental health involves all professionals who work toward strengthening social and emotional development of young children and their families, and it is not synonymous with any specific discipline.

For some, the term infant mental health – if not the idea mental health in infancy – is objectionable. The discomfort may come from several sources: a negative association of mental health with major mental illnesses, a more general cultural issue of stigma related to mental health (e.g., many hospitals now have behavioral health units rather than mental health or psychiatric units), or a belief that the earliest years are carefree and innocent.

It is likely that even those who object to the term can agree on a shared goal of fostering healthy development for our youngest and most vulnerable citizens. Nevertheless, there are those who find it difficult to imagine that infants and toddlers can have mental health problems. They discuss risk factors for later disorders rather than disorders *per se*, or prefer to focus on problem behaviors rather than psychiatric symptomatology. Some suggest using the term infant well-being as a strengths-based approach to describe early childhood social–emotional development. Well-being, however, does not capture the actual experience of many young children who do suffer, nor is it particularly helpful in guiding us in how to enhance early experience. Thus, this article is written from the perspective that the construct of infant mental health is both clinically useful and developmentally important.

Further definition of some terms is necessary to facilitate this discussion. In infant mental health, infancy is considered the first 3 years of life or so. Typically in American culture, infancy is considered to be the first year of life, so infant mental health requires a broadening of that view. While we recognize that influences on the child's early development begin prior to birth, and extend through adolescence, the first 3 years represent the period of the most rapid developmental gains in the human life span. The term developing capacity refers to the enormity and rapidity of growth and development during the first 3 years of life. Finally, we emphasize that an exclusive focus on the infant alone is untenable, as the needs of parent and child in their many family, environmental, and cultural contexts are all a part of the focus of infant mental health.

Development

As noted above, the developmental gains during the first three years of life are exceptional. Normal newborns are capable of recognizing their caregiver (at a sensory level), and have basic modes of communicating with their caregiver. Over the first few months of life, they begin to discriminate caregivers, express a variety of emotions, and are increasingly able to communicate needs. By age 3 years, they have developed strategies for learning, and are able to engage in complex interactions with peers, including cooperating with and showing empathy for others, and have some abilities to initiate and to resolve conflicts.

Though there is a wide range of what is considered normal, there is also increasing understanding of how delays and deviations impact the pathway for normal development, and the implications for current and future mental health. For example, research shows that infants in the first few years of life who experience serious adversity (i.e., exposure to violence, trauma, or multiple medical procedures) are more likely to show abnormal patterns in the expression of emotions, unusual or deviant behaviors including increased motor activity, distractibility and inattention, disruptions in feeding and sleeping patterns, and/or developmental delays in motor and language skills. Many of these problems are not transient but herald the onset of longstanding problems.

Contexts of Infant Mental Health

Context refers to all of the many factors that influence infants' development. Intrinsic, or internal, factors include biological, genetic, and constitutional make-up. Extrinsic, or external, factors include the infants' caregiving relationship, family, culture, and social class. These intrinsic and extrinsic characteristics are risk and protective factors that dynamically interact with each other. Risk factors increase the probability of adverse outcomes, and protective factors decrease the probability of adverse outcomes.

Biological Context

The biological context includes all of the intrinsic factors that affect an infant's development: genetic influences, temperament, constitution, physical health, and physical attributes. These factors are considered 'within the individual'; they may or may not be modifiable. Much of primary healthcare is devoted to ensuring that the infant is off to a healthy start and addresses some of the modifiable intrinsic factors by using interventions such as nutritional education, developmental surveillance, and early intervention for various health and developmental problems. Clearly, development depends in part on biological dimensions of the individual's experience of the world.

Important contributors to the infant's mental health are evident in the biological context. In addition to genetic dispositions, many nongenetic biological factors may be important. From the third trimester of pregnancy to the second year of life is the most rapid period of brain development in the human life cycle, though brain development begins in the first few weeks after conception and continues well into adulthood. Much of the structural development of the brain occurs prenatally, but circuitry continues to be elaborated after birth, as a result of experiences. Functional development depends on making connections between distal and local neural circuits through the formation and pruning of neuronal synapses – believed to occur in part as a result of prenatal and postnatal experiences. Thus, numerous prenatal experiences such as poor nutrition or poor maternal health may directly affect brain growth. Prenatal exposure to pharmacological agents may result in the newborns showing withdrawal symptoms at birth, and prenatal maternal stress has

been associated with changes in infants' stress-regulation abilities.

Physical health impacts the type of care needed by the infant, how his caregivers respond to him, and his capacity for normal physical as well as mental growth and development. The infant's temperament (e.g., behavioral inhibition or effortful control), as well as the infant's physical attributes (e.g., resembling a family member or disfiguring anomalies) can powerfully impact the caregiver's perceptions of and responses to the infant. Physical or temperamental characteristics may result in the caregiver feeling drawn to, protective of, or disconnected from the infant. Infants' physical or behavioral attributes may facilitate positive or negative interactions and further exacerbate negative interactions. For example, a fussy infant may be off-putting for a disengaged caregiver leading the infant to cry more in an effort to elicit attention.

Cultural Context

Culture provides norms for parenting beliefs and behaviors, defining how to care for infants and young children, as well as expectations about the roles of mothers, fathers, and extended family members. Although different cultural and ethnic groups develop different child-rearing practices, there are certain values that are evident in cultures around the world: (1) ensuring the child's safety and health, (2) ensuring the child becomes capable of economic self-maintenance, and (3) ensuring the child will be able to maximize societal values. Finally, the family exerts a strong influence on the day to day experience of the infant, particularly the type and availability of support for the parent. Culture also influences the parents' expectations, hopes, and values regarding the infant, and in turn, how the parent cares for and experiences the infant.

Social Context

Social class confers access to resources. Increasing availability and use of external supports for families with young children are associated with higher social classes. Living environment impacts the needs of the infant and the family as well as the prioritization, type, and availability of resources. Rural or isolated areas, inner cities with crowded living conditions and unhealthy living spaces, and even extreme climate or physical terrain, all confer unique needs and limit families' access to resources. Lower social class also is associated with probability of the individual encountering environmental risk factors. For example, poverty exerts a strong negative influence on the early experience of many young children because of the myriad of associated environmental and psychosocial stresses, including an increased risk of community violence and mental health issues.

Relationship Context

The most crucial interpersonal context for the developing infant is the small number of caregiving relationships that the child encounters. Through these relationships the infant begins to understand his world, learns how to interact with others, and begins to develop a sense of his competence and self-worth. After all, the impact of infant's experiences of environmental risk factors, such as poverty, maternal mental illness, and partner violence is primarily via their effects on the infant–parent relationship. Further, intrinsic risk factors, such as biological difficulties, are moderated by the infant–parent relationship. For example, infants with complications of prematurity have better outcomes when their caregiving environments are supportive, and more problematic outcomes when their caregiving environments are less supportive. Also, difficult temperaments can be moderated through a responsive, nurturing, and consistent caregiving experience.

The attachment relationship is a biologically based process that motivates the young child to seek comfort, support, nurturance, and protection in times of distress from discriminated attachment figures – providing the basis for psychological security as well as physical safety. The attachment relationship develops over the course of the first year of life through the myriad of daily interactions between the infant and the primary caregiver(s). The quality of the infant–caregiver relationship is a risk or protective factor for infants' later development. A warm, nurturing, sensitive, responsive, and consistent pattern of interactions between the infant and caregiver leads to a 'secure' attachment; through these interactions, the infant learns that he is worthy of being taken care of, that he can count on his caregiver to be there when he needs her, and he develops a sense of self-competence in that his actions (i.e., signals, cues, behaviors, communications) can be understood and are effective in getting his needs met. Conversely, interactions that lack these positive qualities and are inconsistent, unpredictable, harsh, or punitive lead to insecure or disorganized attachments. Preferred attachment appears in the latter part of the first year of life, heralded by the appearance of separation protest and stranger wariness. Infants become attached to caregivers with whom they have a significant number of interactions. If more than one attachment figure is present, infants develop a hierarchy of preferred caregivers to whom they turn for comfort, support, nurturance, and protection.

During these early months, the infant appears to develop a set of expectations, termed 'working models', of what it is like to be in an intimate relationship with another person. These models are relationship specific, so that the infant's experiences with each caregiver determines the nature of the expectations that the infant develops for his or her relationship with each caregiver. This relationship specificity has significant implications for assessment and treatment.

Psychopathology in Infancy

The idea of psychiatric diagnoses of infants and young children often makes us uncomfortable. We prefer to think of infancy as a carefree time with unlimited possibilities for the future. Faced with infants who are distressed or who have impairments in functioning, we may prefer to think about them as having risks for subsequent disorders rather than discrete psychiatric disorders. Nevertheless, in clinical practice, examples of patterns of severe psychopathology are impossible to avoid. Young children present with consistent patterns impairing symptoms which affect their functioning and development.

As early as the first year of life, some infants demonstrate significant behavioral or emotional problems, including odd behaviors or unusual social or emotional responses in certain situations. Even when an infant has a mild or subclinical problem, the dynamics of the interaction between caregiver and child may be altered: the caregiver may become more or less attentive, more nurturing or annoyed at the difficulties the infant presents. While such problems may not be disorders they do affect the relationship between the infant and caregiver, and when the relationship is altered or stressed, the infant is likely to react.

Of course, real challenges exist in the psychiatric diagnosis of disorders in young children. Because infants and preschoolers develop social, emotional, communication skills at such a rapid rate, there are developmental differences in presentation of disorders across this age range. Furthermore, the major nosology-describing criteria for psychiatric diagnoses, the DSM-IV-TR, was developed without attention to young children. Many researchers and clinicians have been concerned about the usefulness of DSM-IV-TR diagnostic criteria in evaluating the symptoms of infants and toddlers because the diagnoses were primarily derived from studies of adults and used limited empirical data related to children, much less very young children. Alternative diagnostic systems have been proposed and the field continues to finetune the definition of disorders in young children.

Diagnostic Classification Systems

Specific symptoms or symptom clusters become problematic in children when they interfere with normal development or functioning; for example, in infants and young children, this may include disturbances in interactions between peers or with caregivers, impediments to play and learning, or negative impacts on health, growth, emotional, or behavioral development. Diagnostic classifications allow effective communication with parents and colleagues about our understanding of the problem and provide a common foundation for research to understand the validity, prognosis, intervention effects of the identified symptom constellations.

An alternative to the DSM approach was first developed in 1992, when the Zero to Three organization published the *Diagnostic Classification of Mental Health and Developmental Disorders of Infancy and Early Childhood (DC:0–3). DC:0–3* was revised in 2005. It uses a clinically driven set of developmentally derived criteria and a multidimensional approach to diagnostic classification to attempt to capture both developmental issues and contextual features of psychopathology. The diagnostic classifications include descriptions of relationship psychopathology as well as the infant's functional emotional level.

A third diagnostic approach was created in 2003, when a group of investigators developed the Research Diagnostic Criteria – Preschool Age (RDC-PA) to facilitate communication and additional research on the reliability and validity of early childhood disorders.

Although only preliminary data exist, it appears that overall prevalence of disorders in young children is similar to rates in older children, that is, roughly 10–20%. Disorders with prominent externalizing symptoms, such as inattention/hyperactivity, oppositional defiant disorder, and aggressive behavior disorders are common diagnoses in most referred and nonreferred populations in mental health settings. Trauma-related disorders also are prominent, though the rates of other internalizing disorders, such as depression and anxiety disorders, vary in different reports, perhaps a reflection of limited data related to their use. In primary care settings, on the other hand, regulatory problems, such as feeding and sleeping problems, are most commonly reported particularly in infants.

Types of Disorders

Disorders of regulation

The earliest-appearing disorders in infancy are those that disrupt basic regulatory functions such as feeding and sleep.

Feeding disorders

In early infancy, feeding is a major activity involving parent and child, and feeding continues to be central in the lives of toddlers. In some diagnostic classification systems, feeding disorders are grouped under a single heading but in others they are split into many types. Most feeding disorders involve an inability to eat or food refusal, sometimes associated with an inability to maintain appropriate weight gain. Feeding disorders can present in the context of caregivers who are disengaged from the infant during feedings, or with intense conflict between infant and caregiver during feedings. Although some feeding disorders can be related to specific events (e.g., nasogastric feedings or traumatic intubations), most feeding disorders appear to have multifactorial etiologies. Sensory-processing abnormalities, attachment-relationship disturbances, state-regulation difficulties, and complicated medical conditions all may play a role in the development or perpetuation of feeding disorders. Regardless of the etiology, feeding disorders are generally stressful both for parents and for the parent–child relationship. These disorders often create feelings of inadequacy in parents. Of most concern is when feeding problems impair growth (failure to thrive), since malnutrition is particularly pernicious as an influence on brain development.

Sleep disorders

Sleep is a central index of infant state regulation. Newborns spend up to 18 h of every 24 h sleeping. As children get older, they begin to develop a diurnal sleep pattern, sleeping in the evening and being awake during the daylight. This developmental process provides for the opportunity of a varied developmental course, and some researchers have suggested that sleep patterns be classified specifically by their frequency and duration, as some sleep problems are part of a normal developmental course. Disorders of sleep in young children can occur around sleep onset (primary insomnia or sleep refusal) or during sleep in the form of night wakenings or parasomnias (nightmares and night terrors). In toddlers and preschoolers, enlarged tonsils and adenoids can lead to obstructive sleep apnea symptoms, including night-time snoring and daytime drowsiness and sometimes irritability. Sleep disturbances may affect children's attention and behavior, as well as impact family sleep practices and relationships.

Behavioral disorders

Behavioral disorders are characterized by externalizing symptoms, such as aggression, tantrums, oppositional/defiant behavior, and inattention/hyperactivity. They are uncommon in the first 18 months of life but are commonly described in preschool children. Aggressive behavior is the most common presenting sign in children in the third year of life who are brought for mental health evaluations. It is important to distinguish true signs and symptoms of disorders from variants of normal development. The challenge of diagnosing these disorders in young children involves determining the developmental appropriateness of some of the symptoms. As children develop an enhanced sense of autonomy and they test the limits of their emotional and physical dependence, parental report of oppositional behaviors often increases. Parental reports of aggression and externalizing behaviors peak at about age 2 years and then begin to decrease to some extent. Even in the context of developmentally typical behaviors, parental distress in response to these behaviors must be acknowledged and addressed. However, there are also clearly cases in which a child's behaviors reflect an impulsivity and dysregulation out of proportion for the normal developmental phase.

The three major behavior disorders described the diagnostic classification systems include attention deficit hyperactivity disorder (ADHD), oppositional defiant disorder (ODD), and, less commonly, conduct disorder (CD). These diagnoses are among the best-validated disorders in the preschool age group, and they show significant stability over time.

Attention deficit hyperactivity disorder

ADHD is defined as a maladaptive and developmentally inappropriate level of inattention, hyperactivity, and impulsivity. Like older children with ADHD, preschoolers with ADHD present primarily with hyperactive, impulsive symptoms or with notable inattention and disorganization, or both. Because of the diagnostic challenges of assessing young children with these symptoms, it is especially important to obtain information about the child's behavior in multiple settings and from various caregivers, especially day care providers to rule out differential diagnoses like anxiety disorders, learning disorders, or relationship-based disorders.

Oppositional defiant disorder

In most clinical settings, aggressive and negativisitic behavior problems are commonly seen, especially in boys. ODD is characterized by a pattern of negative, hostile, and defiant behaviors including arguing with adults, losing temper, refusing to follow directions and seeming angry, resentful, or spiteful. Children with ODD often have associated ADHD. In those cases, the outcome 2 years later is significantly less favorable than in children with ADHD only.

Conduct disorder

Conduct disorder, a more extreme disorder of disruptive, aggressive, and destructive behaviors, is less common in the preschool population. Nevertheless, not only have signs and symptoms associated with conduct disorder been identified in young children (e.g., aggression, bullying, and cruelty to others), but also dispositions associated with conduct disorder symptoms at older ages, such as callous unemotional traits, also have been identified in preschoolers.

Not all children who present with aggression or negativistic and defiant behaviors as their chief complaints have a disruptive behavior disorder. Assessing the biological, emotional, relationship, and environmental contexts of the symptoms can guide the diagnosis. Children presenting with externalizing behaviors may have mood or anxiety disorders, including post-traumatic stress disorder (PTSD).

Emotional disorders

The category of emotional disorders includes disorders of mood, that is depressive disorders, and anxiety.

Depression

Depression in young children looks similar to depression in older children and adults. In young children, irritability or sadness can be the core symptom of depression. In addition, depressed children can have notable sleep, appetite or concentration disturbances, as well as preoccupation with death or excessive guilty feelings. Unlike adults, preschoolers with depression may not demonstrate the consistent presence of daily symptoms for 2 weeks. Recent data indicate that somatic symptoms may occur, but depressive symptoms and anhedonia (lack of interest in usual activities) dominate the clinical picture.

Anxiety

Anxiety symptoms normally are prominent in early childhood, with the fears peaking in the toddler years and then usually decreasing over time before entering school. It is during this time that young children can develop fears of the dark and of monsters. However, it is also possible for children to present with impairing anxiety symptoms. Young children can present with specific phobias during this period. It is not yet clear if young children present with social phobia (though they may be extremely shy, or behaviorally inhibited), panic disorders or acute stress disorders. It is clear that young children can experience post-traumatic stress disorder (PTSD) after traumatic events such as witnessing violence, being in motor vehicle accidents, or experiencing physical or sexual abuse. Among preschoolers, trauma reactions commonly include re-experiencing symptoms such as distress in response to a reminder of the trauma and/or repetitive play related to the traumatic event; avoidance of reminders of the trauma (e.g., not wanting to go in the car); and increased arousal as evidenced by increased irritability and temper tantrums, hypervigilance (increased scanning and attention to perceived threats in the environment), and increased startle response. The context of the traumatic event is an important mediator in the development of PTSD. Children who experience a single major traumatic event are more likely to develop PTSD than those who experience chronic traumas, such as ongoing abuse or neglect, although chronic traumas increase children's risk for other disorders. The ability of the child to feel safe and return to normal activities after a traumatic event can help to minimize the child's reactions. A secure, supportive parent–child relationship may provide the most important way to ameliorate children's symptoms related to a traumatic event.

Relationship disorders

Although psychiatry and psychology traditionally have considered disorders to be within-the-individual, the unique dependence of infants on their caregiving context have led some to suggest that disorders may exist between individuals – in this case, infant and parent. This approach is bolstered by clinical observations and research evidence of relationship specificity. What this means is that the young child may be symptomatic in the context of one relationship but not others.

In young children, a relationship with a nurturing, sensitive, responsive caregiver is one of the most important contributors to healthy development. In nonreferred children, the formal attachment classifications based on the strange situation procedure provide a way to understand various relationship patterns. A secure attachment is found in children who have had warm, sensitive, responsive caregiving, and can be observed when young children are able to seek and respond to comforting in a stressful situation. Three types of insecure attachment have been described. Insecure–avoidant is seen when young children respond to stress by not seeking, or actively avoiding, help from their caregiver. Insecure–resistant attachment is characterized by the young child who can signal his distress but has great difficulty getting effective comfort from the caregiver. The disorganized attachment classification is found in dyads in which the young child does not have coherent, reliable ways of signaling distress to the caregiver, often associated with bizarre or unusual behaviors.

The insecure attachment classifications can be predictive of later psychopathology, but these classifications do not necessarily indicate current pathology. For example, children who exhibit avoidant attachment behaviors in the strange situation are at risk of developing anxiety disorders, and those children with disorganized attachments have an increased chance of developing preschool behavior problems. These characterizations of the parent–child relationship also are associated with later behavior problems and social–emotional difficulties.

In some dyads, disordered patterns of behaviors as well as distortion of perceptions about the other in the relationship can impair the child or dyadic functioning at the level of a disorder. Attachment disorders are considered to reflect a significant disturbance in the relationship between the infant and his or her primary caregiver, such that it interferes with the child's ability to develop normally in other domains, including cognitive, physical, behavioral, as well as social–emotional development.

Controversy remains about how best to diagnose attachment disorders. The DSM-IV-TR contains only criteria for the diagnosis of reactive attachment disorder (RAD). The diagnosis requires a total lack of an attachment relationship and requires a known history of maltreatment to make the diagnosis. However, even in situations of profound deprivation, it is rare for a child not to develop some type of attachment with a caregiver, most likely to be a disturbed type of relationship. In contrast to DSM-IV-TR, the RDC-PA provides an alternative means of concretely operationalizing the concept by clearly describing behaviors of disordered attachment, even in the context of an attachment relationship. Unlike the DSM IV, the RDC-PA does not mandate that the child has been maltreated. DC:0–3R

has similar criteria for attachment disorders as RDC-PA, but also uses Axis II for diagnosis of problematic relationship patterns which do not meet the standards for reactive attachment disorders and/or which are not focused specifically on the attachment portion of the relationship.

Whatever the specific diagnostic criteria used, it is clear that clinically relevant disturbances in children's attachment behaviors exist. A healthy attachment allows for a balance between the toddler's developmentally appropriate exploratory drive and need for emotional reassurance and support. Children with healthy attachments to a caregiver or parent can use that person in an effective manner for comfort and are able to successfully begin to explore their environment in a safe way. Children with attachment disorders generally demonstrate two major patterns of behaviors: inhibited and disinhibited behaviors. Children with the inhibited form of RAD tend to be emotionally restricted, are overly cautious, and do not seek out comfort effectively, if at all. In the disinhibited type, children do not have the usual wariness of new situations and new people. They are excessively and indiscriminately friendly with unfamiliar adults and rarely check back with their parent, even in new environments where they may not know anyone. These two patterns of attachment disorders are not mutually exclusive; children can present with features of both patterns. Indiscriminate behaviors, but not inhibited behaviors, appear to persist in young children who have been raised in institutions such as orphanages, even after a child has been adopted and has developed a new attachment relationship with a committed caregiver. Although it is clear that disturbances of attachment may continue to put children at risk for other disorders, attachment disorders have not been studied in children older than 5 years, and the current descriptions of these disorders may not be helpful in the older age group.

Summary of disorders

While different categories of diagnosis for infants and toddlers exist, significant psychopathology can exist within children and their relationships with their primary caregivers. The field continues to move toward further validation of the disorders of early childhood. These disorders can impair children's emotional, physiologic, and diurnal regulation as well as children's abilities to function within the structured rules of family and school and peers. Because of the critical role of the primary caregiving relationship, recognition of disorders of this relationship – whether because of parent psychopathology, child disorders or a relationship disorder – should be evaluated and, if necessary, diagnosed to provide intervention.

Assessment of Infants and Caregivers

We use the term assessment to describe the process of gathering data about an individual child and family for purposes of determining if intervention is needed and what the nature of that intervention should be. In this framework it subsumes diagnosis and includes an inventory of strengths and stressors that may affect both caregivers and child. Although we diagnose disorders, we assess individuals and families as a way of developing a comprehensive and coherent plan of intervention.

Infant mental health assessments are multimodal evaluations which often take place over a number of appointments and in different settings. A thorough history, careful observations, and collateral information are critical components of the assessment. Formal assessments including structured questionnaires, observations, and interviews, developmental assessments, and relationship assessments can add additional understanding to the child and the relationships which define his or her world.

One of the most important principles of assessment in infant mental health is that the infant–caregiver relationship is the most important focus of assessment rather than the infant as an individual. This principle derives largely from the extraordinary dependence of the human infants on their caregivers in the first several years of life and is bolstered by research demonstrating the following: (1) relationship patterns are more stable than individual characteristics of infants and they are important predictors of individual characteristics in later childhood and beyond, (2) the infant–caregiver relationship moderates the effects of intrinsic biological risk factors (e.g., complications of prematurity or adverse temperamental characteristics) on the infant, (3) the infant–caregiver relationship mediates the effects of extrinsic risk factors (e.g., poverty or partner violence) on the infant, and (4) there is often a remarkable degree of relationship specificity in signs and symptoms of disturbance in young children, suggesting that many problems in early childhood are most usefully conceptualized as relationship disorders rather than within the individual disorders. For all of these reasons, the usual assessment of the individual must be supplanted by a more comprehensive relationship assessment of young children in all of their important contexts.

Conventionally, two components of the relationship are assessed. These are (1) the recurring patterns of observable interactions between infant and parent, and (2) the subjective experience of each member of the dyad with regard to the 'other' and the relationship. Assessment of these two components allows one to evaluate both patterns of behavior and also of the meaning of behavior for the dyad.

Interactions between young children and their caregivers may be observed in unstructured, in naturalistic settings, such as during home visits or visits to child-care settings, or they may be observed in structured clinic visits during which prescribed tasks are given to the dyad. Common activities in more structured assessments are free play, problem-solving tasks, feedings, and brief separations and reunions. Most useful, even among more structured tasks, are those which do not overconstrain or prescribe parental behavior in order to allow the dyad to reveal to the evaluator how they negotiate different situations and challenges. Different paradigms of interaction have been used in clinical assessments and these are usually modified based on infants' ages or cognitive levels.

Parents' subjective, or internal, experience of the dyad may be assessed directly but the infant's perceptions must be inferred. Several structured interviews for assessing parents perceptions of their infants exist. Although these typically have formal coding systems for use in research, some have been used extensively in clinical settings without strict use of the formal coding system. An important contribution of these structured interviews was the demonstration that qualitative features of the parents' narrative accounts of their infants are important predictors of their behavior with their infants; that is, what the parent says about their infant may be important, but how they say it may be even more important. Of course, a parent's subjective experience of their infant also may be assessed in less formal ways, such as through listening carefully to parents' descriptions of their infant's behavior or personality or how the baby makes them feel, during the assessment process.

Domains of the parent–child relationship are the usual targets of assessment in both history taking and observations. These domains include parent characteristics that are conceptually linked with emerging infant behaviors and qualities. Thus, parents' emotional availability is associated with infants' patterns of emotion regulation. Parents' nurturance and warmth are associated with infants' sense of trust and security. Parents' response to distress is related to infants' learning to seek comfort for distress. Further, parents' protection of their infants is related to the infants' feelings of safety and the later development of the capacity for self-protection. Parents are important play partners for their infants, and play is an important domain of the infant–parent relationship. Parents also are teachers of their infants, and these efforts relate to infants' curiosity, sense of mastery, and interest in learning. Parents provide structure, routines, and instrumental care in order that their infants develop a sense of predictability and the capacity for self-regulation.

Finally, parents set limits and discipline as needed to assist young children to develop self-control and a reasonable degree of compliance and cooperation. Parents may have strengths in some areas, but difficulties in other areas of parenting; likewise, infants may experience difficulties in one or more domains, but not others. By assessing all of these domains of parent–infant relationship using both the external, observable pattern of interaction and the internal, subjective experience of who the infant, it is possible to construct an understanding of the relationship. Once the strengths and concerns of the relationship have been identified, it is important to appreciate them within contexts of caregiver functioning, and family, community, and environmental resources, including culture and class.

A comprehensive infant mental health assessment includes assessment of the caregivers' abilities to care for and understand the infant. Issues such as depression, substance abuse, a history of trauma, abuse, or significant losses, ongoing domestic violence, and isolation and/or lack of a supportive family system can all contribute to the caregiver's ability to engage in treatment and care for the infant. Furthermore, any other environmental factors that could contribute to difficulties in the relationship or that could interfere with treatment, such as lack of stable housing, also must be identified as part of the assessment process.

A comprehensive assessment must also include identification of the strengths of the infant, caregiver, and family. Including strengths in the assessment gives a fuller perspective of the infant's experience and can help build the treatment alliance between family and professional. Knowledge of strengths also can provide the building blocks for intervention.

Finally, any interventions must be congruent with a parent's cultural belief system. Because social class typically determines access to resources, enhancing a family's access to needed services is a critical step toward enhancing the young child's development. The overall goal is to design an intervention that is appropriate for whatever problems exist, uses the family's strengths, and will be acceptable and useful for the family.

Intervention in Infant Mental Health

Levels of intervention in infant mental health vary from the level of treating the individual infant/family through more comprehensive systems approaches aimed at changing policies to better address the needs of our most vulnerable citizens. They also may be arrayed along a continuum from universal, to focused, to selected (i.e., treatment). The overall goals of infant mental health services across universal, focused/targeted, and selected approaches are similar. They involve enhancing the ability of caregivers to nurture young children more effectively, expanding the ability of nonfamily caregivers to identify, address, and prevent social–emotional problems in early childhood, and minimizing or averting suffering, and ensuring that families in need of more intensive services can obtain them.

Preventive Interventions

Universal approaches are aimed at improving child development, parenting knowledge, and behavior. These approaches often are applied in primary healthcare settings, in early childhood education and childcare, and in family support settings. Strategies generally include health and behavioral promotion, screening and assessment, education and guidance, and referral for more intensive assessment and intervention services when needed.

Focused, or targeted approaches are aimed at specifically identified groups considered at risk for developing potentially serious social or emotional problems. These approaches may be administered in any setting serving at risk infants and their families. Examples include early intervention for premature or low birthweight babies, home visiting services for first-time mothers, or preventive interventions for abused or neglected children. Family support interventions include income assistance, adult basic and secondary education, parenting education to promote positive parent–child interaction, and interventions that address other environmental risk factors associated with poverty. The nurse home visiting program developed by David Olds, for example, has shown longlasting effects on children's emotional well being, child abuse, and even adolescent delinquent behaviors, even though the intervention extends only from late pregnancy to the child's second birthday.

Intensive, or selected services serve infants and caregivers experiencing current difficulties, and also attempt to prevent or lessen future problems. These services are most likely to develop from mental health programs, and may be provided for those infants currently experiencing distress, such as those who have experienced significant trauma, or for whom there are serious parent–infant relationship problems.

Treatment (Selected Interventions)

Treatment of infant mental health disorders may be focused primarily on changing the infant's behavior, the parents' behaviors, or the infant–parent relationship. Although each of these therapeutic 'targets' use different strategies, all are concerned with changing the infant–parent relationship as a way of changing infant behavior and ensuring that the changes are enduring.

Working with parent and infant together on changing their relationship requires the establishment of a good 'working alliance' between parents and therapist. This is a shared commitment to work together in the best interest of the child. The relationship between the therapist and the parent becomes an important component of treatment. In the context of this relationship, therapy focuses on appreciating the parent's emotional experience of the young child, and the young child's experience of the parent. Examples of effective treatment strategies in infant mental health include infant–parent psychotherapy, in which patterns of intimate relationships and communication are explored using a psychodynamic approach, and interaction guidance, which uses videos of the dyad to identify and strengthen positive interactions within the dyad.

All successful treatment strategies with infants require active parent participation. Furthermore, caregivers must be able to function effectively in order to care appropriately for the child. Thus, it is often the case that treatment of the caregiver for problems such as maternal depression, substance abuse, domestic violence, or other issues occurs simultaneously with dyadic treatments. Coordination of services, as well as availability of services for caregivers, can be impediments to effective infant mental health treatment.

Finally, treatment of established problems aims to resolve current symptoms and distress and to prevent or minimize the detrimental effects of the symptoms on infants' later development. For these reasons, infant mental health treatments are concerned simultaneously with present and future adaptation of the child, and treatment of infants is always concerned with prevention.

Systems Intervention

When considering how to support infant mental health through a comprehensive system of services, it is important to think strategically. One important strategy is the development of a workforce with a continuum of expertise. A growing consensus holds that infant and early childhood mental health requires specialized training and that there are far too few mental health clinicians with requisite skills given the number of young children who could benefit from provision of services. It is equally important to better equip healthcare and other nonmental health service providers, such as child-care providers and preschool teachers, to promote infant mental health and serve as efficient and effective sources of screening and referral. Tertiary providers, such as adult mental health or substance abuse services, may not be familiar with the impact of such disturbance on the parenting ability of their client, and thus, they also need education to work effectively with such clients.

Another set of strategies focuses on the environmental factors that impact infant mental health. For instance, improving the financial well-being of families and communities will help to relieve the myriad of stresses associated with poverty and other environmental factors. The data are clear that the negative consequences of poverty are cumulative, pervasive, longlasting, and impact all aspects of physical, cognitive, and socioemotional development. Relief of poverty-related stressors can directly improve the health and social situations of young children and their families, ease stress on the parent–infant relationship, and directly and indirectly improve the social and emotional development of young children.

Summary of Principles of Infant Mental Health

Infant mental health is considered synonymous with healthy social and emotional development. Warm, nurturing, protective, sensitive, stable, and consistent relationships provide the fundamental building blocks to

infant mental health. Important indicators of infant mental health include the young child's capacity for emotion regulation, the ability to communicate feelings and needs to caregivers, and active exploration of the environment. These behaviors lay the groundwork for later social and emotional competence, readiness to enter school, and better academic and social performance.

Risk and protective factors have been clearly identified that relate to current and later function. Risk factors predispose to subsequent psychopathology, but most clinicians also believe that infants can experience psychological disorders in the first 3 years of life. Protective factors are important especially when they can be mobilized to prevent or minimize adverse outcomes in high-risk infants.

The central focus of infant mental health assessment is on the infant–parent relationship. Any factors that impact the relationship between the infant and caregiver have the potential to impact the infant's mental health. The strengths perspective, as well as inclusion of cultural influences, provides a full picture of the infant's experience, and can provide the foundations for intervention. For these reasons, the usual infant-focused assessment must be supplanted by a comprehensive assessment of infant and young children that examines functioning across physical, developmental, environmental, family, and relationship contexts.

A continuum of services is needed to address prevention and treatment in infant mental health. Programs that address infant mental health must focus on relationships, be based in current developmental knowledge, and be supportive of the family. It is important that whenever possible, families are involved in the planning and delivery of infant mental health services.

See also: ADHD: Genetic Influences; Autism Spectrum Disorders; Depression; Failure to Thrive; Feeding Development and Disorders; Sensory Processing Disorder; Separation and Stranger Anxiety; Shyness.

Suggested Readings

American Psychiatric Association (2000) *Diagnostic and Statistical Manual of Mental Disorders,* 4th edn. – Text revision (DSM-IV-TR-TR Washington, DC: Author.

Gleason MM and Zeanah CH (2006) Infant mental health. Comprehensive handbook of personality and psychopathology. In: Hersen M and Thomas JC (eds.) *Child Psychopathology,* vol. 3, pp. 173–191. Wiley: New York.

Sameroff A, McDonough S, and Rosenblum K (eds.) (2003) *Treatment of Infant–Parent Relationship Disturbances.* New York: Guilford Press.

Task Force on Research Diagnostic Criteria: Infancy and Preschool (2003) Research diagnostic criteria for preschool children: The process and empirical support. *Journal of the American Academy of Child and Adolescent Psychiatry* 42: 1504–1512.

Zeanah CH (ed.) (2000) *Handbook of Infant Mental Health,* 2nd edn. New York: Guilford Press.

Zeanah PD, Stafford B, and Zeanah CH (2005) *Building State Early Childhood Comprehensive Systems Series, Vol. 13: Clinical Interventions in Infant Mental Health: A Selective Review.* Los Angeles, CA: National Center for Infant and Early Childhood Health Policy.

Zeanah P, Stafford B, Nagle G, and Rice T (2005) *Building State Early Childhood Comprehensive Systems Series, Vol. 12: Addressing Social–Emotional Development and Infant Mental Healthin Early Childhood Systems.* Los Angeles, CA: National Center for Infant and Early Childhood Health Policy.

Zero to Three (2005) *Diagnostic Classification of Mental Health and Developmental Disorders of Infancy and Early Childhood,* revised edition. Washington, DC: Zero to Three.

N

Neurological Development

M C Moulson, Massachusetts Institute of Technology, Cambridge, MA, USA
C A Nelson, Harvard Medical School, Boston, MA, USA

Glossary

Axon – A long projection from a neuron that transmits information to other cells by conducting nerve impulses away from the cell body.

Dendrite – A protrusion from a neuron that receives information from other neurons.

Developmental plasticity – The ability of the brain to be modified by experience during development. A normative process that involves the formation and elimination of synapses.

Glia – Cells in the brain that perform supporting functions such as guiding neurons to their correct locations in the developing brain and speeding up the transmission of information between neurons. There are many different types of glia.

Myelin – A lipid protein substance composed of glial cells, which forms a sheath around axons to insulate them and speed transmission of nerve impulses.

Neural induction – The genesis of the nervous system approximately 18 days after conception, whereby cells of the dorsal ectoderm are specified to become neural tissue, forming a flat structure called the neural plate.

Neurulation – The process by which the neural tube, which gives rise to the central nervous system (CNS), is formed from the neural plate. It occurs between 3 and 4 weeks after conception.

Progenitor – A cell that gives rise to neuronal and glial precursors through cell division.

Programmed cell death (PCD) – A normative event in which approximately 50% of all neurons in the developing brain die.

Synapse – The miniscule gap between axons and dendrites through which information flows in the form of neurotransmitters.

Introduction

Over the course of development, the central nervous system (CNS) grows from a single sheet of undifferentiated cells into our most complex organ, the brain, and the processes by which it does so are nothing short of miraculous. Brain development begins approximately 18 days after conception and experiences an explosion of growth during the prenatal period. During this period, the brain takes on both the rudimentary form and function of the mature organ, but its development is not complete at birth. Rather, the brain undergoes a protracted period of development. Whereas other bodily organs are mature at birth, the brain continues to develop at least through the adolescent period. There is even some evidence that certain aspects of brain development continue into middle age.

The brain is composed of two major classes of cells: neurons and glia. In the mature brain, there are approximately 100 billion neurons and many more glia. Neurons communicate information throughout the brain by forming connections called synapses. Glia are the support cells of the brain, and perform numerous functions, including guiding neurons to their correct locations in the developing brain, and speeding up the transmission of information and stabilizing connections between neurons in the brain.

Neurological development, though heavily constrained by genetics, is not predetermined. Rather, the developing brain is an open system that is shaped by both genetic and epigenetic factors. That is, although genetically programmed influences induce the events that give rise to the mature nervous system, this does not mean that these events are impervious to exogenous influences. For example, it is well known that exposure to certain agents during prenatal development (e.g., mercury, alcohol, rubella) can have deleterious effects on the developing fetus. These agents are said to have teratogenic effects and are a clear example that the developing brain, even during very early stages of prenatal development, is not immune to the outside world. Moreover, during the later stages of brain development (e.g., circuit formation) the developing brain actually requires normative experiences in the form of sensory input in order to customize its connections and, correspondingly, to increase its information processing efficiency. The ability of the brain to be modified by experience is called plasticity, and different processes during the development of the brain are more or less plastic. Specifically, early events are less amenable to experience (i.e., less plastic), whereas later events including circuit formation are more amenable to experience (i.e., more plastic). Importantly, the major vehicles of plasticity during later stages of brain development are in fact regressive events, including programmed cell death (PCD) and the loss of synapses. These regressive events allow the brain to capture experience, an ability that will be described in more detail in the final section of this article.

An understanding of plasticity in the developing brain holds promise for researchers studying child development. We know that early experiences alter the course of behavioral development in both positive and negative ways depending on the nature of the specific experiences a child has; understanding neural plasticity will lead to an understanding of how these early experiences exert their effects. Thus, a thorough understanding of neurological development will permit researchers to move beyond the historical nature–nurture debate, and to address multifaceted questions regarding which behavioral systems are modifiable by experience, the nature of experiences required to alter the brain circuitry underlying these behavioral systems, and when these experiences must occur in order to have their effects.

Thus, the purpose of this article is to review the typical development of the human brain by describing the series of events that give rise to the mature nervous system and to investigate the role that experience plays in brain development. These events include neural induction and neurulation, proliferation, migration, and circuit formation. Each event will be discussed in terms of the timing and course of typical development and the resulting morphological changes of the developing brain. Additionally, errors that may occur during each major event and their consequences will be described. In the final section of this article, developmental plasticity will be discussed. It is important to note that although the events of brain development are described in sequence, they represent overlapping waves of development. That is, later processes are initiated before earlier processes are completed, which creates a complexity that is often difficult to study, especially in the human. This brings us to a significant limitation in our understanding of neurological development. Much of our knowledge of brain development in humans is extrapolated from work with animals and based on postmortem studies of small numbers of human brains. Thus, a full description and understanding of brain development has not yet been reached for humans, especially with regard to the molecular events that give rise to brain development. With this caveat in mind, we turn to a discussion of the major events that give rise to the mature brain, a summary of which can be found in **Table 1**.

Neural Induction and Neurulation

The human nervous system begins to form by day 18 postconception. Prior to this, the cells of the embryo have

Table 1   Timeline of neurological development

Developmental event	Timing	Description of event
Neural induction	Prenatal day 18	Dorsal side of ectoderm becomes specified as neural tissue
Neurulation	18–26 prenatal days	Neural tube is formed
		Cells within the neural tube become the CNS
Proliferation	6–20 prenatal weeks	Progenitor cells within ventricular zone give rise to neuronal and glial precursors
		* In some areas of brain, neurogenesis continues until adulthood
Migration	6–24 prenatal weeks	Neurons migrate out of the ventricular zone along radial glia
		Six-layered cortex is formed in an inside-out manner
Programmed cell death	2nd and 3rd trimesters	On average, 40–60% of neurons undergo programmed cell death
		Helps establish optimal connectivity
Axon and dendrite growth	15 prenatal weeks – 2nd postnatal year	Chemical signals guide axons and dendrites to their correct targets
		Synapses are formed between outgrowing axons and dendrites
Synaptogenesis	23 prenatal weeks – 2nd postnatal year	Synapses are strengthened through neural activity
		* Experience-dependent synapse formation continues throughout life
Synaptic pruning	1st postnatal year – adolescence	Inactive and aberrant synapses are eliminated
		* Mechanism whereby brain 'captures' early experience
Myelination	3rd trimester – middle age	Glial cells form myelin sheath around axons
		Results in increased speed and efficiency of neural transmission

differentiated into three different layers. The endoderm is composed of cells that give rise to the gastrointestinal system, liver, and lungs; the mesoderm gives rise to the vascular system, muscle, and connective tissue; and the ectoderm gives rise to the nervous system and epidermis (skin). Neural induction is the process by which the dorsal side of the ectoderm becomes specified as neural tissue. The mesoderm, although not composed of neural tissue itself, plays a vital role in this specification; proteins secreted from the organizer region of the mesoderm determine differentiation of the ectoderm into neural vs. epidermal tissue. Initially, this newly specified neural tissue forms a flat structure called the neural plate. Soon after the neural plate has formed, the process of neurulation begins. First, a crease is formed along the longitudinal axis of the neural plate. The neural plate buckles along this crease, the neural groove, causing the edges of the neural plate to rise up. Starting at gestational day 22, the edges of the neural plate begin to fuse together, forming the neural tube. Cells inside the neural tube become the CNS while cells trapped between the outer wall of the neural tube and the overlying ectoderm form the autonomic and peripheral nervous systems (ANS and PNS, respectively). The midsection of the tube fuses first, proceeding toward the rostral and caudal ends of the tube. The rostral end of the tube, which later becomes the brain, closes by gestational day 24, and the caudal end of the tube, which becomes the spinal cord, closes by gestatorial day 26.

Errors in neurulation, collectively called neural tube defects, have devastating consequences on the developing fetus. Craniorachischisis totalis, or the complete failure of neurulation, most often results in spontaneous resorption of the embryo, and therefore its incidence cannot be estimated. More common are defects in neural tube closure. Anencephaly, which has an incidence of approximately 0.2 per 1000 births, occurs when the rostral end of the neural tube (the part which later becomes the brain) fails to close. Of fetuses that suffer anencephaly, 75% are stillborn and the others generally die within several weeks of birth. Myelomeningocele, which has an incidence of approximately 1 per 1000 births, occurs when the caudal end of the neural tube (which later becomes the spinal cord) fails to close. Also called spina bifida, this defect results in portions of the spinal cord protruding unprotected from the back of the fetus. Infants affected by myelomeningocele generally survive, and the defect can be fixed surgically. However, myelomeningocele results in paralysis, with the extent of paralysis being determined by the location and size of the spinal lesion. Although genetic factors may predispose a fetus to neural tube defects, the environment can also play a pivotal role. For example, neural tube defects have been associated with a deficiency of folic acid in the maternal diet, and supplementing the maternal diet with folic acid seems to reduce the incidence of neural tube defects.

Proliferation

As the neural tube closes, cell proliferation within the tube takes off at an astonishing rate. Between the second and fifth month of prenatal life, the vast majority of all neurons that make up the adult nervous system are born in a process called neurogenesis. Prenatal cell proliferation also gives rise to glial cells, the support cells of the brain, on a timeframe that lags somewhat behind neurogenesis (although radial glial cells, discussed in a later section, are among the first cells to be produced). As one might imagine, cell proliferation dramatically alters the anatomical form of the developing nervous system.

Initially, the cells within the neural tube are all progenitor cells, meaning that they undergo mitosis (cell division) and can give rise to either neurons or glia. These cells reside in the innermost layer of the neural tube, an area called the ventricular zone. During mitosis, progenitor cells migrate from the luminal (inner) surface to the pial (outer) surface of the ventricular zone through a process called interkinetic nuclear migration. As they travel to the pial surface, they undergo DNA replication. They then migrate back to the luminal surface of the ventricular zone where they undergo cell division. Progenitor cells can divide either symmetrically or asymmetrically. During symmetric cell division, which starts at approximately the sixth prenatal week, progenitor cells give rise to two identical daughter cells that are themselves progenitors capable of undergoing cell division. Thus, symmetric cell division causes an exponential increase in the number of progenitor cells (i.e., after only 10 rounds of cell division, one progenitor cell gives rise to 1024 new progenitor cells). Asymmetric cell division on the other hand results in two daughter cells that are not identical. Rather, one daughter cell is a progenitor, as in symmetric cell division, whereas the other daughter cell is now a precursor to a neuron or a glial cell. These daughter cells that are destined to become neurons or glia are postmitotic (they do not undergo further rounds of cell division), and begin the process of migration and differentiation (see the following section). Between prenatal weeks 8 and 10, an additional zone of cells forms above the ventricular zone. This zone, called the subventricular zone, also contains progenitors that give rise to neurons and glia through the prenatal period and into the second year of postnatal life.

Neurogenesis, through asymmetric cell division, is largely complete by the end of the fourth postnatal month, while glial cell production continues until at least the second postnatal year. However, in certain regions of the brain, including the olfactory bulb and the dentate region of the hippocampus, neurogenesis continues into adulthood. Be that as it may, the vast majority of the 100 billion neurons that comprise the human brain are prenatal in origin.

This exuberant proliferation beginning in the sixth week of prenatal life in the human leads to considerable morphological change in the developing CNS. As the neural tube closes, uneven cell division along different parts of the tube leads to three distinct swellings at the rostral end of the neural tube – the prosencephalon (forebrain), mesencephalon (midbrain), and rhombencephalon (hindbrain) – that are apparent by 22 days postconception (see **Figure 1(a)**). Further subdivisions occur by approximately day 29 (see **Figure 1(b)**); the prosencephalon subdivides into the telencephalon and diencephalon, while the rhombencephalon subdivides into the metencephalon and myelencephalon. This creates five subdivisions, which give rise to all parts of the brain from the cerebral cortex to the brainstem, while the rest of the neural tube becomes the spinal cord (see **Figure 1(c)** for a micrograph of a chick neural tube at this stage in development). At this point in development, the neural tube has also acquired several bends (flexures) between these distinct swellings, which leads to the distinct curvature seen from the spinal cord to the brain in the mature nervous system (see **Figure 1(d)**). By the end of proliferation, at approximately 4.5 months prenatally, the brain is more comparable in shape to

the mature brain, although the gyri (folds) and sulci (grooves) present on the surface of the mature brain are not fully formed until the end of the prenatal period (see **Figure 2**).

Unlike errors in neural tube formation, which are often lethal and lead to frank anatomical defects, errors in cell proliferation result in more subtle abnormalities. These errors result in two broad categories of disorder: microencephaly, in which the brain is grossly undersized, and macroencephaly, in which the brain is grossly oversized. The term microencephaly subsumes a heterogeneous group of disorders in which the proximal cause of the significantly smaller brain is a deficit in either symmetric or asymmetric cell proliferation, engendered by either genetic or environmental factors. Often, the ultimate cause of the deficit in cell proliferation is unknown, although environmental factors such as rubella, HIV, maternal alcoholism or drug abuse, and exposure to radiation or mercury have been shown to result in microencephaly. The significantly larger brain characteristic of macroencephaly results from excessive cell proliferation, although it is unknown whether this

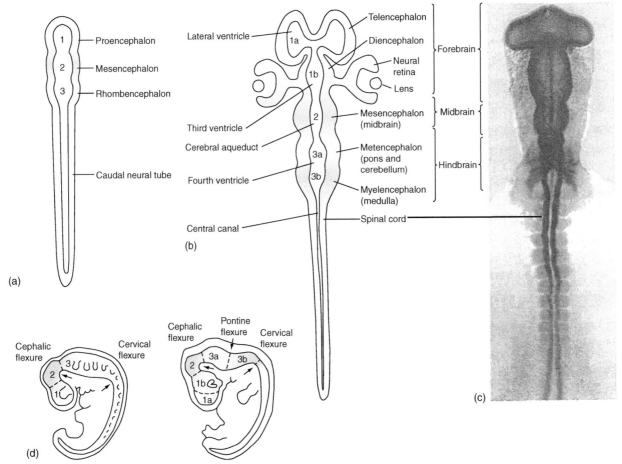

Figure 1   Stages in the development of the neural tube. (a) Three-vesicle stage of the neural tube; (b) five-vesicle stage of the neural tube; (c) micrograph of a chick neural tube at the five-vesicle stage; and (d) flexures of the neural tube. Reprinted from Kandel ER, Schwartz JH, and Jessell TM (eds.) (2000) *Principles of Neural Science*, 4th edn. New York: McGraw-Hill Companies.

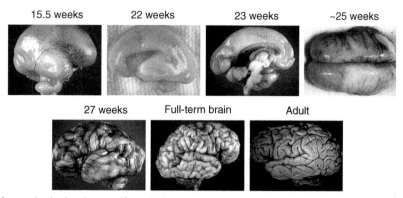

15.5 weeks   22 weeks   23 weeks   ~25 weeks

27 weeks   Full-term brain   Adult

Figure 2 Overview of gross brain development from 15.5 prenatal weeks to adult. Reprinted from http://www-medlib.med.utah.edu/kw/sol/sss/subj2.html – Spencer S. Eccles Health Science Library, National Network of Libraries of Medicine, University of Utah Health Sciences Center, Salt Lake City, Utah.

excessive cell proliferation is due to a faster rate of proliferation, an extended period of proliferation, or decreased incidence of cell death (see later section on PCD). The ultimate cause of macroencephaly is frequently unknown, although it can be genetic in origin. Both microencephaly and macroencephaly generally result in mental retardation with accompanying seizures.

Migration

After neurons are born, they must find their way to their correct locations in the developing nervous system, in order to give rise to the intricate organization of the mature nervous system. The mature cerebral cortex consists of six horizontal layers of cells oriented parallel to the surface of the brain. Other areas of the brain, such as the hippocampus and cerebellum, contain only two layers, while still other areas, like subcortical structures such as the amygdala, are not arranged in a layered formation at all. Layer I is the outermost layer of the cortex, and layer VI is the innermost layer. Vertical columns of related cells span all six layers. The processes by which neurons find their correct home is incredibly intricate, and occurs through two distinct types of migration: (1) radial migration, and (2) tangential migration.

Radial migration occurs when cells migrate from the ventricular and subventricular zones out to the surface of the brain along perpendicular tracts. Radial migration depends upon specialized glial cells, aptly named radial glia, which are among the first cells to be produced by asymmetric division and to differentiate during proliferation. Radial glia contain projections that extend from the ventricular and subventricular zones to the outer surface of the brain. Neurons produced through asymmetric cell division form close associations with radial glial fibers and use them in order to 'crawl' to their correct locations in the cortex.

The first wave of migration out of the ventricular and subventricular zones creates the marginal zone at the surface of the brain, which contains sparsely distributed neurons and becomes layer I in the mature brain (see **Figure 3**). The intermediate zone, between the marginal and subventricular zones, contains the processes (axons and dendrites) of these newly differentiating neurons and in-growing axons from subcortical structures. After this scaffold composed of the ventricular, subventricular, and marginal zones is formed, the second wave of migration begins. The cortical plate, located between the marginal and intermediate zones, is formed by neurons migrating in this second wave (see **Figure 3**). Neurons that come to reside in the cortical plate, which later becomes layers II through VI of the cerebral cortex, migrate in an inside-out fashion. What this means is that neurons with earlier 'birthdays' settle in deeper layers of the cortex (e.g., layers VI, V, IV), whereas neurons with later 'birthdays' migrate over the earlier-born neurons to settle in more superficial layers of the cortex (e.g., layers II and III). Because widespread neurogenesis does not continue beyond a certain point in development, the ventricular and subventricular zones are not present in the mature brain. Radial glia are also not present in the mature brain, and there is some evidence that they differentiate into astrocytes (another type of glial cell) once they are no longer needed for migration. Migration in the cerebral cortex begins during the sixth prenatal week, and continues until approximately 24 weeks, although glial cells continue to migrate throughout the brain until at least the second postnatal year of life.

Although the majority of neurons migrate radially to their final destination, tangential migration also plays a role in the establishment of the mature organization of cerebral cortex. Unlike radial migration, which involves cells moving perpendicular to the surface of the brain, tangential migration involves migration parallel to the surface of the brain through the subventricular or

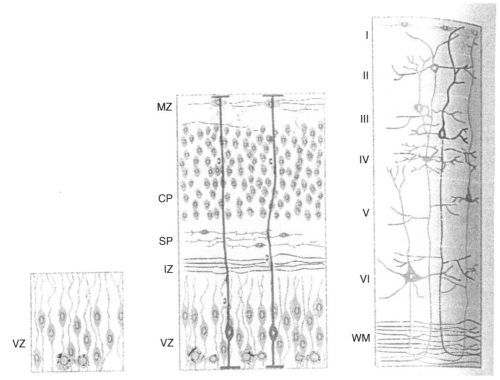

Figure 3 Migration in the developing cerebral cortex, showing the ventricular zone (VZ), intermediate zone (IZ), subplate (SP – a transient population of neurons not present in the adult), cortical plate (CP), marginal zone (MZ), white matter (WM), and layers I–VI. Adapted from Zigmond MJ, Bloom FE, Landis SC, Roberts JL, and Squire LR (eds.) (1999) *Fundamental Neuroscience*. San Diego, CA: Academic Press.

intermediate zone. It is estimated that approximately 20–30% of cells reach their destination via tangential migration. Although it is still unclear what factors determine which populations of cells will migrate tangentially, radial and tangential migration each seem to be associated with particular types of neurons. There is also some evidence that progenitor cells engage in lateral dispersion through tangential migration.

Proliferation and migration cause the surface area of the cortex to expand rapidly. The resultant pressure exerted on the brain contributes to the formation of gyri, the folds on the surface of the brain. Thus, errors in cell migration often lead to abnormalities of the gyri. If neuronal migration to the cortical layers is aberrant in some way, the gyri do not form correctly. In lissencephaly, all cortical layers fail to receive the appropriate number of neurons, and so the surface of the brain is completely smooth. Poly-microgyria refers to an excess of gyri, due to a much larger surface area of the outer cortical layers compared to the inner cortical layers. Defects in the corpus callosum often accompany errors in cell migration, with agenesis (failure to form) of the corpus callosum being the most severe case. These anatomical abnormalities due to errors in cell migration are usually accompanied by mental retardation, seizures, and motor problems.

Circuit Formation

Through the processes involved in neurulation, proliferation, and migration, the crude anatomical organization of the brain is laid down. However, it is not until connections between neurons (i.e., synapses) are formed that the brain begins to assume its mature function. The formation of precise connections between neurons is crucial to normative functioning. It is estimated that there are approximately 100 trillion functional synapses in the mature brain, and the processes by which the neurons of the brain form these connections are astounding in their complexity.

Much more than earlier stages of brain development, circuit formation involves progressive cycles of organization and reorganization. Initially, the connections formed in the brain are only a coarse approximation of the eventual organization of the adult brain; with each progressive cycle of reorganization, the brain becomes more finely tuned until it finally attains its mature organization. Unlike the earlier stages of neurological development (neurulation, proliferation, and migration), the formation and refinement of circuits in the brain are less tightly controlled by genetics. Rather, they are influenced by epigenetic events and external signals from the environment – indeed, external input is necessary for the proper refinement of most circuits in the human brain – although always within the constraints imposed by genetics. Circuit formation involves several steps, including the formation of specialized neural processes, the formation of synapses between neurons, and myelination. Importantly, fine-tuning is largely dependent upon regressive events, including PCD, synaptic pruning, and process retraction.

Programmed Cell Death

PCD (the term apoptosis is often used interchangeably with PCD; however, apoptosis refers to only one well-studied mechanism of PCD, characterized by segmentation of DNA into fragments of a characteristic length) is the earliest initiated of the major regressive events that contribute to the final organization of the adult brain. Importantly, PCD is now known to be a normative part of development (i.e., its root cause is not damage to the brain, nor are the neurons and glia that undergo PCD defective). On average, somewhere between 40% and 60% of neurons produced within the brain die, although this number varies widely across brain regions – in some regions of the brain, as many as 85% of the neurons produced undergo PCD. Neurons can undergo PCD at any phase in their development, although there seem to be two major waves of cell death: an early phase that occurs during proliferation and axonal growth, and a later phase that occurs after the formation of synapses.

PCD is mediated by growth factors produced during cell–cell interactions. Growth factors, also called neurotrophins, are produced in a limited supply in the brain by both neurons and non-neuronal cells, and there is competition among neurons for access to them. Neurons that make inappropriate or nonfunctioning connections with other neurons, or make no connections at all, will not gain access to neurotrophins, and therefore will undergo PCD.

Although the functional significance of PCD is not fully understood, it seems to help establish optimal connectivity in the brain by eliminating aberrant connections.

Growth of Axons and Dendrites

Axons and dendrites are the specialized processes that neurons develop as they differentiate (see **Figure 4**). They mediate communication between neurons at junctions called synapses; generally, axons are on the transmitting end and dendrites are on the receiving end of the signals passed between neurons. Astonishingly, axons can grow up to several centimeters in length, and both axons and dendrites can contain multiple branches so that one neuron can make connections with numerous others.

Growth cones, located at the end of axons, are responsible for both growth of axons and connection with their correct target neurons in the brain. Growth cones are composed of specialized structures called lamellipodia and filopodia. Lamellipodia are thin fan-shaped structures, and filopodia are spiky protrusions from lamellipodia. In order to extend its length, the growth cone attaches to an external substrate in the brain (e.g., the extracellular matrix, or axons of neighboring neurons) and modifies its internal structure – in this way it 'crawls' through the tissue of the brain to its final destination. Growth cones are also responsible for directing the axon to the correct target in the brain. This function is crucial, given the need to form precise connections among the billions of neurons in the brain. The growth cone accomplishes this through receptors that are sensitive to molecular cues in the external environment (e.g., in the extracellular matrix, or located on nearby neurons). Numerous molecules serve to attract or repulse growing axons by promoting or inhibiting growth of the growth cone, thereby directing it in one direction or another. Dendrites begin as thick protrusions from the cell body of the neuron. With the

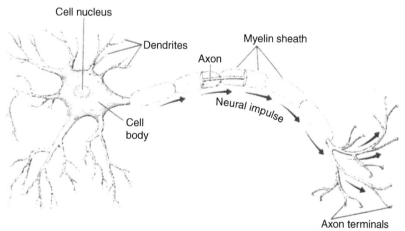

Figure 4 Schematic diagram of a neuron. Adapted from Cole M, Cole SR, and Lightfoot C (2005) *The Development of Children*, 5th edn. New York: Worth Publishers.

growth of incoming axons and the afferent activity that they provide, dendrites expand, form branches, and develop spines – small protrusions at which synaptic contacts generally occur.

Not surprisingly then, the timings of the development of axons and dendrites closely parallel each other. The first axons are apparent at approximately 15 weeks prenatally, although the timing of their development varies widely across brain regions. Crude dendrites also appear at approximately prenatal week 15. Dendritic spines, the sites of synaptic contact, are first apparent by the prenatal weeks 25–27. Both axon and dendrite development continues postnatally until at least the second year of life. There is an initial overproduction of both axons and dendrites, followed by a regression. This elimination is largely driven by competition, and will be discussed in more detail in the section on synaptic pruning.

The formation of axons and dendrites causes further increases in cortical surface area and density, thereby contributing to the establishment of gyri and sulci on the surface of the brain. Thus, the formation of axons and dendrites contributes to an overall increase in brain size and a more mature appearance of the brain.

Errors in axon and dendrite formation often arise as a secondary consequence of other problems in neurological development, such as problems in cell migration. Genetic and environmental factors can both play a role in aberrant axonal and dendritic development. In certain genetic syndromes, such as Down syndrome and fragile X syndrome, dendrites demonstrate reduced branching and reduced number and density of spines. Prematurity and prenatal and perinatal insults can also result in abnormalities in axon and dendrite formation. The most common phenotypic consequences of errors in the development of neuronal processes are mental retardation and seizures. In many cases of severe mental retardation with unknown etiology, postmortem analyses reveal significant abnormalities in dendritic formation, including a paucity of dendritic branches, decreased length of dendritic branches, and decreased number of dendritic spines.

Synaptogenesis

Synapses refer to the points of contact between neurons where information is passed from one neuron to the next. Synapses most often form between axons and dendrites, and consist of a presynaptic neuron, synaptic cleft, and a postsynaptic neuron. In electrochemical synapses an electrical impulse (called the action potential) travels down the length of the axon. Once it reaches the end of the axon, it causes the release of neurotransmitters into the synaptic cleft. These molecules travel across the synaptic cleft, where they interact with receptors on the postsynaptic neuron. As a result of this interaction,

the postsynaptic neuron is either potentiated (i.e., more likely to fire an action potential and 'pass on' the message) or inhibited (i.e., less likely to fire an action potential). (Gap junctions are another type of synapse found in the brain. They are electrical synapses, in which the information is passed directly from one neuron to another through an electrical impulse. As less is known about their development and functional significance, they will not be discussed further.) Although it is difficult to determine when the first synapses form in the human brain, some areas of the brain may form functional synapses as early as prenatal week 15. By prenatal week 23, synapses have started to form in the cerebral cortex. Synaptogenesis continues throughout the prenatal period and peak levels of synapses are not reached until the postnatal period. This article focuses on synapse production and elimination during development. However, it is important to note that synapse formation and elimination occur throughout the lifespan, and are the mechanisms by which new learning occurs.

Peter Huttenlocher and colleagues have thoroughly described a key feature of normative synaptogenesis – specifically, that there is a massive overproduction of synapses across all regions in the human brain. Approximately 40% more synapses are produced during development than are present in the adult brain, and the quantity of this overproduction is remarkably consistent across brain regions. Topographical differences do exist, however, in the timing of synapse overproduction. For example, the rate of synaptogenesis in the visual cortex peaks between 2 and 4 months postnatally, and the peak number of synapses is reached by approximately 8 months. On the other hand, the peak number of synapses in the middle frontal gyrus does not occur until sometime between 12 and 15 months of age. There is compelling evidence that this massive overproduction of synapses seems to be largely under genetic control. For example, when a monkey's eyes are removed prior to birth so that no sensory stimulation can reach the visual cortex, the peak number of synapses in the visual cortex is not different from typical development. Thus, it does not seem as if experience is playing a role in driving the formation of synapses during this initial overproduction phase of development.

Given that the infant brain contains 40% more synapses than the adult brain, how and when is the mature number of synapses reached during development? The adult number of synapses is reached through a process called synaptic pruning, which refers to the loss of synapses in the absence of cell death.

Synaptic Pruning

Initially, the synapses that are formed in the infant brain are labile. Whether or not a synapse is stabilized or weakened and eventually pruned depends in large part on the activity of that synapse. Specifically, synaptic pruning follows the Hebbian principle of use/disuse; that is, synapses that are more active are strengthened, whereas synapses that are less active are weakened and eventually pruned. Activity at a synapse involves both the pre- and postsynaptic neuron, and both neurotransmitters and neurotrophic factors (and their receptors on the pre- and postsynaptic cells) are involved in producing the coordinated activity between neurons that is necessary for the stabilization of synaptic contacts. Thus, neurotrophic factors play a role in both neuron and synapse survival. When synapses are eliminated, this also involves the withdrawal of the axon that participated in that synapse, thereby leading to the competitive elimination of axons that was mentioned in a previous section.

Like the timing of synapse overproduction, there are differences among brain regions in the time course of synaptic pruning, although it generally follows a much more protracted time course than synapse overproduction. As mentioned earlier, synapse production reaches its peak in the visual cortex at approximately 8 months of age. Pruning of these synapses continues until approximately 6 years of age, when the adult level of synapses is reached. On the other hand, synaptic pruning in the prefrontal cortex, where peak levels of synapses are not obtained until sometime in the first year of life, is not complete until adolescence.

Synaptic pruning, thought to be common to all neuronal systems, allows for fine-tuning of the connections in the brain based on experience. Although spontaneous, endogenous neural activity does contribute to synaptic stabilization, activity due to exogenous events impinging on neural systems (e.g., sensory stimulation) plays a crucial role in synaptic stabilization. Earlier events in the development of the brain are under tight genetic control and, although influenced by the local environment, are relatively impervious to all but the most dramatic of outside influences (e.g., teratogens). However, synaptic pruning depends largely upon the experiences that the developing child has with the world around him/her, and is the mechanism whereby the brain 'captures' experience. The incredibly precise organization of the mature brain is the instantiation of the interaction between the brain and the external environment throughout development. Thus, normative experiences during development lead to the maintenance of proper connections and the elimination of aberrant ones, whereas aberrant experiences during development will lead to a failure to maintain appropriate connections and maintenance of inappropriate connections. The last section of this article will further explore two main mechanisms by which the brain captures experience during development, although the final step in the development of mature connections within the brain is discussed first.

Myelination

Myelin is a lipid protein substance composed of glial cells that wraps around certain axons, creating an insulation effect that allows for more rapid conduction of action potentials. Thus, myelinated axons transmit information much faster than do unmyelinated axons. Myelination begins prenatally and continues, in some areas of the brain, into middle age. The time course of myelination, like synaptogenesis and pruning, varies widely across brain regions. As a general rule, myelination occurs first in neural systems that underlie behaviors that are present early in life. For example, primary sensory and motor areas are myelinated before association areas, and the neural systems involved in postural control and the vestibular sense are fully myelinated before birth. On the other hand, areas of the prefrontal cortex do not become fully myelinated until middle age.

Although not all areas of the nervous system are myelinated (e.g., the ANS is not myelinated), myelination is critical for proper behavioral functioning. Genetic and environmental factors can result in deficiencies in myelination, and myelin is also the target of certain adulthood diseases (e.g., multiple sclerosis). Demyelination results in decreased conduction velocity and increased conduction failures, leading to an overall slowing of information transmission in the brain. As one might imagine, errors in myelination often lead to mental retardation and movement disorders.

Thus, circuit formation involves PCD, the growth of specialized neural processes (axons and dendrites), synaptogenesis and synaptic pruning, and myelination. The timing of these processes during development varies across neural systems (see **Figure 5**); earlier maturing neural systems (e.g., primary visual areas) reach peak levels of synapses, undergo synaptic pruning down to adult levels, and myelinate sooner in development than later maturing systems (e.g., prefrontal cortex). Regressive events play a pivotal role in fine-tuning the connections in the brain based on experience, and it is to this topic that we turn next.

Developmental Plasticity

The early events in neurological development are under tight genetic control and therefore do not depend on the external environment for elaboration (although they are not completely impervious to experience). However, once these building blocks of the brain are in place, there is a continuous reciprocal interaction between the brain and the external environment. Through sensory input, the external environment impinges on brain circuitry, which causes progressive refinement of connections until some optimal level of organization is attained. This ability of the developing brain to adapt based on interactions with

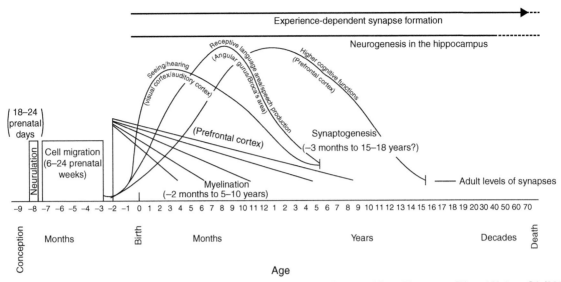

Figure 5 Developmental trajectories of mechanisms of brain development. Reprinted from Thompson RA and Nelson CA (2001) Developmental science and the media: Early brain development. *American Psychologist* 56: 5–15. American Psychological Association.

the external environment is referred to as developmental plasticity and is rooted in the regressive events (e.g., synaptic pruning) that were described previously. (The term plasticity is also used to describe the extent of recovery following brain damage (e.g., stroke) in the adult. It is important to note that the process of developmental plasticity described here is a normative part of development. The adult brain is also capable of normative plasticity, e.g., new learning causes the formation or elimination of synapses.) The extent of plasticity observed during neural development varies across brain regions. Different systems in the developing brain are more or less open to input from the environment, and are sensitive at different times across development.

William Greenough and colleagues have proposed a model of neurological development that distinguishes between two forms of plasticity: experience-expectant and experience-dependent plasticity. This model is an attempt to explain the mechanisms by which experience 'gets inside' the brain, as there is ample evidence that behavior and its underlying neural circuitry are influenced by experiences throughout life. Experience-expectant and experience-dependent plasticity differ in terms of their mechanisms (synaptic pruning vs. synaptogenesis), the characteristics of the environmental input that drive these processes, and whether or not they are associated with sensitive periods. However, both types of plasticity can lead to long-lasting changes in the brain.

Experience-Expectant Plasticity

Experience-expectant plasticity occurs via the massive overproduction and the subsequent pruning back of synapses in the developing brain. Synapses that are more active are more likely to be preserved, whereas synapses that are less active are weakened and eventually eliminated; as such, the experiences that occur during developmental periods of synaptic pruning play a critical role in determining which synapses are strengthened vs. eliminated. In this way, experience-expectant plasticity can take advantage of experiences that, through evolutionary history, have become species-typical and occur at defined points in time during development (e.g., patterned visual input). Experience-expectant plasticity follows the time course of synaptic pruning, and therefore varies across different regions of the brain that have different developmental trajectories of synapse overproduction and pruning (e.g., visual cortex vs. prefrontal cortex). Because synaptogenesis and pruning occur at defined periods during development, this gives rise to a phenomenon called a sensitive period, which is a window of time during development in which specific experience(s) must occur for the normative development of the system in question. If typical experiences do not occur during that time window, or the quantities of specific experiences are not sufficient, development does not proceed in a normative fashion, even if those same experiences occur later in life.

Experience-Dependent Plasticity

Conversely, experience-dependent plasticity is a lifelong process by which the brain adapts to experiences that are unique to the individual. As in experience-expectant plasticity, experience-dependent plasticity involves synaptic changes; however, it involves the creation of new synapses and changes in the morphology of synapses, rather than the pruning of unnecessary or aberrant synapses. Synaptogenesis based on experience continues to occur throughout the lifespan, and thus, this mechanism of plasticity is responsible for learning and memory in adulthood as well as during development. As the underlying neural mechanism of this type of plasticity occurs across the lifespan, it is not associated with sensitive periods. That is, learning unique to the individual can occur at any point in time. It is important to note that human behaviors can rarely be explained entirely in terms of only one type of plasticity; most complex behaviors involve both mechanisms of plasticity.

Conclusion

In summary, neurological development follows a protracted course that involves both progressive and regressive events. These events occur in overlapping waves beginning at prenatal day 18 and continuing through adolescence, and their timing varies widely across brain regions. The brain does not develop in a vacuum; as such, it is affected by interactions with the external environment, although earlier events in the development of the brain (i.e., neural induction, proliferation, migration) are less amenable to change based on exogenous influences than are later events (i.e., axon and dendrite outgrowth, synapse formation, and retraction). Indeed, one of the hallmarks of human brain development is plasticity, or the ability of the brain to adapt in accordance with environmental influences.

See also: Down Syndrome; Intellectual Disabilities; Teratology.

Suggested Readings

Cole M, Cole SR, and Lightfoot C (2005) *The Development of Children,* 5th edn. New York: Worth Publishers.

Greenough WT, Black JE, and Wallace CS (1987) Experience and brain development. *Child Development* 58: 539–559.

Huttenlocher PR (1994) Synaptogenesis, synapse elimination, and neural plasticity in human cerebral cortex. In: Nelson CA (ed.) *Threats to Optimal Development: Integrating Biological, Psychological, and Social Risk Factors,* pp. 35–54. Hillsdale, NJ: Lawrence Erlbaum Associates, Inc.

Kandel ER, Schwartz JH, and Jessell TM (eds.) (2000) *Principles of Neural Science,* 4th edn. New York: McGraw-Hill Companies.

Monk CS, Webb SJ, and Nelson CA (2001) Prenatal neurobiological development: Molecular mechanisms and anatomical change. *Developmental Neuropsychology* 19: 211–236.

Nelson CA, de Haan M, and Thomas KM (2006) Neural bases of cognitive development. In: Damon W, Lerner R, Kuhn D, and Siegler R (eds.) *Handbook of Child Psychology: Vol. 2. Cognitive, Perception and Language,* 6th edn., pp. 33–57. Princeton, NJ: Wiley.

Rakic P, Ang ESBC, and Breunig J (2004) Setting the stage for cognition: Genesis of the primate cerebral cortex. In: Gazzaniga MS (ed.) *The Cognitive Neurosciences,* 3rd edn., pp. 33–49. Cambridge, MA: MIT Press.

Thompson RA and Nelson CA (2001) Developmental science and the media: Early brain development. *American Psychologist* 56: 5–15.

Volpe JJ (1995) *Neurology of the Newborn,* 3rd edn. Philadelphia, PA: Saunders.

Webb SJ, Monk CS, and Nelson CA (2001) Mechanisms of postnatal neurobiological development: Implications for human development. *Developmental Neuropsychology* 19: 147–171.

Zigmond MJ, Bloom FE, Landis SC, Roberts JL, and Squire LR (eds.) (1999) *Fundamental Neuroscience.* San Diego, CA: Academic Press.

Obesity

C F Bolling, Children's Hospital Medical Center, Cincinnati, OH, USA
S R Daniels, University of Colorado Health Sciences Center, Denver, CO, USA

Glossary

Adipocyte – Individual fat cell.
Adiposity (or body mass index, BMI) rebound –
The period between 4 years and 8 years when a
child's BMI is at its nadir.
At-risk for overweight (AROW) – 85th or greater
and less than 95th percentile BMI for age and
gender.
Body mass index (BMI) – A mathematical formula
to assess relative body weight. The measure
correlates highly with body fat. BMI is calculated as
weight in kilograms divided by the square of the
height in meters ($kg\,m^{-2}$).
Energy density – A general description of calories
per volume. A high-calorie, low-volume food is
generally high in fat or sugar content and is low in
fiber or water content.
Ideal body weight (IBW) – A term describing the
weight that people are expected to weigh based on
age, sex, and height which is the weight for an
individual that results in a body mass index of 20–25.
Overweight – 95th or greater percentile BMI for age
and gender. For adults, this is represented by a BMI
25 or greater. In adults, obesity is defined as having a
BMI 30 or greater.

Introduction

Obesity is a term generally reserved for the study of adult
medicine and is defined by having a body mass index (BMI)
of over 30, historically the 90th percentile for adults. In
pediatric patients, weight status is generally more often described as either overweight or at-risk for overweight
(AROW). Overweight is defined as being at greater than or
equal to 95th percentile BMI for age and gender. AROW is
defined as being greater than or equal to the 85th percentile
and less than the 95th percentile BMI for age and gender.

There are experts in the field of obesity who advocate
for a definition of pediatric obesity consistent with the
Institute of Medicine accepted adult definitions in which
overweight is defined as having a BMI greater than or
equal to the 85th percentile and less than the 95th percentile and obesity is defined as greater than or equal to
95th percentile. Other experts in the field also advocate
for the use of greater than or equal to the 99th percentile
as being obese. Resolution of this occasionally confusing
terminology is expected as the study of overweight
matures as a discipline.

Further delineation occurs between morbid obesity
and super-obesity. Universally accepted definitions are
lacking, but general classifications are accepted. For adults,
morbid obesity or extreme obesity is often defined as being
over 100 lb overweight or having a BMI of 40–50 or
50–100% over ideal body weight (IBW). Super-obesity is
similarly defined as being approximately greater than
200 lb overweight, having a BMI of 50–60 or being 225%
over IBW. Some studies will define persons over a BMI of
60 as being super–super obese. These classifications are
less widely accepted in the pediatric practice.

For reference, the BMI of a 'typical' 12 kg (26.4 lb) and
87 cm (34 in) 2-year-old boy at the 50 percentile for height
and weight is 15.9. The 'normal range' for BMI for a
2-year-old is form 14.8 at the 5 percentile to 19.3 at the
95 percentile. The same 87 cm 2-year-old boy would need
to weigh 14.6 kg (32.1 lb) to be considered 'overweight'.
Minimum BMI is typically achieved between age 5 and 6
when the 50th percentile BMI is 15.4. After this point, BMI
'rebounds'. Early BMI rebound is considered to be a risk
factor for later obesity. Girls' BMI are very similar to boys
with earlier achievement of final BMI reflecting faster
progression through puberty.

Other definitions of overweight are currently under consideration, but are, as yet, not widely accepted. Certain researchers and clinicians advocate for measurements that more accurately measure total body fat as BMI can be elevated by increased musculature. Abdominal circumference is more difficult to measure and is less standardized in technique, body impedance analysis requires additional equipment and can be somewhat inaccurate, and dual X-ray absorptionetry (DEXA) scan exposes patients to radiation and incurs added costs. Displacement techniques of body fat analysis are under development.

Epidemiology

US

Rates of AROW and overweight are on the increase throughout all areas of the US. The commonly accepted rates of 10% between the 85th and 95th and 5% of the population were generated from longitudinal studies carried out between 1967 and 1994. Using these values, subsequent surveys of pediatric height and weight have demonstrated an approximate doubling in the prevalence of both AROW and overweight children.

Highest rates of AROW and overweight come in certain sociodemographic groups. Higher rates are associated with low socioeconomic status. Being African American, Native American, Latino, or Appalachian is also associated. The highest rates of overweight occur in the Southeastern and Midwestern areas of the country.

The prevalence of super-obesity is difficult to describe in younger age groups, but is increasing in adolescents. Approximately, 750 000 American adolescents, or approximately 2.5% of the population, have a BMI greater than 40 and well over 1 000 000 adolescents have a BMI between 35 and 40.

Other Nations

Comparing national rates of pediatric obesity is problematic for a number of reasons. Differing definitions, variations in measurement practice, varying cultural acceptance of weight status, disparities in body composition all conspire to make comparing rates between countries very difficult. In spite of these limitations in comparing country rates, longitudinally following individual country rates has demonstrated a worsening international problem.

Nations with developed economies
While the US has experienced the most profound explosion in overweight pediatric prevalence, many other nations are experiencing a similar phenomenon. The UK, Germany, France, Italy, Spain, Canada, and Australia have closely followed patterns seen in the US. Other industrialized nations in Europe have shown a similar but delayed pattern. Developed nations in Asia have seen a milder but still significant increase in prevalence in overweight.

Developing nations
One of the more concerning epidemiologic occurrences since 2000 has been the spread of pediatric overweight to nations with developing economies. Previously unreported, China, India, and Mexico have all experienced a statistically significant increase in the rates of pediatric overweight. Increasing access to food and access to technology encouraging sedentary behavior is felt to be a major contributor to this rise in these rates and, as a result of increasing economic development, is expected to worsen in these countries.

Etiology

Pediatric overweight may be described as either being endogenous, caused by innate biologic processes, or exogenous, caused by external factors. This distinction does not imply exclusion of behavioral modification for endogenous obesity nor the exclusion of pharmacologic or surgically based treatment for exogenous overweight.

Exogenous Overweight

The relatively fixed number of cases from endogenous causes of overweight implies that the greatest number of cases of overweight is due to an increase in the number of cases of exogenous overweight. Promotion of increased calorie intake and discouragement of activity have combined to create a more obesigenic environment. These factors that may be modified by behavioral and environmental determinants have upset energy balance and led to an increase in weight status.

Increased energy intake
Calorie intake in average American children had remained steady until approximately 1990. Since 1990, studies have indicated an increase of approximately 10–15% in daily caloric intake across most pediatric age groups. The source of this increase in calories is likely due to increased intake of simple sugars.

The percentage of daily calories derived from fruit juice and sweetened drinks including soft drinks and sports drinks have doubled from 1994 to 2004 in preschool groups. In other pediatric age groups, soft drink consumption has been accelerating. In recent surveys when describing generally accepted food classifications, soft drinks are the third greatest contributor of calories in 6–8-year-olds, second highest contributor in 9–11-year-olds and greatest contributor in 12–15-year-olds.

Fast food has been linked to decreased fruit and vegetable intake, decreased milk intake, increased sweetened drink consumption, increased calorie intake, increased intake of high-calorie foods, and increased intake of starchy vegetables (potatoes). These are behaviors that have been associated with excess weight gain. Approximately, 25% of children aged 4–8 years eat fast food on any given day. French fries are the most commonly eaten vegetable for children aged 15–24 months.

All groups have experienced a steady decline in the intake of foods low in energy density, namely fresh fruits and vegetables. Large nutritional studies estimate that 25–33% of American preschool children consume no fruits or vegetables. In other studies, the leading vegetable for children in all age groups is identified as deep-fat fried potato products. Other studies have demonstrated increased intake in other high-energy density foods. Various studies have demonstrated increases in snack foods, prepared baked goods, candy, pizza, hamburgers, fried chicken, and Mexican and Chinese fast food.

Portion control studies also demonstrate the increase in portion size seen in American dietary habits. Vended items, fast food promotions, and buffet-style eating habits have all been implicated in elevating calorie intake.

Decreased energy expenditure

Average energy expenditure has also been implicated as a root cause in the increased prevalence of pediatric overweight. In the US example, parental concerns over safety, the proliferation of point to point automobile transport, and limitations of public transit have reduced walking and cycling as transportation methods for children. Studies have shown a decrease in outdoor time and an overall total decrease in time spent in active play. Environmental studies have begun to make a link between green space interconnectivity/accessibility and rates of overweight. The connection between pediatric overweight and urban sprawl associated with a lack of connected and accessible parks is not completely clear.

Excess screen time is also associated with increased overweight. Children who spend more than 2 h daily in front of computer, television programming, video games, or DVD/VHS movies have been shown to have elevated rates of pediatric overweight. Educational academic mandates have also reduced time available in school days for physical education. This has presumably further reduced activity during school time.

Other considerations

Breastfeeding appears to be protective against pediatric overweight. Studies have indicated that children who bottle-feed have significantly higher concentrations of insulin than children who breastfeed. Elevated insulin promotes fat deposition and more rapid development of adipocytes in young children. Breastmilk also contains factors like epidermal growth factor and inflammatory hormones such as tumor necrosis factor-alpha (TNF-α)

that promote fat cell growth. Breastfeeding may also increase levels of leptin which suppresses appetite. It has also been demonstrated that children who breastfeed have lower overall intake of calories and protein than bottle-fed children. Other studies suggest that formula contains higher levels of protein than breast milk and that this may cause increased weight gain in infants.

Children with early adiposity rebound may be at greater risk for overweight at a later age. Adiposity rebound is the period between 4 and 8 years when a child's BMI is at its nadir. Children with an earlier nadir (between 4 and 5 years of age) tend to have a greater risk of obesity, hypertension, impaired glucose tolerance, and diabetes in adulthood. Early adiposity rebound has also been recorded in a number of childhood diseases that are characterized by adult obesity, including congenital adrenal hyperplasia, hypothyroidism, hyperphenylalaninemia, and acute lymphoblastic leukemia. Unfortunately, the mechanism of adiposity rebound leading to these conditions is not well described. These factors make addressing documented early weight gain a priority in reducing pediatric overweight.

Endogenous Obesity

Endogenous causes of obesity are much less common and are usually associated with other obvious medical syndromes. These organic causes of obesity may be mediated by specific hormone deficiencies. Leptin that is secreted by adipocytes crosses the blood brain barrier to influence energy balance and reduce adipose content by increasing heat generation and decreasing appetite. Leptin-deficiency states have been associated with obesity. Likewise, other hormonal deficiencies and hormone receptor dysfunction states have been linked with genetic causes of obesity.

Certain chromosomal anomalies are associated with obesity. The prevalence of overweight in Down syndrome is greater than that in the general population when it has been accurately assessed. Prader–Willi syndrome which is accompanied by characteristic physical features and developmental delay is caused by a chromosomal deletion of a section of chromosome 15. Obesity in Prader–Willi syndrome is likely related to over secretion of the growth-promoting hormone, ghrelin. Sim-1, a syndrome characterized by a balanced translocation between chromosomes 1 and 6, has been associated with obesity. WAGR syndrome (WAGR – Wilm's tumor, anorexia, ambiguous genitalia, and mental retardation) is associated with obesity through an apparent chromosome 11 deletion.

Other polygenic syndromes are associated with obesity. These syndromes are likely to be mediated hormonally. Patients who are carriers for the genetic enzyme deficiency, pro-opiomelanocortin (POMC) deficiency, and relatives of patients with this defect appear to have lack of neural regulation of appetite, excess eating and resulting obesity. A deficiency in certain cellular hormone receptors, melanocortin-4 receptor deficiency, is likely a cause for obesity in heterozygous family members due to hyperinsulinism. Bardet–Biedl syndrome is a polygenic, autosomal recessive condition characterized by central obesity, mental retardation, underdeveloped gonadal tissue, and kidney abnormalities. Albright's hereditary osteodystrophy is an autosomal dominant disorder in which patients demonstrate short stature, obesity, round facies, extremity abnormalities, and nonfunctional soft tissue transformation into bone. Patients with fragile X-syndrome often have obesity accompanied by mental retardation, large testes, large ears, macrocephaly, large mandibular jaws, and high-pitched speech. Borjeson–Forssman–Lehman syndrome is characterized by mental retardation, epilepsy, underdeveloped gonadal tissue, and obesity. Cohen syndrome is an autosomal recessive disorder and is characterized by obesity, mental retardation, small head size, unusual facial features and disorders of eye and neural tissue that impair vision. Alström syndrome is inherited in an autosomal recessive pattern and is characterized by high insulin and glucose as well as sensory neurologic deficits. An extremely rare syndrome associated with excess weight gain is MOMO (macrosomia, obesity, macrocephaly, ocular abnormalities) syndrome. Acromegaly and growth hormone excess may result in increased weight but is generally accompanied with increased height growth.

Obesity as a Complication of Medical or Surgical Therapy

Obesity may also present as a side effect of medical therapy. Cushing's syndrome from chronic steroid use for asthma, juvenile rheumatoid arthritis, or other disease processes may result in overweight. Central nervous system procedures may result in disturbance of the hypothalamic appetite regulation center that may prevent satiety.

Pathophysiology

While the basic pathophysiology of overweight and obesity involves a simple mismatch between energy intake and energy expenditure with resulting fat deposition, the effects on the body are far reaching and potentially devastating.

Cardiovascular Effects

Dyslipidemias
Increased intake of dietary fats contributes to elevated circulating triglycerides and cholesterol through direct absorption and can lead to overweight. However, the relation between overweight and circulating levels of agents associated with atherosclerosis is not completely understood.

Hyperlipidemias are multifactorial in origin and are regulated by genetic, exercise, and dietary factors. High-density lipoprotein (HDL) or 'good cholesterol', which increases with increasing activity, is associated with decreased atherosclerosis. HDL is involved in the clearing of agents that cause clot formation and the transport of them to the liver. Low- and very low-density lipoproteins (LDL and VLDL) or 'bad cholesterols' are elevated in part by increased lipid and cholesterol intake and are associated with an increase in these clot-forming agents. Inflammatory processes associated with elevated circulating triglycerides and lower density lipoproteins have also been implicated with atherogenesis. C-reactive protein has also implicated as mediating this clot-formation process.

Hypertension
The relationship of obesity and overweight to hypertension is well established. The prevalence of overweight in hypertensive patients combined with the response in blood pressure to weight loss speaks to a causative relationship between weight status and hypertension. Unfortunately, the pathophysiologic mechanism is still poorly defined.

Renal Effects

Renal complications of obesity include hypertension as described above and complications associated with the development of diabetes. The pathogenesis of these processes is, again, incompletely understood but likely related to inflammatory processes.

Endocrine Effects

Hyperinsulinism
Weight status has a demonstrable impact on the development of insulin resistance. In particular, adipocyte-derived hormones, TNF-α and adiponectin, are potent inducers of insulin resistance through cell membrane mechanisms. This increase in insulin resistance ultimately can lead to type II diabetes. The mechanism is unknown, but there is also an association with obesity in patients with type 1 diabetes.

Cytokines in obesity
A variety of hormones have been implicated in the development of obesity and the complications seen in it. **Table 1** summarizes the source, mechanism, and probable effect of some of the more understood hormones. It should be noted that the interaction between these hormones is unclear and the identification of other cytokines are areas of needed research.

Gastrointestinal Effects

Adipocytes, long felt to be merely storehouses of fat for use in times of limited food, have become more understood as inflammatory cells. Some of the most dramatic activity as inflammatory cells occurs in the liver. Nonalcoholic fatty liver disease and the more severe

Table 1 Hormones important in appetite and weight regulation

Agent	Source	Other	Mechanism	Effect
Insulin	Pancreas	Postprandial	Facilitates cellular uptake of glucose	Growth, energy metabolism
PYY	GI	Postprandial	Decreases release of orexigenic hypothalamic neuropeptide Y (NPY) via arcuate nucleus	Induces satiety and decreases food intake
Ghrelin	GI	Preprandial	Increases expression of NPY	Stimulates food intake
GLP-1	GI	Postprandial	Increases postprandial insulin release	Inhibits food intake
PP	GI		?	Inhibits appetite and promotes energy expenditure
Leptin	Adipose		Inhibits NPY, melanin concentrating hormone, orexin A, agouti-related peptide, cannabinoid systems Upregulates pro-opiomelanocortin/ mela-nocortin, cocaine and amphetamine regulated transcript and corticotropin-releasing hormone	Suppression of food intake
Orexin A(&B)	Hypothalamus	Affects sleep wake cycle	Integration of metabolic and circadian sleep debt influences	Promotes wakefulness and increases appetite
Adiponectin	Adipose	Inversely related to BMI; female > male	1. Bind to receptors affecting AMP kinase 2. Complementary to leptin	Promotes gluconeogenesis, glucose uptake, TG clearance, weight gain and insulin resistance
TNF-α	Adipose	Lipolysis and apoptosis (cell death)	Acute phase protein which initiates a cascade of cytokines and increases vascular permeability	Induction on insulin resistance

GI, gastrointestinal tract

nonalcoholic steatohepatitis are both felt to be mediated through the local inflammatory effects of adipocytes that secret TNF-α and other agents.

Psychological Effects

Children who are overweight perceive their different weight status usually by age 6 years. This perception of difference may interfere with assimilation and self-image. Depression and poor school performance have been linked to overweight in childhood. Degree of overweight is positively correlated with poor school performance, lessened self-esteem and depression.

As the average weight of children continues to increase, this perception of 'being different' may subside. This may reduce the stress certain children feel about being different. Unfortunately though, this increasing average population weight may reduce the recognition of abnormally high weight in other patients by making it less physically obvious.

Neurologic Effects

Idiopathic intracranial hypertension or pseudotumor cerebri is a potentially life-threatening swelling of the brain. It has symptoms that resemble the symptoms of brain tumor due to increased pressure. It has been linked in repeated studies with obesity. This condition is also increased in diseases which are characterized by coagulation disorders. The inflammation-mediated coagulation disorders seen in obese patients have led to the theory that thromboembolic events in the cerebrospinal fluid reabsorption system in the central nervous ventricular system in overweight patients is the instigating factor in pseudotumor cerebri for them.

Hematologic Effects

Venous stasis, inactivity, and microvascular injury associated with diabetes create a milieu more favorable to thromboembolism formation in overweight and obese patients.

Pulmonary Effects

A relatively common complication of obesity is hypoventilation syndrome with sleep. This process is likely related to anatomic obstruction and to altered central control of respiration. While the pathogenesis of this syndrome is not completely understood, the resulting cardiac effects are likely due to ongoing high carbon dioxide levels and low oxygen levels.

Orthopedic Effects

Overweight patients have an increased likelihood of having slipped capital femoral epiphysis (SCFE) or Blount's disease (progressive bowing of the proximal tibia). Both processes are felt to be mechanical complications of excess weight. The fact that the incidence of these disorders increases with increasing weight lends support to the acceptance of this mechanism.

Clinical Picture and Diagnostic Testing

The clinical picture of obesity and overweight can be varied. This variability stems from the multiple possible comorbidities and the unpredictable expression of those comorbidities.

Some of the more common historical presentations include behavior problems, sleep difficulties, snoring, depression, lethargy, shortness of breath on exertion, ankle sprain, asthma, sleep apnea, headache, abdominal pain, leg pain, back pain, vomiting, and diarrhea. Common physical examination findings include limited mobility, shortness of breath, flat affect, large tonsils, premature height growth, hypertension, abdominal discomfort, acanthosis nigricans (excess neck pigmentation from high circulating insulin levels), generous suprapubic fat pad and bowing of the proximal tibia.

Table 2 describes a suggested inventory of historical questions and physical examination items to document during a clinical visit.

Laboratory evaluation is not necessary in most cases. However, poor response to therapy or extreme overweight requires diligent exclusion of organic causes of overweight. The implications of certain laboratory values, such as fasting insulin and oral glucose tolerance, are not fully understood and therefore not universally recommended. Table 3 lists labs to consider in the evaluation of an overweight patient.

Treatment

A basic principle of treatment has been the use of a graduated approach guided by severity of overweight

Table 2　History and physical exam template for a visits with overweight preschoolers

History (should be complete, but the following lists all needed areas of focus)

Chief complaint	What are your feelings about your/your child's weight status?
Present illness	What is the course of your child's weight over the past 6 months?
	What are your feelings about your child losing weight?
	Have you tried to help your child lose weight before?
	If so, how did it work?
Diet	What are your child's three favorite vegetables?
	What does your child like to drink?
	What does your child eat that makes him gain weight?
	What are your and his good habits?
	What are your and his bad habits?
Exercise	Tell me about your child's activity level.
	Tell me about your feelings with exercise.
	Explain to me what it is like to bike and walk in your neighborhood.
Child-care	Where and how often?
	Does the child-care promote physical activity? Explain how or why not.
Primary doctor	Who is your family doctor or pediatrician? What has he/she told you about your weight?
Family history	Document at least the following processes in all first and second degree relatives: obesity, hypertension, cardiovascular disease, dyslipidemias, diabetes, thyroid disease.
Past medical	Medications, allergies, surgeries, hospitalizations, other chronic illnesses such as attention deficit with hyperactivity disorder.
Review of systems	Headache, hot/cold intolerance, sleep problems, joint symptoms, back pain, depression, sleep problems shortness of breath, leg pain, polyuria, polydipsia, snoring.
Social history	Living arrangement.

Physical exam (a complete examination is required, but the following lists all needed areas of focus)

Height	
Weight	
Calculated BMI	
General	Affect, general comfort level, acute distress
Head	Facies, appearance
Eyes	Optic disks
Throat	Posterior pharynx
Neck	Thyroid palpation, acanthosis
Heart	Murmur
Lungs	Rales, wheezes
Abdomen	Liver size
Genital	Tanner stage
Skin	Rash, axillary or intertrginous
Orthopedic	Proximal knee and ankle exam, scoliosis check

and age. Generally, the level of complexity of intervention increases with degree of overweight and increase in age. The continued increase in obesity prevalence across all age groups has called into question all approaches to weight management, but there is a general consensus among experts that the intensity of intervention has typically not been adequate.

Although uniformity in treatment is lacking, guidelines for targeting specific behaviors to prevent obesity do exist. In 2005, the American Heart Association recommended the following for healthy weight promotion in preschoolers (**Table 4**).

Feeding Habits for Obesity Prevention

The most appropriate approach for young children is establishment of good eating habits. Young children should be fed on demand and be allowed to self-regulate intake, particularly in the neonatal period. 'Plate clearing' should be discouraged. Meal times should be predictably and consistently scheduled. Limited options are felt to promote trying new foods since children will often eat previously untried foods if previously selected options are not available. Similarly, foods should be presented repeatedly. It is estimated that children will try a food seven times before determining if they like the taste. Meal times should be of a finite length. Making multiple 'on demand'

meals and allowing late night snacks may promote excess caloric intake and promote behavioral problems associated with food. Going to bed with an empty stomach is not contraindicated in young children. Healthy foods should be prepackaged for easy access and should be readily available on countertops and in the refrigerator.

Behavioral Options for Overweight Children

There are many proposed and promoted behavioral options for dietary change in adults, but relatively few options for children. Even inside major medical centers, organized evidence-based and clinically effective programs for overweight children are lacking. Research in this area suggests certain approaches show more promise.

Readiness to change in parental behavior is critical. Historically, the didactic approach of most physicians to parents has been ineffective in bringing about dietary change. Practitioners have tended to address behavior change in the same way other health recommendations were made, that is, prescriptively. Behavioral studies indicate that parents are unlikely to regard even demonstrably overweight children as being overweight. This mismatch between parental perception and practitioner perception has impaired parents' willingness to implement behavior changes. A movement to address readiness, a principle long used in substance abuse work, promises to improve adherence. Behavioral techniques such as motivational interviewing, readiness based tailoring of materials, and more intensive follow-up hold promise.

Behavior modification has been the most commonly used behavioral technique in weight management and remains the central approach of most organized programs. Reward for implementation of healthy habits and redirection from unhealthy habits are common techniques. Teaching parents goal-setting techniques and using nondietary rewards has shown efficacy. Limitation to two to three goals, frequent follow-up, and inclusion of positive activity goals, as opposed to purely dietary denial goals, appears appropriate.

The setting of these programs is nearly as varied as their content. Physician offices, tertiary care centers,

Table 3 Laboratory evaluation of an overweight patient

Consider often
Fasting: Glucose, total cholesterol, high-density lipoprotein cholesterol, low-density lipoprotein cholesterol, triglycerides
Not necessarily fasting: AST, ALT, γ-GT, alkaline phosphatase, total and direct bilirubin, total protein, albumin

Consider if indicated
Fasting: Insulin
Not necessarily fasting: CBC, calcium, sodium, potassium, chloride, bicarbonate, blood urea nitrogen, creatinine, free thyroid hormone, thyroid stimulating hormone, body composition analysis (body impedance analysis, DEXA scan, displacement techniques)

Table 4 American Heart Association Guidelines for healthy weight in preschoolers

Parents chose meal times, not children

Provide a wide variety of nutrient-dense foods such as fruits and vegetables instead of high-energy–density/nutrient-poor foods such salty snacks, ice cream, fried foods, cookies and sweetened beverages
Pay attention to portion size; serve portions appropriate for the child's size and age
Use nonfat or low-fat dairy products as sources of calcium and protein
Limit snacking during sedentary behavior or in response to boredom and particularly restrict use of sweet/sweetened beverages as snacks (e.g., juice, soda, sports drinks)
Limit sedentary behaviors, with no more than 1–2 h per day of video screen/television and no television sets in children's bedrooms
Allow self-regulation of total caloric intake in the presence of normal BMI or weight for height
Have regular family meals to promote social interaction and role model food-related behavior

community health centers, and schools all deliver these and other forms of intervention. Since pediatric overweight is a heterogeneous illness in both origin and treatment, the most appropriate location for delivery is expected to vary with patients and families.

A common concern expressed by practitioners is hesitance to deliver dietary interventions to pediatric patients for fear of unmasking or promoting anorexia nervosa, bulimia or other eating disorders. This risk appears to be small particularly in younger children. In fact, allowing progression to heavier weights may be a greater risk for eating disorders. Eating disorders, in most instances, represent a different psychopathology than that seen in pediatric overweight and practitioners should not avoid discussion of weight with respect to these fears.

The treatment of the extremely overweight infant and toddler is an area of needed research. Approaches to treating extreme overweight, BMI over the 99.5 percentile for age and gender, appear to require very intensive and specialized treatment regimens to bring about normalization in BMI. Children in these categories often come from families with markedly disordered parenting skills. These families often demonstrate a dysfunctional preoccupation with food and disordered parenting and behavioral enforcement.

Successful interventions are rare. Some experts suggest handling cases of extreme overweight similarly to cases of failure to thrive due to undernutrition because of the similar risk to long-term health and the inability of the caregiver unit to provide appropriate nutrition. This approach, which is associated with significant stress for patients, families, and caregivers should be undertaken with great caution and with close involvement of a consistent social worker.

Pharmacologic Options

Pharmacologic intervention for pediatric weight management is not readily accepted nor has it been adequately studied for efficacy or safety due to concerns with side effects in young children. Certain agents have demonstrated limited efficacy in adults and may have a role in certain older pediatric patients over age 12 years with extreme overweight (BMI percentile >99th percentile). These agents include orlistat, bupropion, rimonabant, topiramate, and sibutramine.

Surgical Options

As with pharmacologic agents, surgical options such as gastric bypass and laparoscopic band placement have a therapeutic role in adolescents with comorbidities and extreme overweight but are not applicable to young children who are growing.

Prognosis

As described above, the complications of pediatric overweight are many and range across a variety of organ systems. Unfortunately, a singular effective approach to the management of pediatric overweight is not present and is unlikely due to the multifactorial etiology of pediatric overweight. There are few effective interventions at present. Consequently, the progression to adolescent and subsequent adult overweight and obesity has been unrelenting. Children who are overweight at any time in the first 5 years of life are at 5 times greater risk of being overweight in early adolescence and being overweight on early adolescence is a significant risk factor for adult obesity. Recent studies suggest that a child who is overweight or AROW (BMI percentile >85th percentile) at age 3 years is six times more likely to be overweight by age 9 years. A child who is overweight by age 9 is 11–30 times more likely to be a clinically obese young adult. While the treatment of pediatric overweight is not, as yet, uniform or effective, the urgent need for effective interventions is obvious.

See also: Endocrine System; Feeding Development and Disorders; Fragile X Syndrome.

Suggested Readings

Barlow S and Dietz W (2002) Management of child and adolescent obesity: Summary and recommendations based on reports from pediatricians, pediatric nurse practitioners, and registered dietitians. *Pediatrics* 110: 236–238.

Bowman SA, Gortmaker SL, Ebbeling CB, Pereira MA, and Ludwig DS (2004) Effects of fast-food consumption on energy intake and diet quality among children in a national household survey. *Pediatrics* 113: 112–118.

Farooqi S (2005) Genetic and hereditary aspects of childhood obesity. *Best Practice and Research: Clinical Endocrinology and Metabolism* 19(3): 359–374.

Gidding SS, Dennison BA, Birch LL, *et al.* (2006) Dietary recommendations for children and adolescents: A guide for practitioners. *Pediatrics* 117(2): 544–559.

Hedley AA, Ogden CL, Johnson CL, Carroll MD, Curtin LR, and Flegal KM (2004) Prevalence of overweight and obesity among US children, adolescents, and adults, 1999–2002. *JAMA* 291(23): 2847–2850.

Thompson D, Obarzanek E, Franko D, *et al.* (2007) Childhood overweight and cardiovascular disease risk factors: The national heart, lung, and blood institute growth and health study. *Journal of Pediatrics* 150(1): 18–25.

US PreventiveServices, Task Force (2005) Screening and interventions for overweight children and adolescents: Recommendation statement. *Pediatrics* 116: 205–209.

Whitlock EP, Williams SB, Gold R, Smith P, and Shipman S (2005) *Screening and Interventions for Childhood Overweight: Evidence Synthesis.* July 2005, Agency for Healthcare Research and Quality, USA.

Parental Chronic Mental Illness

T Ostler and B Ackerson, University of Illinois at Urbana–Champaign, Urbana, IL, USA

Glossary

Alogia – A poverty of thinking inferred from observing language behavior and speech.

Anhedonia – An inability to experience pleasure.

Catatonia – A motionless, apathetic state or certain types of excessive motor activity.

Delusions – False beliefs based on incorrect inferences about external reality. The belief is sustained despite clear evidence or proof to the contrary.

Dual diagnosis – A term used to refer to an individual who has both a psychiatric disorder and a substance abuse or addiction problem.

Externalizing behaviors – A term used to refer to aggression, delinquency, and hyperactivity in children and adolescence as opposed to internalizing behaviors such as depression and anxiety.

Folie a deux – A rare psychiatric condition in which a symptom of psychosis (usually a delusional or paranoid belief) is transmitted from a parent to a child. The Diagnostic and Statistical Manual of Mental Disorders (DSM-IV) refers to this syndrome as shared psychotic disorder.

Hallucinations – Sensory perceptions that have a compelling sense of reality of true perception but that occur internally, that is, without external stimulation of a sensory organ.

Hypomania – A persistently expansive, irritable or elevated mood associated with an unequivocal change in functioning that does not cause marked impairment. It is accompanied by some of the following symptoms: grandiosity, pressure of speech, flight of ideas, inflated self-esteem, psychomotor agitation, and excessive involvement in pleasurable activities that have a high potential for painful consequences.

Kindling effect – Kindling effect refers to what happens with recurring manic episodes over time.

The individual may experience manic episodes more frequently over time due to changes in the brain caused by previous episodes. It is similar to what occurs in seizure disorders. Kindling specifically refers to the repeated triggering of certain nerve cells over time.

Mania – An abnormally and persistently expansive, irritable or elevated mood that lasts at least 1 week. It causes marked impairment in the individual and is accompanied by some of the following symptoms: grandiosity, pressure of speech, flight of ideas, inflated self-esteem psychomotor agitation, and excessive involvement in pleasurable activities that have a high potential for painful consequences.

Negative symptoms – Symptoms that involve a diminution or loss of functioning, such as blunted affect, apathy, self-neglect, loss of motivation, difficulty with abstract thinking and social withdrawal. Negative symptoms usually occur first and may be present during periods of remission (i.e., periods when there are no symptoms) as the illness progresses.

Positive symptoms – Symptoms that involve an excess or distortion of normal functions, such as hallucinatory behavior, conceptual disorganization, and delusions.

Psychotic disorders – Psychiatric disorders involving severe impairment to thought and perception. Such disorders can include positive symptoms of schizophrenia such as disorganized speech, grossly disorganized or catatonic behavior.

Stress-diathesis theory – A theory whereby a genetic predisposition or vulnerability (diathesis) interacts with stresses from life events in the environment (stressors) to trigger psychiatric disorders. The greater the underlying predisposition is, the less stress is needed to trigger the disorder. In cases where there is a smaller genetic contribution, greater levels of stress are required to produce psychiatric illness.

Wrap around services – Comprehensive mental health services designed to help individuals with severe and persistent mental illness. They are often home based and include case management, psychiatric treatment, and rehabilitation services.

Introduction

Individuals who are diagnosed with a mental disorder experience clinically significant distress or impairment in social, occupational, and other important areas of functioning. The individual also shows a pattern of symptoms that is characteristic of a specific psychiatric disorder in the Diagnostic and Statistical Manual of Mental Disorders (DSM-IV), the standard manual that is used for diagnosing disorders in the US. Mental illness symptoms vary greatly across individuals even with the same diagnosis and they may be mild or severe. Several mental illnesses have a chronic course and symptoms wax or wane over time.

About one-third of women in the US and one-fifth of men show evidence of psychiatric disorder. The majority of these individuals are parents. For these individuals parenting is a central and highly valued role. However, when an individual's illness is both chronic and severe, parenting is usually compromised to some degree. While many individuals are able to care for their children either alone or with the support of others, others struggle in the parenting role as they confront the dual challenges of dealing with a mental illness while meeting the stresses associated with raising children. In some cases, mental illness symptoms can interfere with an individual's judgment, behavior, feelings, and energy to the point that they seriously compromise the individual's ability to recognize risk or to provide for their child's basic needs and safety.

Children of parents with mental illness are also vulnerable and exposure to parental mental illness can compromise a child's development and well-being in a variety of ways. Problems are likely to be more enduring if a child is exposed to parental mental illness in the early years of life, a sensitive developmental period in which a child is highly dependent on the parent for survival. During this period, early environmental stimulation and emotional responsiveness from a caregiver are essential in influencing how well an infant or young child fares in his or her development and well-being.

This article provides an overview of the effects of mental illness on parenting and on infants and young children. Fathers with chronic mental illness can be and are primary caregivers. At the same time, women with chronic mental illness are far more likely to be involved in caring for children. For this reason, focus is given to women as parents. Focus is also given to chronic mental illnesses and to parenting in the peripartum period, a time period when women are especially prone to either develop a mental illness or to experience illness exacerbations. In the sections that follow, the article describes major types of chronic mental illness, discusses the challenges that individuals with chronic and severe mental illness face in the parenting role, and outlines how different mental illnesses symptoms can affect parenting. The article then addresses factors that can increase parenting risk in individuals with mental illness and presents a model for understanding how chronic parental mental illness can affect children's development. Literature on the outcomes of infants and young children of parents with mental illness is then synthesized followed by a description of approaches for developing effective, multifaceted interventions that can address the needs of children and their parents.

Types, Symptoms, and Course of Chronic Mental Illnesses

Schizophrenia

Schizophrenia and other psychotic disorders are some of the most severe mental illnesses. Schizophrenia is characterized by severe disruption in cognitive functioning and perceptions. The most pronounced symptoms, sometimes referred to as positive symptoms, are hallucinations, delusions, disorganized thought process, and grossly disorganized behavior. Hallucinations are false perceptions (e.g., hearing voices) that are not based upon any external stimulus. Persons with schizophrenia do not imagine hallucinations. They actually experience the perception (hear, see, etc.), but it is caused by abnormal activity in their brain rather than an external stimulus. Delusions are false beliefs that are not consistent with a person's culture or religious beliefs and are caused by a disruption in reasoning abilities. Disordered thought content seen in delusions often accompanies impairment in thought processes. Examples of disorganized thought process are flight of ideas, loose associations, tangential thinking, disorganized speech, and incoherent speech. In addition to impairments in cognitive abilities and perceptions, individuals with schizophrenia may also experience disorganized behavior manifested as agitation, catatonia, or an inability to perform goal-directed behavior, such as caring for oneself. The extent that any of these symptoms are present varies according to the subtype of schizophrenia and the severity of the disorder in a particular individual. Any or all of the positive symptoms may be present during an acute phase of the illness.

Schizophrenia also consists of negative symptoms, which include flat affect, social withdrawal, ambivalence, alogia, and anhedonia. These symptoms may be present in the residual phase of the illness as well as in the active phase. Because the side effects of antipsychotic medication can also contribute to lethargy and withdrawal, it may be difficult to determine the extent to which these behaviors are due to medication or the negative symptoms of the illness. It is important to understand that withdrawal, ambivalence, and other negative symptoms are a function of the illness and not personal traits of the individual. Schizophrenia is best understood as a chronic psychiatric disability that impacts social functioning as well as cognitive abilities.

Bipolar Disorders

Bipolar disorders are marked by extreme mood swings, from depression on one end to mania or hypomania on the other end. Formerly called manic-depression, bipolar disorder is now categorized as having two forms. Bipolar I disorder is classic manic-depression. Individuals experience highly euphoric moods, referred to as mania, that impair their reasoning and judgment. These mood states, which may include feelings of grandiosity, flights of thought and speech, and impaired judgment, may last days, weeks, or months but eventually subside. When not in a manic state, individuals may experience normal moods for a period of time or may go directly into a major depressive episode.

In bipolar II disorder individuals more often experience a depressed mood, but they still alternate between depression and elevated moods. However, their elevated mood states never escalate past hypomania, a milder form of mania that lasts for at least 4 days, but unlike mania it is not severe enough to cause impairment in functioning. In both mania and hypomania individuals may have very little sleep, talk excessively, and engage in excessive pleasure seeking behavior. At times manic states may not be easily recognized because the individual's mood may be irritable or agitated instead of euphoric. However, they still experience a reduced need for sleep and other excessive behaviors seen in mania.

Bipolar disorder is considered a chronic mental disorder and it often results in psychiatric disability. The fluctuating nature of the disorder contributes to difficulties in social and occupational functioning. Many people with bipolar disorder are able to hold jobs, engage in social relationships, and raise families. However, their ability to function in any of these roles is compromised when they experience an episode of either major depression or mania/hypomania. Rapid cycling, or the frequent shifting from one mood episode to another, may occur in more severe cases. The longer an individual has had the illness, the greater they are at risk for developing rapid cycling, similar to the kindling effect in seizure disorders.

Major Depression

Depression is the most common mental disorder. It affects about 10% of people in the US in a year and about 17% experience it during their lifetime. Individuals with major depression, also referred to as clinical depression, are at much higher risk for having another mental disorder, such as anxiety or substance abuse.

Major depression is more than just feeling sad or 'blue'. It is defined as experiencing one or more major depressive episodes. Symptoms include feeling chronically sad or depressed, anhedonia, changes in eating or sleeping, lack of energy, feeling helpless or hopeless, having problems with memory or concentration, and being socially withdrawn. Individuals with recurring major depressive episodes have a psychiatric disability that may impair their ability to work and to function socially.

Major depression may begin at any developmental period. Depressive episodes typically last 6–9 months in children and adolescents. About half of the children who experience major depression will experience another episode within 2 years. Adolescent depression often continues into adulthood. Other individuals may not experience their first depressive episode until well into adulthood. For some, depressive episodes are episodic, with long periods of normal mood during which time they are able to fully engage in life. Other individuals experience a severe form of the disorder where depressive moods are more frequent and have a longer duration.

Fortunately, depression has proved to be a very treatable illness. A variety of antidepressant medications have been shown to be effective, all of them working in some way on the neurotransmitters serotonin and epinephrine. Several forms of psychotherapy have also been shown to be very effective, with research showing strong support for various forms of cognitive therapy (understanding how people perceive, attribute, and interpret meaning) and interpersonal therapy. The most effective treatment strategy is a combination of psychotherapy with antidepressant medication, especially if a person has had two or more major episodes of depression.

Anxiety Disorders

Anxiety, a vitally important physiological response to dangerous situations, prepares an individual to evade or confront threats. In some individuals, the mechanisms that regulate anxiety break down and the individual experiences excessive anxiety. There are several anxiety disorders, all characterized by clinical levels of excessive anxiety. An individual who is diagnosed with panic disorder has repeated panic attacks, high intensive episodes of anxiety that occur without a precipitating cause. During a panic attack, an individual may experience shortness of breath, rapid heart rate, trembling, restlessness, lightheadedness or dizziness, perspiration, as well as cold hands and feet.

An individual who is diagnosed with generalized anxiety disorder (GAD) experiences pervasive worries for at least 6 months about a variety of events or activities. It is difficult for the individual to control these worries and he or she experiences ongoing tension and restlessness. The duration, intensity, and frequency of the anxiety are out of proportion to the actual likelihood that the feared event will occur.

Obsessive-compulsive disorder (OCD) is another severe anxiety disorder characterized by recurring and intrusive thoughts or images (obsessions) and repetitive behaviors or mental acts (compulsions) that an individual feels compelled to perform in response to the obsession. Some compulsive behaviors are very obvious, such as excessive hand washing, while others are more internal and not easily observed, such as mental checking or counting. These obsessions and compulsive behaviors are very time consuming, cause great personal distress and significant functional impairment. Unlike obsessive-compulsive personality disorder, these behaviors are not merely signs of an overly perfectionistic personality. Adults with OCD are aware that their behavior is abnormal and dysfunctional, but they feel as if they have little or no control over these thoughts and behaviors. OCD has a strong biological basis. It is very persistent and requires extensive treatment involving medication and psychotherapy.

Individuals who are exposed to a life-threatening event or a threat of serious injury may develop a severe anxiety disorder in response to their trauma. There are two types of severe anxiety disorders that may occur as a result of trauma, acute stress disorder, and post-traumatic stress disorder (PTSD). Acute stress disorder occurs within the first month after experiencing trauma. PTSD is the more chronic of these disorders. Symptoms persist for more than 1 month and may last for many years.

PTSD symptoms can be grouped in three categories: re-experiencing of the event, avoidance of stimuli associated with the trauma and numbing, and increased arousal. In adults and adolescents re-experiencing may take many forms which include recurring and intrusive images and thoughts, distressing dreams or nightmares, flashbacks, and other feelings as if the trauma were recurring. Avoidance behaviors may be related to avoiding thoughts and feelings as well as avoiding places, people, and activities and a sense of detachment may also be experienced. Arousal symptoms are both physical (autonomic nervous system) and psychological (irritability, hypervigilance). Because many of these symptoms may also be seen in depression or other anxiety disorders, PTSD may be missed or confused with another mental disorder. In addition, individuals with PTSD are at risk for developing other mental disorders and substance abuse.

Personality Disorders

Personality traits are normal variations of human behavior and personal characteristics. Personality disorders reflect rigid, inflexible, and maladaptive forms of behavior that lead to personal distress or functional impairment – social and/or occupational. To be diagnosed with a personality disorder, maladaptive behavior must be seen in at least two of the following areas: cognition (how the person sees themselves and others), affect (range and intensity of moods), interpersonal functioning, and impulse control. While some inflexible traits or maladaptive behaviors may emerge during adolescence, personality disorders are not diagnosed until early adulthood.

The DSM-IV lists 10 personality disorders that are categorized into three clusters. Cluster A consists of paranoid, schizotypal, and schizoid personality disorders. These three disorders share the common trait of odd and eccentric behavior, social aloofness, and milder forms of symptoms that are associated with schizophrenia. Cluster B consists of antisocial, borderline, histrionic, and narcissistic personality disorders. These disorders are all characterized by dramatic, emotional, and erratic behavior. They also have a high comorbidity with mood disorders and substance use disorders.

Cluster C consists of avoidant, dependent, and obsessive-compulsive personality disorders. Individuals with these disorders all exhibit anxious or fearful behaviors and the disorders appear to be closely associated with anxiety disorders. In recent years there has been special attention given to borderline personality disorder, which is diagnosed more frequently in women. Once considered extremely difficult to treat, dialectical behavior therapy, a psychosocial treatment that combines behavioral theory with components of cognitive therapy, and other forms of cognitive therapy have been shown to be effective.

Mental Illness and Parenting: Dual Challenges

Mothers with severe and persistent mental illnesses (e.g., schizophrenia, bipolar disorder, depression) face a dual challenge. They have to manage a chronic illness that causes impairments in judgment and social functioning while also dealing with the stress and complex demands of parenting. However, even the severe and persistent mental disorders are typically episodic in nature. The symptoms and behaviors that pose risk for a mother's children, then, fluctuate over time and are amenable to a variety of treatment interventions.

The special challenge these mothers face is that while most of them express a strong desire to be good mothers, the stress of parenting can exacerbate their symptoms. Therefore, these mothers need help both with learning how to manage their psychiatric disability as well as with learning effective parenting techniques. They require special interventions that address the interaction between the demands and stress of being a parent and the symptoms of their particular illness.

Mothers with depression, bipolar disorder, and schizophrenia experience negative or depressed mood symptoms. In depression and bipolar disorder these occur as major depressive episodes, which may be of limited duration or may extend for months or years. In schizophrenia these negative moods are part of the negative symptoms of the disorder. These negative symptoms may exist even when other symptoms such as delusions and hallucinations are not prominent. When a parent experiences depressive moods they may be emotionally unavailable or exhibit maternal insensitivity to their children. They may also withdraw and exhibit lower levels of energy which may impair their ability to provide for their children's basic needs. Discipline of their children may also be erratic or ineffective during these periods of negative moods. It is important to note that these mood symptoms are typically episodic and are often amenable to treatment with medication. Mothers can be trained to recognize when these symptoms occur and to seek treatment and social support for their family. Services for these parents and their families should address emotional and social support needs.

Another common symptom of severe and persistent mental illnesses is lack of sustained motivation. This can result in inadequate care of children's hygiene, failure to provide appropriate clothes and adequate nutrition, and inconsistent child discipline. This apathy and amotivation may be misunderstood as a lack of desire to engage in the parenting roles.

When mothers with a chronic mental illness have been interviewed about their roles as parents, they report a strong desire to be effective parents and they derive a great deal of pride and self-esteem from being parents. Several studies have found that many of these mothers are aware of their difficulties in performing the parenting role. Therefore, it is important to distinguish between the symptoms of their illness and a lack of desire to function as parents. Similar to episodes of negative moods, they need to learn effective coping strategies for dealing with periods of lower motivation and how to appropriately seek assistance during these times.

Mothers with psychiatric disabilities may also experience cognitive deficits that impair their ability to accurately interpret or understand their children's behavior. In fact, unrealistic expectations of children's behavior along with impaired problem-solving abilities are more reliable indicators of risk for child maltreatment than psychiatric diagnosis.

Cognitive deficits are a key symptom of schizophrenia and other psychotic disorders. Severe deficits are easily recognized in the form of delusions and problems with forming coherent thoughts. Fortunately, these symptoms can be managed with appropriate medication. More subtle deficits may not be as easily recognized. In these cases the parent may misinterpret a child's behavior and overreact. Mothers with severe mood and anxiety disorders may also have unrealistic expectations of their children. This is caused both by their illness and by a tendency at times to rely on older children to help care for the house and younger siblings. For these reasons, parent skills training is an important component of treatment for many parents with chronic mental disorders. Education regarding developmentally appropriate behavior and parental expectations should be an important component of this training for these parents.

Parenting and Chronic Mental Illness in the Peripartum Period

Women are especially vulnerable to developing a psychiatric illness and to experiencing symptom exacerbations during the childbearing years, that is, in the time when they conceive, carry, and give birth to children. This section examines how parenting is affected by different chronic mental disorders and their symptoms in the period during pregnancy and after birth.

Depression

About 10% of women develop clinical depression during pregnancy. New mothers (10–20%) develop depression after giving birth to their babies. These rates double in low-income mothers and in adolescent mothers.

Although the symptoms of depression in pregnancy are the same as the symptoms that occur in depression at other phases in life, they often go unrecognized because normal pregnancy changes cause similar symptoms such as difficulties in sleeping, tiredness, changes in body weight, and strong, emotional reactions.

Clinical depression in pregnancy can pose formidable problems for the mother and baby to be. A mother who becomes depressed during pregnancy may fail to seek out prenatal care. In addition, she may not eat properly, lose weight, and increase her use of addictive substances, particularly smoking and alcohol use. If a mother develops suicidal thoughts as part of her depression, there is a risk that she may overdose on medications, posing a substantial risk for herself and her fetus.

There is growing evidence that depression in pregnancy can negatively affect fetal and infant well-being. Untreated maternal depression in pregnancy has been associated with premature labor and with low infant birth weight. Maternal smoking and substance abuse can all exert a negative effect on fetal and infant development. Pregnant mothers who are depressed also experience high levels of stress. Their babies, in turn, show high levels of activity during pregnancy and high stress hormone levels after birth.

Recognizing factors that increase the chances that a pregnant woman will develop depression can help in preventing depression in this critical phase of life. **Table 1** lists several factors that increase the risk that a pregnant mother will develop depression.

Postpartum depression is not the same as the postpartum 'blues', which is a normal experience for many women in the immediate postpartum period. Women experience the blues within the first 10 days after birth. They alternate between feeling irritable, having an elated mood, and having increased crying spells. Women who develop postpartum depression, by contrast, experience sleep and appetite disturbances, impaired concentration, feelings of inadequacy, and a sad mood. These symptoms occur within 6 months after a woman has given birth to her child.

Postpartum depression can greatly affect how a mother feels about herself as a parent and how she perceives and responds to her newborn baby. A mother who becomes clinically depressed after giving birth may develop a negative attitude toward her baby or harbor negative feelings and thoughts about her ability and desire to parent. She may be emotionally unavailable to her baby and have difficulties in responding to her baby's cues. Some mothers feel that their baby hates them. Most women with postpartum depression feel guilty about these thoughts and are anxious about their ability to parent.

The exact etiology of postpartum depression is unknown, but the lack of sleep, stress, and new responsibilities that are part of having a baby can contribute to its development. **Table 2** summarizes factors that increase the risk that a woman will develop depression in the postpartum period.

Depression in the postpartum period often remains unrecognized by mothers, family members, and mental health professionals alike. In about 50% of cases, however, episodes of postpartum depression are continuations of a depressive episode from pregnancy. Mothers may be reluctant to acknowledge that they are depressed after giving birth to their child because it may seem incongruous with the happiness they feel they should experience in the mothering role. Given the negative repercussions that it can have on parenting, recognizing symptoms of depression in the postpartum period as early as possible and helping mothers to seek treatment is essential.

There is some evidence that prolonged interventions may be needed to achieve positive outcomes for parenting. A significant proportion of women who are vulnerable to postnatal depression, however, refuse to engage in treatment. Understanding the barriers to engaging in services is therefore essential for achieving better outreach and care for these women and their babies.

Bipolar Disorder and Schizophrenia

Bipolar disorder and schizophrenia can pose risks to parenting at any time in the life span, but there are specific risks that can be recognized during the prenatal period. Impaired judgment and hypersexuality, both symptoms of mania, can contribute to high rates of unplanned pregnancies and HIV infection in women with bipolar disorder. High rates of substance use, including nicotine, that are characteristic of individuals with both bipolar disorder and schizophrenia, can increase the risk to the fetus in the first trimester of pregnancy. In addition, women with schizophrenia are more prone to have higher rates of unplanned or unwanted pregnancies and to recognize their pregnancy later than nonmentally ill mothers.

Psychotic denial of pregnancy is a complication that can co-occur with some chronic psychiatric disorders and, though rare, can lead to a high level of risk to the mother and unborn baby. A woman who psychotically denies pregnancy is unaware that she is pregnant. She may misinterpret or ignore symptoms of pregnancy. She may attribute fetal movements to gas or interpret labor as signs of menstruation. As delivery approaches, she may not seek out help or go to a hospital, placing both the women at risk for precipitous delivery of the baby, and, in some cases, for fetal abuse or neonaticide.

Psychotic denial of pregnancy is more common in women with schizophrenia than in women with bipolar disorder or severe personality disorders. Treatment involves integrating comprehensive obstetrical and psychiatric care, medication, and supportive psychotherapy with an evaluation of a mother's parenting skills.

Postpartum psychosis is a rare condition that typically starts within the first few days to 2–3 weeks postpartum. It has a rapid onset and is characterized by hallucinations and/or delusions. Having bipolar disorder or severe

Table 1   Factors that increase risk of clinical depression during pregnancy

A past history of depression or substance abuse
A family history of mental illness
Anxiety about the unborn baby
Problems with a past pregnancy or birth
Young age
Marital or financial problems
Little social support

Table 2   Factors that increase the risk for postpartum depression

A previous history of depression
A family history of mood disorder
Little social support
Anticipating a separation from the unborn baby after birth
Prior custody loss of a child

postpartum depression are major risk factors for postpartum psychosis.

If untreated, postpartum psychosis can greatly affect a mother's ability to parent her baby. Some mothers with postpartum psychosis experience a loss of love for their babies, a feeling which they often experience as painful. Others may develop bizarre beliefs about their babies, thinking, for instance, that the baby is still in the uterus, or that the baby is deformed or dead. Some mothers with postpartum psychosis try to harm their infants. The short-term prognosis for parenting is usually good if a mother responds to medication and is in treatment.

Anxiety Disorders

Little is known about how anxiety affects parenting during pregnancy. However, mothers with GAD apparently experience higher levels of distress when their young child is engaged in routine activities and in structured play tasks than nonanxious mothers. Obsessional rituals associated with OCD, another anxiety disorder, can interfere with childrearing responsibilities. A parent with OCD, for instance, may be overmeticulous and demand too much from a young child. Similarly, obsessive self-doubting can contribute to a young child doubting his or her abilities. In some cases, obsessive symptoms may lead to repetitive checking to ensure a young child is safe. Clearly, to the extent that they are communicated to a child, obsessive worries and compulsions can burden the child emotionally and increase his or her anxiety level.

There is little systematic research on the parenting capabilities of individuals with PTSD. Parental PTSD has, however, been found to be a salient risk factor for PTSD in offspring. Clinical evidence suggests that parents with PTSD may have difficulty in expressing emotions and in recognizing a young child's cues, especially if the child is distressed. There is evidence for interactive effects between child and parent. Studies, for instance, show that if a child is traumatized, the child's trauma symptoms may reactivate PTSD symptoms in a parent.

Personality Disorders

Mothers with personality disorders have serious problems in social and occupational functioning which can make it difficult for them to sustain a safe, predictable environment for their babies. Since many are victims of childhood abuse and neglect, they are often vulnerable in intimate relationships, including those with their young children. This vulnerability may make it difficult for a mother with a personality disorder to distinguish her own needs from those of her baby and for her to tolerate her baby's distress. A mother with a personality disorder may also project feelings she canot tolerate in herself onto her young child. Change can occur for individuals with this

diagnosis, but it usually takes considerable time to engage a parent in the treatment process which the parent may perceive as threatening.

Assessing Parenting Risk in Individuals with Chronic Mental Illness

Many individuals with mental illness raise their children to adulthood, either alone or with the support of others. Some protective factors that ameliorate risk and are associated with good enough parenting are listed in **Table 3**.

Risk for serious parenting problems is especially high in individuals whose illness is chronic and severe. As many as 60–80% of women with chronic and severe mental illness may relinquish or lose custody of their children at some point in their lives. There is some evidence that custody loss may occur more frequently right after birth or in the early years of parenting, probably because women are at high risk in these periods for developing a major mental illness or for experiencing illness exacerbations.

Some factors that can signal risk for serious parenting problems during pregnancy for mothers with a chronic mental illness include: a marked ambivalence about wanting a baby, delusions about the pregnancy or baby, a denial of pregnancy, significant family tension prior to delivery, refusal of prenatal care, thoughts of harming the baby to be, a suicide attempt during pregnancy, poor support, and lack of compliance with treatment.

Only two mental disorders, depression and substance abuse, have been specifically linked to child maltreatment and their overall contribution is small. Overall, illness dimensions and symptoms appear to be more important predictors of parenting risk than psychiatric diagnoses. **Table 4** provides an overview of illness dimensions and symptoms that increase parenting risk in individuals whose illness is chronic and severe.

While mental illness symptoms can increase risk, maltreatment is multiply determined. It results from a broad range of environmental and familial factors that interact with each other to compromise a parent's ability to nurture and provide adequate care and protection for a child. **Table 5** summarizes factors, beyond the parent's psychiatric symptoms, that can contribute to parenting risk.

Table 3 Protective factors for parenting in individuals with psychiatric disorders

Good coping skills
A supportive network of friends and relatives
Compliance with treatment
Responsiveness to treatment
Good insight into illness symptoms and the need for treatment
Will power and motivation to change

Table 4   Psychiatric factors that can increase parenting risk

Dual diagnosis
A comorbid substance abuse problem
Active psychotic symptoms
Aggressive or violent behavior
Poor insight into the mental illness
Including a child in delusions
Parent has command hallucinations
Lack of response to treatment
Noncompliance with treatment
Low level of adaptive functioning

Table 5   Nonpsychiatric factors that can increase parenting risk

Neglect of the baby's basic needs
Apathy or hostility toward the baby
A projection of feelings onto the baby (e.g., 'he hates me')
A refusal to hold and engage the baby
Parent has an intrusive or hostile interactive style
Parent has expectations that the child should provide the parent with comfort and support
Parent lacks basic knowledge about the child or holds unrealistic expectations about child
Parent has difficulties in meeting their own basic needs
Parent utilizes extreme disciplinary measures
Parent has a small or unviable support network
Parent has difficulties in establishing and maintaining supportive relationships
Parent denies he or she has problems
Domestic violence
Marital disharmony and conflict

How Parental Mental Illness Affects Infants and Young Children

Young children who experience parental mental illness are often characterized as a high-risk group of youngsters. Some of the risk to children is due to biological and genetic factors, but risk also results from environmental influences, including poor parenting, marital discord, socioeconomic disadvantage, and the increased stresses that result from living with a parent with mental illness. Child factors, including temperament, intelligence, and gender can also contribute to risk.

Parental mental illness may affect children's well-being and development in different ways. Risk may be transmitted genetically to a child. There can also be a direct impact on the child's development and well-being through exposure to the parent's illness. Parental mental illness can also impact a child's development indirectly via poor parenting or through its impact on the parent's interpersonal behavior. The effect on children's development may also occur through factors that are associated with chronic mental illness such as poverty, social adversity, and disadvantage. Marital discord, for instance, can result in part from living

with an individual who has a chronic mental illness and can impact children's development and well-being. Genetic factors can also interact with environmental factors to affect child outcome.

Child factors can interact with parenting in an individual with chronic mental illness, thereby affecting child outcome. In early development, for instance, perinatal and medical complications, prematurity, or a low birth weight, conditions more common in infants of mothers with chronic mental illness, may contribute to severity of postpartum depression in a mother, and thereby influence how she cares for her baby and how the baby fares developmentally.

A young child's temperament is another factor that can contribute to parenting, thereby affecting a child's developmental pathway. A baby with a difficult temperament, for instance, may elicit different responses from a parent with a chronic mental illness than a baby with an easy temperament, thereby contributing to a more difficult parenting pathway and to a less favorable outcome for the child. Having a child with disabilities or a chronic illness can also contribute to the overall stress that a parent experiences in the caregiving role. Supporting the view that child factors interact with parenting to influence child outcome is the finding that children with is behavioral disorders or disabilities are more likely than other children to experience maltreatment by a caregiver.

The stress-diathesis theory helps to explain how risk develops. In this theory, child vulnerability due to genetic or to early environmental stresses interacts with later stresses to precipitate risk or the onset of illness symptoms in the child. For instance, if the child's parent has a heritable psychiatric disorder, the child may have an elevated genetic vulnerability for developing a disorder under adverse environmental conditions. This child may be particularly susceptible to poor parenting. Under adverse conditions, including stress and poor parenting, the child's disorder may be expressed. Whether risk in a vulnerable child is actualized, however, will turn on the degree to which the child is vulnerable biologically to begin with, how the mother fared during pregnancy, how the child has been parented and cared for after birth, and by the larger environment in which he or she lives including the stresses the child experiences.

Effects on Children's Development and Well-Being

Studies have documented that parental mental illness can affect various aspects of young children's well-being and development. Studies show increased rates of externalizing problems, delays in cognitive development, particularly in boys, and interpersonal difficulties, including attachment insecurity and feelings of guilt.

Children of parents with mental illness are also at increased risk for developing a psychiatric disorder over the course of their life. By age 10 years, over 20% of children born to a mother who has major depression are likely to develop a major episode of depression or dysthymia, a low-grade form of chronic depression, twice the amount of children born to mothers who had never been depressed. A child with a parent with major depression has a 40% chance of developing an episode of depression by age 20 years. This rate increases to 60% by age 25 years. If a parent has a dual diagnosis, risk is increased further. Problems are more enduring if the child is exposed to parental mental illness in the early years of development, a period when vulnerability emerges and is maintained.

The next section reviews recent findings on the outcomes of infants and young children of parents with mental illness. Since much research attention has been given to major depression in mothers, this work is emphasized. However, when available, findings on the effects of other disorders are discussed. Emphasis is also given to identifying areas and sources of strength in children, an area that has, until recently, been neglected.

Infancy

Maternal depression in the postpartum period affects mothers' ability to respond in a sensitive and contingent manner to a baby's cues and to show delight in the baby's presence. Their babies in turn show limited engagement, poor eye contact, and muted affective expressions. They are also more prone than babies whose mothers are not depressed to develop insecure attachment patterns to their mothers as assessed in the Ainsworth Strange Situation procedure, a standard observation that is used to classify mother–infant attachment quality when the baby is 12 months of age.

Babies of mothers with postpartum depression are most prone to develop an insecure-disorganized attachment pattern, a pattern which has been linked to frightened or frightening maternal behavior. This pattern is viewed as an at-risk pattern and is associated with high levels of insecurity in the mother–child relationship.

Several studies show effects of postpartum depression on early cognitive development. Infants of mothers who have postpartum depression, for instance, have been found to be significantly delayed in their language development and on the development of object permanence, a key measure of early representational capacities in infants when compared to infants of nondepressed mothers. Object permanence is constructed over the first 18 months of life and involves the child coming to grasp that what is out of sight is not out of mind.

Infants of mothers who develop depression in the postpartum period are also disadvantaged in their behavior and in their social and emotional development. They show more negative responses with other adults, less

sharing, and less concentration than infants whose mothers are not depressed in the postpartum period. They are also more prone to act out in order to obtain a response from an adult, and have more eating and sleeping problems, more temper tantrums and more difficulties with separations.

Studies on the attachment quality and cognitive development in infants of mothers who are depressed in the postpartum period have found that development is more compromised when the mother has a severe rather than mild episode of depression and if her illness is chronic and occurs in the context of other adversities. Poor outcomes in behavior and cognitive development may persist even after the mother's depression has abated. In the early years of life, the mother is the baby's primary environment. Small wonder, then, that the adverse effects of maternal depression on infant development are mediated through the quality of the mother–child attachment bond.

Young boys of mothers with postpartum depression may be at particular high risk for adverse effects in attachment, behavior, and cognitive functioning. One explanation for this difference is that girls appear to hold a maturational advance which may protect them more than boys from the experience of postpartum depression. Another explanation is that mothers who are depressed may treat their sons and daughters differentially.

Less is known about the effects of chronic psychotic disorders in a parent on infant well-being and development. Interactions between mothers with psychosis and their babies have been found to be more deviant and negative than those of mothers and infants in a control group. Mothers with schizophrenia show greater deficits while interacting with their babies than mothers with mood disorders. They are more insensitive to their babies' cues, more remote, intrusive, and self-absorbed. Their babies in turn are more avoidant and have poorer interaction quality than babies of mothers with mood disorders. Babies of mothers with psychotic disorders lag in their cognitive functioning, including the development of object permanence and show more anxiety in exploring objects. One study found that at age 12 months, babies of mothers with postpartum psychoses showed no fear of strangers, a development which appears on the average at about age 8 months and is observable in almost all infants by age 12 months. The findings suggested aberrance or delays in the infants' social development.

Early childhood

Maternal depression can exert a strong negative effect on the self-system of young children and on their social and emotional development during toddlerhood and the preschool years. For instance, young children of depressed mothers are more prone than children of nondepressed mothers to express negative views about their own worth and performance.

According to John Bowlby, the father of attachment theory, young children construct so-called 'internal working models' of self and other based on their day-to-day experiences with their primary caregiver. These internal or representational working models include children's notions of self and others – how worthy and able the self is and how caregivers are likely to respond if the child is in need. With increasing development, children's internal working models are generalized to other important relationships.

If the primary caregiver is experiencing chronic severe depression, she may not focus on the child's needs, grow irritated at the child's bids for attention, or tell the child her behavior is 'too much' or is making the parent 'ill'. A young child may conclude from these experiences that she is not lovable and that she is responsible for the parent's illness. The child may also have a working model that expects others to respond to the child's needs with irritation or lack of concentration.

Postpartum depression is linked to behavior problems in toddlers and to distractibility and antisocial behavior in the preschool years. The risk of a child developing behavior problems is increased if there is marital conflict and if the family is economically disadvantaged. Choice of play can also be affected, with children of depressed mothers being more prone to avoid more personally challenging creative play and to engage in simple physical play than children of mothers who are not depressed.

A substantial number of young children with depressed caregivers do not evidence dysfunction. Such findings point to the need to look at protective factors in the broader social context in which young children develop and are raised. If a mother is not experiencing current difficulties or conflict with the child's father, for instance, the child may fare better in his development.

Separation and custody loss

Between 60% and 80% of mothers with chronic mental illness may lose temporary or permanent custody of their children at some point in their lives. Some studies suggest that custody loss may occur early on, either at birth or in the first years of life. If a parent with a chronic mental illness is hospitalized, the child may stay with the nonmentally ill parent, or with relatives or friends until she stabilizes and recovers. Others may be placed in foster care.

Infants and young children who experience a separation are at higher risk in all areas of development as they experience not only the loss of a healthy mother and loss of a normal family life, but a loss of stability and confidence that the mother is available. How well they fare will turn not only on their own vulnerabilities and constitution, but on the care they receive from their mother and from alternate caregivers. If a child has already established an attachment bond to the biological mother who is mentally ill, he or she may experience profound changes in their feelings toward the mother during and after the separation.

Long-term effects

The impact of chronic parental mental illness on family members is referred to as a 'burden'. Children are confronted not only with the objective burden of coping with the parent's symptoms, the stigma of the illness, and with additional caregiving responsibilities, they may also grieve for a lost childhood, or for a parent they knew and loved before the illness set in. This burden is stressful and contributes to the sense of isolation and loneliness that many of the children experience.

Several long-term patterns can be identified in children who grow up with a parent with a chronic mental illness. Many children, for instance, experience difficulties in deciphering which of their family experiences are normal and which are not. Some children may feel guilty that they are healthy or feel embarrassed at the odd behaviors their parent may engage in. Many do not have someone with whom to talk to about what they are going through. Children who experience these feelings need advice and help from adults so that they can come to terms with the illness, and understand and acknowledge how the illness affects themselves and their family.

Role reversal and intensified self-sufficiency are other patterns that may be evidenced in children of parents with chronic mental illness as they grow older. Children who evidence these patterns have adapted their behavior to make things work within a family which is under considerable strain. Even very young children may show these patterns. Role reversal and intensified self-sufficiency often build on a child's need to control situations to obtain some outward security about what she can expect. While sometimes viewed as mature, if extreme, these patterns can come at a high emotional cost to a child. Children who are parentified or highly self-sufficient, for instance, have great difficulties in relying on others for help or support. In addition, they may miss out on being a child and their own capacity to feel and to learn may be constricted.

Family members may fail to acknowledge a mental illness or minimize or distort its effects on the individual and family. As a result, children may learn to keep the illness secret as they grow older. Secretive and distorted communication patterns in turn can contribute to a child feeling a need to hide her own feelings and needs from others. In extreme cases, children who hide their own feelings and thoughts develop a false sense of self. Such children try to do or be what they think is right for others in the family. Underlying this outward appearance of perfection, however, is a fundamental fear that the child is not good enough.

If a child lives alone with a parent who has a chronic mental illness, the child may become enmeshed in the

Table 6 Heritability of major mental illnesses: Child's lifetime risk of becoming ill

	General population rates if neither parent is ill (%)	Risk if one parent is ill (%)	Risk if two parents are ill (%)	Risk for other monozygotic twin if one twin is ill (%)	Risk for dizygotic twin if one twin is ill (%)
Schizophrenia	1.5	10	40	18–60	15
Major depression	10	20–25	30–50	50–60	20
Bipolar disorder	1	5–10		40–70	10–20

Reproduced from Brunette M and Jacobsen T (2006) Children of parents with mental illness. In: Hendrick V (ed.) *Psychiatric Disorders in Pregnancy and the Postpartum: Principles and Treatment*, p. 200. Totowa, NJ: Humana Press, with permission from Humana Press.

parent's symptoms. Children in this situation may become the parent's confidant and be burdened with too much information to the detriment of their own development. Children in this circumstance often experience high levels of anxiety and keep their worries to themselves. Some children enter their parent's psychotic world and accept their beliefs as their own so as to feel close to a parent who is hard to reach, a condition that is called a 'folie a deux'.

Risk for psychiatric disorders

While environmental context is important in the etiology of mental illness in a child, genetic factors also contribute to risk and interact with environmental factors in the expression of vulnerability. The genetic risks for children of parents with schizophrenia, major depression, and bipolar disorder are summarized in **Table 6**.

Recent work on anxiety disorders also shows both genetic and environmental contributions. There are higher rates of anxiety disorders among children of anxious parents, but only when the child's mother has the disorder. A maternal history of anxiety disorder doubles the risk that a child will develop an anxiety disorder. If a mother has both an anxiety and a depressive disorder, the risk that her child will develop an anxiety disorder is tripled. This high risk of transmission is thought to be linked to genetic factors, but also to the higher levels of general pathology that mothers with dual diagnoses are likely to exhibit. Studies on transmission from fathers to children need further study. Fathers may be less likely than mothers to report symptoms of anxiety.

Factors that ameliorate risk

Risk to children is cumulative. The more risk factors present, the greater the likelihood that the child will fare poorly in his or her development, especially if the risks occur in the early years of development. Some important protective factors that can ameliorate risk and influence young children's outcomes favorably include help and understanding from family members and relatives, a stable living environment, feeling loved by parents, including the parent who has a mental illness, and psychotherapy, either individual or within the family. Understanding that they

have not caused the illness and that they are not to blame for the parents' symptoms is also essential.

Conclusions

Parents with mental illness face the dual and challenging demands of managing their disability while meeting the many stresses associated with raising children. When the illness is chronic and severe, parenting is usually compromised to some degree. How well an individual fares as a parent, however, will turn on many factors, including the parent's responsiveness and compliance with treatment and the social support he or she receives in the parenting role. To ensure positive outcomes, parents with chronic mental illness need a comprehensive range of multifaceted interventions. In designing such interventions, individual strengths should be considered as well as the needs of the children. Interventions should be closely informed by an assessment of parenting and children's needs. They may include medication management, pregnancy decision making, trauma and abuse therapy, substance abuse treatment, marital and family counseling, comprehensive case management, self-help, parenting mentoring, assistance with housing, and independent living. Assessment of the home environment and the parent's social support system is crucial. Building support networks for the parenting role and meeting the needs of affected children are other essential aspects of such interventions. Community mental health services targeted specifically for parents with chronic mental disorders and their families may include: intensive case management, psychiatric rehabilitation day programs that include parent skills training and day care for preschool children, psychoeducation classes that include information about child development and parenting skills along with information about mental disorders and symptom management, and crisis nurseries and other types of respite care for young children when the mother's symptoms become acute. Because children of mothers with chronic mental disorders are at risk, they need interventions that provide wrap-around services and linkage with schools and healthcare providers. These children may also benefit from education about their parent's mental illness along with community support services.

See also: Depression; Mental Health, Infant; Postpartum Depression, Effects on Infant; Separation and Stranger Anxiety.

Suggested Readings

Ackerson B (2003) Coping with the dual demands of severe mental illness and parenting: The parents' perspective. *Families in Society* 84: 109–118.

Ackerson BJ (2003) Parents with serious and persistent mental illness: Issues in assessment and services. *Social Work* 48: 187–194.

American Psychiatric Association (2000) *Diagnostic and Statistical Manual of Mental Disorders DSM-IV-TR Fourth Edition* (Text Revision). Washington, DC: Author.

Brunette M and Jacobsen T (2006) Children of parents with mental illness: Outcomes and interventions. In: Hendrick V (ed.) *Treatment of Psychiatric Disorders in Pregnancy and the Postpartum*, pp. 197–227. Totowa, NJ: Humana Press.

Cleaver H, Unell I, and Aldgate J (1999) *Children's Needs – Parenting Capacity. The Impact of Parental Mental Illness, Problem Alcohol and Drug Use, and Domestic Violence on Children's Development.* London: TSO.

Göpfert M, Webster J, and Seeman MV (eds.) (2004) *Parental Psychiatric Disorder: Distressed Parents and their Families,* 2nd edn. Cambridge: Cambridge University Press.

Holley TE and Holley J (1997) *My Mother's Keeper: A Daughter's Memoir of Growing Up in the Shadow of Schizophrenia.* New York: Morrow.

Murray L and Cooper PJ (eds.) (1997) *Postpartum Depression and Child Development.* New York: The Guilford Press.

Nicholson J, Biebel K, Hinden B, Henry A, and Stier L (2001) *Critical Issues for Parents with Mental Illness and Their Families* (KEN01–0109). Rockville, MD: Center for Mental Health Services, Substance Abuse and Mental Health Services Administration.

Ostler T (2007) *Assessing Parenting Competency in Individuals with Mental Illness.* Baltimore, MD: Paul H. Brookes Publishing Co.

Relevant Websites

http://www.aacap.org – American Academy of Child Adolescent Psychiatry.

http://www.nmha.org – Mental Health America.

http://www.nami.org – National Alliance on Mental Illness.

http://www.niaaa.nih.gov – National Institute on Alcohol Abuse and Alcoholism, National Institutes of Health.

http://mentalhealth.samhsa.gov – National Mental Health Information Center, Center for mental health services.

http://www.nida.nih.gov – The National Institute on Drug Abuse, National Institutes of Health.

http://www.lookingglass.org – Through the Looking Glass.

Postpartum Depression, Effects on Infant

D M Teti and N Towe-Goodman, The Pennsylvania State University, University Park, PA, USA

Glossary

Comorbid – Term used by diagnosticians to describe an illness or condition that coexists with another illness or condition (e.g., depression is frequently comorbid with anxiety).

Depressogenic – A term describing an event or process that may be causal in the development of depression.

Goodness-of-fit – The quality of the 'match' or 'fit' between the characteristics of an individual and the environment. This term is frequently used to describe the quality of fit between infant characteristics (e.g., temperament, gender) and personality attributes of a parent. Theoretically, the better the fit, the better the adaptation of the parent and infant to each other and, in turn, the child's adaptation to the wider world.

Infant–mother attachment classifications – Infant–parent attachments are based on a scoring system developed by Mary Ainsworth and Mary Main for infants between 12 and 18 months, with particular attention to infant behavior during infant–mother reunions in the Strange Situation. Secure infants typically greet the parent, approach the parent to achieve contact, soothe quickly after contact is achieved, and are eventually able to resume toy play. Insecure-avoidant infants do not greet and conspicuously avoid the parent following reunion and appear to prefer toy play to achieving contact with or interacting with the parent. Insecure ambivalent/resistant infants overtly express anger toward the parent during reunions and have great difficulty soothing and returning to toy play. Insecure-disorganized infants appear to lack a coherent strategy in gaining access to the parent and show fear and/or confusion in response to the parent's during reunions.

Major depressive disorder (MDD) – As defined by the American Psychiatric Association's Diagnostic and Statistical Manual – 4th edition (DSM-IV), a diagnosis given for a single major depressive episode (nonrecurrent), or for multiple episodes (recurrent). MDD should be distinguished from other mood disorders that have depressive features but whose cause can be traced to a medical condition, substance use, dementia, or psychosocial stressor, or whose patterning of depressive symptoms cannot be clearly linked to the postpartum period (e.g., bipolar disorder or dysthymia).

Major depressive episode – A period of at least two consecutive weeks of depressed mood or loss of interest or enjoyment in most activities, accompanied by at least four of the following symptoms lasting 2 weeks or longer: loss of energy; difficulties in concentrating, thinking, or making decisions; a change in weight, appetite, psychomotor activity, or sleep; feelings of worthlessness or guilt; and recurrent thoughts of death or suicide, or suicide plans or attempts.

Maternal self-efficacy – Mother's beliefs or judgments about their competency in the parental role. Depressed mothers commonly report feeling less efficacious in the parenting role than do nondepressed mothers.

Negative affective bias – The tendency of depressed individuals to view oneself, others, or events in a negative or pessimistic light. Depressed women tend to hold negative cognitions about their children and themselves, which may impact their behavior in the parenting role.

Postpartum – Of, or pertaining to, the period of time, typically the first year, following an infant's birth.

Still face paradigm – An observational procedure composed of three 2 min phases: (1) free play phase – the caregiver engages the child in face-to-face play, talking and engaging the infant in a playful manner; (2) still face phase – the caregiver is instructed to maintain a flat or emotionally neutral facial expression (a 'still face') and does not respond to the infant in any way; (3) free play 'reunion' phase – the caregiver re-engages the infant in face-to-face play.

Strange situation procedure – A 21 min procedure, conducted in a laboratory playroom with toys, developed by Mary Ainsworth to assess quality of infant–parent attachment. The procedure enables one to observe infant behavior in the presence of the parent and a (typically) female stranger during a series of separations from and reunions with each. The pattern of infant behavior is then classified into one of four attachment categories (see above).

Transactional perspective – A conceptualization of development in which individual development is viewed as a dynamic process in which individual and environment mutually and reciprocally influence each other over time.

Introduction

Depression is particularly common among women of childbearing age, and approximately 13% of women can be expected to experience at least one bout of significant depression during the early postpartum period. Postpartum depression is similar in symptom profile to depressions that occur at other points in life. It is characterized by sadness or an inability to experience pleasure, accompanied by several additional symptoms, including negative cognitions (poor self-worth, perceptions of failure, guilt, and/or suicidal thoughts), somatic dysfunction (loss of appetite, sleep disturbance, fatigue), and impairment in daily functioning (e.g., inability to make decisions and to work effectively). The American Psychiatric Association's Diagnostic and Statistical Manual – 4th edition (DSM-IV) identifies a major depressive episode in terms of the symptom profile outlined above, which persists for at least a 2-week period. A DSM-IV diagnosis of major depressive disorder (MDD) may be given for a single major depressive episode, or for multiple, recurring episodes, and should not be confused with other mood disorders that have depressive features but whose etiology can be traced to a medical condition, substance use, dementia, or psychosocial stressor, or whose patterning of depressive symptoms cannot be clearly linked to the postpartum period (e.g., bipolar disorder or dysthymia). Postpartum depression is also not to be confused with the 'postpartum blues', a mild depressive condition that occurs early in the postpartum period, is not associated with significant impairment, and resolves quickly. Some postpartum depressions can also be accompanied by psychotic symptoms, such as hallucinations, delusions, and excessive psychomotor disturbances. Psychotic postpartum depressions are rare, however, and most discussions of postpartum depression are with reference to nonpsychotic depression.

Postpartum depression can have insidious effects on the mother and her family. Because of its high prevalence rate, it has become a major public health concern. Prevalence estimates vary as a function of the nature of the assessment and the window of time during which assessment takes place. Depressive symptoms can be assessed either through self-report questionnaire assessments, or by more formal clinical interviews. Self-report assessments include such well-known measures as the Beck

Depression Inventory, the Center for Epidemiological Studies – Depression Scale, and the Hamilton Rating Scale for Depression, each of which taps the frequency and severity of such symptoms and provides overall score cut points that, when exceeded, identify individuals with clinical levels of symptom severity. Clinical interviews, by contrast, use a more comprehensive interview format to inquire about current and past symptoms of depression that can be used to diagnose a depressive disorder, past or present. Not surprisingly, prevalence rates of postpartum depression are somewhat lower when comprehensive clinical interview assessments are used than when mothers are asked to complete self-report questionnaires.

The effects of postpartum depression are broad-based, with consequences not only for individual functioning but also for the quality of the mother's relationships with other family members. Marital discord in families with depressed mothers is common, as are troubled relationships between the depressed mother and her children. Indeed, children of depressed mothers are at significant risk for maladjustment and cognitive delays. Infants of depressed mothers are more likely than are infants of nondepressed mothers to be fussy, irritable, or withdrawn, to deploy attention ineffectively and manifest developmental delays in significant cognitive milestones such as object permanence, and are at risk to become insecurely attached to their mothers. Among older children of depressed mothers, rates of psychiatric disorder are as much as four to five times those among their same-aged counterparts of nondepressed mothers. Although maternal depression appears to predispose children to become depressed, these children are also at elevated risk for the full spectrum of externalizing disorders, including oppositional-defiant disorder and conduct disorder. Not surprisingly, these children are also at risk for poor academic performance, and for difficulties in interpersonal relationships, depressive and anxiety disorders, substance abuse, and delinquency over the long term.

Mechanisms for the transmission of psychopathology from depressed parent to child are poorly understood. Depression appears to be at least partially heritable, which may account in part for the elevated psychiatric risk status among children of depressed women. Other biologically based influences may also be at work. Recurrent bouts of significant depression among women are common. It is not unusual that women suffering from postpartum depression have experienced depressive episodes during pregnancy and pre-pregnancy. Interestingly, infants born to mothers suffering prepartum depression manifest a biochemical profile (i.e., levels of cortisol, catecholamines, and serotonin) that is similar to that of their mothers, but different from infants born to nondepressed mothers. The potential impact of genetically and biologically based factors on the psychiatric risk status of children of depressed women has been given relatively short shrift among researchers who study parental depression and its effects. We will return to this point later.

Most research examining mechanisms of transmission of psychopathology from depressed parent to child has focused on the kinds of environments depressed parents create for their children, and the impact such environments have on the developing child's interpersonal, cognitive, and emotional life. Depressed mothers indeed create pathogenic child-rearing environments to which even very young (3–4 months old) infants are reactive. Importantly, the degree to which maternal depression singly influences child outcomes, however, depends on the chronicity and severity of the mothers' illness. A single, isolated, nonrecurrent bout of major depression, albeit debilitating to the mother while it occurs, is much less likely to affect children's adjustment over the long term than is chronic, severe depression, involving multiple, recurrent bouts of depression during the early postpartum period and beyond. Unfortunately, a woman who experiences postpartum depression is likely to experience at least one additional depressive episode sometime during her child's first 5 years of life.

Also important to note is that depression is more likely to occur under adverse environmental circumstances, such as poverty and single parenthood, and it may also be but one feature of a broader spectrum of psychiatric symptoms. It is common to find, for example, that depression is comorbid with anxiety, and that depression, broadly speaking, is a salient feature of a variety of other psychiatric disorders. Interestingly, recent research suggests that depression that is chronic and severe may be comorbid with some personality disorders, as outlined in DSM-IV, axis II diagnoses. Indeed, some have proposed that chronic, severe depression is almost always comorbid with personality disorder, and that the depression is a by-product of the significantly impaired interpersonal relationships, problems in living, and emotional volatility that characterize personality disorders. This has raised significant concerns about whether chronic, severe depression without features of personality disorder can be distinguished from the effects of personality disorder alone. The ability to address these concerns rests on whether mothers with recurrent MDD that is not comorbid with an axis II disorder can be identified and compared, in terms of features of the mother–child relationship and child developmental outcomes, with mothers whose recurrent depression is paired with personality disorder. Most research to date has not systematically addressed the effects of maternal depression with vs. without comorbidity with other psychiatric problems.

Depressed Women as Parents

Depressed Mothers' Cognitions

Because cognitive distortions feature so saliently in depression, we begin a discussion of depressed mothering with a focus on what is known about depressed mothers' thoughts about themselves as parents and their thoughts about their children. Put simply, depressed women hold decidedly negative cognitions about their children and themselves. Depressed mothers are more likely than are nondepressed mothers to perceive themselves as inadequate parents, and to enjoy parenting less. Depressed mothers are also more likely to view their children negatively, in terms of their overall social competence and adjustment. Because children of depressed mothers are indeed at risk for maladjustment, it is unclear if depressed mothers' negative views of their children are accurate, or if they represent depression-induced cognitive distortions. Some studies suggest that the difference between depressed and nondepressed mothers' perceptions of their children is not based on the negative affective bias associated with depression, but on the tendency of nondepressed mothers to be more positive about their children than is actually warranted (i.e., a 'positive affective bias'). Indeed, when depressed and nondepressed women's perceptions of their children were compared with perceptions obtained from nonfamilial sources such as teachers, there is some evidence of greater concordance between depressed mothers' perceptions and teacher perceptions of the same children than between nondepressed mothers' and teachers' perceptions. However, because of depressed women's tendency to dwell on and exaggerate problems of all types, it is likely that depressed mothers' negative perceptions of their children are in part driven by a negative affective bias, the strength of which is probably directly proportional to the severity of their depressive symptoms.

It is reasonable to expect that a depressed mother's tendency to dwell on the negative, or to perceive a perfectly normal, developmentally appropriate behavior or accomplishment as problematic, may have its own impact on a developing child's emotional well-being. A child whose mother repeatedly labels her/him in negative terms is likely, at the least, to be at risk for low self-esteem, and possibly for a host of internalizing and externalizing problems. The negative affect and negative cognitions that define depression, however, are intimately tied to action tendencies. It is thus not surprising that depression takes a toll on the quality of mother–child interactions. The symptoms associated with depression challenge the ability of mothers to interact with their children in a developmentally supportive manner, and many studies now available describe depressed mothering as noncontingent and unresponsive, irritable and intrusive, insensitive, asynchronous, and incompetent. Difficulties observed in

depressed mothering may stem from deficiencies in the depressed mother's awareness and interpretation of her child's behavior (i.e., a 'signal detection' deficiency). For example, a depressed mother's rumination and self-absorption can influence her attention to and awareness of her children's needs and social signals, and can also interfere with her ability to process social information efficiently and accurately. Her negative affective bias may create tendencies to misinterpret child behavior, and depressed mothers may be inclined to attribute negative intentions and motives to their children's behavior. Further, a depressed mothers' own need for support and comfort may lead her to expect more support and comfort from her child than the child is able to provide. Parenting difficulties among depressed mothers may also stem from the general slowing effect depressed affect has upon one's capability and motivation to act. Lack of energy and indecisiveness are hallmark features of depression, which in turn would be expected to influence a mother's motivation to respond promptly and contingently to child signals that she does comprehend. Thus, the problems observed in depressed parenting may arise from the debilitating effect depression has on mothers' capacities for processing social information (awareness and interpretation of child cues), and from the dampening effect of depression on a mother's capacity and motivation to respond contingently.

Depressed Mother–Infant Interactions

In infancy, the emotional climate of parent–child interactions may be particularly important for the development of self-regulation, secure attachments, and the promotion of other social and emotional competencies. Unfortunately, the disturbances associated with depression have a clear impact on the emotional quality of early mother–child interactions. Depressed mothers interact less with their infants, are less aware of their infants' signals, and are less contingently responsive to their infants' bids for attention. The joint attention, shared positive affect, and appropriate scaffolding that characterizes warm, nurturant parent–child relationships are often missing in depressed mother–infant dyads. Further, depressed mothers show less emotional availability and affection toward their infants, display less pleasure and positive emotion during interactions, and express more negative affect overall. Some depressed mothers may alternate between being disengaged and then overly stimulating, the latter of which can be so intrusive that they appear disorganizing to the infant. In turn, their infants' behavior is conspicuously devoid of positive affect, and is also characteristically high in distress or protest, unresponsiveness to maternal bids, avoidance, and withdrawal, and this behavior sometimes generalizes to other, nondepressed adults. The infant's distress and unresponsiveness in turn may increase the mother's feelings of inadequacy or rejection, thus creating a vicious cycle of negative, dysregulated affect in the mother–infant relationship.

Experimental evidence underscores the premise that depressed mothers' emotional unavailability and lack of responsiveness is emotionally dysregulating to infants. In 1978, Edward Tronick and colleagues developed the still face paradigm, a procedure that requires mothers to mimic the flat affect and unresponsive behavior commonly seen in depressed mothers. The procedure is composed of three very brief episodes: In the first episode, the mother engages the child in face-to-face play, talking and engaging the infant in a playful manner; in the second episode, the mother is instructed to maintain a flat or emotionally neutral facial expression (a 'still face') and does not respond to the infant in any way; and in the final 'reunion' episode, the mother re-engages the infant in face-to-face play. Infants of nondepressed mothers are typically very positive and engaged during the face-to-face play, but show a heightened level of arousal and distress to their mothers' sudden emotional unavailability and unresponsiveness during the still face. Typical reactions on the part of the child include attempts to re-engage the mother through smiling, vocalizations, or fussing, and distressed facial expressions such as frowns or grimaces. Infants may use a variety of methods to try to regulate their discomfort during the still face, such as turning their head away from the mother and averting their gaze, or engaging in self-soothing behaviors such as sucking on their thumb. The effects of the still face often linger even when the mother re-engages the infant, with infants often continuing to show distress afterwards. Research with the still face paradigm demonstrates that even very young infants (i.e., as young as 3 months of age) are emotionally attuned to maternal affect and can become emotionally dysregulated when mothers' normally positive affect is withdrawn.

Interestingly, when the still face procedure is conducted with depressed mothers and their infants, clear differences emerge between these dyads and nondepressed mother–infant dyads. First, when the mother is depressed, there is less distinction in the behavior of both the child and the mother across the three episodes. There are often less shared positive emotions during face-to-face play, with more neutral affect and withdrawn behavior in both the mother and infant. Second, during the still face phase, infants of depressed mothers show less active attempts at regaining their mothers' attention than do infants of nondepressed mothers. Instead, infants of depressed mothers become more quiet and withdrawn, and devote more energy toward self-comforting or distraction. Such behavior has led some to suggest that the still face episode is similar to the normative behavior of the depressed mother, and that infants of depressed

mothers are more likely to make attempts at managing their distress without maternal assistance. The inability of infants to gain comfort and support from their mothers when distressed may have serious consequences for the formation of secure attachments, as well as in the development of healthy strategies for regulating emotions.

Tronick's work with the still face paradigm prompted the development of his 'mutual regulation model' as an integrative framework for understanding how mother and infant affective states become mutually and reciprocally regulatory. Among typical, nondepressed mothers with very young infants, mothers' use of contingently responsive, positive affect during interactions with their infants significantly exceeds their use of negative affect. Maternal positive affect in turn elicits similarly positive affective responses (smiles, coos, laughs) from the infant, and both mothers and infants find each others' positive affective signals to be mutually rewarding and reinforcing. Over time, mutually reciprocal positive affect predominates in interactions between nondepressed mothers, which carries developmental benefits for the infant's socioemotional development over the long term. By contrast, mutually reciprocal, negative affect predominates in interactions between depressed mothers and their infants. Depressed mothers may be unresponsive to or critical of their infants' behavior and social cues, leading their infants in turn to withdraw and become distressed. Depressed mothers' lack of sufficient use of contingently responsive positive affect may render them less capable than nondepressed mothers to soothe their infants when distressed (indeed, depressed mothers' negative affect may be, in many instances, the cause of their infants' distress). The infants in turn may become dysphoric and overly reliant on self-soothing and self-stimulatory behaviors to regulate their negative emotions, placing them at risk for psychopathology.

Depressed Mothering and Infant–Mother Attachments

Attachment theory would predict that depressed mothers' interactional difficulties with their infants, if prolonged, will predispose infants to become insecurely attached. Indeed, maternal sensitivity during infancy, which can be defined as an empathic awareness of and appropriate responsiveness to infant needs and social cues, is taken by attachment theory as the single most important predictor of attachment security in infancy. Research that has examined linkages between maternal depression and infant–mother attachment security typically employs the Ainsworth Strange Situation procedure, a brief, 21–24 min seven-episode procedure used for infants between 12 and 18 months of age. The procedure, which almost always takes place in a small room that is novel to the infant, puts the infant through a series of 3 min episodes of separations and reunions with the mother, a (typically) female stranger, and one episode in which the infant is alone.

Specific attention is given to the infant's behavior during the two Strange Situation reunion episodes with the mother. Secure infants typically greet the mother during infant–mother reunions, approach the mother and seek her out for comfort (if the infant experiences separation distress), and are ultimately able to return to toy play and exploring their environment in the mothers' presence. Sensitive mothering during the infant's first year would be expected to promote secure infant–mother attachments, which, as many studies now attest, predicts healthy adjustment in the preschool years and beyond in terms of empathic awareness, child compliance, and peer relations. Insecure-avoidant infants, by contrast, typically do not greet the mother during reunions. They do not approach the mother except in the context of toy play, and it is not uncommon for insecure-avoidant infants to prefer to play with toys rather than interact with their mothers. Maternal insensitivity characterized by intrusiveness and rejection would be expected to predict insecure-avoidant infant–mother attachments, which some attachment theorists propose is developed as a defense against maternal rejection. Insecure-ambivalent/resistant infants direct overt expressions of anger toward their mothers during reunions and typically do not soothe in response to maternal attempts to do so. Mothering characterized by unresponsiveness and/or inconsistency in responsiveness would be expected to predict insecure-ambivalent (resistant) infant–mother attachments. Both insecure-avoidant and insecure-ambivalent/resistant attachments, albeit not adaptive to the infant over the long term, are viewed as 'strategies' the child has developed to maintain access to the attachment figure (the mother) in times of stress. Insecure-avoidant infants learn not to seek out their mothers because doing so in the past has led to rejection. Thus, they employ a 'close, but not too close' strategy to maintain some degree of proximity to the mother. Insecure-ambivalent/resistant infants have learned that overt expressions of anger and prolonged distress is 'what works' to keep their mothers focused on them. This strategy, although maladaptive to their development over the long run, is functional in the short term to maintain access to their mothers. Both insecure-avoidance and insecure-resistant/ambivalent infants are at risk for difficulties in later mother–child relationships and peer relationships, compared to secure infants.

Elevations in insecure infant–mother attachments (i.e., insecure-avoidant and insecure-ambivalent resistant attachments) have been reported in several studies of depressed mother–infant dyads. Further, when mothers' depression is chronic and severe over the infant's first year, infants are at risk for developing insecure-disorganized attachment to their mothers, which some attachment

theorists cite as the most insecure of all of the insecure attachment classifications. Unlike the insecure-avoidant and insecure ambivalent attachment patterns, which appear to be governed by clear-cut strategies (albeit not ideal) for accessing the attachment figure, insecure-disorganized attachment is identified by conspicuous absence of a clear-cut strategy. Disorganized attachment is instead hallmarked by fear and confusion about how to access the attachment figure (the mother) at times when it is in the infant's best interests to do so. In the Strange Situation, insecure-disorganized infants are identified by any of a variety of behavior patterns signifying fear and/or confusion during the infant–mother reunion episodes. For example, disorganization is identified when the infant manifests clear-cut expressions of fear (e.g., infant brings hand to mouth and has a fearful expression) of the mother when she enters the room to begin the reunion episode. It is also identified when the infant freezes or stills in the mother's presence for a substantial period of time, or when the infant, upon approaching the mother, repeatedly veers away from her. These are but a few of a variety of indicators of disorganized attachment, all of which reflect a state of fear or confusion about how to access the attachment figure in times of stress. Rates of disorganized infant–mother attachment are found to be elevated among infants of alcoholic parents, substance abusing parents, and parents with significant psychopathology. Of the three insecure infant–parent attachment classifications, children identified as insecure-disorganized are at highest risk for the development of behavior problems in the preschool years.

Attachment theory proposes that, over time, children develop working models of relationships that spawn from their early attachments with their caregivers, models that are carried forward and applied in subsequent relationships. Such models can be thought of as a set of affectively laden cognitions or expectations about relationships that develop as a result of repeated interactions with attachment figures and that guide behavior and the processing of social information. Attachment theory predicts that children with secure working models develop expectations that their caregivers will be appropriately responsive to them when needed, and such children in turn come to believe that they are worthy of love and support. Such expectations are consistent with a history of sensitive, responsive caregiving. Children who develop insecure working models, by contrast, do not expect their caregivers to be appropriately responsive, and insecure working models may serve as a foundation for low self-worth. Importantly, attachment theory also proposes that children internalize not just the child's role in their early attachment relationships, but the role of the parent as well, and that they are likely to carry forward and enact the parent's side in subsequent relationships with others. Indeed, it is the development of these working models that provides the theoretical link between the insecure attachment patterns infants develop to their depressed mothers and the adjustment problems these children present later in development.

It is important to emphasize, however, that the link between maternal depression and insecure infant–mother attachment is most clear when mothers' depression during the infants' first year is prolonged. A single maternal depressive episode during the postpartum period that resolves and does not recur is unlikely to have long-term negative effects on security of infant–mother attachment, nor on other aspects of infant and preschool-child functioning.

Depressed Mother–Toddler Relationships

Emergent social, emotional, and cognitive capabilities in the toddler years create new opportunities for change and growth, but may also place new demands on the depressed mother. Although the affective connection between the toddler and mother is clearly still important, the inability to appropriately structure and build upon the child's activities may be especially damaging during this developmental period. Depressed mothers are less able to follow the child's interests or facilitate joint attention, making mutual engagement in activities challenging. Further, depressed mothers' lack of verbal communication and reduced responsiveness in interactions with their toddlers may impact the acquisition of linguistic and cognitive skills, important developmental tasks during this time. Similar to the difficulties seen in infancy, depressed mothers often display sad, anxious, or irritable affect with their toddlers, and their interactions lack the shared positive affect and coordination of their nondepressed counterparts. In turn, their children appear to have difficulty regulating negative emotions, showing less positive emotions and more frequent depressed, anxious, or angry behavior.

Toddlers' growing desire to assert their independence often increases parent–child conflict during this period, and depressed mothers may be less able to provide the gentle guidance and limit setting necessary to successfully negotiate these conflicts. Some mothers experiencing depression are more likely to avoid confrontation with their toddlers, expressing fears over their child's willful behavior and their inability to assert appropriate authority. Conversely, some mothers experiencing depression resort to harsh discipline, showing greater hostility toward their children and utilizing more physical punishment than their nondepressed counterparts. Maternal feelings of helplessness and lack of control over their children's behavior increases the likelihood that they will employ coercive or punitive tactics in disciplinary encounters. In fact, maternal depression may be considered a risk factor for physical abuse and maltreatment of young children. In either case,

these ineffective socialization techniques employed by depressed mothers are often met with dysfunctional behavior on the part of the toddler. In some cases, children of depressed mothers show more frequent defiance, hostility, aggression, and externalizing behavior. Alternatively, the toddlers of depressed mothers may show more depressed affect and withdrawal themselves, as well as helplessness in the face of challenges. Notably, the behavior of these toddlers often matches that of their mother, such that the affect and symptoms of the mother are mirrored in her child's actions.

Interestingly, disorganized attachment in infancy is predictive of two rather sophisticated yet very maladaptive preschool behavior patterns directed toward the mother, and both of these patterns have been linked to chronic maternal depression. One of these patterns is characterized by the child's repeated attempts to take care of and nurture the mother (i.e., a role-reversing 'caregiving' pattern). Such a pattern, on the surface, does not present with any outward signs of trouble or hostility between the child and mother. However, a role-reversed caregiving pattern that develops in a child at such an early developmental stage has been identified by some as representing attempts on the part of the child to repair a damaged relationship, with consequences for the child's emotional well-being. Insecure-disorganized infant–mother attachment is also associated with a second maladaptive preschool behavior pattern, characterized by repeated, overt attempts by the child to embarrass and punish the mother. These 'coercive' child behavior patterns are thought to develop in response to a caregiving history characterized by unresponsiveness and inconsistency, perhaps particularly in the area of appropriate limit-setting. The coercive and caregiving preschool patterns may be different manifestations of an overarching 'controlling' strategy of accessing mothers in times of stress. Not surprisingly, these caregiving and coercive patterns have straightforward links to child behavior problems.

Maternal Depression and Child Outcomes in Middle Childhood and Adolescence

There tend to be fewer studies of the effects of maternal depression on developmental outcomes of school-aged children and adolescents, but the data that are available indicate that such children are at high risk for depression, anxiety disorder, conduct disorder, delinquency, attention deficits, and academic failure. Similar to younger children with depressed mothers, interactional difficulties are common between children of depressed mothers and their parents, with withdrawal, poor limit setting, and criticism being central features of depressed mothering for children in this age range. School-aged children and adolescents develop stable representations of themselves in relation to others, and they are more likely than are children of nondepressed mothers to develop negative attributional styles and low self-worth. Peer relations may also suffer, with children of depressed mothers being more likely to suffer peer isolation, loneliness, and rejection. It is not uncommon for teachers of children of depressed mothers to rate them as being more aggressive and disruptive, in comparison to children of nondepressed mothers.

Individual Differences in Depressed Mother–Child Relationships and Child Outcomes

Despite the well-documented associations between postpartum depression and difficulties within the mother–child relationship, it is important to emphasize that problematic interactions are not seen in all cases in which the mother is experiencing depression. Further, the association between maternal depression and relationship disturbances is less clear in samples that are not also considered 'at risk' due to factors such as poverty or high interparental conflict. Some mothers experiencing depression appear quite normative in their interactions with their infants, and environmental sources of stress or support may play a large role in altering the effects of depression on the mother–child relationship. Although postpartum depression is clearly a risk factor, the numerous individual differences in the way postpartum depression may impact parent–child interactions should not be overlooked.

The Role of Maternal Self-Efficacy

One important source of individual differences in depressed mothering may be variations encountered in maternal self-efficacy, or a mother's beliefs in her own competencies as a parent. Maternal self-efficacy is a construct that has grown out of Albert Bandura's social-cognitive theory. Bandura defines self-efficacy as a set of beliefs or judgments about one's competency at a particular task or setting. Self-efficacy beliefs are viewed as the final common pathway in predicting the degree of effort one expends to succeed at a particular task. Self-efficacious individuals are strongly motivated to marshal whatever resources (personal, social, economic, etc.) that are available to them to succeed at a given task. Self-inefficacious individuals, by contrast, are likely to give up prematurely, despite the fact that success may be within reach. Whereas the strongest predictor of self-efficacy is the degree of prior success at that task, self-efficacy beliefs are also sensitive to social persuasion, vicarious experiences (e.g., modeling), and affective state.

Given the link between self-efficacy and affect, it is not surprising that depressed mothers feel less efficacious in the parenting role than do nondepressed mothers. At the same time, social-cognitive theory would predict that maternal self-efficacy should also be sensitive to support for their mothering provided by intimate support figures (social persuasion), by previous learning experiences about mothering by watching other competent mothers (modeling), and by mothers' perceptions of how 'easy' or 'difficult' their infants are to care for (perceptions of infant temperament, which should be linked with mothers' histories of prior successes and failures with the infant). Thus, variation in maternal self-efficacy is not a simple, direct function of variations in maternal depression, but also of variations in other social influences in the environment. Self-efficacy theory would also predict, however, that any influences of mothers' affective state, social persuasion, or prior experiences with their infants on parenting should be mediated by maternal self-efficacy, which is the final common pathway in the prediction of behavioral competence.

Douglas Teti and Donna Gelfand tested this hypothesis in 1991 in a study of 86 mothers (48 with clinical depression, and 38 nondepressed) of first-year infants. Maternal self-efficacy was assessed with a scale developed by the authors that tapped mothers' self-efficacy beliefs in nine parental domains relevant to mothering an infant in the first year of life (e.g., soothing, maintaining infant attention, diapering, feeding, changing), with a tenth item asking mothers to report on their overall feelings of competence in the mothering role. Ratings of mothers' behavioral competence (e.g., sensitivity, warmth, disengagement) with their infants were conducted from observations of feeding and free play by 'blind', highly reliable observers. Standard, well-established measures were used to assess severity of maternal depressive symptoms, social marital supports, and infant temperament.

As predicted, mothers' parenting efficacy beliefs were negatively associated with maternal depressive symptoms and perceptions of infant temperament, such that mothers felt less efficacious in the maternal role when they were more depressed and when they perceived their infants as more difficult. Mothers' self-efficacy beliefs, by contrast, were positively associated with perceived quality of social-marital supports and with observer judgments of maternal behavioral competence with their infants. In addition, as expected, mothers' behavioral competence was significantly related to perceptions of infant temperamental difficulty (negatively) and with social–marital supports (positively). Importantly, maternal self-efficacy beliefs continued to predict maternal behavioral competence even after maternal depressive symptoms, social–marital supports, and infant temperamental difficulty were statistically controlled. Further, when maternal self-efficacy was statistically controlled, the linkages between maternal behavioral competence and maternal depression, infant temperament, and social–marital supports were substantially reduced in magnitude. Taken together, these findings identified maternal self-efficacy beliefs as a central mediator of relations between mothers' behavioral competence with their infants and the severity of maternal depressive symptoms, perceptions of infant temperamental difficulty, and social–marital supports.

These findings indicate that depression is more likely to debilitate parenting quality when maternal self-efficacy is also compromised. This is likely to be the case in many depressed mothers because of the strong linkage between affective state and self-efficacy beliefs. However, maternal self-efficacy is also sensitive to infant temperament and social–marital supports, and thus it is possible for depressed mothers to have more positive self-efficacy beliefs about parenting, and in turn to parent more effectively, when their infants are temperamentally easy and when they receive consistent encouragement from intimate support figures. Conversely, the combination of significant depression and difficult infant temperament and/or inadequate social–marital supports may be particularly devastating in their joint effects on maternal self-efficacy beliefs. In their 1991 study, Teti and Gelfand found this to be the case when examining the single vs. joint impact of maternal depression and infant temperamental difficulty on mothers' parenting efficacy beliefs. Maternal self-efficacy was much more compromised among mothers who had high levels of depressive symptoms and who also perceived their infants to be difficult. Further, the joint 'impact' of severe maternal depression and infant temperamental difficulty on maternal self-efficacy was significantly greater than what would have been expected from an additive model of effects.

Maternal Depression in Transactional Perspective

Interestingly, studies that examine the impact of maternal depression in the context of other risk and resilience factors are not common. The dearth of such research is surprising, given that developmental scientists now embrace the spirit of the Transactional Model of development, articulated by Arnold Sameroff over 30 years ago. This model posits that development is a complex function of ongoing, mutually occurring influences between the child and the environment, such that, at any given point in time, one must take into account the impact of the environment on the child as well as the impact of the child on the environment in order to understand individual differences in developmental trajectories. The Transactional Model is a vast conceptual improvement over the more static 'main effects' models, which purport to predict development on the basis of knowledge of a single

environmental event or child characteristic measured at a specific point in time, and over 'interactional models', which improves upon main effects models by taking into joint consideration single environmental events and single child characteristics, again measured from a single time point. Although we feel that a fair test of the Transactional Model, in terms of predicting development across several years, may not be possible, it should govern our thinking about how individual differences in depressed mother-child relationships and in child outcomes can be explained by examining how maternal depression's effects are moderated by specific child characteristics and by features of the maternal environment. We believe such an emphasis is long overdue, because the links between maternal depression, parenting, and child outcomes are far from uniform.

Such a perspective was represented in some ongoing work by the first author, who examined predictive relations between postpartum maternal depression and maternal sensitivity during interactions with infants, maternal self-efficacy, and infant behavior problems, assessed at different points during the infants' first year in a sample of approximately 120 African American, premature infants (56% female) and their mothers. Interestingly, maternal depressive symptoms, assessed prior to infant hospital discharge, did not predict maternal sensitivity toward the infant in the home when infants were 4 months and 12 months of age (corrected for prematurity), nor were they predictive of maternal self-efficacy at 4 months infant corrected age. They were, however, predictive of mother reports of infant behavior problems at 12 months, but only modestly.

When specific child characteristics, assessed either prior to infant discharge or at 4 months of infant corrected age, were taken into account, more specific linkages between early postpartum depression and later mother–infant outcomes emerged. For example, depressed mothers who perceived their infants to have unsettled, irregular states of arousal prior to discharge were observed, by raters who were blind to all other data, to be less sensitive during interactions with their infants at 4 and 12 months of infant corrected age than were mothers without postpartum depression but who also saw their infants as unsettled and irregular. No link between postpartum depression and maternal sensitivity at either age point was observed among mothers who did not perceive their infants as having problems in state regulation. In a separate analysis examining the role of infant gender in linkages between maternal postpartum depression and mother-reported child behavior problems at 12 months, significant longitudinal linkages were only observed for male infants, but not female infants. Thus, the main effect of maternal postpartum depression on 12 month infant behavior problems, reported above, appeared to be accounted for in mother–male infant dyads, but not mother–female infant dyads. This finding is consistent with a large literature documenting that male children tend to be more vulnerable to environmental stressors, including parental psychopathology, than are female children. Very few of these studies, however, document such vulnerability in male children during the first year of life.

What this work emphasizes is that the impact of maternal depression on child outcomes is at least in part dependent on the quality of fit between the mother's illness and characteristics of the children themselves. Goodness-of-fit, of course, is a construct that is well-understood among child temperament theorists, who argue that fit between parental and child characteristics, and not each individual's characteristics alone, is ultimately the driving force that underlies the quality of the relationship that develops between parent and child and, in turn, individual differences in children's outcome. We do not mean to imply that there are certain circumstances under which the effects of maternal depression on child development are nonexistent or not worth pursuing. Indeed, even in cases of a better fit between a depressed mother and a specific child, the mother's depression may be influencing the child in ways that may not be evident at a particular time or in terms of the measures used to assess such effects. The construct of fit, however, has not been systematically employed to understand individual differences in depressed mother–child relationships and maternal depression's effects on child outcomes. We believe such an emphasis is long overdue.

The role of partner involvement in families with depressed mothers, both in terms of the quality of support provided to mothers, and as a potential buffering or exacerbating influence on child development, is also poorly understood. What little work that has been done examining fathers in depressed mother households suggests that these fathers are also likely to be distressed, although it is unclear to what degree such distress is a product of coping with a spouse with an affective illness. Of course, children growing up in households with two parents with affective disorders would likely be at even greater risk for maladjustment than would children with only one affectively disturbed parent, but there is little prior work that documents how much greater this risk might be.

It does appear, however, that the quality of support fathers provide to depressed mothers may be an important buffering influence on the effects of maternal depression. It is quite common for mothers to report high levels of marital distress. Marital distress, in turn, has well-known deleterious effects on child adjustment, and some have speculated that the marital distress that is so common in depressed mother households may actually mediate the effects of maternal depression on child development. Indeed, Robert Emery and colleagues, in a paper published in 1982, found that the degree to which fathers adjusted to their depressed wives disorder was a significant predictor of children's rates of psychiatric symptoms. Specifically, Emery found that the negative effects of mothers' depression on children's adjustment were practically negligible after controlling for marital distress, suggesting that maternal depression's effects may operate via its impact on the larger family system. Low levels of marital distress in depressed mother households is rare; however, when fathers have some insight into their partners' illness, they may be better able to provide appropriate emotional support, which in turn may help mothers parent more effectively and, in turn, the quality of children's attachments to their mothers. In addition, fathers who adapt better to their wives' depression are likely to be better, more engaged parents with their children, which may buffer any direct negative effects of mothers' depression on children. We believe that an important goal in intervening in families with depressed mothers is not simply to work to alleviate mothers' depression and (if needed) promote competent parenting skills, but also to help other family members cope with the mother's illness more effectively by promoting a better understand and appreciation of the nature of the mothers' illness. Indeed, research on the impact of maternal depressed on children as filtered through the larger family system is sorely needed and may foster a better understanding of why some children, in the face of maternal depression, fare better than others.

Conclusions

Maternal depression can have serious consequences for children in social, emotional, and cognitive developmental domains, and children of depressed parents are four to five times as likely as children of nondepressed mothers to be at risk for behavior problems. Children's risk for behavioral disturbances appears to be directly proportional to the chronicity and severity of mothers' depression. Even very short bouts of maternal depression appear to have an emotionally dysregulating effect on infants as young as three months of age, and postpartum depression that is recurrent places infants at risk for insecure attachment. Children who grow up in depressed mother households are at risk for elevated psychiatric symptoms, both internalizing and externalizing, and to develop psychiatric disorders along a broad spectrum, including depressive and anxiety disorders, oppositional defiant disorder, and conduct disorder. Mechanisms of parent-to-child transmission have focused primarily on the impact of depressogenic mothering, although there is also evidence that depression is partially heritable. Importantly, depression's effects on mothering, and on children's development, are heterogeneous and may be buffered or exacerbated by a variety of additional parent, child, and environmental influences. Understanding the effects of maternal depression in the context of other risk and protective factors is a worthy goal for the field.

Fortunately, depression ranks as one of the more treatable psychiatric disorders. Women who suffer from postpartum depression can avail themselves of a variety of treatment approaches, including pharmacological, psychotherapeutic (e.g., cognitive-behavioral, psychodynamic, and support-based 'talking' therapies), or some combination. In addition, approaches that target mother–child interactions have also been successful, in particular when maternal depression co-occurs with skill deficits in mothering. All of these treatment approaches have been effective, to varying degrees, in reducing symptom severity and improving quality of mothering. Pediatricians are likely to be the first health professionals to identify postpartum depression. It is thus important to equip pediatricians with the training and assessment tools to screen for postpartum depression, and to refer mothers to the appropriate mental health facilities for further evaluation and treatment.

Mothers who suffer from depression clearly need help, not just for themselves but for their children. Continued research is needed to understand more clearly the heterogeneous nature of maternal depression and its effects, what role maternal, child, spousal, and family characteristics play in this regard, and to develop effective interventions. Efforts to increase public awareness of postpartum depression and its effects on children are also critically important, if only because such awareness could lead to more mothers seeking treatment.

See also: Depression; Mental Health, Infant; Parental Chronic Mental Illnesses.

Suggested Readings

Elgar FJ, McGrath PJ, Waschbusch DA, Stewart SH, and Curtis LJ (2004) Mutual influences on maternal depression and child adjustment problems. *Clinical Psychology Review* 24: 441–459.
Embry L and Dawson G (2002) Disruptions in parenting behavior related to maternal depression: Influences on children's behavioral and psychobiological development. In: Borkowski JG Ramey SL,, and Bristol-Power M (eds.) *Parenting and the Child's World: Influences on Academic, Intellectual, and Social–Emotional Development. Monographs in Parenting*, pp. 203–213. Mahwah, NJ: Erlbaum.
Gelfand DM and Teti DM (1990) The effects of maternal depression on children. *Clinical Psychology Review* 10: 329–353.
Goodman SH and Gotlib IH (1999) Risk for psychopathology in the children of depressed mothers: A developmental model for understanding mechanisms of transmission. *Psychological Review* 106: 458–490.
Nylen KJ, Moran TE, Franklin CL, and O'Hara MW (2006) Maternal depression: A review of relevant treatment approaches for mothers and infants. *Infant Mental Health Journal* 27: 327–343.
O'Hara MW (1997) The nature of postpartum depressive disorders. In: Murray L and Cooper PJ (eds.) *Postpartum Depression and Child Development*, pp. 3–31. New York: Guilford.
Radke-Yarrow M (1998) *Children of Depressed Mothers: From Early Childhood to Maturity.* Cambridge, UK: Cambridge University Press.
Speranza AM, Ammaniti M, and Trentini C (2006) An Overview of maternal depression, infant reactions, and intervention programs. Clinical Neuropsychiatry: Journal of Treatment Evaluation 3(1): 57–68.
Teti DM and Gelfand DM (1991) Behavioral competence among mothers of infants in the first year: The mediational role of maternal self-efficacy. *Child Development* 62: 918–929.

Relevant Websites

http://www.aafp.org – American Academy of Family Physicians.
http://healthyminds.org – Healthy Minds. Healthy Lives.
http://www.nimh.nih.gov – National Institute of Mental Health, National Institutes of Health.
http://www.4woman.gov – National Women's Health Information Center.
http://www.nlm.nih.gov – United States National Library of Medicine, National Institutes of Health.

R

Reflexes

F S Pedroso, Universidade Federal de Santa Maria, Santa Maria, Brazil

Glossary

Agonist muscle – A muscle that on contracting is automatically checked and controlled by the opposing simultaneous contraction of another muscle – 'prime mover'.

Athetosis – A derangement marked by ceaseless occurrence of slow, sinuous, writhing movements, especially severe in the hands, and performed involuntarily; it may occur after hemiplegia, and is then known as 'posthemiplegic chorea'. Called also 'mobile spasm'.

Automatism (self-action) – Aimless and apparently undirected behavior that is not under conscious control and is performed without conscious knowledge; seen in psychomotor epilepsy, psychogenic fugue, and other conditions. Called also 'automatic behavior'.

Cephalocaudal – Proceeding or occurring in the long axis of the body especially in the direction from head to tail.

Clonus – A series of alternating contractions and partial relaxations of a muscle that in some nervous diseases occurs and is believed to result from alteration of the normal pattern of motor neuron discharge.

Distal to proximal – Maturation process that follows the direction from the trunk to the limbs.

Extrasegmental – Involvement of other segments of the spinal cord beyond primary stimulated.

Lower neuron – Motor neurons that belong to the anterior horn in the spinal cord or brainstem, when compromised, these cause atrophies, weakness, and muscular hypotonia.

Myelination – The process of acquiring a myelin sheath around the axons of neurons by oligodendrocytes or Schwann cells.

Ontogenesis – The development or course of development of an individual organism.

Pyramidal injury – Injury of cortex cerebral or the central motor way responsible for the body voluntary movements.

Tone – The normal degree of vigor and tension; in muscle, the resistance to passive elongation or stretch.

Introduction

Reflex is defined as an involuntary motor response, secretory or vascular, elicited shortly after a stimulus, which may be conscious or not. The response to the stimulus is unalterable, it cannot be changed or adapted according to needs or circumstances. It can be concluded, thus, that the response is stereotyped and has a fixed reflex arc, whose response is also fixed. The reflex arc – stimulus reception and motor response to the same stimulus – is a physiological unit of the nervous system (NS).

In its most simple form, the reflex arc comprises: (1) a receptor which corresponds to a special sensory organ, or nerve terminations in the skin or neuromuscular spindle, of which stimulation initiates an impulse; (2) the sensory or afferent neuron, which carries the impulse through a peripheral nerve to the central nervous system (CNS), where it synapses with an internuncial neuron; (3) an internuncial neuron relays the impulse to the efferent neuron; (4) the motor or efferent neuron conducts the impulse through a nerve to the effector organ; and (5) the effector can be a muscle, gland, or blood vessel that manifests the response.

Despite this narrow definition of segmental integration, the polysynaptic involvement of other NS segments is common, constituting intra-, extrasegmental, and contralateral reflexes to the stimulus origin. For the reflex motion to occur, it is necessary to contract the agonist muscles and relax the muscles that perform the opposite motion (antagonist), regarding the latter, instead of causing the muscle to contract, inhibitory synapses will prevent muscle contraction. An example is the knee jerk reflex or patellar reflex: contraction of the quadriceps and extension of the leg when the patellar ligament is tapped (**Figures 1** and **2**).

However, reflex manifestations are typically diverse after a specific stimulation, as occurs with most primitive reflexes (PRs). **Figures 3** and **4** show the complexity of responses to hand-compression stimulus.

The newborn is endowed with a set of reflex and automatic movements, which makes his NS apt to react to the environment where he lives in; the responses necessary to his adaptation and subsistence, such as suction, crying, deglutition, defense, and escape reactions, cannot be simply defined as reflexes in the strict sense of the definition, since these can be subject to alteration or adapted to needs and circumstances, and are therefore alterable, as the responses elicited by a given excitation do not manifest themselves in a clearly predeterminate way, nor are exactly identical over time. These responses express the neurophysiological state upon stimulation, constituting reflex reactions or automatisms; hence, these motor manifestations have been named differently by different authors, such as: PRs, primary reflexes, archaic reflexes, reflex responses, special reflexes, automatic reflexes, neonatal reflexes, primary responses, and developmental reflexes. Without a denomination of their own, some authors have included them among reflexes in general; in this article we call them PRs.

In order to define a reflex, we also need to specifically know its stimulation area, its integration center, and its response. Regarding PRs, it is still necessary to associate a functional concept that accounts for their ontogenetic and phylogenetic purpose. Although it is didactical to study each reflex isolately, we should bear in mind that this is a theoretical abstraction, convenient for the analysis of nervous phenomena, which does not exist in real life, since the PRs constitute a harmonic ensemble and are closely intertwined with one another, depending on the child's physiological needs and environmental conditions at the moment they are elicited.

Origin

Reflex activities are inherited, ranging from one species to another and oscillating according to life conditions

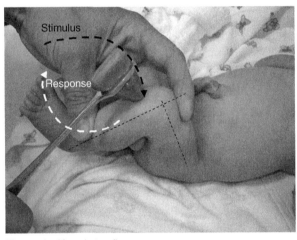

Figure 1   Knee jerk reflex.

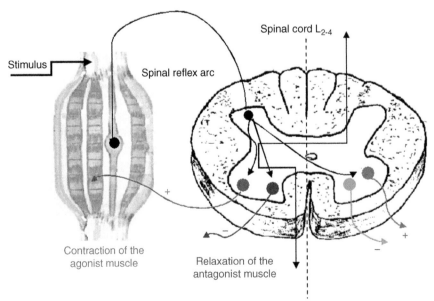

Figure 2   Spinal reflex arc.

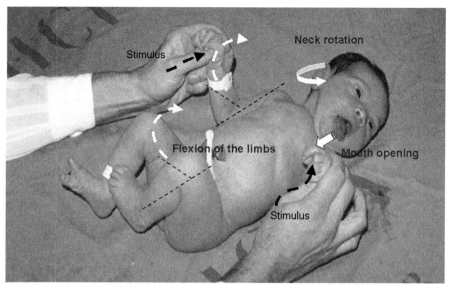

Figure 3 Babkin reflex and other responses to hand compression stimulus.

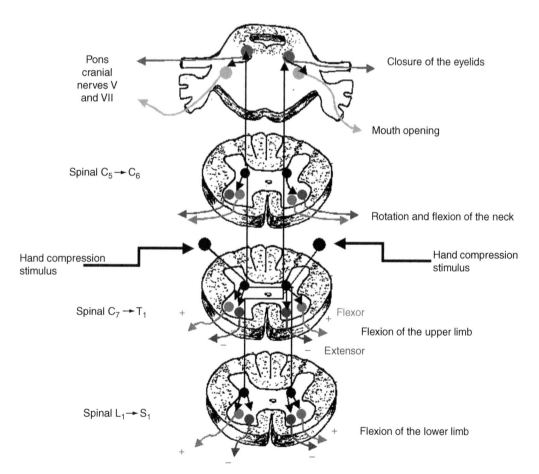

Figure 4 Babkin reflex and other responses to hand compression stimulus – diagram.

peculiar to each one. During human development, reflex, automatic, and voluntary motor control appear consecutively, which are anatomically processed respectively in the spinal cord/brainstem, basal ganglia, and cerebral cortex. The maturation process (cell organization and myelination) of these structures occurs at first in the caudocephalic direction, starting with reflex motor activity, which is exclusive until the 24th week of pregnancy.

Thereafter, neural activities of reticular formation begin in the brainstem, enabling tonic movements of the head and neck and, subsequently, of the root of limbs. Later, with the maturation of the extrapyramidal prosencephalic nuclei, more complex motions appear, such as those of feet and hands. From the 37th to 40th week of gestation on, it is already possible to observe the early manifestation of cortical functioning, often evident via visual attention, sensory habituation, and first voluntary movements.

Classification

In function of the possibility of a diversity of names for the same reflex activity, one becomes useful to present here the classification of the consequences under different aspects as: place of origin of the stimulus, time of permanence during the development, by purpose evolution landmarks, and clinical significance.

By Stimulus Location

Superficial or exteroceptive reflexes
Those that originate in external parts of the organism, elicited by noxious or tactile stimulation of the skin, cornea, or mucous membrane, exemplified by the following reflexes: corneal, palatal, abdominal, cremasteric, and anal (**Table 1**).

- *Corneal.* Closure of the eyelid when the cornea is touched.
- *Palatal.* Contraction of the pharyngeal constrictor muscle (causes swallowing) elicited by stimulation of the palate or touching the back of the pharynx.
- *Abdominal.* Contractions of the abdominal muscles on stimulation of the abdominal skin (**Figure 5**).
- *Cremasteric.* Stimulation of the skin on the front and inner thigh retracts the testis on the same side.
- *Anal.* Contraction of the anal sphincter on irritation of the anal skin.

Proprioceptive or deep reflexes
Proprioceptive or deep reflexes originated in receptors within the body, in skeletal muscles, tendons, bones, joints,

vestibular apparatus, etc. They comprise all deep tendon reflexes, postural reactions, and some PRs. The deep reflexes are elicited by a sharp tap on the appropriate tendon or muscle to induce brief stretch of the muscle, followed by contraction. They are examples of the deep reflex (**Table 2**):

- *Glabella or orbicularis oculi.* Normal contraction of the orbicularis oculi muscle, with resultant closing of the eye, on percussion at the outer aspect of the supraorbital ridge, over the glabella, or around the margin of the orbit (**Figure 6**).
- *Oris-orbicularis.* Pouting or pursing of the lips induced by light tapping of the closed lips in the midline.
- *Jaw jerk.* Closure of the mouth caused by tapping at a downward angle between the lower lip and chen.
- *Biceps.* Contraction of the biceps muscle when its tendon is tapped.
- *Triceps.* Contraction of the belly of the triceps muscle and slight extension of the arm when the tendon of the muscle is tapped directly, with the arm flexed and fully supported and relaxed.

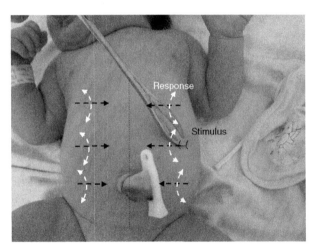

Figure 5   Abdominal reflex.

Table 1   Superficial (exteroceptive) reflexes innervation

Reflex	Innervation
Corneal	Cranial nerves, pons, and VII
Palatal	Cranial nerves IX, medulla, and X
Abdominal	Spinal nerve, spinal cord T_{7-12}
Cremasteric	Ilioinguinal, genitofemoral nerves, spinal cord L_{1-2}
Anal	Inferior hemorrhoidal nerve, spinal cord S_{3-5}

Table 2   Deep tendon (muscle stretch) reflexes innervation

Reflex	Innervation
Glabella	Cranial nerves V, pons, and VIII
Oro-orbicularis	Cranial nerves V, pons, and VIII
Jaw jerk	Cranial nerves V, pons, and V
Biceps	Musculocutaneous nerve, spinal cord C_{5-6}
Brachioradialis	Radial nerve, spinal cord C_{6-8}
Triceps	Radial nerve, spinal cord C_{6-7}
Knee jerk (Patellar)	Femoral nerve, spinal cord L_{2-4}
Thigh adductors	Obturator nerve, spinal cord L_{2-4}
Ankle jerk (Achilles)	Tibial nerve, spinal cord L_5-S_2

- *Brachioradialis.* With the arm supinated to 45°, a tap near the lower end of the radius causes contraction of the brachioradial (supinator longus) muscle.
- *Knee jerk (patellar).* Contraction of the quadriceps and extension of the leg when the patellar ligament is tapped (**Figure 1**).
- *Thigh adductors.* Contraction of the adductors of the thigh caused by tapping the tendon of the adductor magnus muscle while the thigh is abducted.
- *Ankle jerk (Achilles).* Plantar flexion caused by a twitch-like contraction of the triceps surae muscle, elicited by a tap on the Achilles tendon, preferably while the patient kneels on a bed or chair, the feet hanging free over the edge.

Viceroceptive or autonomic reflexes

Those that originate in the viscera and have, as responses, actions on smooth muscles, glands, and vessels, as, for instance, the emptying of the rectum and the bladder by rectal and vesical reflexes, and the increase in gastric juice secretion and contractibility of the stomach during food ingestion. They are examples of the viceroceptive reflex (**Table 3**):

- *Oculocardiac.* Slowing of the rhythm of the heart following compression of the eyes.
- *Carotid sinus.* Slowing of the heartbeat on pressure on the carotid artery at the level of the cricoid cartilage.
- *Vesical.* Contraction of the walls of the bladder and relaxation of the trigone and urethral sphincter in response to a rise in pressure within the bladder; the reflex can be voluntarily inhibited and the inhibition readily abolished to control micturition.
- *Rectal reflex.* Normal response to the presence of feces in the rectum.

Sensory special reflex

These are generated by a distant stimulus in specialized organs of the senses as eyes and ears (pupillary, optical blink, and acoustic blink). They are examples of the sensory special reflex (**Table 4**):

- *Pupillary.* Contraction of the pupil on exposure of the retina to light.
- *Optical blink.* Contraction of the orbicularis oculi muscles (closure of both eyes) after stimuli of the retina to light.
- *Acoustic blink.* Contraction of the orbicularis oculi muscles (closure of both eyes) to an intense sound.

By Development

There are three forms of motor manifestations in this category (**Figure 7**), which coexist and overlap over time, yet they represent distinct stages of the CNS maturation.

Static reflexes

Those that remain stable all life long and represent the most primitive and caudal manifestations of the CNS, predominantly processed at the level of the spinal cord and some in the brainstem, represented by the deep tendon, pupillary and acoustic blink reflexes.

Table 3 Autonomic (viceroceptive) reflexes innervation

Reflex	Innervation
Oculocardiac	Cranial nerves V, medulla, and X
Carotid sinus	Cranial nerves IX, medulla, and X
Vesical and rectal	Sacral autonomic fiber, spinal cord S_{2-4}

Table 4 Sensory especial reflexes innervation

Reflex	Innervation
Pupillary	Cranial nerve II, mesencephalon, and III
Optical blink	Cranial nerve II, mesencephalon, pons, and, VII
Acoustic blink	Cranial nerve VIII, pons, and VII

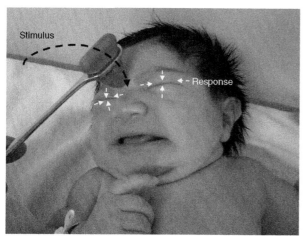

Figure 6 Glabella reflex.

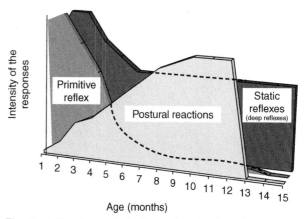

Figure 7 Development of reflex and postural reactions.

Primitive or developmental reflexes

These develop during pregnancy and are processed from the spinal cord to the basal ganglia; hence, they show a greater complexity in their manifestations (automatisms). They are present at birth, and thereafter begin to be integrated with the CNS, most disappearing within the first 6 months of life. There are several tens of these reflexes, the author describes some and illustrates the exam technique of other reflexes of this group.

- *Plantar grasp.* It consists of a flexion response in the toes when the sole of the feet is stimulated (**Figure 8**).
- *Palmar grasp.* Flexion or clenching of the fingers on stimulation of the palm.
- *Asymmetrical tonic neck or Magnus-De Kleijn.* It must be tested with the child at a supine position, eliciting a rotation of the head to one side produces extension of extremities on that side and contralateral flexion – the 'fencer' posture (**Figure 9**).

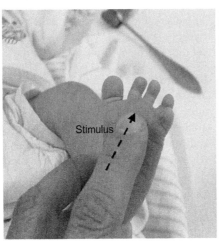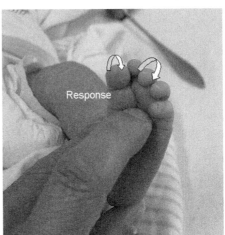

Figure 8   The plantar grasp.

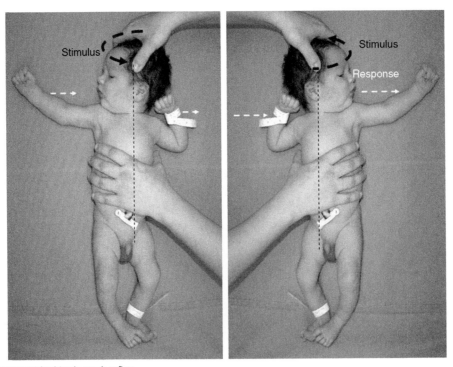

Figure 9   The asymmetrical tonic neck reflex.

- *Babkin.* When the palms of the two hands are strongly pressed, the mouth opens in response, often associated with neck rotation, flexion of limbs, and closing of the eyes (**Figure 3**).
- *Moro.* It is tested by many ways, for example, by displacing the child's gravity center, or by visual or auditory stimulus. As a response, an abduction and extension of the limbs will occur, with extension and opening of the fingers, except for the distal phalanges of the index fingers and thumbs, which remain flexed. Then occurs the aduction and flexion of limbs.
- *Diving.* Stimulation of the face or nasal cavity with water or local irritants produces apnea in neonates. Breathing stops in expiration, with laryngeal closure, and infants exhibit bradycardia and a lowering of cardiac output. Blood flow to the skin, splanchnic areas, muscles, and kidneys decreases, whereas flow to the heart and brain is protected.
- *Sucking.* Sucking movements of the lips of an infant elicited by touching the lips or the skin near the mouth.
- *Rooting.* Reflex consisting of head-turning and sucking movements elicited in a normal infant by gently stroking the side of the mouth of cheek.
- *Magnet.* It is tested by light pressure made upon a toe-pad with the finger causes reflex contraction of the limb extensors; the limb is thus pressed gently against the finger, and when the finger is withdrawn slightly, the experimenter has the sensation that the finger is raising the limb or drawing it out as by a magnet.
- *Galant.* It is elicited by holding the newborn in ventral suspension (face down) and stroking along the one side of the spine. The normal reaction is for the newborn to laterally flex toward the stimulated side.
- *Palmo-mental.* Unilateral (sometimes bilateral) contraction of the mentalis and orbicularis oris muscles caused by a brisk scratch made on the palm of the ipsilateral hand.
- *Withdrawal.* A nociceptive reflex in which a body part is quickly moved away from a painful stimulus.
- *Crossed extensor.* When the reflex occurs the flexors in the withdrawing limb contract and the extensors relax, while in the other limb the opposite occurs. An example of this is when a person steps on a nail, the leg that is stepping on the nail pulls away, while the other leg takes the weight of the whole body.
- *Placing.* Flexion followed by extension of the leg when the infant is held erect and the dorsum of the foot is drawn along the under edge of a tabletop; it is obtainable in the normal infant up to the age of 6 weeks.
- *Positive support or plantar support.* In vertical suspension, the stimulation of the ball of foot produces leg extension to support the weight.
- *Walking.* When the child is held at a vertical position and keeps the feet in contact with a surface, alternate movements of the lower limbs may appear, with a general morphology similar to stepping.

- *Extensor plantar.* Stroking the lateral part of the foot – a sequence of stimuli applied more laterally – (the Chaddock technique) produces extension (dorsiflexion) of the big toe, often with extension and abduction of the other toes. It is not Babinski reflex.

Postural reaction

It is defined as a fixed response or posture from the initiation of the stimulus until its removal, lasting for as long as the stimulus persists. A postural response represents complex motor responses to a plurality of afferences such as the joints, the tendons, the muscles, the skin, receptors (eye and ear), and, of course, the labyrinth. They are characterized by a certain stereotyped posture of the trunk, head, and extremities, when the examiner attempts a strictly defined sudden change of position. The postural reactions are all absent in infancy and appear gradually later, simultaneously with the diminution of PRs. They involve the highest level of motor control that is voluntary, represented by the Landau, parachute, and lateral propping reactions. The Landau' reaction develops at 3 months. When held in ventral suspension, the infant's head, legs, and spine extend. When the head is depressed, the hips, knees, and elbows flex. This reflex continues to be present in most infants during the second 6 months of life, but then it becomes increasingly difficult to demonstrate. The parachute reaction occurs when the baby is suspended ventrally and dropped suddenly with the head directed toward a table. This prompts a defensive reaction in which the upper limbs are extended and the hands are opened in order to prevent the fall. This reflex appears starting at 6 months of age. Lateral propping usually appears between 6 and 8 months of age, when the child is able to sit without assistance. If the infant is pushed sideways with an abrupt shove on one shoulder while sitting, s/he extends the appropriate arm and puts his/her open hands over the support plane near the legs or in the angle formed by them.

By Purpose Evolution Landmarks

Alimentary

These landmarks are involved in oral motor activity, with the purpose of search, capture, and ingestion of food, among them are the rooting, sucking, palmar grasp, and Babkin reflexes.

Defense and escape

These account for the maintenance of the organism's integrity (e.g., withdrawal, diving, and Galant reflexes).

Support and locomotion

These account for a better body positioning in relation to gravity, to objects in the environment, and for grasping these. In this group we find the palmar grasp, plantar grasp, extensor plantar, Moro, plantar support, withdrawal, crossed extensor, walking, placing, and magnet reflexes.

By Clinical Significance

Normal reflexes
Normal reflexes are those for which intensity, location, symmetry, diffusion, onset time, and integration time follow normal physiological patterns.

Pathological reflexes
These are normal reflexes that stop complying with the physiological conditions or are physiopathological manifestations of the CNS, as the Babinski reflex and the reflex of spinal automatism.

Normal Development of Reflexes in Childhood

The ontogenesis of reflexes in the human being contributes to the identification of evolutionary stages in our species. In intrauterine life, the reflexes follow a cephalic to caudal onset pattern, while in the limbs their pattern is from distal to proximal, differing from the muscle tone, which is the opposite – it increases with gestational age from caudal to cephalic. The spinal reflex arc is fully developed by the 8th week of gestation and the deep tendon reflex at the knees and ankles may be elicited in premature infants at 19–23 weeks of gestation, but they all become evident only after the 33rd week of gestation. In examining a 28-week-old preterm infant, we also find the deep tendon, the withdrawal, the cutaneous extensor plantar, and the palmo-plantar grasp reflexes, the extensor phase of the Moro reflex, and the Galant, rooting, acoustic blink, and optical blink reflexes. The pupillary reflex is absent before 28 weeks of gestation and present after 30 weeks of gestation, Glabella around 32 weeks, the neck-righting reflex appears between 34 and 37 weeks; head turning in response to light appears between 32 and 36 weeks. Full-blown walking and crossed extensor reflexes appear only between 35 and 37 weeks.

After birth, the direction of maturation is now only cephalo–caudal, as occurs with the myelination of the pyramidal tract, which enables the voluntary control of more cephalic than caudal segments. It is already possible to observe at the first 3 months of life manifestations of voluntary control of the facial muscles that are used to smile and eat, and subsequently the control of neck muscles, the voluntary use of the hand, the ability of sitting down, the control of the standing position, and finally the control of the sphincter (**Figure 10**). This sequence in maturation allows the muscle tone to decrease and many PRs to be integrated in the CNS.

In preterm infants, the reflexes, as well as the tone and the voluntary movements, show a lagged evolution in comparison with full-term infants. The same does not occur with the sensory function which in the premature

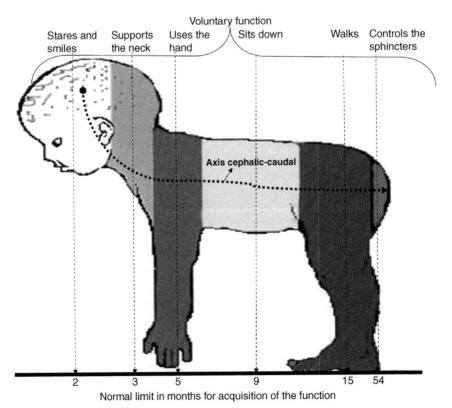

Figure 10 Sequence of voluntary motor control.

child maturates before the motor one. From the 37th week of gestation on, the infant is already capable of performing conditioned reflexes and learning.

This ability of learning is supported by the reflex motor activity, which enables a contact with the external environment in ample and diversified ways, thereby resulting in new sensory inputs that, integrated with cortical levels, will create a feedback able to gradually turn movements that are initially reflex or automatic into voluntary. The predominatly inhibitory synaptic connections of the cerebral cortex to the brainstem (cortico-subcortical integration process) are known to be able to change the reflexes, leading the infant to learn how to use these basic patterns of reaction in his automatic activities, and later in the voluntary activities as well. The reflexes are thus partially discarded and partially incorporated into new patterns of motor expressions (**Figure 11**). The reflex multiplicity, especially the primitive, is, therefore, of paramount importance to neuropsychological evolution.

Despite a few conjectures that some PRs are the precursors to voluntary activities, as the walking and palmar grasp reflexes, for instance, these have not been supported, since the results of studies, including those carried out by us, do not show any relationship between the age of extinguishing of these reflexes and the age at which the first voluntary activities are observed, both being able to coexist.

We should also consider the period of transition from reflex activities to voluntary ones, an intermediate behavior in which many reflexes become more or less conditioned and full of patterns of repetitious movements, which precede the voluntary control (called the rhythmic stereotypes, e.g., the movements of the toes of the feet). Another example are the rhythmic vocalizations, which provoke one feedback auditory which is basic for the development of the hearing and the language. The decline of rhythmic stereotypes is related with the progressive prevalence of voluntary behavior.

Assessment of Reflex Activity in the Child – General Considerations

The reflexes constitute one of the earliest, and most frequently used tools among developmental neurologists and pediatricians all over the world to assess the CNS integrity of infants and young children. The examination of reflexes is far more difficult in children than in adults, since they do not understand, do not collaborate, feel afraid, and, hence, are too agitated, often crying, and do not relax their muscles suitably. In order to increase the chances for a successful examination, we must consider:

- examination location (adverse conditions, as within an incubator);

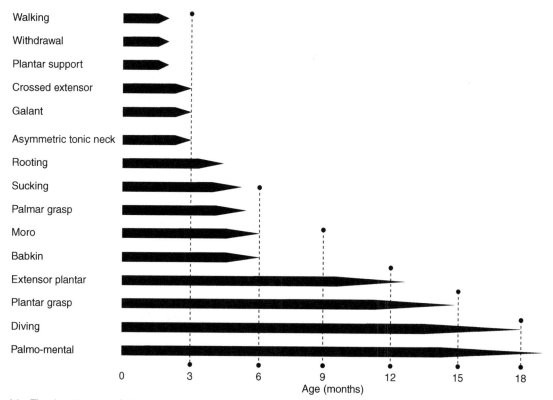

Figure 11 The development of primative reflexes.

- gestational age at birth (if premature, make corrections for age);
- general clinical conditions (temperature, pO$_2$, etc.);
- support therapies (drug use; immobilization, catheter, etc.);
- neurological pathology (coma, convulsions, hemorrhage, etc.);
- time of life ('birth shock' within the first 48–72 h);
- time after last breastfeeding (satisfied or hungry);
- behavioral states of the newborn and breastfed infant (**Figure 12**); and
- physiological properties of reflexes (stimulation site, excitation threshold, latency, fatigue, central inhibition, volitional inhibition, refractory period).

We still have to proceed patiently, applying the exam protocols in an 'accidental' sequence, seizing the opportunities, consoling the child to bring her to more suitable behavioral states and saving for the end of the procedure those maneuvers that may cause the infant to cry, also extracting from the latter the necessary information for a more thorough examination.

The five behavioral states that must be observed in the examination of the newborn and small infant are based on sleeping patterns, respiratory rhythm, changes in ocular opening, alert-state activity, and crying. The assessment of these states via polygraphic tests (brain electric activity, heart rate, and muscle contraction) demonstrates that these are different ways of cerebral activity, each state being a qualitatively different condition, a particular mode of CNS functioning. Therefore, it is of paramount importance to learn about these, especially in the neonatal period, since many reflex and behavioral responses depend on them to be modified. Overall, the best state is the 3rd, next coming the 4th, the 2nd, the 1st, and finally the 5th (crying); however, it is possible that in sound sleep the deep tendon reflexes are enhanced. It is necessary to comment on the time period elapsed from birth to the first 48–72 h of life, when the delivery stress causes a rebound effect of lower neurologic energy in which the reflexes, as well as the muscle tone, are found to be diminished, a period known as 'birth shock'.

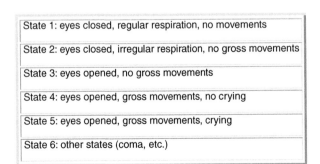

State 1: eyes closed, regular respiration, no movements
State 2: eyes closed, irregular respiration, no gross movements
State 3: eyes opened, no gross movements
State 4: eyes opened, gross movements, no crying
State 5: eyes opened, gross movements, crying
State 6: other states (coma, etc.)

Figure 12 Behavioral states.

Assessment of Deep Tendon Reflexes

The deep tendon reflexes are the elementary unit of the neurological processes based on the reflex arc; they are part of the motor activity exam, along with the muscle tone and muscle strength test, which is useful for the location of NS lesions. Usually, the reflex hammer is used, which must be suitable for the child's age, with a long, flexible handle and a sufficiently elastic and soft percussion area. The stimulus to be used should not be more intense than necessary to elicit a reflex, which may necessitate two or three stimuli of increasing intensity. The assessment of a reflex is mandatorily followed by the assessment of the same reflex on the opposite side for symmetry. The examiner must adapt his technique to the conditions of each case. Maneuvers such as that of Jendrassik (closing the eyes and performing an isometric contraction of untested limbs) in older children can be useful, especially for those with difficulty relaxing and when the reflexes are hypoactive.

The knee jerk reflex is the best known one and is always present in normal children, another reflex of greater clinical significance is the ankle jerk (Achilles) reflex, which is useful in the diagnosis and follow-up of lesions in the lower neuron, such as poliomyelitis, Guillain–Barre syndrome, metabolic disorders as hypocalcemia, etc.

To illustrate just the technique indicated for the knee jerk reflex – with the child sitting up, with legs hanging loosely and relaxed, or lying on her belly, with the knee slightly folded, and supporting the palm of the examiner's hand – the quadriceps tendon (below the patella) is tapped, and the leg is expected to kick out (**Figure 1**).

Deep tendon reflexes can be normal, absent, diminished, brisker, or asymmetrical, largely ranging in intensity from one person to another; in some rare cases they cannot be elicited even by using the best technique under normal conditions. Any asymmetry should be considered pathological, but it may be difficult to say if the abnormal reflex corresponds either to the side that seems brisker or to the side on which it seems diminished.

As a rule, the reflex that most differs from the individual's pattern of reflexes and/or the one that coexists with other anomalies in the motor exam is abnormal. A second element to value is hyperreflexia (range, quickness of response, and increase in the reflexogenic zone), which can be an important pathological sign of a central injury. If the reflexes are hyperactive, we need to test the clonus (there are many responses to a single stimulus) and when it is inexhaustible, it is always a sign of abnormality, and even if it is the only alteration in the reflexes, it is a safe pyramidal sign of CNS injury. The clonus of the patella and foot (Achilles tendon) is the most frequent one. For example, the Achilles reflex is tested by performing sudden flexion movements in the foot and maintaining this position, with the leg partially flexed.

The clinical significance of a pathological hyperreflexia is the loss of the normal inhibition to which the reflex arc is subject; it appears when there is injury in an inhibitory structure, most often in the pyramidal tract. However, in the initial stage of a pyramidal injury by trauma of the spinal cord or stroke, a transitory hyporeflexia or areflexia occurs. The diminution or extinguishing of deep tendon reflexes implies the existence of an injury in any one of the reflex arc components, most often indicating a peripheral injury. The deep tendon reflexes must be rated according to the following scale: 4+ hyperactive with clonus; 3+ hyperactive without clonus, with increase in the reflexogenic zone; 2+ normal; 1+ hypoactive; and 0+ no response.

Assessment of Superficial Reflexes

In this group of reflexes, we are going to illustrate the abdominal reflex, which is elicited with a blunt object stimulating the lateral regions of the abdomen (upper, middle, and lower) toward the middle line, and, when present, a contraction of the stimulated musculature is observed (**Figure 5**). Just like the deep reflexes, the superficial ones must be compared with the opposite side at each of the three levels. The response is normal when a unilateral contraction occurs and abnormal when the reflex is absent or asymmetric. The superficial reflex (abdominal, cremasteric), in the initial stage of a pyramidal injury of acute onset as occurs with a stroke, may disappear contralaterally to the injury, even before a change in strength, and remain absent or hypoactive, as occurs in children with cerebral palsy (CP). In obese individuals or after abdominal surgery, muscle contraction may be absent.

Assessment of Primitive Reflexes

The presence of all PRs during the first weeks of life is indicative of the CNS integrity. They can outlast the usual time, be absent, diminished, or increased in relation to the normal state or disappear when some compromising of the cortical integration occur by pre- or perinatal events. A normal motor development is unlikely with the PR outlasting the usual time, as their disappearance is necessary for the improvement of early voluntary motor activity in childhood.

Studies in an animal model, as those by Sherrington, in 1898, who surgically disconnected the CNS inhibition in order to observe more primitive reflex responses, are in agreement with concepts still used today to explain the outlasting of the PRs or their reappearance in humans with compromised cerebral functions. In these cases, the upper injury liberates the lower centers, more specifically the brainstem, which is the underlying structure of these connections.

Understanding the normal development of motor functions is possible only when the patterns of PRs are known, which are the precursors to those functions, since

they are the best tools to early detect motor disorders in childhood, being one of the early markers for CP. This fact underscores the importance of the assessment of PRs in the newborn and infant, not only for understanding the neuropsychological development of the human being, but also for the neurologic assessment of the child, with the intent to identify possible damage to the CNS in the pre- and perinatal periods. This important semiological tool helps every professional involved in the rehabilitation of children with neurological pathology not only with respect to the prognosis, but also to the planning of more suitable treatment methods. Among these are the therapies based on the Bobath method, which inhibit the PR and stimulate more advanced stages of development.

Primitive reflex activities are closely dependent on the infant's physiological needs upon stimulation and interact with one another, at times facilitating and at other times inhibiting, as can be observed at the moment of hunger when oral reflexes have already been exacerbated, and an increase in the palmar grasp reflex and movements of general flexion of the body concomitantly occur, associated with a diminution of extensor reflexes such as the Moro, plantar support, and crossed extensor. The elicitation of the palmar grasp reflex normally inhibits the Moro reflex, which can make the infant calm down, while conversely labyrinthine stimuli and/or sudden stimuli in general elicit crying and an unstable attitude which is well characterized in the extensor phase of the Moro reflex; even in this situation the lower limbs tend to a flexor predominance and exacerbation of the plantar grasp reflex.

The techniques of examination of some PRs already had been indicated together with the description of the same ones, and in the diagrams of figures in the item of the classification of reflex.

Reflexes and Clinical Significance

Different methods have been used to evaluate the NS of infants: neurological examination, neurophysiological examination, imaging studies, laboratory investigation, and observation of spontaneous and/or provoked behavior. The integrity and maturation of the NS can be evaluated by a structured neurological examination that provides information for diagnosis, follow-up, and prognosis.

The changes found in the reflexes during the development are of paramount importance to the definition of normality.

Several screening tests to assess child development have been recommended, such as the Bayley test, the early language milestones, which is another instrument suitable for office screening that was designed for identifying delays in language in children less than 3 years old, and the Denver II, the latter being the best known among pediatricians. It has a good sensitivity for detection of developmental delays, but only evidences these when the neurologic function expected for the respective age is not present. In these cases, an earlier thorough examination may indicate the existence of dysfunction or neurologic injury, for example, the persistence of PRs and a deep hyperreflexia predominantly involving the lower limbs in an infant less than 1-year-old can indicate a CP of diplegic form and that the walking reflex will not appear at the expected age, although other aspects of the child's development may be normal. Another shortcoming of screening tests is the wide qualitative–quantitative spectrum in the presentation of developmental disorders, which demands detailing in the exam of each child, rendering the aforementioned tests inviable.

The emphasis placed on a reflex or any motor response in a neurological evaluation depends on what is known about this item, and on the possibility of associating it with specific pathologies, as is the case with the plantar support reflex, asymmetric tonic neck reflex, and tonic labyrinth reflex in the early diagnosis, rehabilitation, and prognosis of CP.

The failure in extinguishing PRs such as the Moro, Galant, and plantar grasp reflexes, regardless of postural reactions, indicates a possible CP of the athetoid (extrapyramidal) type, while in the CP of spastic type, when the brain injury is predominantly cortical, the persistent PRs are others, such as the crossed extensor, cutaneous extensor plantar, and Rossolimo reflexes. Evidently, the mixed forms of CP must be considered, when this association loses, then, its specificity.

The situation in which the PRs evolve normally, but not their postural reactions, is more likely to indicate a developmental delay than a CP. The reappearance or nonextinguishing of some PR both in children and in adults may imply a cortical impairment, especially in the frontal lobus, as seen in Down syndrome, degenerative encephalopathies in general (e.g., HIV), Alzheimer's disease, schizophrenia, multiple sclerosis, Parkinson, and hydrocephalus. An exception is made for the palmomental reflex, which may remain in normal individuals all life long; in this case its intensity and the extension of the reflexogenic zone are discreet.

In our study, the cutaneous plantar response was extensor for all infants; however, there are authors that find a prevalence of the cutaneous flexor plantar response in 3% of term newborns. It is known that the cutaneous extensor plantar response will become flexor after a few months as maturation takes place, and that the flexor response does not occur in the newborn, nor in the infant in the first 4 months of life, it is the plantar grasp reflex that occurs, triggered spontaneously or by the Chaddock technique – a sequence of stimuli applied more laterally – as there is a predominance of the grasp reflex over the extensor plantar. Plantar reflexes usually become flexor between 6 and 15 months, and this inversion is not correlated with the ability to walk. The discrepancies observed in the prevalence of plantar reflexes

certainly result from the lack of theoretical–conceptual uniformity and the methodology adopted.

An extensor plantar response may coexist with the normal development up to 15 months of life postnatally in the full-term newborn, and that is not the Babinski's sign. However, it is possible that an injury or any compromising of the CNS during this early period of life can cause the Babinski's sign, which is an exacerbation and/or qualitative change in the normal extensor plantar response.

The result of our exam can show that the reflexes may be: absent, diminished, brisker than normal, asymmetrical, and primitive, outlasting the usual time, or returning after their disappearance. The knowledge of a wide range of PRs also provides the clinician with a sometimes unique, broad spectrum of opportunities for the diagnosis of a pathology, since the range of PRs can vary according to different ages (maturation), the anatomical location of injuries, specific neurologic pathologies, and individual variations for still unknown physiopathological motives. The set of PRs found in a child, associated with deep tendon reflexes, muscle tone, strength, and postural reactions set a motor pattern that makes up, along with the exam of sensitivity, the upper cerebral functions and the clinical history, the 'jigsaw puzzle' of most neurological diagnoses.

To establish that a reflex is absent, one has to know how to look for it, an absent response may have no clinical significance, and a single exam may not suffice to make a decision. An experienced examiner is the best judge of what laboratory investigations should be performed, since the sophisticated neurodiagnostic technology now available for complementary examinations does not preclude the use of neurological examination. A serial clinical follow-up of the development is the safest and most economic way to make long-term predictions, constituting the gold standard for prognosis.

The assessment of neurological functions through a thorough neurologic exam that includes reflexes provides a complement for developmental screening tests, since these are not useful as a diagnosis or for therapeutic planning, being only the first step that will conduct an interdisciplinary evaluation. Despite the recognition of the great usefulness of modern and sophisticated exams in the management of acute neurologic pathology, these are not available in most hospitals in several countries around the world.

See also: Birth Complications and Outcomes; Birth Defects; Cerebral Palsy.

Suggested Readings

Allen MC and Capute AJ (1990) Tone and reflexo development before term. *Pediatrics* 85: 343–399.
Ashwal S, Russman BS, Blasco PA, *et al.* (2004) Practice parameter: Diagnostic assessment of the child with cerebral palsy. *Neurology* 62: 851–863.

Bayley N (1993) *Bayley Scales of Infant Development,* 2nd edn. San Antonio, TX: The Psychological Corporation.

Cans C, Dolk H, Platt MJ, Colver A, Prasauskiene A, and Kkrägeloh-mann I (2007) Recommendations from the SCPE collaborative group for defining and classifying cerebral palsy. *Developmental Medicine and Child Neurology* 49(s109): 35–38.

Capute AJ, Shapiro BK, Accardo PJ, *et al.* (1982) Motor functions: Associated primitive reflex profiles. *Developmental Medicine Child Neurology* 24: 662–669.

Jacobs SE, Sokol J, and Ohlsson A (2002) The newborn individualized developmental care and assessment program is not supported by meta-analyses of the data. *Journal Pediatrics* 140: 699–706.

Paine RS (1960) Neurological examination of infants and children. *Pediatric Clinics North America* 17: 471–510.

Paine RS, Brazelton TB, Donovan DE, *et al.* (1964) Evolution of postural reflexes in normal infants and in the presence of chronic brain syndromes. *Neurology* 4: 1036–1048.

Pedroso FS and Rotta NT (2003) Neurological examination in the healthy term newborn. *Arquivos Neuropsiquiatria* 61: 165–169.

Prechtl HFR (1977) The neurological examination of the full-term newborn infant. *Clinics in Developmental Medicine 63,* 2nd edn. London: William Heinemann.

Sandra Rees S and Inder T (2005) Fetal and neonatal origins of altered brain development. *Early Human Development* 81: 753–761.

Spreen O, Risser AH, and Edgell D (1995) *Developmental Neuropsychology.* New York: Oxford University Press.

Volpe JJ (2001) *Neurology of the Newborn,* 4th edn. Philadelphia, PA: Saunders.

Zafarian DI (2004) Primitive reflexes and postural reactions in the neurodevelopmental examination. *Pediatric Neurologic* 31: 1–8.

S

Sensory Processing Disorder

L J Miller, Sensory Processing Disorder Foundation, Greenwood Village, CO, USA
R C Schaaf, Thomas Jefferson University, Philadelphia, PA, USA

Glossary

Adaptive response – An appropriate action in which the individual responds successfully to a challenging demand.

Occupational therapy using a sensory integrative approach – The use of sensory-rich activities, tailored to individual needs, that are playful yet organizing, and elicit adaptive responses. Usually involves total body movements that are rich in vestibular, proprioceptive, and tactile input. The goal of therapy is to improve the way the brain processes and organizes sensations. Intervention is based on sensory integrative principles that guide the therapist's clinical reasoning skills. The intervention addresses the underlying substrates of dysfunction (e.g., neurological immaturity) rather than difficulties with specific skills. This intervention approach is most commonly utilized by occupational therapists.

Proprioceptive system – The sensory system that detects information from the muscles and joints and perceives sensation about the position or velocity of movement of body parts including force, tension and position. Proprioceptive input tells the brain which muscles are contracting or stretching, when they are doing so, and the amount of resistance on the muscles and joints. The receptors for the proprioceptive system include the muscle spindle, the golgi tendon organ, and the joint receptors.

Sensory modulation disorder (SMD) – This condition is the inability to automatically regulate incoming sensory information resulting in sensory over-responsivity, sensory under-responsivity, and/or sensory seeking/craving.

Sensory processing – The ability to detect information through the senses, organize that information, and interpret the information making a meaningful and appropriate adaptive response. For most people the process of sensory processing is automatic and unconscious.

Sensory processing disorder (SPD) – This complex disorder is a neurological condition that affects children and adults. People with SPD misinterpret everyday sensory information, such as touch, sound, and movement. They may feel bombarded by information, crave intense sensory experiences, be unable to discriminate the fine qualities of sensation, or have awkward responses to sensory input. To be classified as a disorder, the symptoms of SPD must be severe enough that participation in daily life activities is restricted.

Tactile system – Receptors for the tactile system are located in the skin and are responsible for the sense of touch.

Theory of sensory integration – This theory explains the relation between deficits in interpreting sensory input and learning, behavior, or motor difficulties. The theory recognizes brain–behavior interactions and focuses on the role of the senses in creating a foundation for higher level cognitive, emotional, and motor activities. The theory postulates that adequate detection, modulation, discrimination, and responses to sensory information are needed for normal adaptive behavior to occur.

Vestibular system – This sensory system responds to the position of the head in relation to gravity and to the acceleration or deceleration of movement. The receptors for the vestibular system are the semicircular canals and the utricle and saccule that are located in the labyrinth of the inner ear. These receptors detect the pull of gravity and movement of the head.

Introduction

What is sensory processing disorder? Sensory processing is our ability to take in information through our senses (touch, movement, smell, taste, vision, and hearing), interpret that information, and organize a meaningful response. For most children this process is automatic. When we hear someone talking to us or a bird chirping (auditory stimuli), our brain interprets this information as speech or an animal sound, and we respond to the information appropriately (e.g., turning our head to listen). When someone taps us on the shoulder (tactile stimulus) we turn our attention to that individual. When we are standing in a bus or train and it starts to move (vestibular stimulus), we automatically shift our weight so we do not fall. Individuals (both children and adults) who have sensory processing disorder (SPD) do not detect, regulate, interpret, and/or respond to sensory information accurately. SPD symptoms occur along a wide continuum from mild to severe and manifest in a variety of behavioral, motor, and social symptoms.

Seven sensory systems exist and SPD can occur in one or a combination of systems. The five well-known sensory systems are: visual, auditory, olfactory (smell), gustatory (taste), and tactile (touch). Two 'hidden senses' also exist, the vestibular and proprioceptive systems. The vestibular system detects information about the movement of the head in relation to the Earth's gravity through receptors in the vestibules (hence the term vestibular) located in the inner ear. The proprioceptive system detects information in the muscles and joints and provides information about the location and movement of the parts of the body (i.e., you can feel where your little toe is located without looking at it).

History

Dr. A. Jean Ayres, an occupational therapist (OT) and neuroscientist, pioneered the theory of sensory integration, expanded primarily in the field of OT. Sensory integration theory describes the underlying brain mechanisms hypothesized to cause SPD, defines a set of behavioral characteristics indicative of SPD, and also suggests intervention methods for remediating the disorder. Ayres called the disorder sensory integrative dysfunction and termed the intervention sensory integration treatment. Her theory discusses the relation among the neural processes of receiving, modulating, and integrating sensory input and the resulting output that Ayres called adaptive behavior. The theory postulates that adequate processing of sensory information is needed for normal adaptive behavior to occur.

Ayres developed two assessment batteries, the Southern California Sensory Integration Test in 1972 and the Sensory Integration and Praxis Test (SIPT) in 1989. The SIPT includes 17 subtests evaluating children ages 4 years 6 months to 8 year 11 months. It measures the ability to detect and interpret sensory information by responding to tactile, proprioceptive, vestibular, auditory, and visual stimuli. The results provide detailed information about underlying sensory factors that may affect a child's learning and behavior.

Although Ayres originally outlined the central theoretical tenets of the theory in her book *Sensory Integration and Learning Disorders* in 1972, she recognized that the theory would evolve and change as new scientific findings informed the field. This evolution is exactly what has happened over the 35 years since the original book was published. For example, Ayres originally identified six subtypes of sensory integration dysfunction: postural and bilateral integration dysfunction, developmental apraxia, form and space perception, tactile defensiveness, unilateral disregard, and auditory-language disorders. She later revised her theory and, based on new data, renamed some of the subtypes. However, as she predicted, new research has emerged and her theory has evolved. Thus, an update to Ayres' original taxonomy is presented.

Signs and Symptoms of Sensory Processing Disorder

The newest taxonomy encompasses and expands Ayres' original ideas based on new research. Dr. Lucy Jane Miller and colleagues note that delineating specific subtypes is crucial so that homogenous groups can be identified for intervention and research purposes. They have proposed a set of classic patterns with subtypes based on physiological research and behavioral studies. The new taxonomy utilizes the term SPD to identify the condition and includes all the subtypes identified by Ayres. The Ayres' classification scheme is reorganized into a new nosology that includes subtypes that were not labeled previously. The current diagnostic taxonomy is delineated in **Figure 1** Definitions and behaviors observed in each subtype follow.

Sensory Modulation Disorder

The first classic pattern is sensory modulation disorder (SMD), defined as difficulty regulating and responding to sensory input in a graded manner. Almost all people experience SMD to some degree, at some point in their life. For example, when you get home after a long tiring day, any sensation can be 'too much' such as a loud radio or someone touching you. Because your stress level is high and your usual methods of coping with stimuli is poor, you experience normal levels of sensation as uncomfortable. However, poor modulation of sensation is a disorder only when it disrupts a person's ability to take part in daily life routines and self-care activities on a routine basis. Children and adults with the disorder demonstrate severe and frequent over or under-responsivity and/or

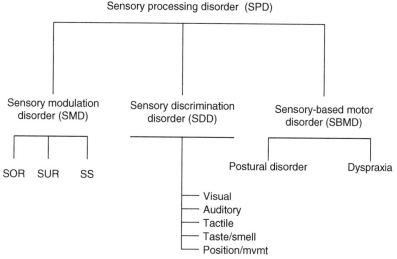

Figure 1 Current taxonomy of sensory processing disorder. SOR, sensory over-responsivity; SS, sensory seeking craving; SUR, sensory under-responsivity.

sensory-seeking behaviors in response to levels of sensory stimuli in their environment that most of us would automatically process without effort.

Screening for SMD can be completed using parent, teacher, and self-report scales such as the 'sensory profile', the 'infant toddler sensory profile', and the 'adult sensory profile' developed by Dr. Winifred Dunn and colleagues, by the 'sensory processing measure' by Dr. Diane Parham and colleagues or by other similar report measures. Diagnosis of SPD also involves testing and observations by well-trained clinicians, usually OTs or other professionals with advanced training in sensory processing. In Miller's taxonomy, three types of SMD are proposed: sensory over-responsivity, sensory under-responsivity, and sensory-seeking.

Sensory over-responsivity

Children with sensory over-responsivity respond to sensation more quickly and intensely than most people. Their responses appear to be fight or flight reactions and are sometimes labeled sensory defensiveness. They often try to avoid or minimize sensations by withdrawing from the situation (e.g., covering their ears, pushing a person who touches them away, or closing their eyes) or they respond with aggressive behavior. For example, a child touched unexpectedly may punch the person who touched him. Many of the common sensory symptoms and the behaviors that accompany sensory over-responsivity are described by Miller. A few examples of the sensory symptoms and accompanying behaviors are shown in **Table 1**.

Sensory under-responsivity

Children with sensory under-responsivity do not respond to typical levels of sensation and, as a result, are lethargic and unaware of stimulation. They may seem oblivious to

their environment and often do not respond to typical stimuli such as hearing their name called. Common behaviors associated with sensory under-responsivity are noted in **Table 1**.

Sensory seeking craving

A third type of SMD is sensory seeking craving. Children with sensory seeking/craving are hypothesized to have a high threshold to sensory stimuli, and compensate by constantly seeking stimulation that is more intense or prolonged than most children prefer. Children who seek sensation often take part in extreme activities or move constantly to provide the sensory input their brains seem to crave to feel normal. They may make unsafe choices in play such as jumping from the top of a slide, play music or talk very loudly, and/or constantly intrude upon other people's space, touching people, and handling their objects. Other behaviors associated with sensory seeking are noted in **Table 1**.

Many children have more than one type of sensory modulation problem and their symptoms include behaviors from several subtypes. To be diagnosed with SMD the child's responses to sensation must be extreme, well outside of the range typical responsiveness. The responses must be seen in a variety of settings such as school, daycare, home, and in the community. The child must exhibit these behaviors in 'ordinary' daily situations to receive a diagnosis of SMD (e.g., not just at the end of a tiring day or a long trip).

Sensory Discrimination Disorder

The second classic pattern is sensory discrimination disorder (SDD), difficulty interpreting sensory input. When a child has this problem, he or she can detect the stimuli

Table 1 Characteristics of sensory over-responsivity, sensory under-responsivity, and sensory seeking

Sensory over-responsivity
Sensory symptoms – Frequently bothered by
- Having his hair, fingernails, or toenails cut
- Food textures
- Noise in a restaurant, mall, or large gymnasium or loud, unexpected sounds
- Being upside-down, as when turning a somersault
Behaviors include being
- Aggressive or impulsive when overwhelmed by sensory stimulation
- Irritable, fussy, moody
- Unsociable; avoids group activities and has trouble forming relationships
- Upset by transitions and unexpected changes

Sensory under-responsivity
Sensory symptoms
- Does not cry when seriously hurt and is not bothered by minor injuries
- Nearly always prefers sedentary activities like computer time to active physical games
- Often seems unaware of what's going on around him (e.g., does not hear his name being called)
- Often seems unaware of body sensations such as hunger, hot or cold or need to use the
Behaviors include being
- Passive, quiet, withdrawn
- Hard to engage in conversation or other social interaction
- Apathetic and easily exhausted
- Exhibits no inner drive to get involved in the world around himself (e.g., uninterested in exploring games or objects)

Sensory seeking/craving
Sensory symptoms
- Is on the move constantly, crashing, bashing, bumping, jumping and rough-housing
- Constantly touches objects and/or intrudes on people
- Seems unable to stop talking and has trouble taking his turn in conversations
- Frequently fixates visually on objects such as reflections of the sun in the side-view mirrors of the car
Behaviors include being
- Described by others as hyperactive
- Angry or explosive when he is required to sit still or stop what he's doing
- Intense, demanding, hard to calm, excessively affectionate
- Prone to create situations others perceive as 'bad' or 'dangerous'

From Miller LJ (2006) *Sensational Kids: Help and Hope for Chi; dren with Sensory Processing Disorder*. New York: Putnam.

Table 2 Characteristics of sensory discrimination disorder

Difficulties with these sensory tasks
- Distinguishing exactly what is touching him and/or where on his body
- Judging how much force is required for a task (e.g., how firmly to hold onto a pencil)
- Detecting whether he is in motion or not
- Identifying and distinguishing between different sounds
- Difficulty differentiating textures of food and smells
Behaviors include
- Difficulty following directions; gets lost easily
- Aversion to playing with puzzles or other visual games
- Frustration when unable to differentiate visual or auditory signals
- A need for directions repeated
- A need for more time than other children to perform assigned tasks

From Miller LJ (2006) *Sensational Kids: Help and Hope for Chi; dren with Sensory Processing Disorder*. New York: Putnam.

but does not recognize the precise details of sensation, including the quantity, location, duration, size, and/or shape of stimuli. This interpretation of sensory qualities is needed to execute fine and gross motor skills. SDD can occur in visual, auditory, tactile, olfactory, gustatory, proprioceptive, and/or vestibular systems. Some children with SPD can respond adequately when only one sensory modality is presented; however, when two or more stimuli are present (as is the case in many typical daily activities), they are unable to organize appropriate responses.

As a result, they have difficulty successfully participating in learning, play, and social activities. Tactile, vestibular, proprioceptive, and visual discrimination can be assessed using the 'sensory integration and praxis test' battery. Common sensory symptoms and behaviors associated with SDD are noted in **Table 2**.

Sensory-Based Motor Disorder

The final classic pattern type of SPD is sensory-based motor disorder. There are two types: postural disorder and sensory-based dyspraxia. Each is described below.

Postural disorder

Postural disorder includes problems with core body positions, for example, stability and mobility. Whenever the child is required to move against gravity (such as when lying on stomach and extending arms and legs into an airplane position, or lying on back and curling up into a ball or doing a sit up), the child with postural disorder has difficulty contracting muscles and using core stability. As a result the child may be slow to sit, crawl, walk, and run. This child frequently has difficulty using the two sides of the body in a coordinated manner, called poor bilateral integration. In addition, because they cannot contract the muscles needed for stability, they may exhibit poor balance. It is hypothesized that difficulty with these postural issues is related to poor detection of vestibular and proprioceptive stimuli resulting in poor muscle tone. Postural disorder is most frequently assessed using the 'clinical observations of sensory integration' by Dr. Erna Blanche, or by using a standardized motor development assessment that allows for observation of posture and balance. For example, the Miller assessment for preschoolers, The Miller function and participation scale, and the DeGangi-Berk test of sensory integration contain

Table 3 Characteristics of postural disorder and dyspraxia (motor planning difficulties)

Postural disorder
Sensory symptoms
- Has poor muscle tone and/or seems weak compared to other children
- Often slumps over at a desk when writing
- Has difficulty crossing the middle of his body to complete a task (e.g., uses his left hand to write on left side of a piece of paper and his right hand for the right side of paper)
- Has poor endurance and gets tired easily
Behaviors include
- Appearing lazy, unmotivated, or indifferent
- Appearing weak and limp, tires easily
- Difficulty holding his own in competitive games like tug of war
Dyspraxia
Sensory symptoms
- Has difficulty with motor activities that require more than one step (e.g., opening a carton and then pouring a glass of milk)
- Has difficulty learning new motor skills, for example riding a bicycle, tricycle, big wheels
- Is clumsy, awkward, and/or accident-prone, tripping or bumping into other people or things
- Has difficulty keeping personal spaces such as a school desk or bedroom organized
Behaviors include
- Preference for fantasy games, talking or sedentary games rather than 'doing' things
- Messy or sloppy eating
- A disheveled appearance
- Frustration when unable to complete tasks due to poor motor skills

From Miller LJ (2006) *Sensational Kids Help and Hope for Chi; dren with Sensory Processing Disorder*. New York: Putnam.

structured observations that are useful in the evaluation of postural disorder. The primary features of postural disorder are provided in **Table 3**.

Dyspraxia

The second type of sensory-based motor disorder is dyspraxia, also called motor planning problems. Children with this problem have difficulty utilizing tactile and proprioceptive information to plan and carry out motor activities. Dyspraxia is different from developmental coordination disorder, a diagnosis included in the Diagnostic and Statistical Manual (DSM)-IV because the core problem is based upon deficits in sensory awareness and planning. In contrast, the core issue in developmental coordination disorder is poor motor execution. Children with sensory-based dyspraxia appear clumsy and awkward in movements and are delayed in acquiring complex motor skills such as riding a bike or tying shoes. They have problems in particular with new motor actions or activities that require a series of motor steps to perform. The 'sensory integration and praxis test' battery provides an extensive series of subtests evaluating dyspraxia. Common characteristics associated with sensory-based dyspraxia appear in **Table 3**.

Diagnosis and Diagnostic Classification of Sensory Processing Disorder

There is controversy regarding whether SPD is a valid diagnosis because, in the past, it was not listed in diagnostic classification references such as the DSM. Recently, however, it was accepted into two diagnostic classification resources. Both focus on one classic pattern of SPD, SMD, sometimes referred to as SPDs of regulation. While the differences in terminology may be confusing, important is that, for the first time, disorders of sensory processing are now recognized across professional disciplines. As a result, children with these problems have more formal justification for receiving treatment.

Research and advocacy efforts are underway to have SPD recognized by the DSM and the International Classification of Diseases (ICD). Only when SPD is formally recognized by these standard diagnostic manuals will third party payers likely be willing to consider benefits for children with this disorder. Formal recognition will also aide in efforts to receive federal funding to research this disorder.

Prevalence of Sensory Processing Disorder

Although clinicians and educators have speculated that a large number of children are affected by poor sensory modulation, prevalence data have been nonexistent until recently. Miller and colleagues recently conducted a survey to estimate rates of SPD in incoming kindergartners from one suburban US public school district. A conservative estimate of prevalence was made, assuming that all nonrespondents failed to meet positive criteria for SMD. This cautious estimate suggested that approximately 5% of the kindergarten enrollment met screening criteria for SPD. These percentages are consistent with hypothesized estimates published in the literature.

Other Clinical Populations of Children with Sensory Processing Disorder

In addition to children with SPD and no other diagnosis, children with other clinical disorders also have characteristics of SPD. These children are described in *The Nature of Sensory Integration with Diverse Populations*, a book by Smith Roley, Blanche, and Schaaf, as well as in other publications. These populations include children from 'at risk' environments or with low birth weight, cerebral palsy, visual impairments, fragile X syndrome (FXS), or autism spectrum disorder (ASD). Given the multiple and often complex nature of the needs of this group of children, treatment of their SPD provides an excellent complement to their comprehensive program of therapeutic and educational services.

Of particular note, children with ASD and FXS demonstrate a high incidence (80–90%) of SPD, contributing to their maladaptive behavioral profile and limiting their participation in daily life activities. They demonstrate significantly more sensory symptoms than typically developing children and children in other clinical groups. Their SPD leads to a restricted range of behaviors including self-stimulation, avoidance, or fearfulness. Children with autism often demonstrate stereotypic behaviors and repetitive behaviors that are sensory seeking in nature such as spinning, hand flapping, or tapping that limits their ability to participate in the activities with their family and peers. Recently, there has been a surge in research on SPD in ASD and FXS. Given the unique cluster of behaviors and their inherent heterogeneity of children with ASD and FXS, this research is challenging, yet it promises to provide useful data to improve behavior and learning in these children.

Children diagnosed with attention deficit disorders show a range of responses to sensory stimuli with about two-thirds of those studied demonstrating some symptomatology suggestive of poor sensory processing. SPD and attention deficit hyperactive disorder (ADHD) appear to be comorbid diagnosis in approximately 40% of children. Critics of the diagnosis of SPD comment that SPD is 'just another form of ADHD'. However, children with ADHD and SPD have been compared on physiological measures such as sensory habituation and response inhibition and found to differ significantly. Thus, evidence suggests that SPD and ADHD, while frequently co-occurring, are different conditions.

Proposed Mechanisms of Sensory Processing Disorder

Ayres' theory of sensory integration is based on principles from neuroscience, biology, psychology, and education. Noting that many children with learning disorders also demonstrated difficulty with perceptual-motor and sensory processing skills, Ayres theorized that their behavior and learning problems were, in part, due to faulty processing of sensory information and an inability of higher brain centers to modulate the information for lower brain sensory centers. In contrast to other learning-based theories, Ayres' theory was based on the relations among the underlying mechanisms and inadequate learning, behavior, and motor function. Ayres proposed that the integration of vestibular, proprioceptive, and tactile inputs provides a foundation for learning and behavior.

Ayres proposed that dysfunction occurred primarily in the brainstem, viewed as the primary integrator and modulator of sensory information. Specifically, she focused on the vestibular system and the reticular formation, an area in the brainstem, as centers for regulating responsiveness, for example, alerting, arousing, or suppressing sensory input. She believed that the cerebellum and the thalamus played major roles in sensory processing, the cerebellum through the processing of proprioception and the integration of sensory and motor stimuli, and the thalamus through integration of sensory information. Finally, Ayres viewed the limbic system as an important system that contributed to the emotions associated with sensory dysfunction. As her theory evolved, Ayres later included a focus on the role of the cerebral cortex in processing and integrating sensory information, particularly for praxis (motor planning).

Ayres' theory included a set of postulates about nervous system functioning that guided her development of an intervention model. She proposed that the nervous system has an innate drive to seek out the input that it needs for organized interactions with the environment, and that stimuli from one sensory system has the capacity to affect every other system. In addition, she outlined several key principles:

1. sensorimotor development is an important substrate for learning;
2. the interaction of the individual with the environment shapes brain development;
3. the nervous system is capable of change (plasticity); and
4. meaningful sensory–motor activity is a powerful mediator of plasticity.

Since Ayres outlined her theory of sensory integration, several advances in science have shaped the further evolution of the theory. Much of the evolution has been in the domain of SMD where significant scientific advances have occurred since the mid-1990s. Miller and colleagues completed a series of studies examining autonomic nervous system functioning in children with poor sensory modulation. The evidence suggests that children with severe over-responsivity to sensory stimuli have sympathetic dysfunction as evidenced by increased electrodermal activity compared to typically developing controls. Electrodermal activity is a psychophysiological measure that evaluates how much you respond to stimuli by measuring electrical changes in the skin. Your skin conducts more electricity because of eccrine sweat gland activity. Eccrine sweat glands are innervated by cholinergic fibers of the sympathetic nervous system. Thus, measuring electrodermal activity provides an index of sympathetic nervous system activity in the brain.

The research showed that children with sensory oversensitivity during functional activities in daily life also had significantly increased amplitudes, more frequent responses and less habituation of electrodermal responses compared to matched controls suggesting that SMD is

Table 4   Research question and method

Research question	Method	Primary researcher
Do individuals with poor sensory modulation demonstrate metabolic differences compared to controls?	Proton magnetic spectroscopy study	Dr. Sinclair Smith Drexel and Temple Universities
Can physiologic correlates of early perceptual processing in individuals with poor sensory modulation determine subtypes of the disorder?	Auditory and somatosensory evoked potential study	Dr. Barbara Brett-Green University of CO Health Sciences Center
Does the sensory gating evoked potential (P50) discriminate children with over-responsivity from matched controls?	Auditory ERP study	Dr.Patricia Davies CO State University
Are there genetic factors that relate to the etiology of SPD?	A twin study	Dr. Hill Goldsmith University of Wisconsin at Madison
Is there a difference in dopamine D2 receptor binding availability, presynaptic dopamine synthesis and serotonin receptor availability in SPD?	A positron emission tomography (PET) study using a primate animal model	Dr. Mary Schneider University of Wisconsin at Madison
Are selective serotonin reuptake inhibitors and GABA agonists pharmacologic agents effective in affecting sensory gating?	Rat model	Dr. Edward Levin Duke University
Is low parasympathetic activity a marker of over-responsivity to sensation?	Vagal tone study	Dr. Roseann Schaaf Thomas Jefferson University
Do children with SPD show changes in cortisol levels during the Sensory Challenge Protocol?	Salivary cortisol study	Dr. Stacey Reynolds Virginia Commonwealth University
Can a reliable performance assessment be developed to characterize sensory over-responsivity?	Psychometric child and adult study	Dr. Lucy Miller and Dr. Sarah Schoen Sensory Processing Disorder Research Institute

GABA, gamma-aminobutyric acid; SPD, sensory processing disorder; ERP.

associated with sympathetic overactivity. In addition, evaluation of parasympathetic markers suggests that children with SMD also have low parasympathetic activity.

Additional work on the mechanisms of SPD is being completed by two national workgroups: (1) the Sensory Processing Disorders Scientific Workgroup, a multidisciplinary group of established leaders in neuroscience and developmental psychobiology and (2) the Alpha research group, a national group of occupational therapy sensation processing researchers. Current research questions under study are noted in **Table 4**. Future studies will provide additional data about the mechanisms of SPD, the accurate identification of those with SPD and treatment of disorder.

Intervention for Individual's with SPD

The intervention for SPD is called occupational therapy with a sensory integrative approach. The goal of intervention is to improve the ability to process sensory information, providing a basis for improved independence and participation in daily life activities, play, and school tasks. The approach focuses on maximizing adaptive behavior and functional skills, and is most frequently utilized by OTs though some other professionals also have training in this intervention technique (e.g., physical therapists,

speech/language therapists). Mastery of this intervention requires advanced clinical training that includes didactic coursework and mentoring as the trainee actively participates in supervised treatment.

Professionals who use the sensory integrative approach follow a set of principles, based on sensory integration theory, that guide their clinical reasoning skills. Clinical reasoning is a creative and flexible way of looking at a child's personal characteristics and context and then deciding what modifications will help the child function more successfully, in the moment. Rather than a rigid formula for what to do, clinical reasoning is an elastic way to think.

These principles are described in detail in several books that are designed to guide therapists through the clinical reasoning process using sensory integration theory. The primary principles of this intervention approach are described as follows: (1) the intervention is rich in sensory opportunities especially tactile, proprioceptive, and vestibular sensations; (2) activities are tailored to provide the 'just right challenge' for the child's developing skills; (3) intervention is 'child directed', for example, the therapist reads and follows the child's cues guiding him/her to seek the needed sensory activities; (4) intervention supports the child's arousal level, self regulation, and organization of behavior; and (5) the context of intervention is play; (6) the focus of intervention is on obtaining 'adaptive responses', identified by Ayres as a 'purposeful, goal-directed response to a sensory experience'. Therapy consists of fun activities that range from very simple (responds to passive stimuli or maintains organization during multisensory activities), to moderately challenging games (initiates and sustains an activity requiring familiar movements), to quite complex activities (initiates and executes a complex activity requiring unfamiliar complicated movements requiring exact timing and multiple adaptations). The focus on the adaptive response ensures that each activity is challenging (a little hard for the child) but also that the child succeeds (often with help or scaffolding from the therapist). These activities that meet these criteria provide the 'just right challenge', and provide the best chance of facilitating learning and development.

OT with a sensory integration approach is a unique intervention because it addresses the underlying substrates of dysfunction (e.g., neurological immaturity) rather than just difficulties with skill performance. The therapeutic environment resembles a huge playroom or gymnasium with suspended swings, pillows, mats and large balls, and the equipment taps into the child's inner drive to play. Therapy provides opportunities for engagement in sensory and motor activities rich in tactile, vestibular, and proprioceptive sensations. The therapist uses keen observation skills to detect and interpret the child's behaviors and interests, and then creates a constantly changing playful environment in which the child actively pursues achievable challenges. For example, occupational therapy using a sensory integrative approach for a child with over-responsivity to tactile and vestibular input might include an activity such as climbing up a rope ladder to access a hanging trapeze swing, swinging across the room while holding the trapeze bar, and then 'crashing' into a large ball pit (surrounded by mats and pillows for safety). During this activity, the child is enticed into play that is rich in vestibular (swinging), proprioceptive (climbing), and tactile (ball pit) input and thus through play his or her over-responsivity to sensory stimuli is modulated. The therapist focuses on the specific adaptive responses needed by each individual – evolving from tolerating the sensory demands, to adapting to the challenges by beginning to organize motor responses. Play serves as the medium to engage the child so that even though the child may be hesitant initially, the urge to play in a colorful, fun environment outweighs hesitation and encourages participation. Ayres called this 'the art of therapy' or the careful process whereby the therapist actively adapts activities to match the child's emerging skills always ensuring that the child has fun. Thus, the child is guided through challenging but fun activities designed that stimulate the sensory systems, challenge the motor system, and facilitate performance of cognitive, attentional, social, and emotional tasks. Ultimately, the child begins to process sensory information in more typical ways and this improved 'sensory integration' provides the foundation for more organized and competent play, self regulation, self esteem, learning, and participation in daily routines. In addition to direct intervention with the child, the therapist also collaborates with and educates the parents, teachers, and others who are involved with the child.

Recent developments in the field have advanced and refined the protocol for using OT with a sensory integrative approach in part because defining intervention in a manner that is replicable is required for treatment effectiveness studies. The existing literature that addresses the effectiveness of intervention is fraught with methodological problems that limit interpretation and utility including the lack of replicable intervention (e.g., a manualized approach). Recently, the collaborative multisite group of occupational therapy clinicians and researchers developed a 'Fidelity to Treatment' measure. This scale outlines the core principles and philosophy of the intervention, and also provides a mechanism to evaluate whether the intervention uses a sensory integrative approach. This tool will be useful in future studies examining the effectiveness of intervention.

Another effort to define the intervention in a replicable, valid manner is the work of Miller and colleagues who have operationalized the principles of the sensory integrative approach into an intervention protocol that guides therapist's clinical reasoning and parent education. This model, 'A SECRET', provides an organizational framework to guide treatment sessions.

A SECRET has seven elements:

A Attention
S Sensation
E Emotion regulation
C Culture
R Relationships
E Environment
T Tasks

The first three elements – attention, sensation, and emotion regulation – are the individual characteristics that influence children internally. The last four – culture, relationships, environment, and tasks – are the contextual elements that influence children externally.

Using 'A SECRET', the therapist tries out and then provides a 'toolbox' of strategies for the parent and child using the therapy 'secrets' that increase the child's performance, social participation, and self-confidence/esteem. Finally, other specific goals and priorities of the family are addressed.

Intervention by OTs and other professionals using this approach is not a quick 'fix'. It is a therapeutic program designed to improve the child's ability to neurologically process sensory information improving the quality of the child's life by enhancing his or her ability to learn and play. Treatment can take place in a number of settings:

public schools, hospitals and outpatient clinics, and private practices. In all these settings, the role of intervention is to improve the child's ability to interact socially, to regulate him or herself, to maintain self-esteem, and to be independent in their daily living skills. Therapeutic methods in a school-based program compared to a direct service private therapy program are different. The child's treatment experience is significantly influenced by the setting of the therapy.

Evidence Evaluating Effectiveness of Intervention

Although controversy regarding the effectiveness of OT using a sensory integration approach exists, over 80 studies have been conducted that measure some aspect of the effectiveness of this approach to intervention. About half of the studies demonstrate some type of treatment effectiveness. Two meta-analyses and four research reports have been published summarizing the outcomes of these various studies; some of the syntheses conclude that the approach is effective and other syntheses suggest the intervention was equally effective as other approaches or not effective.

At this point in time, interpretation of the findings of these 80 studies is difficult due to three methodological limitations. The first limitation is defining the independent variable (the treatment) in a manner that is replicable. As this intervention approach is individualized (similar to the way psychotherapy is individualized), standardization of treatment has been a challenge to the researchers. With the development of the 'fidelity to treatment' measure and A SECRET, future intervention studies will be more able to adhere to a manualized treatment approach.

A second limitation is the outcome measures utilized. Previous research used outcomes not specifically related to the proposed changes from intervention. In addition, a quantity of research has been conducted on sensory stimulation rather than embedding it in the context of a full OT program as was originally intended. Ayres always used an 'occupational frame of reference' in providing intervention (e.g., the goals of therapy were functional abilities and routines, including the 'occupations' of childhood such as sleeping, eating, dressing, playing, interacting with others, learning, and active participation). Studies that do not use this frame of reference do not inform evidence-based practice related to OT using a sensory integrative approach.

Few studies establish a theoretical basis for their hypotheses, asking a global question instead, for example, 'does sensory integrative treatment work?' can be seen as a simplistic and atheoretical question. The last limitation of previous studies is that multiple outcome measures are utilized with no good explanation of how the outcomes relate to the suspected effects of treatment, for example, a 'fishing expedition' approach, hoping to find 'something'

that might be statistically significant. This results in low power to detect significant changes.

The collaborative multisite occupational therapy research team that developed the 'fidelity to treatment' measure is also working on a systematic way to apply goal attainment scaling (GAS) as a primary outcome measure for effectiveness studies. GAS provides a means to establish intervention goals that are specifically relevant to individuals and their families and allowing comparison of achievement across diverse functional outcomes. GAS in combination with physiologic outcome measures is envisioned to provide a method of measuring effectiveness that will increase the integrity, strength, and replicability of effectiveness studies.

The final limitation relates to the homogeneity of the samples studied. Previous researchers have not defined a homogenous sample. The heterogeneity of samples in previous research increased the within group variability and again the probability of finding significant group differences was reduced. Now with the 'short sensory profile' and the physiologic paradigm, the 'sensory challenge protocol', highly selective inclusion criteria, can be utilized to select specific sensory processing subtypes for study samples. Building on this work, future studies can define samples in a manner that allows replication across sites.

The limitations in previous studies have resulted in a lack of consensus regarding the effectiveness of OT using an SI approach. Given the current constraints of research, diverse findings are not surprising. This inconsistency is predictable, given the variation in sample characteristics, intervention methods and duration, and outcomes measured. The knowledge base in this field is in its infancy and additional work is needed before valid conclusions about the effectiveness of this intervention approach can be derived.

Conclusion

In conclusion, significant progress has been made in defining homogenous subgroups for analysis, in describing a replicable treatment, and in choosing valid outcome measures. However, gaps exist in knowledge related to the effectiveness of occupational therapy in ameliorating SPD. Hence, a clear and exciting call to action exists. We and others are implementing a series of studies to elucidate the underlying mechanisms of the impairment, to define the phenotypic characteristics of the disorder, to discriminate the disorder from other developmental disorders (ADHD and autism), and to evaluate the effectiveness of OT in remediating the dysfunction. New research with stronger empirical standards is forthcoming. We are on the cusp of an explosion of knowledge in this area that will increase rigorous scientific data and move the field forward. Scientists and practitioners are collaborating to conduct research that leads to more specific diagnoses and more effective interventions, thereby improving the lives of children with SPD and their families.

See also: ADHD: Genetic Influences; Autism Spectrum Disorders; Developmental Disabilities: Cognitive; Fragile X Syndrome.

Suggested Readings

Ayres AJ (1972) *Sensory Integration and Learning Disorders.* Los Angeles: Western Psychological Services.
Ayres AJ (1979) *Sensory Integration and the Child.* Los Angeles: Western Psychological Corporation.
Bundy AC, Lane SJ, and Murray EA (2003) *Sensory Integration Theory and Practice.* Philadelphia: F.A. Davis.
Kranowitz C (2005) *The Out of Sync Child.* (Revised). New York: Penguin.
Miller LJ (2006) *Sensational Kids: Help and Hope for Children with Sensory Processing Disorder.* New York: Putnam.
Miller LJ, McIntosh DN, McGrath J, *et al.* (1999) Electrodermal responses to sensory stimuli in individuals with fragile X syndrome: A preliminary report. *American Journal of Medical Genetics* 83(4): 268–279.
Parham D and Mailloux Z (1995) Sensory integrative principles in intervention with children with autistic disorder. In: Case-Smith J, Allen AS, and Pratt PN (eds.) *Occupational Therapy for Children*, pp. 329–382. St. Louis, MO: Mosby.
Schaaf RC and SmithRoley S (2006) *Sensory Integration: Applying Clinical Reasoning to Diverse Populations.* Tucson, AZ: The Psychological Corporation.
Smith Roley S, Blanche E, and Schaaf RC (eds.) (2001) *Understanding the Nature of Sensory Integration with Diverse Populations.* San Antonio, TX: The Psychological Corporation.

Relevant Websites

http://www.abilitations.com – Abilitations.
http://www.aota.org – American Occupational Association.
http://www.icdl.com – Interdisciplinary Council on Developmental and Learning Disorders.
http://www.KIDFoundation.org – KID Foundation.
http://www.neurolearning.com – Neurological Concepts.
http://www.out-of-sync-child.com – Out of Sync Child.
http://www.sierf.org – Sensory Integration Education and Research Foundation.
http://www.sensory-processing-disorder.com – Sensory Processing Disorder Resource Center.
http://www.sensorycomfort.com – Sensory Products.
http://www.sensoryresources.com – Sensory Resources.
http://www.genjereb.com – Sensory Tools.
http://www.southpawenterprises.com – Southpaw.
http://www.spdnetwork.org – SPD Network.
http://www.seriweb.com – Special Education Resources on the Internet.
http://www.Slfocus.com – The international magazine dedicated to improving sensory integration.
http://www.spinkids.org – This site raises awareness of sensory processing disorder.

Separation and Stranger Anxiety

A Scher and J Harel, University of Haifa, Haifa, Israel

Glossary

Anxiety – The psychological and physiological reaction to an anticipated danger, real or imagined.
Distress – An intense negative reaction to adverse events. The reaction may be emotional and/or physical.
Person and object permanence – The understanding that people and objects continue to exist when they are not directly observed.
Separation anxiety – A distress reaction in response to separation from the primary caregiver.
Separation anxiety disorder (SAD) – Developmentally inappropriate and excessive anxiety concerning actual or anticipated separation from the caregiver, most often the parents.
Stranger anxiety – The fearful, distressed response that infants exhibit when approached by an unfamiliar person, in the second half of the first year.

Introduction

In the second half of the first year, infants show signs of distress when approached by an unfamiliar person and when their primary caregiver leaves. The study of these phenomena underscores the link between advances in the child's ability to mentally represent people and events, along with changes in the emotional tie to the caregiver. Separation anxiety is an important psychological construct within a number of emotional development theories. While the reaction is normative, some children develop a separation anxiety disorder.

Reactions to the Approach and Disappearance of People

The second half of the first year of life is a time of major cognitive and emotional discoveries and challenges.

In this period, infants not only explore and manipulate the environment more actively, but they also start expressing clear social preferences and apprehensions. While infants happily exchange smiles with strangers during the first months of their life, in the second half of the first year they begin to exhibit a clear preference for specific social partners, typically their parents. Moreover, at this stage when parents leave the room, even for a short time, babies often become distressed and start crying. Another trigger for distress during this period is the approach of an unfamiliar person. Upon encountering strangers, infants of this age observe the unfamiliar face intently, turn their heads away, and sometimes cry. In the developmental literature, the emergence of these distress responses – to separation and to strangers – is considered a major developmental milestone. When describing the reaction to the approach of an unfamiliar person, researchers use the terms wariness, apprehension, distress, fear, and anxiety depending, partially, on the theoretical perspective they are using to explain the response. In psychoanalytic theory, the reactions to the disappearance of the familiar caregiver and to the approach of an unfamiliar person are conceptualized as anxiety: separation anxiety and stranger anxiety.

Stranger Anxiety

Around 6–8 months, when infants are approached by an unfamiliar person, a new response appears: the expression of wariness and distress. At this stage, infants react to encounters with unfamiliar people who try to engage them in ways they are not used to, including becoming sober and quiet, staring and frowning, lowering the gaze or turning the head away, getting a frightened expression, or even starting to cry or scream. These responses are particularly striking when they show up with family acquaintances or relatives who were greeted with smiles a month or so earlier. While there is variation in the form, intensity, and duration of the response, infants across diverse cultures show some degree of wariness toward strangers which tends to peak toward the end of the first year of life and generally decreases thereafter.

The contextual variables that affect the intensity of the stranger anxiety response include proximity and accessibility to the mother. More distress is shown when the mother is not present in the room; when the mother is holding the infant, the reaction is least intense. A sudden and abrupt approach of the stranger, as opposed to a slow warm-up period, also intensifies the distress reaction. Research on stranger characteristics is mixed, suggesting that infants react more favorably to child than adult strangers (presumably because children are perceived as more like themselves), while findings regarding stranger gender are inconclusive.

The emergence of the anxious response to strangers, which is widely acknowledged in child development textbooks and often discussed in the popular parenting media, was a topic of focused research during the 1960s and 1970s, but has received less attention in recent years. A review of the empirical studies reveals discrepancies and disagreement as to the prevalence of the behavior, the age at which it is first observed, and how it fades across time. In a number of reports, the reaction to strangers is described as emerging between 6 and 8 months or even earlier, while others conclude that the phenomenon is first evident only toward the end of the first year. There is also considerable discrepancy concerning the specific ages in which the response peaks (9–10 months according to some reports, 12–15 months according to others) and diminishes (toward the end of the first year vs. during the course of the second year). The different timetables described in these studies partially reflect differences in methodology. Still, a fairly consistent finding is that sometime in the second part of the first year infants display a noticeable new response to unfamiliar people – showing signs of distress when approached by strangers. What makes this response particularly interesting is that it underscores the important links between emotion and cognition.

Cognitive Advances Underlying the Response to Strangers

Object permanence

In the latter part of the first year infants are capable of evaluating situations and responding to them in a more complex way. Advances in sensory–motor capacities allow more regulated attention to relevant components of novel situations and more awareness of violated expectations. The examination of these evolving capacities is the hallmark of Jean Piaget's theory of cognitive development. Piaget was interested in how infants develop an understanding that objects are independent of themselves, occupy physical space, and continue to exist even when they do not see them. Piaget used the term object permanence to describe this capacity and suggested that the concept of people as permanent develops before the understanding of the permanence of objects. This is important for conceptualizing the infant's developing discrimination of the mother from the other. However, the prediction that the anxious reaction to strangers would occur only after the achievement of object permanence (typically around 12 months of age) is not supported, given that this phenomenon may appear as early as 6 months.

Research on the maturation of distance vision has indicated that it is not until 6 months of age that infants reach adult-like discrimination, allowing them to identify familiar faces from different angles and distances, and across a wide variety of situations. Nonetheless, we know that infants learn to recognize and differentiate between their parents and other people at a much earlier age; for example, it has been shown that newborns are able to identify the face, voice, and smell of their mothers already in the first weeks of life. Extensive research over the past few decades suggests that infants learn to recognize the invariant features of people and objects, as well as the concepts of appearing and disappearing and occupying different locations, earlier than Piaget claimed. Using internalized schemes and representations to bring past experience to bear on the present, young infants engage in detecting regularities and discrepancies in stimuli, and form expectations about events. Through repeated exposures during the early months, infants come to distinguish between the familiar and the unfamiliar. But why do they start expressing apprehension, avoidance, and distress when encountered by a less familiar or a strange person?

Incongruity between the familiar and the unfamiliar face

A number of investigators have argued that the reaction to unfamiliar people results from an incongruity between the stranger and the internalized schema of the familiar caregiver. Donald Hebb's cognitive theory, which links perception and behavior to the neuronal network, offers insight into infants' fearful response to strangers. Hebb argued that perceptual experiences establish memory traces in the form of neural circuits, and that these are activated when a new perceptual experience is sufficiently similar to a previous one. But when the new stimulus is not similar enough to maintain continued smooth transmission in the neural circuit, the ensuing disruption produces a distress reaction. According to this explanation, an approaching adult could seem somewhat familiar to an infant at first, but then turn out to be different from the well-established mental representation of the familiar caregiver, and this disruption stirs up emotional distress. The intensity of the reaction to novel experiences depends on the extent to which the child has developed an internal representation of the stimuli and the degree of discrepancy between the new situation and the internalized schema. According to the incongruity principle, it is the discrepancy between the novel face and the internalized standard (e.g., the caregiver) that is responsible for the distress reaction, not social interaction with the stranger *per se*. However, as noted earlier, infants can discriminate between their mothers and strangers already in the first weeks of life, but they do not show fear of strangers until 6 or 8 months of age.

Jerome Kagan, who has been studying the links between children's cognitive capacities and emotional reactivity for over 30 years, maintains that perceptual experiences and memory traces yield interest rather than fear in infants younger than 6 months; in older infants, who are better able to generate explanations about new and unexpected events, a discrepant event that they cannot explain generates emotional distress. This developmental account adds to the incongruity

model in that it links the newly acquired capacity to explain the discrepancy between the familiar and the strange to distress when the explanation fails. Although this concept is plausible, it is difficult to test.

Brain maturation

During the latter part of the first year, the ability to retrieve knowledge from memory and use this information for performing tasks improves dramatically. Adele Diamond, who studied the development of memory functions and their neural basis, provided evidence that links the improvement in infants' search for hidden objects to the maturation of the prefrontal cortex, including the growing differentiation of gamma-aminobutyric acid (GABA), an inhibitory neurotransmitter known to play an important role in the regulation of anxiety and behavioral reactivity. Another critical development during this period is the integration of the limbic and endocrine systems into the memory networks. The capsula interna, which links the cerebral cortex with the amygdala, develops mature myelin around 10 months of age, allowing increased connectivity and efficient integration between the two systems. As the amygdala is also linked to the hypothalamic–pituitary–adrenal (HPA), or the stress axis, the improved connectivity between stimulation, interpretation, and emotional processing also increases the involvement of the stress axis in the processing of experiences.

Fear and Anxiety as Indicators of Emotional Advances in the First Year

The 8-month anxiety

Although distress reactions to strangers were described by the pioneers of infant observation at the turn of the nineteenth century, the first systematic study of the phenomenon was conducted by Rene Spitz. As a psychoanalyst working with infants in group care, he methodically observed and recorded behavioral patterns that marked the changing relations between infants and the social environment. The observations were documented in a film entitled *Anxiety: Its Phenomenology in the First Year of Life*, and discussed in a 1950 paper on the manifestation of anxiety in the first year. The naturalistic observations showed that between 6 and 8 months, infants no longer responded with smiles when unfamiliar visitors approached them, and instead showed apprehension and distress. While the specific behaviors of different children varied (e.g., turning the head away, covering the face, or screaming), the common denominator was an avoidant response, refusal to contact, and distress. Spitz called this pattern the 8-month anxiety and considered it the earliest manifestation of psychological anxiety.

According to Spitz, the 8-month anxiety is unique and differs from earlier expressions of fear, for instance, a fearful reaction to repeated inoculation. In reacting to a stranger, the infant is responding to a person with whom no previous unpleasurable encounters have been experienced. So why manifest wariness and anxiety? Using psychoanalytic reasoning, Spitz argued that the response to approaching strangers is triggered by the realization that, since the unfamiliar person is not the mother, mother has left. The anxiety results from an inference process involving the comparison of the stranger to an internal representation of the mother, and the fear of losing her. In attributing the 8-month anxiety to the infant's wish for the mother and the disappointment that the approaching person is not her, Spitz underscored the role of the infant's affective communication in the caregiving process, and attributed to the 8-month anxiety a major organizing role in the evolving psychological self.

Fearfulness as a marker of a new level of emotional organization

Inspired by Spitz's work, Robert Emde and colleagues conducted a longitudinal investigation of emotional development in the mid-1970s. Following a sample of 14 infants throughout their first year, at home and in the laboratory, the researchers collected an elaborate database that included naturalistic behavioral observations, interviews with mothers, structured tests, as well as EEG recordings. Emde, like Spitz, identified two organizing principles of emotional development that emerge in the course of the first year: the social smile and stranger distress.

Around 2 months of age, infants typically show the milestone of social smile, which is a marker for inquisitive, active engagement with their surroundings. At this age, infants' curiosity is on the rise as they develop and master new ways to maintain and increase interesting stimulation (e.g., shaking a rattle). Whereas Piaget viewed sensory–motor schemas of exploring and understanding the world (e.g., hand–eye coordination, mouthing) as the major organizers of experiences in the first year, Emde and colleagues emphasized the role of emotionality as a key organizer. The appearance of the social smile marks a new way of interacting with the world. Whereas crying, the key organizer in the first weeks of life, conveys an urgent need for change and a plea for alleviating discomfort, smiling signals positive engagement, an invitation for the continuation of a pleasurable exchange. Emde observed that by 2.5 months, infants smiled regularly in response to the faces of their parents, as well as the faces of unfamiliar individuals. By 4 months, the infants in the study showed more smiling and motor responsiveness in the presence of their mothers than with other people. At around 5 months, some infants curiously studied and compared their mother's face with that of strangers, and between 5 and 7 months, they stared soberly at strangers faces.

Around 8 months, the infants in Emde's study manifested a distress reaction to unfamiliar people which, according to his model, marks the second shift in emotional expression. While the average age was 8 months, considerable variation among the infants was observed; as to the duration of the response, 11 of the 14 infants manifested distress for 2 consecutive months and eight continued to show stranger distress into the third month. In their attempt to explain the roots of the fearful response to strangers, Emde and colleagues acknowledged the importance of the infant's changing relationship to the mother and the cognitive advances of the second part of the first year, but also suggested a new focus: the emergence of the capacity for fearfulness.

Evidence from numerous studies shows that around 7–9-month infants not only show distress to strangers and unfamiliar surroundings, but also start to manifest wariness of heights, mechanical toys, masks, etc. Before this age, distress was nonspecific, mostly a reaction to physical discomfort, whereas the new distress responses are linked to specific stimuli in the environment, as evidenced by the fact that infants look and evaluate before displaying distress. Cardiac measurements support the idea of a developmental shift in the capacity for fear. At 5 months of age, the approach of an unfamiliar person led to heart-rate deceleration in the infant, accompanied with a facial expression of delighted curiosity, but at 9 months, the stranger's approach was associated with cardiac acceleration, frowning, gaze aversion, and crying. Emde argues that from a social communication perspective, the fearful reaction to the approach of a stranger conveys a clear message to the mother: a preference for her company and a plea not to be left alone with unfamiliar people. This new message to the primary caregiver is linked to another major emotional milestone of infancy: separation anxiety.

Separation Anxiety

Sometime in the middle of the first year, when infants understand that people exist even when they are out of sight (person permanence), they react to the everyday recurring disappearances of their parents by attempting to maintain proximity through the behaviors available to them, including crying, cooing, and crawling. In manifesting these responses, infants not only indicate their desire to stay in proximity with the caregiver but also the development of ways to control distance and separation. During this stage, infants increasingly initiate interaction with their parents and actively protest when their primary caregiver departs, even for a moment. By the first birthday, behaviors that indicate separation distress are even more clearly detected, with infants tending to become agitated and upset upon separation.

The Normative Course of Separation Anxiety

Separation distress, signaled by crying in response to parental separation, may be observed as early as 4 or

5 months of age, but most accounts identify 8 months as the age when separation anxiety emerges. Distress from brief separations continues to characterize toddlers' behavior well into the second year of life; the normative response typically peaks around 12–18 months and then fades after 2 years of age. In diverse cultural contexts, such as the Kalahari Bushmen, the Israeli Kibbutz and Guatemala, infants display distress in response to separation from their mothers; this is considered a normative part of development and its emergence is viewed as a major milestone in the formation of the emotional tie between the child and primary caregiver. The reaction to separation from the mother appears to be a universal phenomenon; however, specific parenting practices and cultural experiences may impact the timing and the intensity of the response. For example, in cultural settings where infants experience constant physical contact with their mothers distress to separation was observed earlier than 8 months; Japanese, as compared to Western toddlers were found to express more intense reactions to separation from their mothers. The use of an inanimate companion such as a blanket or doll (also known as a transitional object) is one of the ways toddlers attempt to alleviate separation distress. While separation anxiety gradually fades for the majority of children after the second birthday, some children will continue to express extreme distress in the face of parental separation. In many cases, these children will be subsequently diagnosed as suffering from separation anxiety disorder (SAD), a psychological disorder briefly discussed in the final section of this article.

The role of cognitive and social factors

The emergence and decline of separation distress has been linked to the cognitive advances of the first and second year. As with stranger anxiety, object permanence has been suggested as one of the determinants of the response to the disappearance of the familiar caregiver. In a series of experiments on infants' early representational capacities, Chris Moore and colleagues demonstrated that while infants younger than 6 months are able to detect violation of identity of objects (characteristics of the objects), they only appear to understand the concept of permanency of objects at 9 months. However, Piaget suggested that understanding person permanence comes earlier, and Mary Ainsworth's observation of infants and mothers in Uganda revealed that around 4–6 months, when mothers left the infants and went out of sight, some of the infants appeared distressed and cried. Silvia Bell, who compared object vs. person permanency, confirmed that indeed the concept of persons as permanent objects appears before infants understand the permanency of inanimate objects.

The understanding that the parent continues to exist when out of sight, together with advances in motor control, are believed to shape the process of active searching for the caregiver (e.g., crawling). In the same vein, advances in

cause–effect reasoning shape infants' responses; they begin to grasp that calling or crying increases the likelihood of the parent's reappearance. The establishment of an integrated and enduring representation of the caregiver plays a critical role in the formation of the emotional tie between the child and parent, but it is less clear why infants at this stage show distress when separated from their primary caregivers.

Drawing on the concept of discrepant event, discussed earlier with respect to stranger anxiety, Kagan maintained that the infant is likely to display separation anxiety when the sight of the mother leaving is a discrepant event which the child is unable to prevent and/or integrate with previous experiences. It was found that infants showed less distress in a home setting when the mother departed through a door she used frequently, compared to when she exited through a door she rarely used. The decline of separation distress in the latter part of the second year is believed to be associated with the toddler's increased cognitive capacity to understand the circumstances of the separation and maintain the expectation that the parent will return. For example, when the mother left the room through a door rarely used, it was found that some of the toddlers approached the door and engaged, on and off, in play with toys, but did not cry.

In the second half of the first year, as infants gain better control of posture and movement and become more active explorers of their environment, they appear to pay extra attention to the location of other people, both caregivers and strangers. Infants at this stage frequently monitor their relative proximity to the caregiver; while venturing away from their mothers, they tend to frequently look toward their mother's face. Social referencing, an active search for others' emotional expression as a source of information to help clarify uncertain events, begins around 8–9 months. At this age, infants can understand that facial expressions have emotional meanings and they make use of others' emotional expressions to guide their own behavior with reference to specific situations and events. By monitoring their parents' facial expression, infants obtain information as to the danger or safety of their planned actions. When infants encounter a potentially dangerous setting, such as a visual cliff (a glass-covered table with an illusionary deep drop), they make use of parents' facial information to regulate their actions; when mothers smile, infants typically cross the deep part whereas when mothers show fear, infants avoid crossing.

The Developmental Significance of Separation

In psychoanalytic theorizing, separation anxiety in infancy is viewed as a consequence of, on the one hand, the capacity to mentally represent the mother, and on the other hand, the interpretation of her absence as 'losing' her. In other words, the cognitive ability to keep the mother in mind even in her absence not only triggers feelings of longing, but also stirs up the distress of separation. To understand the anxiety produced by separation, it is essential to conceptualize the significance of the absence and its implications from the perspective of the infant. When separated from the primary caregiver, infants lose a significant regulator of their needs, not only physical but, just as crucially, emotional.

Consequences of Separation in Animals

Significant insights into the formation of the emotional bond between infant and mother, and the detrimental consequences of maternal separation, come from studies of animal behavior, specifically the work of Harry Harlow and Stephen Suomi with monkeys, and Myron Hofer's studies with rats. For example, rat pups emit initial separation calls and their heart rate falls significantly after separation, regardless of supplemental heat. By studying a number of systems, such as those controlling sleep and arousal, activity level, and sucking, Hofer and colleagues identified changes in the activation of these systems that resulted from maternal separation and concluded that through ongoing interactions, mothers regulate their offspring, and that the loss of the maternal regulators has serious consequences, including a decrease in growth hormone secretion. In demonstrating the regulatory function of mother–infant proximity, animal models have significantly advanced our understanding of the neurobiological nature of separation distress, and provided important clues as to how proximity-maintenance shapes the well-being of mammals, including humans.

Physiological and Behavioral Correlates of Emotional Distress

Studying emotional distress among infants and young children presents many challenges of measurement and interpretation. Since fear and distress involve complex neural interactions and coordinated activities of psychobehavioral, physiological, and hormonal systems, measurement can take place at different levels. Facial expressions provide one avenue. Charles Darwin underscored the innateness, universality, and survival value of children's fear and distress responses when he documented, in a series of photographs, facial expressions displayed by different youngsters in circumstances of pain, hunger, and discomfort. Since then, a number of researchers have devised detailed measurement systems for coding facial expressions that index specific emotions (e.g., Izard's MAX coding system and Baby FACS, which is based on Ekman's Facial Action Coding System). In the MAX, for example, criteria of distress/pain expression include closed eyes and a squared and angular mouth, whereas in the fear expression, eyelids are lifted and the mouth corners are retracted straight back. Vocal response is another way to study the expression of distress, but there is still a debate whether infants cry distinctively when they are physically as opposed to emotionally distressed.

Measuring cortisol, a blood-borne hormone that increases under stress, has significantly advanced our understanding of children's responses to daily normative challenges, as well as the long-term effects of poorly regulated stress levels. For more than two decades, Megan Gunnar has been studying children's stress by measuring cortisol; she showed that the quality of the mother–child tie regulates levels of cortisol secretion. Children who experience secure relationships with their mothers show stable cortisol levels even when emotionally upset, whereas in insecure mother–child relationships, even minor challenges raise cortisol levels.

The way different children react to stress-producing stimuli has been studied within the conceptual framework of temperament. Kagan, who longitudinally studied children with different reactivity levels to unfamiliar stimuli, found that inhibited infants were more fearful as toddlers and were more likely to manifest symptoms of anxiety at school-age compared to uninhibited infants. Together with other studies, these findings point to a relative stability across time in children's reactivity. Temperamental disposition is one source of individual variability in the ways children cope with fearful events. Mothers' behavior is another determinant. For example, recent findings from Nathan Fox's laboratory show that infants who received insensitive caregiving display higher levels of right frontal electroencephalogram (EEG) asymmetry and fearfulness to unfamiliar stimuli compared to infants whose mothers were more responsive and sensitive in their daily caregiving behavior. The ways in which temperament, social learning, and caregiving variables jointly modulate stranger and separation anxiety during infancy have yet to be comprehensively investigated. The focus of the subsequent section is separation anxiety from the standpoint of the psychoanalytic and the attachment perspectives.

The Mother–Child Dyad and Separation Anxiety

Freud's description of his nephew playing with a reel of string is the first account in psychological literature describing a toddler coping with separation and anxiety. The child, in his crib, was throwing the reel and pulling it back again. Freud maintained that for the playing child, the reel represented his mother, who had to leave him several times. The play sequence helped the child gain control over his mother's disappearance and return, which in real life was an experience he endured passively, anxiously, and as beyond his control. Since then, many theoreticians have tried to describe children's reactions to separation and differentiate between the normative and disturbed variations.

The concept of separation is central to two influential theories of emotional development: John Bowlby's Attachment theory, and Margaret Mahler's Separation–Individuation theory. Both of these theories had a major impact on the way we understand separation reactions and separation anxiety today. Both these theories emphasize the relationship between the child and the parent (especially the mother) as the regulating factor of separation reactions, both normative and pathological.

Attachment as a window on separation anxiety

John Bowlby, the founder of attachment theory, was among the first to emphasize the human infant's biological disposition to participate in relationships, and proposed that the formation of the mother–child tie is controlled by mechanisms that evolved as a result of evolutionary adaptedness. This tie – the attachment relationship – is shaped through interactions in which proximity to the caregiver plays a significant role. In his book, *Separation: Anxiety and Anger*, Bowlby discusses the situations that trigger fear in children and lists four main categories: noise, strange people/objects/places, animals, and darkness. He also notes that being alone significantly increases the likelihood that fear will be aroused by these stimuli. In studies of infants' fear of strangers, the presence of the mother served as a moderator of the intensity of the distress: in the absence of the caregiver, infants were more fearful. It was found that the proximity to the mother was particularly significant around 12 months of age; Bowlby explains that as their emotional tie to mother becomes better consolidated, their knowledge of objects and situations becomes more sophisticated, and their ability to move in space becomes more skillful, infants are better able to coordinate moving away from a fearful situation toward the comforting proximity of the attachment figure, usually mother.

From an evolutionary perspective, proximity to the parent allows protection and thus provides a survival advantage; a predisposition to seek the protection of caregiver is particularly advantageous in times of danger and distress. According to Bowlby, attachment behavior – responses that aim to keep the caregiver in proximity to the baby – evoke caregiving behavior that promotes infants' sense of security. Attachment is a primary survival system, akin to other instinctual systems like feeding and sexual behavior, and is irreducible to other drives. Infants are born with the motivation and capacity to form emotional ties with their caregivers, and to use them as a source of comfort in times of danger and stress. During the first 6 months of life, the infant learns to prefer the primary caregiver as a source of comfort and security, thus creating an attachment bond. The attachment system is activated by external danger conditions (for instance, darkness, loud noise, sudden movements) and by internal conditions (such as illness, fatigue, pain). When the

system is activated, the child seeks proximity to the caregiver to attain a sense of security. The caregiver can alleviate the child's distress by different means, depending on various factors including the child's age and the level of anxiety aroused. With young children, physical contact is the most effective response; with older children, more distal means like talking are also effective. When the danger is serious, even older children (and adults) may need physical contact to relieve the distress and anxiety.

Attachment theory explains why situations of separation or threats of separation arouse anxiety in people of all ages, but since children are more dependent on the protection provided by the caregiver, they suffer more intense separation anxiety. Bowlby and his coworkers described the sequence of typical reactions when young children are separated from parents. Children first protest, then show despair, and if the caregiver does not return, they subsequently show detachment. When the child perceives a threat of separation, she/he protests by crying, clinging, expressing anger, and looking for the parent; the protest is often expressed around sleep, at bedtime, and in the course of the night. When in despair, babies looks sad, move slowly and sometimes cry persistently, withdraw, and even act hostile. In the detachment phase, the child seems to return to normal behavior and is willing to accept comfort from unfamiliar adults. The problematic behavior shows up upon the parent's return: the child ignores the parent, or avoids and walks away. These behaviors might alternate with crying and extreme clinging, showing the child's suffering and anxiety regarding a possible future separation from the parent.

A key principle in attachment theory is the interrelation between the attachment, fear, and exploration systems. For example, the activation of the fear system generally heightens the activation of the attachment system and deactivates the exploration system. Bowlby maintained that the biological function of the fear system, like the attachment system, is protection. Because the two systems are inter-related, frightened infants increase their attachment behavior and seek protection; the fear not only triggers a desire to escape from the frightening stimulus but also a search for the anticipated security provided by the attachment figure. Separation anxiety occurs when attachment behavior is activated by the absence of the attachment figure, but cannot be terminated because the caregiver is not available to provide security. With the cognitive advances of the latter part of the first year, infants become capable of expectant anxiety in situations that seem likely to be threatening or in which the attachment figure is likely to become unavailable. As discussed, the presence or absence of the mother was found to attenuate or enhance the fear of strangers – in attachment terms, the proximity and trust in the availability of the attachment figure makes the infant less fearful. As the attachment and exploratory systems are linked, a child who is anxious about separation or does not have a secure relationship with the caregiver is expected to be inhibited in exploration and learning.

Separation anxiety in secure and insecure children

Attachment research identified different patterns of relationships between the infant and the attachment figure. Empirical studies, particularly those that use Ainsworth's Strange Situation procedure, differentiated between secure and insecurely attached infants. Secure children represent their relationship with mother as providing a sense of security, while insecure children encounter difficulties in attaining a sense of security, developing unique strategies to counteract this. Avoidant children tend to minimize their signals of needing mother, while anxious ambivalent children tend to exaggerate them; they have learned which strategies are most effective in eliciting caregiving from their mothers. The different attachment patterns are schematically represented in the child's mind as internal working models, guiding the child's behavior in relationships and specifically in stressful and emotionally charged situations. For secure children, the represented relationship with the attachment figure potentially provides security and alleviates anxiety, even in the absence of mother. Children with secure attachments are better equipped to cope with situations evoking negative emotions, including separation anxiety, than children with insecure attachments. For example, in Bell's study of person and object permanence, it was found that infants with secure attachment more actively searched for their mothers.

The separation–individuation process

Margaret Mahler was the first psychoanalyst to observe nonpatient mothers and infants as a source of information about emotional development, making her an innovator at a time when the accepted investigation method in psychoanalysis was the reconstruction of infancy from adult patients' narratives. In Mahler's opinion, the human infant's physical birth does not coincide with his or her psychological birth. The psychological birth involves a separation–individuation process, which is based upon the child's maturation and dependent not only on the child, but on the mother and eventually the father too. The process has two components which usually develop at the same pace: separation, the attainment of an experience of separateness from mother as opposed to nondifferentiation from mother (a different body), and individuation, the attainment of a sense of having specific, individual characteristics (being somebody).

Mahler describes several stages in the infant's journey from a state of nondifferentiation between infant and mother to a state of differentiated representations of self and mother, as well as in the attainment of differentiation between inner and outer worlds. Grasping these differentiations is an important step in the child's ability to

function independently from mother without experiencing too much separation anxiety. The child who successfully goes through the separation–individuation process is one who can separate from the actual mother since he/she has an internally represented mother who is available to comfort the child when distressed, frustrated, and anxious.

The first two stages, labeled by Mahler as the 'normal autistic' and the 'symbiotic', span the first half-year of life. The infant's emergence from what Mahler referred to as 'symbiosis' marks the beginning of the separation–individuation process proper; the infant is 'hatching' from the mother–infant unit and turning his or her attention toward the world out there. In the differentiation phase, the infant, still in his mother's arms, starts exploring mother, pushing his body away from her and looking at her from a distance, pulling her hair, and fingering her face. The infant is comparing the mother who is known to the unfamiliar elements in the environment. The peek-a-boo game, much enjoyed at this age, is an exercise in separation, a way of facing this basic fear in a controlled, pleasurable atmosphere.

When the child is able to move away from mother (e.g., by crawling), the 'practicing' phase begins, peaking with the attainment of walking. With the achievement of this milestone, children are able to move further away from mother, and new cognitive abilities enable them to further explore the world outside them and enjoy new experiences. The child is at the height of feelings of omnipotence, in love with the world and with his or her own skills. Still, periodically the child will return to mother for emotional support when he momentarily becomes aware of being alone and anxious.

During the second half of the second year the toddler enters the phase of 'rapprochement' (approaching again) which lasts to about 2 years of age, considered one of the most sensitive, difficult periods of the separation–individuation process. During this phase, the toddler experiences the need to explore and function without mother, but at the same time, the need for mother is rediscovered because the growing awareness of separateness is anxiety-arousing. Reapproaching the mother is, on the one hand, a source of comfort to the infant, but it also triggers fear of regressing to earlier states of less differentiation and loss of independence and identity. Mothers find it difficult to adjust their behavior to the changing moods of the child who is clinging one moment and pushing her away the next. Mahler contends that both mother and toddler experience the loss of earlier ways of being with each other during this phase. The toddler experiences anger and sadness, and expresses these feelings by separation protest and temper tantrums. As the child explores separation from the mother, the father becomes a valuable alternative, a less conflicted caregiver figure for the child.

One of the main achievements of the rapprochement phase is the mastery of separation anxiety. Toddlers who have successfully resolved the conflicts of rapprochement enter the next phase, beginning around the third year of life: consolidation of identity and the beginnings of integrated self and other representations. The integration of the maternal representation, including positive and negative aspects of mother, establishes in the child's mind an 'internal mother' who is always with him/her and available to comfort the child when separated from his or her parents, or feeling anxious or distressed.

Although Mahler's theory, and mainly her first two subphases came under severe criticism, it is a rich source of insights and understanding of normative separation anxiety, as well as the more pathological separation reactions. Toddlers at risk for developing problems, including different degrees and forms of intense separation anxiety, are those with developmental limitations (e.g., regulatory disorders), those whose mothers have failed to respond sensitively to the child's needs during the separation–individuation process, and those experiencing an inordinate number of separations.

Separation anxiety as a marker of emotional development

Both Bowlby and Mahler underscored separation-related experiences and theorized about their developmental significance. Bowlby focused more on the observable aspects of the behavior, whereas Mahler emphasized the implicit, subjective experiences of the child. Both theories provide a detailed description of the child's development from a state of needing the actual, physical presence of the parent and experiencing distress and anxiety when separated from the parent, to a stage when the parent and the relationship with the parent are represented in the child's mind, consequently lessening the need for the parent's actual presence. In both theories, the representation of the caregiver takes the role of the comforting parent when anxiety is aroused. The qualities of the representation, and thus its effectiveness in reducing anxiety, are dependent on the child's experiences with the parent. Children who have had more positive experiences, whose parents are more attuned to their needs, are expected to form more positive representations of themselves, their caregivers, and their relationship. Whereas Bowlby gives more room to the real, objective aspects of the relationship, and assumes a closer correspondence between the real relationship and the child's representation of it, Mahler adds the child's subjective experience of the relationship, and the child's own drives and fantasies, as an additional formative factor of the representation. In both theories, the separation and reunion of the child and the caregiver, as well as the anxiety induced by the separation and its regulation, serve as key theoretical constructs for explaining child development in general, and emotional development in particular.

Maternal separation anxiety

The way in which mother and child negotiate separations has been a topic of continued developmental research. While separation anxiety has been typically addressed from the perspective of the child, mothers also experience distress when separation occurs. Bowlby postulated that caregiving is governed by a behavioral system which is reciprocal to attachment and is biologically predisposed to protect the child. The system is activated by the child's distress, for example, when separated from the parent, or by the caregiver's perception of danger to the child (e.g., at night); when the caregiving system is strongly activated, the parent seeks proximity to the child in order to insure protection. In situations of danger, real or imagined, when separated from the child, and the provision of care and safety cannot be maintained mothers experience anxiety.

Maternal separation anxiety has been studied by Ellen Hock, who defined it as an unpleasant emotional state that reflects concern and apprehension about leaving the infant. Maternal separation anxiety involves feelings of guilt, worry, and sadness that accompany short-term separation from the child. As mothers' separation concerns are likely to shape their tolerance of staying apart and their behavior upon return, it has implications for child behavior and development. For example, it has been found that high levels of maternal separation anxiety was linked to infants' sleep difficulties as well as to SAD in older children.

Separation Anxiety Disorder in Young Children

While SAD occurs most frequently after age 5 years (and is thus outside the age group addressed in this article), it is nevertheless important to include a brief description of the characteristics and correlates of the disorder as in some cases children as young as 2 years old are diagnosed. SAD is one of the most common disorders in childhood; prevalence estimates for SAD in community samples range from 3% to 13%. Though it is common and causes much distress to child and family, in most cases it is not severe and does not predict future emotional disorders. The clinical presentation of SAD includes a variety of signs of anxiety; it is not easy to differentiate between severe normal separation anxiety and the pathological variety, or among the different types of anxiety disorders (panic disorder and general anxiety disorder).

Differentiating Separation Anxiety Disorder from Normal Separation Reactions

SAD is suspected when the child expresses excessive anxiety upon actual or anticipated separation from the caregivers, most often the parents. Age is one criterion in diagnosing pathological separation anxiety. Although children older than 3 years are not supposed to show separation anxiety under regular circumstances, when ill, fatigued, or in a strange environment, they might exhibit signs of anxiety even at later ages. In diagnosing SAD, clinicians need to observe whether the child regresses to behaviors that were present at earlier ages; for example, children who stopped wetting the bed might begin bedwetting again as part of a SAD. An additional criterion in diagnosing SAD is the severity of the anxiety reaction. Children often cling, protest, and cry when separated from their parents and/or appear sad and distressed when their caregiver is away. However, children who throw up, cry for hours, and cannot be soothed, exhibit severe nightwaking and bedtime settling problems, and/or suffer from persistent depressive mood might be suffering from SAD. Another criterion often used in diagnosis is the pervasiveness of the reaction. Children who react anxiously or show physical distress in every situation unless they are in close proximity to their parents could be suffering from SAD. Some children express fears that something terrible might happen to them or to their parents, are afraid of being alone, refuse to go to sleep, or express a fear of monsters. Others complain of more diffuse feelings that are disturbing them and have difficulty describing why they are troubled. Children suffering from SAD try to coerce their parents not to separate and may react to separations with anger and aggression. Since some young children suffering from SAD are unable to verbalize their feelings and distress, it is important to look out for physical and somatic symptoms that may be signs of emotional distress. To assess separation anxiety in infants and very young children, the DC: 0–3R (Diagnostic Classification of Mental Health and Developmental Disorders of Infancy and Early Childhood) may be used. Although the DC: 0–3R is intended to diagnose children in the first 3 years of life, it is maintained that SAD is difficult to diagnose at this early age (for reasons we have delineated before).

Clinical and Etiological Consideration

While there is some evidence that secure attachment serves as a protective factor against psychopathology, the link between insecure attachment and anxiety disorders proved difficult to establish. Nevertheless, in the clinical literature on SAD, the child's and parent's failure to develop a secure realtionship is considered a key factor. It is assumed that this failure might arise for different reasons, including the child's temperament or parental mental problems that lead to compromised parent–child relationship. Normal anxiety reactions might become chronic or exaggerated by specific life events or circumstances. Children experiencing prolonged separations,

death of a parent, traumatic events like war, as well as children living with anxious, overprotective, or neglectful parents are more vulnerable to SAD. In young children, even experiences such as vacations or illness might cause difficulties with separation. Bowlby stressed that separation anxiety might be heightened in children who are chronically exposed to actual separations or threats of separation, making them more vulnerable to normally occurring separation events. Clearly, not all children experiencing the above conditions and circumstances develop SAD. So far, risk factors rather than causes of the disorder have been identified. Although the causes of SAD are still unknown, parents who consult with professionals are often told that their own anxiety about separation negatively influences the child's ability to cope with separation. Informed by both the psychoanalytic and the developmental approach, many clinicians view sensitive parental responsiveness to the child's needs and attachment security as protective factors against SAD.

Finally, with respect to intervention and prognosis, clinicians maintain that children who are effectively and timely treated for SAD develop into mentally healthy individuals. When untreated, children with SAD may be at risk for depression and other anxiety disorders. In young children, sleeping and eating problems can be related to SAD; if not treated properly, more complicated problems in these areas might develop. Given the multiple contributing factors, difficulty in diagnosis, and different intervention approaches, there is a need for more research in the field, including longitudinal investigations of the antecedents and consequences of SAD, as well as intervention studies.

See also: Mental Health, Infant.

Suggested Readings

Cassidy J (1999) The nature of the child's ties. In: Cassidy J and Shever PR (eds.) *Handbook of Attachment: Theory, Research and Clinical Applications.* New York: Guilford Press.

Eisen AR and Schaefer CE (2005) *Separation Anxiety in Children and Adolescents: An Individualized Approach to Assessment and Treatment.* New York: Guilford Press.

Emde RN, Gaensbauer TJ, and Harmon RJ (1976) *Emotional Expression in Infancy: A Biobehavioral Study.* New York: International University Press.

Fonagy P and Target M (2003) *Psychoanalytic Theories: Perspectives from Developmental Psychopathology.* London and Philadelphia: Whurr Publishers.

Spitz RA (1965) *The First Year of Life: A Psychoanalytic Study of Normal and Deviant Development of Object Relations.* New York: International Universities Press.

Witherington DC, Campos JJ, and Hertenstein MJ (2001) Principles of emotion and its development. In: Bremner G and Fogel A (eds.) *Blackwell Handbook of Infant Development,* pp. 427–464. Oxford: Blackwell.

Shyness

J B Asendorpf, Humboldt-Universität zu Berlin, Berlin, Germany

Glossary

Behavioral inhibition to the unfamiliar – Tendency to react with wary, inhibited, and sometimes fearful behavior to novel situations and strangers.
Modesty – Tendency to act in a reserved, modest, unassuming way in the presence of others.
Shyness – Tendency in social situations to show inhibited or modest behavior.
Social anxiety – Tendency to react with anxiety to others because of anticipated neglect or rejection.
Social isolation – Being alone because of social neglect or rejection.
Social withdrawal – Being alone because of shyness, social isolation, or unsociability.
Unsociability – Preference to be alone rather than with others.
Wariness to strangers – Wary, inhibited, in older children sometimes also coy behavior to strangers.

Introduction

Shyness is a term deeply rooted in everyday language that, when applied to infants and young children, refers to various forms of modest, reserved, wary, inhibited, anxious, or withdrawn behaviors in social situations, and to a temperamental personality trait. After discussing different facets of shyness (wariness to strangers, behavioral inhibition, social anxiety, and modesty) and distinguishing shyness from related constructs such as social withdrawal, social isolation, and unsociability, a simple developmental model for the development of trait shyness from infancy into early and middle childhood is provided. Finally, the evidence for the long-term outcome of early shyness in adulthood is reviewed.

Shyness: Social Behavior, Affective State, Temperamental Trait

In everyday discourse, 'shy' is used for describing (1) the subjective experience of uneasiness and discomfort in social situations ("I feel shy"); (2) observable modest, reserved, wary, inhibited, mildly anxious, or withdrawn behavior in social situations ("she reacts shy"); and

(3) a recurrent tendency to experience shyness or to react with shyness frequently and intensely ("he is a shy person"). In developmental psychology, shyness in infants and young children refers to (1) an affective state in social situations, characterized by shy behavior and underlying physiological reactions, that may vary from bold disinhibition to a totally inhibiting phobic reaction, or (2) a temperamental personality trait that may vary from boldness to social phobia.

Around 8 months of age, nearly every infant starts reacting shy to adult strangers once in a while, and later most children react shy from time to time in particular situations. Both extreme shyness and the complete absence of shyness indicate problems with social–emotional adaptation. Interindividual differences in shyness to strangers do not show sufficient temporal stability over the first 18 months to be considered a personality trait; only later, they begin to show substantial stability, and this stability increases over childhood. Therefore, shyness can be considered a personality trait not before the second half of the second year. Because this trait refers to an affective state, it is part of children's temperament.

Facets of Shyness and Related Constructs

In this section, four facets of shyness and three psychological constructs that are related to shyness, but not identical with it (see also the glossary for brief definitions), are discussed. These different constructs are used in different research traditions, and the similarities and differences between the constructs are far from clear. Therefore, a careful discussion is in order to avoid confusion of similar but nonidentical constructs.

Wariness to Strangers

When infants and young children are exposed to unfamiliar people, they often react with a specific form of shyness that is called 'wariness to strangers'. Five stages of intensity are commonly distinguished: wary brow (a subtle movement of the eyebrow), wary averted gaze (wary brow plus gaze aversion), avoidance (body movement away from the stranger), cry face (distressed, fearful face without crying), and crying. Wariness to strangers is one of the earliest observable fearful reactions in infants (fear reactions to the visual cliff emerge even earlier). Wariness to strangers can be observed as early as 6 months of age although most infants begin to show this reaction around the age of 8 months.

Wariness to strangers is a normal reaction that peaks in intensity around 12 months of age, and generally lasts into the child's second year. Just as separation anxiety, it is an observable indication that infants are cognitively able to differentiate between familiar and unfamiliar people. Rather than indicating emotional difficulties, the emergence of wariness to strangers and separation anxiety in the second half of the first year is a milestone of mental development.

The setting and way in which the stranger approaches the child can influence how the child may respond. If the stranger approaches slowly when the caregiver is nearby, smiling and speaking softly, offering a toy, the infant will sometimes show interest rather than distress. Experimental variation of stranger characteristics has shown that stronger, more fearful responses are evoked by strangers who approach faster, are taller, and have lower voices. In an intriguing study, infants were exposed either to an unfamiliar adult, an unfamiliar peer, or an unfamiliar midget (small adult). Although the midget was the most unfamiliar type of person, infants responded strongest to the adult, with intermediate intensity to the midget, and with least intensity to the peer. Thus, it is not the discrepancy between a general mental image of human interaction partners and the stranger that evokes wariness of strangers, as assumed by the so-called discrepancy hypothesis, it is the unfamiliarity of the stranger paired with cues that signal danger (fast approach, body size, low voice).

The predominantly negative reactions to strangers in the first and second year of life are later followed by emotionally ambivalent responses that consist of both negative and positive components, particularly a coy smile. A coy smile is a smile during a wary averted gaze, signaling both approach and avoidance motivation. Ambivalent responses to strangers peak around the age of 3 years, and then decrease in intensity.

Detailed analyses of the videotaped behavior of the caretakers that accompany infants and children during encounters with strangers have shown that most caretakers also react with mild forms of wariness, particularly a wary brow, a coy smile, or a brief wary averted gaze. These studies support a 'social referencing' hypothesis according to which the caretaker's reaction is an important cue even for 8-month-olds on how to react to the stranger: The stronger the caretaker responds with wariness, the stronger the infant responds.

The intensity of wariness to strangers varies greatly among agemates. One source of inter-individual differences is the different developmental onset of the wary reaction. For example, some 8-month-olds will not show any wary behavior simply because they are not yet cognitively able to differentiate between familiar and unfamiliar people, and some 15-month-olds may react only slightly

more because their wariness peaked already at 12 months, whereas some of their agemates just reached the peak of their responsivity.

If this source of interindividual differences is controlled in longitudinal studies that compare infants at their individual peak of responsivity, substantial interindividual differences remain that are often considered as an early form of trait shyness or trait fearfulness. However, both the cross-situational consistency and the temporal stability of these inter-individual differences are so low that such a trait interpretation is not valid.

Shy behavior reaches sufficient consistency across different unfamiliar people and sufficient temporal stability, not before the end of the second year of life. At this age, it begins to show consistency not only between adult and peer strangers but also between unfamiliar social and nonsocial situations. For example, a 2-year-old who reacts with strong wariness to a stranger is expected to explore unfamiliar rooms rather slowly, even if no stranger is present. At this age, a first form of trait shyness can be observed which is called behavioral inhibition to the unfamiliar.

Behavioral Inhibition

'Behavioral inhibition to the unfamiliar' is a term introduced by Kagan and associates in 1984 that refers to a temperamental trait of young children. According to both parental reports and behavioral observations in the laboratory, approximately 15% of toddlers react with marked inhibition to novel situations or unfamiliar adults and peers. They cease their play behavior and withdraw to the proximity of their caregivers, remaining vigilant of the situation and rarely approaching novel objects or unfamiliar people.

Behavioral inhibition has been initially studied by comparing extreme groups of young children characterized by very high or very low inhibition. Later research in North America, Europe, and China has shown that interindividual differences in behavioral inhibition are gradually, continuously distributed and show moderate stability over childhood.

Building on neuroscience models of fear, Kagan suggested that high behavioral inhibition in infancy is due to an overactive amygdala, resulting in an enhanced fear response to unfamiliar situations. This hypothesis relates to early forms of behavioral inhibition that are mainly based on initial affective response tendencies. One prediction is that inhibited children should show higher heart rate and heart rate acceleration in response to novel stimuli, another prediction is that inhibited children should show higher salivary cortisol levels. Both predictions have only found mixed support, however.

Concerning precursors of interindividual differences in behavioral inhibition, behavioral inhibition after age 2 years shows only weak correlations with the intensity of wariness to strangers during the first 18 months of life. It seems that the many and profound changes in toddlers' cognitive ability during the second year affect also interindividual differences in reactions to novelty. It is assumed that the ability to understand social norms and rules and the ability to self-regulate one's affective responses according to such rules that both begin to emerge during the second year are important sources of interindividual differences that overlay the earlier developing interindividual differences in wariness to novelty.

Indeed, research on the development of self-regulation in infants and young children has described a gradual transfer of control over affective responses at both the behavioral and the neural level. Whereas infants' responses are initially governed only by affective response tendencies generated predominantly by the limbic system, with age and cortical development, cognitive control capacities such as response inhibition and attentional control increase, allowing for a greater cortical control over the initial response tendencies.

Concerning the later development of behavioral inhibition over childhood, children show an increasing repertoire of behaviors in response to novel situations and strangers, and despite a moderate stability of interindividual differences over shorter time periods, there is much evidence for long-term differential change in behavioral inhibition. Behavioral inhibition is by no means a fixed temperamental trait. The main reason seems to be, again, children's increasing ability to self-regulate their attention and initial affective responses.

For behaviorally inhibited children, the shifting of attention to a different aspect of a situation, or distracting oneself, can be an effective means of regulating their emotional distress in novel situations. Another means of coping with novelty that is more difficult to study in young children is the cognitive re-assessment of the situation as less dangerous or arousing. Indeed, there is increasing evidence that the emerging interindividual difference in self-regulation over childhood moderates the stability of the early temperament-based affective reactions to novel situations.

Research by Eisenberg and colleagues took up the hypothesis originally put forward by Rothbart and Bates that the development of 'effortful self-regulation' leads to important changes in children's temperament-based reactions. Effortful control is commonly defined as the efficiency of executive attention, including the ability to inhibit a dominant response and/or to activate a subdominant response, to plan ahead, and to detect errors. It involves abilities to focus or shift attention as needed, and to activate or inhibit behavior as needed. Eisenberg and colleagues distinguished effortful control from reactive control that is less under voluntary control, such as behavioral inhibition as an immediate reaction to unfamiliarity. They found some evidence that effortful control fosters

the skills needed to get along with others and to engage in socially constructive behavior. Although effortful control seems to be most effective for preventing problems due to reactive undercontrol (high impulsivity), there is also some evidence that the ability for effortful control also helps children disposed to reactive overcontrol (high behavioral inhibition) in self-regulating their initially inhibited response to strangers.

Indirect evidence is also provided by a longitudinal study by Asendorpf who found that social competence as judged by preschool teachers and general intelligence as assessed by standard intelligence quotient (IQ) tests both moderated the long-term outcome of preschool inhibition: more competent and more intelligent children were better able to overcome inhibition in both laboratory and school settings. There is much evidence that more socially competent and more intelligent children are better able to self-regulate their reactivity, and therefore Asendorpf's finding may be interpreted in terms of the enhanced self-regulation ability of the more competent children.

Other studies have focused on interactions between behavioral inhibition and attachment to parents. There is some evidence that infants' early temperamental characteristics influence the development of both behavioral inhibition and anxious-ambivalent attachment. For example, in a 2-year longitudinal study by Fox and colleagues, observed distress to the withdrawal of a pacifier at 2 days of age was related to insecure attachment at 14 months, and reactivity to novelty at 5 months was related to inhibition at 14 months.

Furthermore, anxious-ambivalent attachment to parents may impede the self-regulation of behavioral inhibition. For example, in the above longitudinal study, anxious-ambivalent attachment at 14 months was related to behavioral inhibition at 24 months. In addition, a temperament by attachment interaction was found. Infants who were classified as anxious-ambivalent with their mother at 14 months and who had not cried to an arm restraint procedure at 5 months were the most inhibited at 24 months.

The few studies of attachment–temperament interactions over the first years of life suggest neither a main effects model for temperament (later inhibition is due to early temperament independent of attachment) nor a main effects model for attachment (later inhibition is due to early attachment independent of temperament). Instead, these studies suggest a transactional model such that early differences between infants in temperament, together with differences between parents in the sensitivity to their child's needs, give rise to insecure attachment to the parents which, in turn, interacts with infants' increasing self-regulation ability in unfamiliar situations.

More recently, behavioral inhibition has found increasing attention by clinical child psychologists because a few studies have shown that strong behavioral inhibition in early childhood is a risk factor for diagnosed anxiety disorders later in childhood and in early adolescence, particularly social anxiety disorders. Therefore, intervention programs have been developed that aim at reducing this risk. For example, Rapee and colleagues developed a short-term educational program designed to help parents of preschool-aged children with withdrawn/inhibited behaviors to better understand their child's problem and to better support the child in overcoming inhibition and anxiety. The children were randomly allocated to the education condition, or to no intervention. The children whose parents participated in the educational program showed significantly lower anxiety 1 year after the end of the intervention, as compared to the children in the control condition. However, no effects of the program were observed on measures of inhibition/withdrawal. This pattern of results suggests that the intervention affected children's subjective experience of anxiety but not their temperament.

Social Anxiety

As the more clinically oriented studies of behavioral inhibition show, behavioral inhibition is linked to social anxiety in childhood and adolescence. However, behavioral inhibition should not be equated with social anxiety for three reasons. First, behavioral inhibition is more general because it refers also to nonsocial situations. Second, it refers to observed behavior whereas anxiety refers to both behavior and subjective experience. One important consequence is that studies of social anxiety in older children sometimes include interview data or self-reports of their experience in social situations. Third, and most importantly, social anxiety is the more general concept for social situations because it includes fearful, anxious responses also in response to familiar people or situations.

Studies of social anxiety in adolescence and adulthood show that a main reason for anxious reactions in social situations are concerns of being negatively or insufficiently positively evaluated by others (familiar or unfamiliar). Asendorpf suggested the hypothesis that shy behavior in children might be linked to either behavioral inhibition (thus, to children's temperament) or to acquired fears of being negatively evaluated or ignored by others (thus, to social experiences).

He interpreted this two-factor model of shy behavior in terms of the temperamental theory of Gray. Based on his animal and psychopharmological research, Gray proposed the existence of a behavioral inhibition system at the neurophysiological level that mediates responses to three kinds of stimuli: novel stimuli, conditioned cues for punishment, and conditioned cues for frustrative nonreward. According to Gray, any such stimulus evokes behavioral inhibition, increased physiological arousal, and increased attention. Interindividual differences arise

due to a different sensitivity (strength) of this behavioral inhibition system, and to interindividual differences in learning history (how many and which stimuli become cues for punishment or frustrative nonreward through conditioning).

Asendorpf applied this model to shy behavior in children (see **Figure 1**). According to this model, either strangers or cues for being rejected or ignored by others trigger the behavioral inhibition system in social situations. The resulting inhibitory tendencies are responsible for the reactivity component of both behavioral inhibition to the unfamiliar and social-evaluative concerns.

Whether these inhibitory tendencies result in shy behavior depends on the child's self-regulatory abilities (see **Figure 1**). Furthermore, the child can modify the situation by both self-regulation ability (e.g., when a person that arouses fear is revaluated as being more friendly) and by overt behavior (e.g., by presenting oneself as modest and nonassuming in order to prevent criticism). These abilities to cope with inhibiting situations increase as children grow older and ultimately may be more important than their underlying temperament or earlier experiences with others.

According to this concept of shyness, a child may react shy to a particular person because of a temperamental disposition that may be genetically based or due to early caregiving, or because the child has been often rejected or ignored by this person (a parent, a sibling, or a familiar peer).

Because the second experiential source of shyness also triggers the behavioral inhibition system, it interacts with the temperamental source in a predictable way (amplification of response). Thus, a child with a 'weak' behavioral inhibition system that is often rejected by the parents may nonetheless not become shy whereas a child with a 'strong' behavioral inhibition system that is moderately rejected or ignored by the parents may nonetheless become shy in their presence. First evidence for this two-factor model of shyness in children was provided

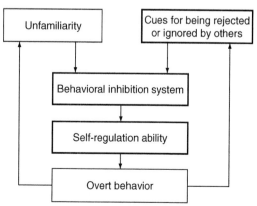

Figure 1 A three-factor model of shyness. Bold lines indicate sources of interindividual differences.

by Asendorpf in 1990. German children were observed in confrontations with adult and peer strangers in the laboratory, in their preschool and kindergarten peer group, and in play situations with a familiar peer in their familiar preschool. As expected, observed shyness was consistent between adult and peer strangers, but inconsistent between unfamiliar and familiar peers. Thus, a child who reacted with strong inhibition to an adult stranger in the laboratory tended to react also with strong inhibition to an unfamiliar peer in the same laboratory setting, but its shyness to a familiar peer was unrelated to its inhibition to peer or adult strangers.

Longitudinal analyses in the classroom showed an increasing influence of peer neglect or rejection on shyness in the classroom. Follow-ups of extreme groups with stable inhibition toward strangers vs. stable shyness in the more familiar peer group in the second and third year in preschool revealed that stable high inhibition toward strangers was unrelated to self-esteem up to age 12 years, whereas stable high shyness in the familiar peer group significantly predicted low social self-esteem between 8 and 12 years of age. Thus, shyness in the familiar peer group which was very likely due to social-evaluative concerns was a risk factor for internalizing problems throughout childhood but not inhibition toward strangers. In line with this finding, a more recent longitudinal study also showed that early peer neglect and rejection in preschool increased the risk of developing stable social anxiety and depression.

Because temperament is more likely stable than experiences of peer neglect or rejection across different peer groups, the consistency between inhibition to the unfamiliar and social-evaluative anxiety is expected to increase with age. This hypothesis was confirmed in another longitudinal study where inhibition to strangers was not correlated with negative peer relationships in late childhood, but in early adulthood. The bottom line of this developmental model of shyness in childhood is that shyness is the outcome of a continuous transaction of stable temperament and fluctuating social-evaluative experiences. During this transaction, the two initially independent factors become more and more correlated, and are hard to distinguish in adulthood. In early childhood, however, shyness due to the temperamental factor and shyness due to social anxiety can and should be distinguished. The former can be identified in its purest form in encounters with strangers, the latter in evaluative situations with familiar people.

Modesty

Shyness is not only used to describe children who react inhibited but also to describe children who act in a reserved, modest, unassuming way in the presence of others, without signs of fear or anxiety. As the model in Figure 1 suggests, modesty can be an outcome of self-regulated inhibition, but this is not necessarily the case; children may be simply socialized to behave in a modest way. It depends then on the cultural norm for modesty – how often modesty is the outcome of self-regulated inhibition and how often it is the result of socialization favoring modesty.

This cultural influence became first obvious to developmental psychologists in a cross-cultural study by Chen who compared the peer reputation of shy-sensitive children, defined as shy, usually sad, and easily hurt by others, between Canada and mainland China in 1990. Whereas these children were less popular among their peers in Canada, they were above-average popular in China and showed superior school adjustment. The authors interpreted this result as the influence of the Confucian norm for modesty in China at the threshold of westernization. In line with this interpretation, studies carried out 8 and 12 years later could not replicate the Chinese results; instead, shy-sensitive Chinese children in large cities today are as low in peer popularity and school adjustment as in Western cultures.

These findings highlight the problem that shy behavior may be due to inhibition but also to self-regulation according to cultural norms favoring modesty, without underlying inhibition. The bottom line is that three different types of shyness in children can be distinguished: stranger shyness (behavioral inhibition to the unfamiliar), anxious shyness (behavioral inhibition to social-evaluative cues), and regulated shyness (self-controlled social restraint characterized by modesty and an unassuming demeanor).

Shyness vs. Social Withdrawal, Social Isolation, and Unsociability

It is important to distinguish shyness from social withdrawal, or solitary behavior, because solitary behavior can be due not only to inhibition and modesty but also to social isolation (sometimes also called social exclusion) and to unsociability, that is, a genuine preference for being alone rather than with others.

Social isolation occurs when children are rejected by their peers. Shy children are neglected by their peers rather than rejected (see also next section). Children are more often rejected by peers because of high aggressiveness. Aggressive-rejected children show a characteristic form of solitary behavior, often called solitary-active behavior, consisting of often-repeated sensorimotor activity and solitary dramatic play. For example, they move a play car back and forth for a long time, run around without any purpose, or pretend to be a famous movie star or a wild animal without interacting with others. Obviously, this would not be called shy behavior.

More difficult is the distinction between shyness and unsociability. Uninformed adults often believe that children are social by nature; therefore, they believe that children who spend much time with solitary behavior have some social or emotional problem. Research by Rubin and colleagues has shown, however, that solitary activity in early childhood is not necessarily problematic. Children's solitary-passive activity defined as exploratory and constructive solitary play in the presence of peers can be the outcome of a successful self-regulation of behavioral inhibition to the unfamiliar (if the peers are unfamiliar) or of social anxiety, of a norm for modesty (they would like to play with others but are socialized to wait until others approach them), or simply because they prefer to explore and play alone.

Indeed, children can be classified in terms of their dominant social motivation as being sociable (they prefer being with others rather than being alone), as being unsociable (they prefer to be alone rather than with others), as shy (they would like to be with others but do not dare to approach them because of inhibition or an internalized norm for modesty), or as avoidant (they avoid others because of experiences of rejection, without any motivation to approach them). From this motivational perspective, shyness is characterized by an approach-avoidance conflict rather than pure avoidance, and shyness is different from unsociability which is characterized by a lack of both approach and avoidance tendencies.

Development of Shyness: Infancy to Middle Childhood

Many cross-sectional and a few longitudinal studies have been conducted on the development of shyness from infancy to middle childhood. The major findings within a simple developmental model that borrows much from similar, more complex models by Rubin and colleagues (see **Figure 2**), are discussed.

Genetic and early environmental risks lead to an infant temperament that was described in the classic work by Thomas and Chess as 'slow-to-warm-up', and that is characterized in the second year of life by behavioral inhibition to the unfamiliar. In terms of the temperamental model shown in **Figure 1**, this early temperament is due to a strong behavioral inhibition system. Behavior genetic studies have supported that a substantial portion of the observed variability in behavioral inhibition in the second year of life is due to genetic differences, but currently the relevant genes are still unknown. Concerning early

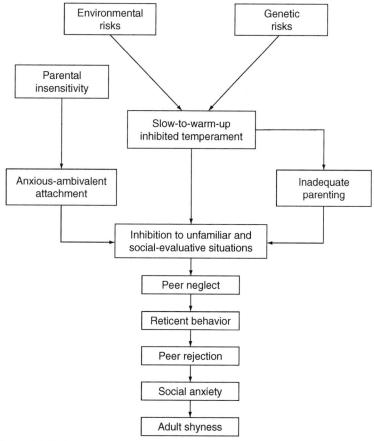

Figure 2 A developmental model of shyness.

environmental influences on behavioral inhibition, only few specific pre- and perinatal risk factors are known.

Interestingly, one is the season of pregnancy. Studies have replicated for both North American and Australian samples that mid-pregnancy at the time of the year with the shortest daylight (December in North America, June in Australia) is a risk factor for behavioral inhibition. This might be less surprising as it seems because hormones such as melatonin and serotonin vary with daylight intensity, and play some role in neuroscience models of fear and behavioral inhibition.

As already discussed in the section on behavioral inhibition, this early temperamental trait, together with parental insensitivity, increases the risk for an anxious-ambivalent attachment to the parents and inadequate responses by the parents to the child such as overprotection or rejection. Anxious-ambivalent attachment as well as inadequate parenting, particularly involving rejection or neglect of the child, reinforce children's inhibitory tendencies, not only to unfamiliar situations but also to familiar social-evaluative situations, resulting at the end of the second year of life in a shy, somewhat socially anxious child who is sensitive to unfamiliar situations and criticism by others.

When such children enter the unfamiliar social world of preschool, they face the risk of being ignored (but initially not rejected) by their peers which, in turn, leads to reticent behavior such as long phases of just looking at others, being unoccupied without playing, and socially wary behaviors, and social-evaluative concerns of being insufficiently accepted by the peers.

Around second grade peers become more and more aware that these reticent children deviate from the age-appropriate pattern of social interaction which increases the risk that they now reject the reticent children. Such peer rejection, in turn, increases social-evaluative anxiety and social withdrawal. If these children later during adolescence also face rejection by their potential dating and sexual partners, adult shyness likely results.

It is important to note that, in line with modern developmental psychology, this is a multifactor model of development where a single factor alone has little to no influence on development; what counts is the interaction between multiple risk factors. Also, personality traits such as early temperament alone are not sufficient for explaining later development; what counts is the transaction between personality and environment over age.

Long-Term Outcome of Early Shyness

The earliest evidence for a predictable long-term outcome of shyness in adulthood came from Kagan's analysis of data from the Fels Longitudinal Study where two measures of observed anxiety in unfamiliar social situations at ages 3–6 years were both significantly correlated with social anxiety in adulthood. The later extensive studies of temperamental inhibition by Kagan and associates did not result in reports about significant predictions from early inhibition toward the unfamiliar to adulthood personality or social–emotional adaptation. However, only a small number of children were followed into adulthood in these latter studies such that firm conclusions about the long-term effects of early temperamental inhibition cannot be drawn.

Much better evidence for the long-term outcome of early inhibition is provided by the Dunedin Longitudinal Study which follows a large, representative New Zealand birth cohort into adulthood. Based on behavioral observations in various situations, 8% of the sample were classified by Caspi and colleagues as inhibited at age 3 years and followed up until age 26 years. Compared to a control group of well-adjusted children (40% of the sample), the inhibited children reported more harm avoidance, less social potency, and positive emotionality at both ages 18 and 26 years, and at age 26 years were described by informants as lower in extraversion but not higher in neuroticism. Psychiatric interviews at age 21 years showed that the inhibited children were not more likely to have anxiety disorders of various kinds, including social phobia, but were more often depressed and had more often attempted suicide.

Thus, the evidence for internalizing disorders in adulthood for formerly extremely inhibited children was mixed. Importantly, social phobia was not related to early inhibition, neither we are aware of any other prospective longitudinal study into adulthood that has shown this, contrary to frequent claims in the clinical literature based on retrospective reports of adults. Thus, despite findings that early inhibition predicts social anxiety and phobia during childhood and early adolescence, early inhibition has not been found to be a risk factor for adult anxieties including social phobia.

With regard to life course sequelae of childhood inhibition, two longitudinal studies reported delays in social transitions for children classified as inhibited in middle childhood. In their reanalysis of the Berkeley Guidance Study, Caspi and colleagues found such delays only for inhibited boys at ages 8–10 years. These inhibited boys married 3 years later, became fathers 4 years later, and entered a stable occupational career 3 years later than the remaining boys. No such delays were found for the inhibited girls; instead, these girls became women who spent less time in the labor force and married men with higher occupational status. This should not be attributed to instability of female inhibition because inhibition as assessed in clinical interviews at ages 30 and 40 years correlated significantly with both boys' and girls' inhibition. The strong sex difference in the outcomes can be attributed to the traditional gender roles for this 1928 birth cohort that required action and social contacts, particularly from men.

In an attempt to replicate these life-course patterns in a 1955–58 Swedish cohort, Kerr and colleagues studied children who were rated as shy with unfamiliar people by their mothers at ages 8–10 years when they were 25 and 35 years old. Self-judgments of inhibition at age 35 years correlated with childhood inhibition significantly for females but not at all for males. Inhibited boys married 4 years later than controls and became fathers 3 years later; shy girls were educational underachievers, that is, reached a lower educational level after controlling for IQ. No effects on the number of job changes or monthly income were observed. Thus, this study replicated the delays for inhibited boys regarding marriage and parenthood as well as the absence of this effect for girls; unfortunately, the age at the time of beginning a stable career was not recorded.

In a recent follow-up of the Munich Longitudinal Study on the Genesis of Individual Competencies (LOGIC), Asendorpf and colleagues replicated the findings of delayed social transitions into adulthood not only for boys but also for girls, and also found a low stability of shyness between early childhood and adulthood. In this 19-year longitudinal study, the 15% most shy children at ages 4–6 years in a normal German sample were targeted by teacher judgments, and were compared with controls who were below average in preschool shyness. As adults, shy boys and girls were judged as shy by their parents and showed a delay in their first stable partnership and their first full-time job. This diminishing of a sex difference found in earlier generations was not unexpected because the LOGIC participants grew up in a culture characterized by more egalitarian gender roles than one or two generations earlier. Only the upper 8% in terms of shyness tended to show internalizing problems, including self-rated shyness; this tendency was of a similar effect size as in the Dunedin Longitudinal Study but not significant because of the smaller longitudinal sample.

Together, these longitudinal studies draw a consistent picture of the long-term consequences of early shyness. There is some stability of the core temperamental trait of inhibition to unfamiliar situations. This temperamental trait makes it more difficult for inhibited persons to cope with social life transitions where they are confronted with unfamiliar people. They are 'slow-to-warm-up' in such situations even as adults when they meet dating partners, enter new educational settings such as university, and apply for jobs which results in delayed social development.

This early temperamental core of shyness interacts so strongly with parental and peer influences over development that it is detectable in adults' self-judgments only in cases of extremely high childhood inhibition. Besides that, according to our present knowledge, early shyness does not lead to any identified psychological problems in adulthood, particularly not to social phobia.

Suggested Readings

Asendorpf JB (1990) Development of inhibition during childhood: Evidence for situational specificity and a two-factor model. *Developmental Psychology* 26: 721–730.

Caspi A (2000) The child is the father of the man: Personality continuities from childhood to adulthood. *Journal of Personality and Social Psychology* 78: 158–172.

Chen X, Cen G, Li D, and He Y (2005) Social functioning and adjustment in Chinese children: The imprint of historical time. *Child Development* 76: 182–195.

Kagan J and Snidman N (2004) *The Long Shadow of Temperament.* Cambridge, MA: Harvard University Press.

Rubin KH and Asendorpf JB (eds.) (1993) *Social Withdrawal, Inhibition, and Shyness in Childhood.* Hillsdale, NJ: Lawrence Erlbaum.

SIDS

T G Keens, Keck School of Medicine of the University of Southern California, Los Angeles, CA, USA
D R Gemmill, California Sudden Infant Death Syndrome Advisory Council, Escondido, CA, USA

Glossary

Apnea – Stopping breathing. This usually refers to a breathing pause at least 20 s in duration.

Bedsharing – An infant sleeping in the same bed with one or more other people.

CHIME study – Collaborative Home Infant Monitoring Evaluation research project. This was a multicenter research study, funded in the National Institutes of Health in 1991–99. The study used custom-designed home monitors to study breathing, heart rate, and oxygen in over 1000 infants in their own homes during the first 6 months of life.

Electrocardiogram (ECG) – A diagnostic test to assess the rhythm and structure of the heart.

Home apnea–bradycardia monitoring –
Commercial devices which monitor breathing and
heartbeat, sounding a loud audible alarm when
breathing stops for a designated time (usually 20 s)
or heart rate falls below a designated rate. These
monitors are designed to alert caregivers when a
baby stops breathing or heart rate falls.

Hypercapnia – Abnormally elevated carbon dioxide
levels in blood or tissues. Blood CO_2 is a measure of
the adequacy of breathing, and hypercapnia
indicates inadequate breathing or respiratory failure.

Hypoxia – Abnormally low oxygen levels in blood or
tissues.

Intrathoracic petechiae – Pinpoint hemorrhages on
the surfaces of organs in the chest. These are
commonly seen in sudden infant death syndrome
victims, but unusual in other causes of infant death.

Overlaying – Smothering an infant by lying on it
during sleep.

Polymorphisms – Variations in gene structure that
occur as variants in a normal population. These
polymorphisms may be associated with quantitative
variations in gene function that may predispose to
disease.

Prone sleeping – Sleeping on the stomach.

Sudden infant death syndrome (SIDS) – The
sudden unexpected death of an infant, under 1 year
of age, with onset of the fatal episode apparently
occurring during sleep, that remains unexplained
after a thorough investigation, including performance
of a complete autopsy, and review of the
circumstances of death and the clinical history.

Supine sleeping – Sleeping on the back.

Introduction

> And this woman's son died in the night . . .
>
> 1 Kings, 3: 19 (∼950 B.C.E.)

Sudden infant death syndrome (SIDS) is the sudden
unexpected death of an infant under 1 year of age, with
onset of the fatal episode apparently occurring during
sleep, that remains unexplained after a thorough investigation, including performance of a complete autopsy
and review of the circumstances of death and the clinical
history. For 3000 years, it has been recognized that apparently healthy infants could die suddenly and unexpectedly during their sleep. Throughout most of history, it was
believed that these infants somehow suffocated, either
by maternal overlaying or by strangling in bedclothes.

Although these explanations have largely been discarded,
one infant per 2000 live births continues to die suddenly
and unexpectedly from SIDS.

A typical clinical course for an SIDS death is that the
parents or caregivers put their infant to sleep, either at night
or during a daytime nap. They return at some later time to
find that the infant has died unexpectedly. Usually, these
infants were healthy prior to death, although some had
evidence of a mild upper respiratory infection. SIDS deaths
have occurred when parents or caregivers have placed their
infants down for a nap, have been within hearing distance of
the infant the entire time, and have returned as briefly as
30 min later to find that their infant has died. Yet, these
parents report hearing no signs of a struggle. Thus, SIDS
deaths appear to occur swiftly and silently.

By definition, the etiology of SIDS is not known. In
approximately 20% of infants who die suddenly and
unexpectedly, a conventionally accepted cause for the
death is found at postmortem examination. These infants
are not said to have died from SIDS, but rather from the
cause of death found by the postmortem examination.
The remainder, in whom no cause of death could be
found, comprises the group called SIDS.

SIDS is the most common cause of infant death between
the ages of 1 month and 1 year. During the 1980s in most
Western countries, SIDS killed approximately 1.5 infants
out of every 1000 live births, or approximately one in every
650 live births. Since 1990, the SIDS rate has steadily fallen,
in conjunction with greater attention to the infant sleeping
environment, and there were approximately 0.5 SIDS
deaths per 1000 live births in 2003. SIDS rates for less
developed countries are probably not accurate, since these
countries have high infant death rates from respiratory,
diarrhea, and infectious disorders, and many SIDS deaths
may be lost in these statistics (**Figure 1**).

By definition, SIDS occurs in the first year of life.
The peak age is 2–4 postnatal months. SIDS is relatively

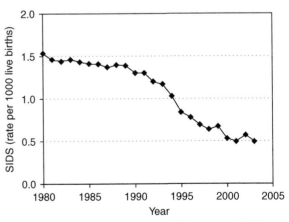

Figure 1   SIDS rates in the US. The SIDS rate per 1000 live
births, is plotted for each year from 1980 through 2003.

less common in the first month of life, and 95% of SIDS deaths occur before 6 months of age. This is a unique age distribution, which differs from that of other natural causes of infant death, where the death rate is usually highest near birth and falls off with increasing age. SIDS tends to be more common in winter months than in summer months. The reasons for these distributions are unknown.

Diagnosis

The diagnosis of SIDS can only be made in an infant who has died. There is no known less severe form of SIDS in a living infant, and SIDS cannot be predicted in any infant prior to death. Many states and countries require that sudden infant deaths must be investigated to determine a cause of death. Ideally, in order to accurately diagnose SIDS, there should be an examination of the death scene performed by a qualified investigator, and an autopsy on the baby performed by a qualified forensic or pediatric pathologist. Death scene investigation protocols and autopsy protocols have been developed, and many authorities urge the use of these standardized protocols in order to improve the accuracy and consistency of diagnosis. The diagnosis of SIDS should be used as the cause of death when an infant meets this definition: (1) under 1 year of age; (2) death was sudden and unexpected; (3) death occurred when the infant was thought to be asleep; (4) examination of the death scene reveals no alternative cause of death; (5) autopsy reveals no identifiable cause of death; and (6) the case history does not indicate a medical problem which could have caused the death.

In some jurisdictions, medical examiners are reluctant to use the SIDS diagnosis if there is a question about other factors that may have contributed to the death, such as bedsharing or dangerous sleeping environments. In such cases, a diagnosis of undetermined cause of death is frequently used. Unless there is convincing evidence suggesting a cause of death other than SIDS, use of the term 'SIDS' is recommended, as this avails parents of SIDS supportive services and makes research dependent on these diagnoses valid.

By definition, an identifiable cause of death is not found at postmortem examination. The autopsy of an SIDS victim shows the absence of other serious illness that could contribute to the death, no signs of severe illness, and no signs of significant stress. However, common postmortem findings in the SIDS victim include: intrathoracic petechiae; pulmonary congestion and edema; minor airway inflammation (not severe enough to cause death); minimal stress effects in the thymus and adrenal glands; and normal nutrition and development. The significance of the latter four of these findings is that these

infants were generally healthy prior to death. Neither epidemiologic studies nor the postmortem findings have resulted in a generally accepted cause for SIDS. The cause remains unknown, though current research efforts are making advances in our knowledge, which may ultimately lead to this answer.

Epidemiology

Epidemiologic studies have been performed in an attempt to identify risk factors for SIDS. When a risk factor is found in a population, the statistical risk of SIDS occurring in those infants who have the risk factor is increased. However, risk factors are not causes of SIDS, although they may provide clues for researchers to the cause of SIDS. Therefore, they are important for research. However, no risk factor, singly or in combination, is sufficiently precise to predict the baby who will die from SIDS. Further, many SIDS victims had few, if any, risk factors prior to death.

Maternal factors associated with a statistically increased risk for SIDS include: cigarette smoking or substance abuse (specifically opiates or cocaine) during pregnancy, teenaged and older mothers, increasing birth order, short interpregnancy intervals, delay in initiating prenatal care, unmarried mothers, low blood pressure during the third trimester of pregnancy, and high or low hemoglobin during late gestation. SIDS is more common in lower socioeconomic groups. SIDS is more common in African Americans, and in indigenous populations around the world (Native Americans, Eskimos, Aborigines, Maoris, etc.). Although these studies do not point to a specific etiology, some investigators believe that they suggest that infants who had a suboptimal intrauterine environment may be at a higher risk of dying from SIDS.

Infant factors that are associated with a statistically increased risk for SIDS include: preterm birth, low birth weight, and multiple gestation (twins, triplets, etc.). Often, SIDS deaths are temporally associated with viral respiratory infections, though often when the infection appeared to be resolving. Recently, many factors associated with the infant sleeping environment have been associated with an increased SIDS risk. Some factors include prone sleeping; soft bedding, pillows, and stuffed toys in the bed; cigarette smoking around babies; overheating; and bedsharing. These risk factors can potentially be modified. Public health programs designed to modify these risks have successfully decreased the number of SIDS deaths by over half.

Epidemiological studies have been invaluable in helping to decrease the number of babies dying from SIDS. However, many infants who died from SIDS had few if any of these risk factors. Therefore, they are not the cause of SIDS.

Research on the Cause of SIDS

The cause of SIDS is not known. There are no tests that can be performed on living infants that will predict SIDS. SIDS appears to be the result of a natural process. SIDS deaths do not occur because of something SIDS parents did or failed to do. SIDS is probably not as simple as one abnormality in one physiological system. Filiano and Kinney suggested that SIDS is likely due to an interaction of: (1) a developmental window of vulnerability; (2) intrinsic physiological differences in infants affecting each one's vulnerability; and (3) environmental factors. An infant's vulnerability may lie latent until the infant reaches a developmental window of vulnerability and is exposed to an external stressor. Thus, it is likely that an understanding of the etiology of SIDS will require a new paradigm for understanding human disease (**Figure 2**).

Cardiac arrhythmias. When one thinks of sudden death, one usually thinks of heart failure or respiratory failure. Some investigators have described genetic abnormalities of cardiac repolarization, which may predispose infants to the sudden development of fatal cardiac arrhythmias. These would not be able to be detected postmortem. However, a large study in Italy, by Schwartz and colleagues, suggests that the prolonged QT interval syndrome may cause a number of SIDS deaths. We now know that several genetic mutations, which can be detected in

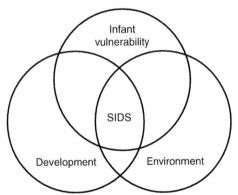

Figure 2 The triple risk model of SIDS. This model visualizes the concept that SIDS is likely due to the interaction of many factors. The risk of an infant dying from SIDS is represented by the area of overlap of all three circles. The top circle represents an infant's vulnerability. Different infants may have different sized circles based on genetic variations or other differences in physiology. The circle on the left is affected by age. Two-to-four months of age represent a developmental window of vulnerability, where the SIDS risk is highest, and the circle would be largest. It would be much smaller for a 1-week-old infant or an 11-month-old infant. The circle on the right represents environment. Prone sleeping, exposure to cigarette smoke, overheating, etc., increase the risk of SIDS. Modified from Filiano JJ and Kinney HC (1994) A perspective on neuropathologic findings in victims of the sudden infant death syndrome: The triple-risk model. *Biology of the Neonate* 65: 194–197.

postmortem tissues by DNA testing, may have been present in some infants who have died. This research indicates that these types of cardiac abnormalities can cause sudden death, which is indistinguishable from SIDS. However, it is unclear if these rare genetic disorders comprise a substantial proportion of SIDS. Since it is not known if these disorders are frequent, there is not enough evidence to suggest that infants should be routinely screened with electrocardiograms (ECGs) to attempt to identify such abnormalities prior to death.

Apnea. Another possibility is that SIDS may be due to a sudden respiratory arrest, or apnea (prolonged breathing pause). This has been a popular hypothesis for many years, but more recently it has fallen from favor. There appears to be little evidence that an isolated apnea is the cause of SIDS. The use of home apnea–bradycardia monitors, which sound an alarm if an infant stops breathing for 20 s or longer or the heart rate drops below set levels, has not resulted in a drop in the SIDS rate, and it is not currently recommended as a strategy to prevent SIDS. Nevertheless, there are significant cardiorespiratory interactions, which may explain SIDS deaths through perturbations of the autonomic nervous system.

Brainstem dysfunction. Most researchers believe that the origin of the cause of SIDS lies in dysfunction of the portions of the brain involved in 'life support'. SIDS occurs during sleep. Sleep disrupts breathing, and this causes hypoxia, even in normal infants not destined to die from SIDS. The low oxygen resulting from an apnea is probably not sufficient to directly cause an infant's death. However, research from postmortem examinations of SIDS victims finds abnormalities in certain parts of the brainstem, which are thought to be important in the control of breathing and/or protective mechanisms when breathing fails. This suggests that many SIDS victims had abnormalities in the way their brains responded to environmental stresses, such as high carbon dioxide (CO_2) or low oxygen. High CO_2 and low oxygen can result from a prolonged apnea.

Arousal (waking up). Arousal is an important defense against danger-signaling stimuli during sleep, and many SIDS researchers believe that a failure to arouse in response to such stimuli may contribute to SIDS. Thus, a great deal of research has been done on a normal infant's ability to be aroused in response to a variety of stimuli, including respiratory stimuli. Infants in the first month of life are better able to be aroused in response to low oxygen than older infants. The decrease in this hypoxic arousal corresponds to the increased risk of SIDS at 2–4 months of age. It is possible that this brainstem-mediated hypoxic arousal response is lost with growth, as cortical development inhibits more 'primitive' brainstem responses. The late Andre Kahn and colleagues performed research sleep studies on thousands of infants in Europe, some of whom subsequently died from SIDS. Kato and Kahn found that those infants who subsequently died from SIDS had fewer spontaneous arousals during sleep than infants who did not die. Further, SIDS victims had more subcortical arousals, detected by electroencephalogram (EEG) criteria. However, these subcortical arousals failed to progress to cortical arousals that would allow an infant to fully awaken and respond to a potentially dangerous situation. Franco and Kahn found that infants with some SIDS risk factors had impaired arousal responses to sound. More research is required in this area. Nevertheless, these results suggest that infants with impaired spontaneous or induced arousals from sleep may be more vulnerable to an SIDS death. Many scientists now believe that anything that inhibits an infant's ability to arouse from sleep may increase the risk of SIDS.

Cardiorespiratory control. SIDS occurs at a peak age of 2–4 months. This is an age when infants are undergoing rapid and tremendous changes in brain development, particularly in cardiorespiratory control. From an engineering point of view, a system in rapid transition is intrinsically unstable. Thus, when the neurologic system controlling breathing is undergoing rapid change, it is also more likely to malfunction, and serious apnea can occur. However, in the 1990s, the Collaborative Home Infant Monitoring Evaluation (CHIME) Study did not find that prolonged apneas occur at the age when SIDS is most common. Thus, apnea alone is not likely to be the mechanism of death in SIDS. SIDS is not as simple as an infant simply stopping breathing during sleep.

Neurologic control of respiration and of cardiac function is linked. We now know that the autonomic nervous system, the life-support part of the central nervous system, links cardiac and respiratory function. Breathing has a profound influence on function of the heart, including its rhythm and blood pressure. The details of this relationship are beginning to be elucidated, but they are not completely understood. Nevertheless, we know that aberrations in breathing can alter cardiac responses to environmental changes. For example, adults with obstructive sleep apnea syndrome (OSAS), a disorder where there are repeated occlusions of the upper airway during sleep, have serious cardiac complications from their primary respiratory disorder, including high blood pressure, cardiac arrhythmias, and sudden death. Similarly, children with other abnormalities in respiratory control (such as congenital central hypoventilation syndrome) have abnormal cardiovascular responses to changes in breathing or in the environment. These are mediated by aberrations in the autonomic nervous system's coupling of cardiac and respiratory function. It is possible that respiratory abnormalities in infants may cause cardiovascular collapse through autonomic nervous system mechanisms, and this cardiovascular collapse may cause sudden death – SIDS.

Do respiratory problems cause cardiovascular collapse in all infants? Do infants need to have abnormalities in the

brain in order to have these abnormal reactions? Can 'normal' mechanisms transform the brain to have aberrant cardiac responses to respiratory perturbations? Imaging studies of the brain's response to hypoxia or hypercapnia performed in children, using functional magnetic resonance imaging (fMRI), show that many parts of the brain are involved in these neural responses to cardiac and respiratory control, not just the brainstem. Harper and colleagues showed that the cerebellum has an important role in neural control of cardiorespiratory function. Similarly, midbrain areas, including areas in the limbic system, also participate in cardiorespiratory control. Thus, lesions or damage to many parts of the brain may affect autonomic function. Some of these areas may be more susceptible to damage from hypoxia than the brainstem, which was traditionally thought to be the anatomic site of cardiorespiratory control.

Hypoxia (low oxygen). Hypoxia may also play an important role in SIDS. The CHIME study showed that normal infants experience significant hypoxia in their own homes during sleep. The Purkinje fibers in the cerebellum are especially sensitive to hypoxic damage. In fact, pathologists often diagnose hypoxia at autopsy when they see damage to Purkinje fibers. These neurons modulate autonomic nervous system control of blood pressure and cardiovascular instability. If Purkinje fibers are damaged by hypoxia, the unchecked autonomic brain structures fire sporadically and erratically, causing highly varying cardiorespiratory function. Specifically, the cardiac response to respiratory perturbations may be unpredictable and potentially dangerous. Thus, hypoxia can make an infant vulnerable to abnormal, exaggerated, and/or life-threatening cardiovascular responses to respiratory stimuli. Removal of this cerebellar modulation of cardiorespiratory control can lead to physiologic crises, perhaps resulting in death. These studies suggest that SIDS may be due to a combination of a respiratory and a cardiac death, with the link being aberrant autonomic nervous system function.

Metabolic disorders. Metabolic disorders are inherited conditions, which decrease the body's ability to generate the energy necessary to sustain life from ingested food. There are thousands of metabolic disorders, but disorders of the β-oxidation of fatty acids are thought to be most relevant to SIDS. These disorders decrease the body's ability to make the energy, especially under conditions of fasting, fever, or other stresses. While some investigators believe that metabolic disorders may explain some SIDS deaths, the proportion of deaths so explained is not known, and most investigators believe it is a small proportion.

Genetic factors. Genetic factors may explain the increased vulnerability for SIDS in some infants. SIDS is not thought to be an inherited disorder. That is, there is no genetic mutation that has been shown to cause SIDS, or even to be present in a large number of SIDS victims.

However, most genes have minor variations in structure (polymorphisms), which do not cause abnormal gene function. However, these polymorphisms may be associated with slight quantitative variations in gene function. For example, promoter polymorphisms of the serotonin transporter gene affect the amount of serotonin, a neurotransmitter thought to be important in cardiorespiratory control, which is available for signaling between neurons. There are two polymorphisms, a short and a long form. The long form metabolizes serotonin more quickly, leaving less available for neurotransmitter function. Narita and Weese-Mayer and their colleagues have found that the long promoter polymorphism of the serotonin transporter gene was more common in babies who died from SIDS than in controls. The long promoter polymorphism of the serotonin transporter gene does not cause abnormal function of the gene, which would cause a disease. Rather it simply promotes more serotonin metabolism than does the short promoter polymorphism of the serotonin transporter gene. Having less serotonin available as a neurotransmitter may make some infants less resilient to coping with environmental changes, or it may slightly alter physiologic protective mechanisms, such that some infants might be more susceptible to environmental or other challenges. Similarly, Weese-Mayer found mutations or polymorphisms in other genes thought to be important in development of the autonomic nervous system that were more common in SIDS victims than in controls. These studies do not prove that SIDS is a genetic disorder. However, such genetic variation may be a partial basis for why some infants are more vulnerable than others in Filiano and Kinney's triple risk model.

In summary, the cause of SIDS is not known. Investigations into the role of cardiac arrhythmias and metabolic disorders must continue. However, SIDS is generally not thought to be due to a single abnormality in a single physiologic system. SIDS is not thought to be due to an infection, environmental toxin, or nutritional deficiency. If there is a pre-existing abnormality in babies who die from SIDS, it must be subtle, as it has eluded identification by researchers for decades. It is more likely that small differences in infant vulnerabilities, such as those caused by genetic polymorphisms that predispose to autonomic nervous system instability, combined with an environmental stressor that occurs in a developmental window of vulnerability, all come together to cause an SIDS death.

Public Health Measures to Reduce the Risk of SIDS

Although the cause of SIDS is unknown, since the mid-1980s, epidemiologists have identified a number of potentially modifiable risk factors, which increase the risk of SIDS. In most cases, the mechanisms by which these risk factors operate are unknown. Nevertheless, a number of countries have established aggressive public health and public education campaigns to reduce the risk of SIDS. These have resulted in a fall in the SIDS rate to less than one-half what it was prior to these campaigns.

Prone Sleeping Position

Beginning in the 1980s, several investigators in several countries found that prone sleeping was associated with an increased risk of SIDS. The increased risk has been reported as being 10–20 times higher than in babies who sleep supine. The mechanism that underlies the danger of prone sleeping is not known. However, several epidemiologic studies from several countries leave no doubt that having babies sleep in the supine position decreases the risk of SIDS. Many countries have instituted public education campaigns to decrease prone sleeping and encourage supine sleeping (**Figure 3**). These campaigns have not only decreased prone sleeping, but they have also been associated with a decrease in SIDS deaths by over 50% (**Figure 4**).

Studies have shown that sleeping on the side is also associated with an increased SIDS risk of three to seven times higher than sleeping on the back, but not as high as prone sleeping. Therefore, all infants should be encouragedto sleep flat on their backs through the first year of life, as this carries the lowest risk for SIDS. Some infant developmental authorities were concerned that the promotion of supine sleeping would hinder infant development, as babies learn many developmental tasks in the prone position. There is no danger to having infants spend waking time in the prone position, where developmental tasks may be mastered. However, they should spend sleeping time on their backs.

Avoid Soft Bedding, Pillows, Stuffed Animals, etc.

Soft bedding, where a baby's head can be nestled in a small air pocket, increases the risk of SIDS. Especially dangerous are beanbags, water mattresses, sheepskins, soft pillows, quilts, comforters, and soft bedding placed under the infant. Studies show that placing pillows and soft objects in the crib with a sleeping infant is associated with a two to three times increased risk of SIDS. Further, infant crib mattresses should be firm, and only covered with a thin sheet. Studies show that soft mattresses are associated with a five-times increased risk of SIDS. Used crib mattresses may be dangerous. If these mattresses are soft and not firm from extensive use, they should be discarded.

Keep soft objects and loose bedding out of the crib. Bedding should be thin and placed in a way that the infant's head cannot be covered. Place the infant's feet at the foot of the

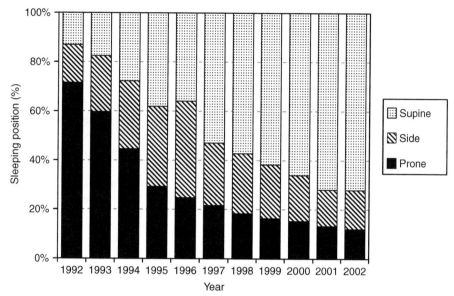

Figure 3 National infant sleep position study (US). The proportion of infants in the US who sleep in the prone, side, and supine positions are shown for each year from 1992 through 2002. There has been a marked drop in the proportion of infants sleeping prone in response to public health campaigns. Data obtained from the National Infant Sleep Position Study, and from Willinger M, Hoffman HJ, Wu K-T, *et al*. (1998) Factors associated with the transition to nonprone sleep positions of infants in the United States: The National Infant Sleep Position Study. *Journal of the American Medical Association* 280: 329–335.

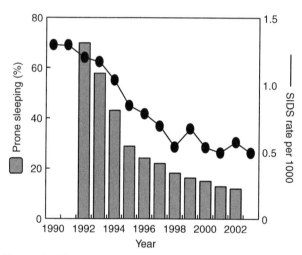

Figure 4 US prone sleeping and SIDS rate. For each year from 1990 through 2003 in the US, the proportion of infants sleeping prone is plotted with the shaded bars (Y-axis on the left); and the SIDS rate per 1000 live births is plotted with the circles connected by a line (Y-axis on the right). As the proportion of infants who sleep prone fell, so did the SIDS rate. Data obtained from the National Infant Sleep Position Study and from Willinger M, Hoffman HJ, Wu K-T, Hou J-R, *et al*. (1998) Factors associated with the transition to nonprone sleep positions of infants in the United States: The National Infant Sleep Position Study. *Journal of the American Medical Association* 280: 329–335.

crib ('Feet to Foot'). Thin blankets should be tucked so they can come up no higher than the mid-chest of the baby. Alternatively, one can use a sleep sack or one-piece clothing designed to keep the infant warm without the possible

hazard of covering the infant's head. Additional blankets or covers are not needed with these sleep clothes. Stuffed animals should not be placed in a crib with a sleeping infant. Infants can play with them when they are awake.

Cigarette Smoking

Mothers should not smoke cigarettes during pregnancy. Infants of mothers who smoke 20 or more cigarettes per day face an eight-times increased risk of SIDS. The specific mechanism by which smoking increases the SIDS risk is not known. However, there are many studies of the harmful effects of maternal cigarette smoking on the fetus, including poor intrauterine growth, autonomic nervous system disturbances, and abnormal lung development. Further, infant exposure to cigarette smoking after birth is also associated with an increased risk of SIDS. No one should smoke cigarettes around any baby. No one should smoke cigarettes in a baby's room, even if the baby is not there. Infants exposed to 8 hours or more per day of environmental tobacco smoke face a tentimes increased risk of SIDS.

Bedsharing

Bedsharing has been the most common sleeping arrangement for mothers and infants for millennia, and it has increased in popularity among Western mothers. However, there has been fear that bedsharing parents could roll onto sleeping infants and smother them, also known as overlaying. The risk of maternal overlaying is thought to increase if the parents' ability to awaken (arouse) is inhibited, as with alcohol ingestion, drug use, or sleep deprivation. But, it is not known how frequently overlaying occurs. A definitive diagnosis of overlaying is difficult, and it can usually only be suggested by observation at the scene of death. Part of the difficulty in being certain about whether overlaying has occurred is illustrated by the following scenario. Suppose a baby is found dead in bed with an adult who has rolled over onto the infant. Did the baby die because the adult rolled onto it and smothered it? If so, why did the baby's movements not waken the adult? Or, did the baby die from SIDS, and the adult roll over on the lifeless baby, who did not move, and therefore did not awaken the adult? Neither a death scene investigation nor an autopsy can distinguish between these two scenarios with certainty.

Some investigators have suggested that bedsharing imparts protection or a survival advantage to the infant. It is clear that there is a great deal of behavioral interaction, which occurs, between a mother and infant during bedsharing. Breastfeeding is increased during bedsharing nights. However, no study has convincingly shown any protective effects of bedsharing on the infant.

A number of epidemiological studies have shown that the risk of SIDS is increased when infants bedshare the entire night. This is especially true if the parents are cigarette smokers, even if they do not smoke in bed. However, many studies show an increased SIDS risk from bedsharing even if the parents do not smoke cigarettes. Most studies indicate that the risk of SIDS with bedsharing is higher in young infants less than 4 months of age. Bedsharing on a couch or sofa is particularly dangerous, and has been associated with a 50-times increased SIDS risk. The issue is further complicated by the nature of the bedsharing. Some families choose to bedshare, but they possibly do so in a safe manner. That is, the mattress is firm, the infant is supine, there is no cigarette smoking, adults' arousal is not impaired, etc. Other families, usually in poor socioeconomic situations, bedshare because they have no choice. Bedsharing may occur in unsafe beds (soft mattresses) or crowded conditions, and there may be multiple bedsharers, including children. In these cases, there may be a number of other risk factors that increase the SIDS risk in addition to bedsharing, and it may be difficult to separate these effects from the effect of bedsharing alone.

Epidemiological studies also indicate that there is an increased risk for SIDS when infants sleep in a separate room from the parents. Therefore, the safest sleeping environment for infants appears to be room sharing without bedsharing. A crib placed in the same room as the parents has the lowest SIDS risk in several studies, and this is currently recommended. The crib should have a firm mattress and conform to safety standards. The baby may be brought into the bed for breastfeeding, but the infant should then be returned to the crib.

Despite this recommendation, many parents are still bedsharing. If parents choose this path, they need to understand that the mechanism for the increased SIDS risk is not known. Therefore, it is difficult to give advice on what to do or not do while bedsharing. However, it is clear that bedsharing is unsafe with: (1) cigarette smoking by the parents; (2) soft or unsafe mattress or bed; (3) quilts, pillows, or soft covers in the bed; (4) covering the infant's head with blankets; (5) prone or side sleeping; (6) parental alcohol or drug use; and (7) parental sleep deprivation, defined as less than 4 h of sleep on the previous night. As a baby frequently disrupts the sleep of new parents, this last condition may be particularly difficult to avoid. In summary, it would be very difficult to avoid all of the above while bedsharing. Therefore, room-sharing, without bedsharing, remains the safest recommendation for infant sleep.

Pacifiers

Pediatricians often discouraged use of pacifiers because it was believed that they caused dental problems and delayed or discouraged breastfeeding. However, a number of studies have shown a marked decrease in the risk for SIDS when infants use pacifiers in the first year of life. The mechanism for this protection is not known. Further, scientific evidence indicating that pacifiers cause dental problems or inhibit breastfeeding is absent. Therefore, it is recommended that infants be offered a pacifier for use during sleep in the first year of life. If an infant does not take the pacifier, it should not be forced. If the pacifier falls out of the infant's mouth during sleep, it need not be reinserted in order to achieve the epidemiologic protective effect. It is recommended that pacifier use be delayed until 1 month of age, so that breastfeeding can be established. There is little evidence that pacifier use will inhibit breastfeeding by this age. Pacifiers should not be coated in sweet solutions in order to avoid tooth decay. Honey, especially, should be avoided because of the risk of infant botulism.

Avoid Overheating

In some epidemiologic studies, there was evidence that SIDS infants were warmer than infants who did not die. SIDS infants were more likely to have more thermal insulation in clothes and blankets, have a heater in the room, use hot water bottles or electric blankets, and wear a hat, compared to controls. It is recommended that parents avoid overheating of infants. Infants should be lightly clothed for sleep, and the bedroom temperature should be comfortable for a lightly clothed adult. Infants should not be dressed so they feel hot to the touch.

Avoid Commercial Devices to 'Prevent SIDS'

A number of commercial devices have been developed and marketed 'to prevent SIDS'. These are designed to fix an infant in a certain sleeping position, or to provide a continuous flow of air through the mattress to make prone sleeping 'safe'. These devices have not been tested for safety or efficacy, and they are not recommended. When infants are placed flat on their backs to sleep, such devices are not necessary.

Home Apnea–Bradycardia Monitoring

Home apnea–bradycardia monitors are devices that monitor an infant's breathing and heartbeat. They sound an audible alarm if breathing stops for a period of time (usually 20 s) or if heart rate falls below a certain specified limit. Trained caregivers are then alerted to a potentially dangerous situation, and they do what is necessary to revive the infant. Although this sounds like a good idea, home monitoring has never been proven to prevent SIDS. Therefore, it should not be used as a strategy to reduce the risk of SIDS.

Breastfeeding

Breastfeeding has many benefits for infant health, and it should be encouraged for these reasons. However, breastfeeding probably does not have a specific effect on reducing the risk of SIDS. Many studies suggest that infants who breastfeed have a decreased risk for SIDS, but some studies show no difference. Many studies show that breastfeeding is associated with a reduced risk of SIDS by univariate analysis. However, when corrected for other co-varying risk factors by multivariate analysis, breastfeeding is not protective. This may reflect the fact that breastfeeding mothers are generally more likely to adhere to other practices known to reduce the risk of SIDS, such as supine sleeping, not smoking cigarettes, using safe bedding, etc. Thus, while breastfeeding should be encouraged for its general health benefits for infants, by itself, it does not appear to reduce the risk of SIDS.

It should be emphasized that none of these potentially modifiable risk factors are causes of SIDS. They have been shown, by epidemiological studies, to reduce the risk of SIDS. Infants without any of these risk factors continue to die from SIDS, and most infants with one or more of these risk factors will not die from SIDS. If an infant with one or more of these risk factors dies, it should not be concluded that these factors caused the infant's death. However, when viewed from a population perspective, adhering to these recommendations has been associated with a substantial decrease in the number of babies who die from SIDS. Therefore, they should be recommended to parents of infants in order to decrease the chances of their infant's dying from SIDS.

Parent Grief

The parents and families of a baby who died from SIDS are no less the victims of this tragedy than their babies.

Although the death of any child is painful, SIDS deaths have some unique characteristics. SIDS deaths come quietly, suddenly, and unexpectedly. These babies were happy and healthy. They were usually tucked safely into their cribs for an overnight sleep or a daytime nap. Sometime during that sleeping period, they died. The death of any child is a devastating loss. The death of an apparently healthy child, with no symptoms or warnings, and no opportunity for SIDS parents to prepare or to say 'good bye', leaves parents with a unique grief.

Because medical professionals cannot tell a family how or why their baby died, parents often search the child's brief life for something they did, or did not do, which may have caused the death. The guilt generated by an SIDS death is tremendous, and it is generally more so than in infant deaths where the cause is known. One mother of an SIDS baby described her reaction: "Even after the autopsy ruled out all other causes of death, assuring us that we'd done nothing wrong, we found little comfort. Our son was dead. He was in my care when he died. Although part of me knew better, it was impossible to not blame myself. What had I missed? What if I had checked on him sooner? It was difficult to accept that my baby had died of no apparent cause."

The death of a child is certainly a stressful event in a family, and marriages are often strained. For many young SIDS couples, this is the first mutual experience with the loss of a loved one, and they are strangers to grief of this magnitude. In some cases, the parent who was with the baby at the time of the death may be blamed for the death by the other parent. Even if this does not happen, the loss of a child, and the individual ways of handling it, may magnify every personality difference between a husband and wife.

While not always the case, fathers (and sometimes mothers) often attempt to handle their grief by immersing themselves in work, sports, or other hobbies. Mothers report their need to discuss their child's life and death, to talk about the details, and to share their grief. This may lead to misunderstandings about one another's feelings, and assumptions about which parent is grieving 'correctly'. Couples may frequently find themselves at different places in their loss and feel worried that they might make each other sad on a 'good' day, and as a result avoid discussing their feelings. When, in the past, they may have been able to discuss most everything, even day-to-day things seem to create conflict.

There have been many unsubstantiated reports that most marriages dissolve following the death of a child from SIDS. This does not seem to be true now. While the sudden and unexpected death of a baby creates a great amount of stress on a family, access to a local SIDS parent peer support group or professional counseling is often a valuable help.

Although friends and family try to help SIDS parents cope with the death, they usually have no better understanding of SIDS than the parents. SIDS is as mysterious to them as it is to the parents. Most people know of SIDS as 'crib death', and many offer explanations based on things they have heard. The most helpful friends are those who sit and listen when parents need to talk, while the least helpful offer theories and advice about planning to have more children. It does not take long for SIDS parents to realize that they have worn out many of their family and friends.

In many families, there are other children in the family when SIDS strikes the youngest infant. Parents are not alone in their grief. The surviving children are suddenly in a family that is different. The parents look the same, but they act very differently. While it may be comforting and helpful for parents to know that their primary role as a parent is still in place, they may question every parenting decision they make. They know it is important to maintain daily routine and security for their surviving children, but at the same time it is difficult to not want to shelter and protect them from everything. Children have many questions that parents are forced to attempt to answer. Why did her brother die? Where was he now? Was she going to die during her nap? Because many young children are at an age where death does not seem final, they may want to know when the baby who died will be coming back. It does not take long for SIDS parents to realize that they are not just grieving parents, they are a grieving family. They often feel isolated, unable to explain or understand how apparently healthy babies can die in their sleep with no warning, and they worry that they will never be happy or whole again.

For most families of SIDS victims, the single best and most important resource is an SIDS parent support group. An SIDS mother said, "We might have drowned in our grief, had we not been put in touch with a local support group for SIDS families. We met with other families who had lost children in this same way, and for the first time, we felt that we were not alone. We found that other couples were grieving in similar ways, and that SIDS didn't have to mean the end of our marriage or our happiness. We were able to discuss current research, and to separate the facts from the myths. While we were unable to learn how or why our son died, we did learn some things that helped diminish our guilt and put us on a path of healing." SIDS parent support groups have SIDS parents who are available to speak with new SIDS parents at any time. While the immediate impact of the SIDS death is devastating to families, the ability to talk with someone who has been through it, who understands how they feel, and who has survived it, is reassuring.

SIDS changes a family's view of the world. One SIDS mother wrote, "It's safe to say that our son's death from SIDS changed the way we looked at everything in our lives. We questioned our marriage, our faith, our friendships, and our work. It felt easier to be cynical than fair, to

be guarded rather than trusting. While we had once talked of having several children, we were now having serious disagreements about the possibility of another baby. My husband was unwilling to risk even the possibility of the death of another child. While I knew it was impossible to replace Tyler, I felt a deep need to mother another child, perhaps to prove to myself that I could, or perhaps simply to fill the empty hole that Ty's death had created. Looking back, I think I mostly just wanted to resume what I could of a normal life. I needed to be happy again. We needed to be happy again."

Many SIDS families do ultimately have subsequent babies, but this brings stress and anxiety that the SIDS death may be repeated. A subsequent child is often born to a still-grieving family, despite their efforts to pretend that everything is normal. This baby's parents may have been the same biological parents as his sibling's, but they certainly are not the same emotionally. They worry more, not just about SIDS, but also about things that had not crossed their minds with their previous pregnancies and babies. This is a time when many SIDS parents turn again to their SIDS support group friends to share their worries and fears. SIDS parents celebrate their subsequent child's first birthday with a big sigh of relief, but also with the quiet realization that, while life is good, it is missing an important member of the family.

Subsequent Siblings of SIDS Victims

When SIDS parents have a subsequent child, they are afraid that this new baby may also die. These SIDS siblings are not at increased risk for SIDS. They have the same risk of SIDS as the general population, which is a risk of approximately one per 2000 live births. There is no testing, such as sleep studies or ECGs, which can predict if a subsequent sibling of an SIDS victim is at increased risk for SIDS. Thus, such tests are not recommended. Nevertheless, SIDS parents frequently ask what they can do to reduce the risk of their subsequent baby from also dying from SIDS. Parents should do everything that any parent does to optimize the health of their baby. Once your baby is born, be sure to follow the 'Back to Sleep' recommendations. These recommendations have been shown to decrease the number of babies dying from SIDS. Find a pediatrician who is sensitive to the fact that you have had a previous baby die, and who will take your concerns seriously.

Summary

SIDS is the most common cause of death between the ages of 1 month and 1 year. It strikes approximately one out of every 2000 live births. The cause of SIDS is unknown. There are no tests currently available that can detect an infant who will die from SIDS. Reduction of SIDS risks for populations has been achieved by public health education, and SIDS rates have dropped by over 50%. Grief in SIDS parents is characterized by guilt. Based on our current understanding, SIDS is a natural cause of death, and there is nothing SIDS parents did, or did not do, to cause their baby's death.

Suggested Readings

American Academy of Pediatrics Policy Statement (2005) The changing concept of sudden infant death syndrome: Diagnostic coding shifts, controversies regarding the sleeping environment, and new variables to consider in reducing the risk. *Pediatrics* 116: 1245–1255.

Byard RW and Krous HF (2001) *Sudden Infant Death Syndrome: Problems, Progress, and Possibilities.* London, UK: Arnold Publications.

Filiano JJ and Kinney HC (1994) A perspective on neuropathological findings in victims of the sudden infant death syndrome: The triple-risk model. *Biology of the Neonate* 65: 194–197.

Ramanathan R, Corwin MJ, Hunt CE, *et al.* (2001) Cardiorespiratory events recorded on home monitors: Comparison of healthy infants with those at increased risk for SIDS. *Journal of the American Medical Association* 285: 2199–2207.

Willinger M, Hoffman HJ, Wu K-T, *et al.* (1998) Factors associates with the transition to nonprone sleep positions of infants in the United States: The National Infant Sleep Position Study. *Journal of the American Medical Association* 280: 329–335.

Relevant Websites

http://www.sidsalliance.org – First Candle/SIDS Alliance.

http://www.ispid.org – International Society for the Study and Prevention of Infant Deaths.

http://www.sidscenter.org – National SIDS/Infant Death Resource Center: Health Research and Services Administration, U.S. Government.

http://www.nichd.nih.gov/ – Research on SIDS. National Institute of Child Health and Human Development, U.S. Government.

http://www.sidsinternational.org – SIDS International.

T

Teratology

R Seifer, Brown University, Providence, RI, USA

Glossary

Behavioral teratology – The study of behavioral occurring in childhood (usually early in life) associated with anomalies feral of exposure to toxic substances.

Developmental embryology – The study of *in utero* development in terms of factors such as of timing, sequence, growth-promotion factors, growth-inhibition factors, and organ systems development.

Developmental psychopathology – A theoretical perspective that simultaneously considers understanding of normative development and understanding of maladaptive development; each is presumed to fundamentally inform the other.

Direct effects model – Explanations of development where single factors are presumed to have causal effect on a specific characteristic, independent of other causal factors.

Direction of effect – Attributions about causality when two or more things are associated.

Effect size – A metric that indicates the size of an association in statistical terms, which can be generalized across specific measurements, and often expressed as a proportion of the variability observed in the measurements.

Interactive effects model – Explanations of development where the effect of single factors on a specific characteristic depends on other causal factors.

Meta-analysis – A statistical approach to combining findings from multiple studies of the same association, designed to provide the best evidence-based estimate an effect size.

Sleeper effects – Behavioral effects not immediately apparent that can only be detected substantially later in development.

Teratology – The study of physical malformations occurring in childhood (usually early in life) associated with exposure to toxic substances.

Toxicology – The study of physiologic processing of substances to which an individual is exposed.

Transactional model – Explanations of development where multiple factors are presumed to have causal effect on a specific characteristic, resulting in transformations of the developmental process.

Translational research – Research that examines phenomena simultaneously at multiple levels of analysis, which might include genetic variation, neurotransmitter action, physiology, behavior, social processes, and health outcomes.

Introduction

Teratology is derived from the Greek noun *teras*, meaning monster, and historically has referred to the study of malformations early in life that result from exposure to chemicals such as mercury, lead, and other complex compounds. The original focus of this work was on gross physical malformations (and hence the borrowing of the Greek noun for monster), and more recently has referred to malformations that result from exposure to chemicals such as lead, mercury, or other compounds. In the period from the 1960s to 1980s, the concept was gradually extended to the domain of behavioral teratology, most clearly articulated by Riley and Voorhees. The key elements of this extension are twofold. First, the focus is on behavioral anomalies, rather than physical malformations. Second, and perhaps more far reaching, is an appreciation that many behavioral anomalies may be subtle in nature and not apparent at all stages of development. Closely aligned with the field of behavioral teratology is the field of toxicology. For the most part, behavioral teratology focuses on variations in behavior that are associated with some known or suspected exposure to a potential toxin in utero.

Like many areas of scientific inquiry, investigation in behavioral teratology was initially inspired by blatant examples of the phenomena. In teratology, severe physical malformation, and in the behavioral realm, frank mental retardation constituted these eye-catching events. By the second half of the twentieth century, several well-publicized events helped establish links between physical and behavioral events and exposure to toxins, and other areas of inquiry subsequently came into play. For example, knowledge from developmental embryology was brought to bear on how and when during embryogenesis the malformations might occur (so we now ask many questions regarding dose, duration, and timing of exposures). Furthermore, the behavioral teratology logic could also be turned on its ear. Instead of pursuing an epidemiologic type of inquiry (how to explain a cluster of congenital malformations), investigators also began inquiries focused on purported antecedents, rather than observed consequences. Thus, substances known or believed to be toxic (though not because of documented links with early malformations) came to be examined with regard to possible physical and behavioral effects. This occurred in the context of widespread public concern about pollutants (in the wake of mercury, polychlorinated biphenyl (PCB) contamination, and identification of lead in many parts of the environment), prescribed and over-the-counter drugs (following the thalidomide exposures), illicit drugs (in tune with increased societal use), and environmental agents such as pesticides (after the publication of books such as *Silent Spring*). The types of malformations and behaviors examined also became far more subtle in nature. Instead of the blatantly negative consequences that drove the field at its outset, investigators began to look for behavioral signs such as attention problems or poor school performance in place of more severe manifestations such as mental retardation.

A large majority of the published papers in behavioral teratology describe studies performed with nonhuman animals. This is quite understandable. Given that the focus is on toxic exposures that can lead to behavioral deficits, intentionally exposing humans to these substances would be unethical. Thus, the ability to investigate basic processes is typically available only in animal models (more about this in the next section). This context of basic research with animals has set the stage for the mostly nonexperimental human research in behavioral teratology that will be the focus of this article. These animal models typically provide excellent starting points for generating and testing hypotheses in humans.

From a broad theoretical perspective, existing models in behavioral teratology in humans parallel those found in the broader field of human development research. A simple tripartite differentiation of common approaches

was articulated by Sameroff and colleagues. Direct effects models examine one-to-one correspondence between antecedents and consequences, with strong causal inferences drawn. In behavioral teratology, for example, a direct effects model would imply that sufficient exposure to a toxin would inevitably result in an identifiable change in a specific developing system. 'Interactive effects models' simultaneously consider multiple antecedents, often a combination of constitutional and contextual factors, in the prediction of developmental outcomes. These effects are linear in nature, easily captured by a typical analysis of variance (ANOVA) interaction model. To exemplify in the behavioral teratology realm, effects of a toxin might only occur when a particular characteristic is present in an individual (e.g., a particular genetic feature). Transactional models, like interactive effects models, consider multiple antecedent factors. Where they differ, however, is in positing developmental transformations in dynamic organism in complex systems – thus making simple predictions from single antecedents to distal outcomes very difficult. In a behavioral teratology example, a particular toxin combined with a particular genetic characteristic might serve to predispose a child to have difficulty with certain types of learning; however, the presence of the learning problems could change the environment, so to speak, so that the learning context is enriched enabling the child to overcome those obstacles, such that the predisposition no longer has developmental consequences. Existing studies in the behavioral teratology literature exemplify these generic models, and the framework will be used to integrate the current knowledge base.

Human and Animal Studies

Behavioral teratology is one area where the contrast between animal studies and work with humans is at its sharpest. In a sense, this contrast highlights the fundamental obstacle in studying teratology in human populations. Put simply, owing to ethical concerns, we cannot conduct the relevant experiments with humans that would allow for less ambiguous understanding of phenomena than we currently possess.

Human Studies

There are two research strategies that characterize virtually all work in human teratology. The first is natural experiments. Although not truly experiments (e.g., there is no random assignment of people to experimental conditions), researchers rely on identification of discrete populations where individuals were exposed *in utero* to a potential teratogen. A classic example of this strategy was examination of mercury exposure in populations living proximal to an industrial discharge site in Minamata,

Japan. The second strategy is naturalistic observation studies. In these studies, populations are examined for naturally occurring levels of prenatal exposure to a particular potential teratogen, and follow-up studies are conducted of the children to identify postnatal effects – this design has been the staple of studies of prenatal tobacco exposure. Often, the study group is chosen because it is known to be proximal to the potential teratogen under study, and this represents a hybrid of the two research designs described above – studies of PCB exposure in communities near Lake Michigan exemplify this hybrid approach. In all of these human research designs, however, the defining characteristic is that the researchers do not have control over the exposure (amount, timing, duration) that is examined with respect to outcomes in young children.

Animal Studies

In contrast to human studies, with animal models we can ethically introduce the presumed toxins in order to study their effects on developing organisms. Differences in animal and human work, however, do not end with variation in how substances are introduced to individuals. Another critical feature of animal studies is the degree to which nonexperimental features of the individuals' circumstances are controlled. In animal work, the contexts of the individuals, ranging from housing, to activity levels, to environmental resources, to nutrition can be held relatively constant. In humans, however, researchers rarely have any degree of control over these factors. More troublesome yet is that some important factors in the studies of humans are systematically biased in those populations prone to various types of substance exposures.

Features of the populations of animals can also be systematically varied. Strains of animals may be employed because they have been bred to express specific physical and/or behavioral characteristics of interest as potential consequences of the exposure. For example, tumor-prone animals may be employed if an outcome under study is carcinogenic effects; propensity to prefer alcohol may be used if behaviors related to substance use are of interest as outcomes.

As technology has improved in recent years, questions regarding interaction of exposure to potential teratogens with genetic factors have become feasible, with different models being used. One of these models is 'knockout' designs, where specific gene sequences have been removed or inactivated in a strain of animals to examine how the absence of the genes interacts with exposure to affect behavior. Alternatively, animals with known gene polymorphisms (individual differences in specific gene sequences) can be examined to identify which variants might interact with a teratogen to yield a developmental effect.

In all of these animal models, dose, timing, and duration of exposure can be carefully controlled and systematically varied. In similar fashion, the timing, frequency, and method of subsequent behavioral and physical testing of offspring can be systematically varied and controlled as well. It is also feasible to replicate findings and to develop research programs that proceed through the testing of theoretical models in a rational and stepwise manner.

Implications of Animal Studies for Research with Humans

The experimental controls just described for animal studies are not available for humans (e.g., we cannot breed genetically altered strains). The question then becomes: how can animal models inform studies of humans? The answer is threefold. First, potential human teratogens and their mechanisms of action can be identified in animals to generate hypotheses for human studies. Second, possible thresholds regarding dose, timing, and duration of exposure can be identified in animals and extrapolated to humans to again generate testable hypotheses. Third, potential genetic interactions can be identified in animals that could again generate hypotheses for studies with humans.

These efforts at translational research represent cutting edge efforts in scientific inquiry, but enthusiasm must also be tempered by the realities of translating animal models to human experience. First, animals, while they have similarities to humans in many ways, also differ in important ways. These differences become more pronounced as we move further away from humans in terms of phylogenetic similarity (e.g., rodent brains have far less in common with human brains than do primate brains). Perhaps more important for the agenda of behavioral teratology, the behavior of nonhuman species does not match the complexity and organization of human behavior. For many behaviors of interest (e.g., math or reading), there is simply no equivalent or analogous animal behavior. The variety of social and contextual influence in humans is far more influential in behavioral outcomes than anything that could be modeled in an animal laboratory. It is thus essential that even well-established animal models of teratogenic effects be clearly replicated in humans before making scientific claims with any confidence. Finally sleeper effects may occur, which in humans can take very long periods to detect. A well-known physical example is diethylstilbestrol (DES; a synthetic estrogen) exposure in pregnancy, which did not reveal itself until reproductive problems occurred in offspring decades later. In the behavioral realm, certain types of cognitive processes do not emerge until middle childhood, which precludes their detection earlier in life.

Behavioral Teratology in Infancy and Early Childhood: Timing of Exposure, Timing of Outcome

The focus of this volume is on infancy and early childhood. In behavioral teratology, however, only part of the story has emerged by the time children enter elementary school (one traditional marker for the end of early childhood). As will become evident in subsequent sections, many of the concerns around potential toxins are in behavioral domains that do not emerge (at least in well- or fully developed form) until middle childhood. Some examples include executive function, school failure, and antisocial behavior.

In a related vein, the timing of exposure to potential toxins is an important factor when considering infancy and early childhood. The strict definition of teratology includes only prenatal exposures (and that will be the focus of this article). Of course, exposure to toxins at any point in development resulting in changes in behavior would be of concern. Early exposure, however, is generally of most concern because of the increased developmental vulnerability of maturing neurological systems.

Prenatal exposures are typically indirect. Exposures to the mother are mediated in various ways before the child is affected. Some examples are the speed at which mothers metabolize substances or the degree to which a substance (or its metabolites) crosses the placental barrier. As such, the nature and extent of exposure may be less certain than with certain types of postnatal exposures. Finally, the rapidity of development during the prenatal period makes the timing of exposure important when considering the expectable type of developmental consequences.

An important characteristic of exposure to most toxins is that they cross the boundary of pregnancy to infancy. Thus, in many research studies the teratogenic effects are occurring in the context of postnatal exposures. Unlike prenatal exposure, postnatal exposures are typically direct – they affect the child via direct experience with the teratogen, and perhaps are more potent as a result. One postnatal route of exposure that mimics some of the qualities of prenatal exposure (see below) is breastfeeding. Although the developing infant is exposed directly, this type of exposure is again mediated by maternal amount of exposure, metabolism, and expression in breast milk, all of which affects the actual experience of the child. This important research confound needs to be considered when attributing findings to the prenatal period.

Many Types of Substances in Many Types of Conditions Are Evaluated as Potential Teratogens

Potential teratogenic effects have been studied in many types of foods, pollutants, drugs, and naturally occurring elements and compounds. Although we have well agreed upon conceptualizations of these categories, the boundaries often become very blurry when examining the association of organismic exposure and developmental sequelae. Mercury, for example, occurs naturally in the environment, occasionally in areas where it runs off into lakes and streams.

In addition, mercury has been an important mining resource and used in many industrial applications because of its unique properties of being a metallic element that is liquid at normal temperatures. Because mercury evaporates when exposed to air, it can travel widely from mining and industrial sites; it is also ubiquitous in aquatic environments in compound form as methylmercury, which makes its way into the human food chain via fish consumption. Finally, mercury has been used in dental amalgam fillings and vaccine stabilizers at various points in history. Thus, it is difficult to distinguish between the category of food, pollutant, drug, or naturally occurring substance when discussing mercury exposure.

Leaving the niceties of clean categorization aside, one can identify many different types of substances thought to be potential teratogens. Environmental pollutants have been a consistent focus in behavioral teratology. Examples include heavy metal exposure (including mercury and lead), PCBs, and dioxins. Pollutants can be found in air, in water, in foods, and in consumer products (ranging from stone-age ceramics to electronics-age microchips). Exposures may occur proximal to pollution sites (as in waste or runoff from manufacturing processes) or very distal from those sites (as in mercury distributed atmospherically throughout the world and absorbed by fish, thereby becoming part of the food supply).

Non-natural substances used for one purpose may have unintended results. This is most apparent in the domain of pharmaceuticals. Perhaps the most notorious example of a teratogenic drug is thalidomide. Prescribed as a sleep aid and antiemetic for pregnant women, the drug ultimately proved to have strong association with limb deformities among children exposed prenatally. One result of the thalidomide experience is that the US Food and Drug Administration (FDA), and other regulatory bodies around the world, now require explicit testing and labeling of pharmaceuticals regarding their teratogenic risk during pregnancy. Most testing is done in laboratory animals, often at doses far exceeding the human-equivalent dose, and it is very difficult to extrapolate such findings to human teratology potential. It is the case, in fact, that few drugs are actually tested in humans during pregnancy, but are simply labeled with generic warnings that risks are unknown; phase III clinical trials almost exclusively prohibit pregnant women and women not using effective contraception from participation. As a result, most newer drugs used by pregnant women for purposes unrelated to pregnancy and childbirth are prescribed without benefit of clear evidence as to safety to the developing fetus, and most knowledge is gained from *ad hoc* postmarketing studies among women and offspring who have chosen to use the drug in question.

Drugs given directly to children may also have unintended effects. Compared with adults, children are relatively in better health and thus have fewer prescribed medications. One class of medications used far more often in children than adults is vaccines. Most immunization strategies focus on children in the first years of life, with attempts to have universal coverage. Although strictly speaking not teratogenic because of their postnatal administration (but still useful for appreciating how to interpret teratogenic effects), the vaccines have become a focus of interest being potentially harmful, particularly in relation to the documented rise in rates of autism spectrum disorders. Most attention has focused on the mercury-based stabilizers commonly used until recent years, while some attention has focused on less-specific components of vaccines.

Use of pharmaceuticals for recreational purposes during pregnancy, either licit drugs used for nontherapeutic purposes or street drugs, may have similar teratogenic potential. Interest has focused on opiates, synthetic opiates, cocaine, marijuana, and methamphetamine among other recreational drugs. These substances are of particular interest because of their psychoactive effects, which in turn lead to suspicion that they may pose particular hazard to the developing central nervous systems. In this vein, two legal substances are important to note: tobacco and alcohol. Both are marketed and used specifically for their physiologic and psychoactive effects, and both have been the focus of intense scrutiny regarding their teratogenic sequelae.

Problematic Developmental Phenomena

Our environments, food supplies, and pharmaceuticals contain many natural and synthetic substances. Only a very small number of them have received any attention as potential teratogens. On a daily basis, people eat, drink, swim, breathe, and otherwise have contact with many facets of their environments. It is typically the case that when unexpected clusters of adverse developmental events or illnesses occur, that a search for proximal causes leads to suspicion of teratogens of some sort. In a minority of cases, very probable cause–effect relationships can be established. These typically occur when exposures are high, when groups exposed are relatively isolated or otherwise clearly distinguishable, and when well-defined syndromes are associated with the exposure.

More frequently, the situation is far more ambiguous. Interest in a teratogen may result from hypotheses derived from the well-identified high-exposure relations described above, which are generalized to lower levels of exposure. Examples include examination of low levels of lead or mercury, capitalizing on well-established associations noted in high-level exposures. Another route to identifying potential teratogens is from clusters of children exhibiting non-normative developmental pathways. Such clusters may be geographically proximal or temporally proximal – the interest in vaccines in regard to autism spectrum disorders is a good example of inquiry motivated by temporal clustering of cases. In general, these types of associations have been far

more difficult to demonstrate in unambiguous fashion. Furthermore, because of the ambiguity inherent in the inquiry, advocacy positions (intellectual beliefs, parents advocating for their children, etc.) often enter into the progress of the science and the interpretation of data.

Normative Phenomena with Specific Problematic Instances

Behavioral teratology examines inherently developmental phenomena. Outcomes of interest are typically in the standard domains of interest to developmental scientists. Timing of exposures *in utero* is of prime interest. Many of the mechanisms proposed target interruptions of complex developmental pathways in attempting to explain the sequelae of interest. It is still the case that behavioral teratology is often not well integrated with other developmental theories.

Of particular note is that the developmental psychopathology approach, which has proven useful in many other domains of atypical development, has only been applied to some portions of the research on behavioral teratology, as noted by Wakschlag and colleagues. In this developmental psychopathology vein, which emphasizes the continuum of normative to pathological development, nutrition may be viewed as a normative phenomenon that under some circumstances is relevant to teratology. Healthy diet is believed to be characterized by a wide variety of foods with high nutritional content. But fish (a good source of high-quality protein) may enter into the behavioral teratology equation when it contains superthreshold levels of environmental contaminants. In similar fashion, breast milk may also contain substances because of mother's diet or substance use/exposure.

Exposure to potential teratogens must always be considered in the larger developmental context. We know that broad variations in social context have profound effects on normative developmental patterns. Often, poverty and minority racial/ethnic status are associated with lower levels of achievement measures on standard metrics and poor developmental outcomes in general. Furthermore, when contextual adversities co-occur, the association with poor developmental outcomes is especially strong. In some circumstances, what may be relatively small effects of substance exposures are dwarfed when compared to those of contextual influences (such that they are difficult to detect or difficult to appropriately interpret). In other circumstances, the confounding of substance exposures with contextual characteristics may mislead investigators as to the source of variation in children's outcomes. Dilworth-Bart and Moore's recent commentary highlights the fact that exposures are not equitably distributed in the population, but are more likely to occur in those from economically distressed and racial/ethnic minority groups.

While emphasizing the importance of context, it is also important to note that the same developmental context will not affect all children in the same way. The notion of individual-by-environment interaction, which has been well articulated by Wachs, is particularly applicable in the realm of behavioral teratology. The complex of substance exposure, other contextual characteristics, and individuals' constitutional characteristics will together help explain variation in children's developmental outcomes. The example of asthma in children succinctly illustrates this point. Some children are constitutionally prone to bronchoconstriction and airway inflammation, in part by virtue of family history and perhaps maternal exposure to air pollutants during pregnancy. Symptoms of asthma, however, are not simply a function of a child's propensity to these physiologic processes. Rather, the presence of triggers that are somewhat specific to individual children (e.g., allergens, mites, rodent droppings, cockroach) will exacerbate symptoms. Furthermore, such triggers are more likely to occur in housing conditions found more frequently among families living in poverty; medical control of symptoms is also less likely when poverty restricts access to healthcare. Finally, chronic activation of these biological responses, from the combined effects of environmental conditions and lack of optimal healthcare, can result in long-lasting increase in propensity of the physiologic responses that underlie asthma symptoms. This combination of prenatal exposure, constitutional propensities, environmental exposures, and promotive contexts should always be considered when attempting to understand the effects of potential behavioral teratogens. Many will recognize this scenario as a classic example of (cumulative) risk and resilience interpretations of human development.

In addition to the broad theoretical conditions on interpreting the behavioral teratology literature, there are specific research concerns as well. Perhaps the most important is the issue of effect size. The interpretation of exposures at very high levels is typically relatively easy – effects on children follow regular patterns that are easily identified and occur in a large proportion of those exposed; this is the usual route by which we become interested in particular teratogens. Most current work, however, is concerned with lower-level exposures where the effects on children are far less pronounced. Typically, children are affected in different ways (many are apparently not affected at all), and the overall sizes of the effects are small. This set of circumstances makes interpretation very difficult. From a pure research perspective, small effects will be statistically significant only in large samples, and it is often the case that some degree of data mining has occurred before the effects are detected (owing to the expense of compiling this difficult-to-obtain data). It is thus important to consider the functional implications of statistical differences that may have small effect size.

We now turn to summarizing results in several specific domains of behavioral teratology. The first sections concern environmental pollutants, followed by sections on substances used by pregnant women. This is not a comprehensive review of all potential behavioral teratogens relevant to infants and young children, but rather a sampling of some of the most notable domains of work.

Environmental Teratogens

Lead Exposure

Lead, which is ubiquitous in the environment, is the teratogen that receives the most attention from a public health perspective. Although much of the attention with regard to lead is on postnatal exposure of children, there are prenatal exposures as well. Exposures can occur in paint, soil, and ceramics; it is a common pollutant in air as well, with gasoline being one historical source (although banned in recent years). Lead exposure at high levels has demonstrable effects on child development. Physical health can be affected in areas as diverse as growth, fertility, hearing, and renal function (even leading to death at very high exposure levels); effects extend to the behavioral realm as well, including intelligence, attention, memory, and self-regulation. To combat these known effects, testing for lead levels is widespread, and therapeutic interventions to reduce levels in the body and in the environment are common when high levels are detected.

The effects of low levels of lead (typically examined between 10 and 20 $\mu g\ dl^{-1}$) are less clear. It has been widely presumed that low levels of lead would have similar, albeit smaller, effects on young children – assumptions reflected in public health policies. Data supporting this assumption are far from conclusive. A large number of published studies identify effects on a wide variety of behavioral outcomes. Many other studies, however, have found little or no effects on the same behavioral parameters. In the case of intelligence quotient (IQ), for example, some argue that small effect sizes (3 IQ points or less) are both of limited practical significance and conceptually suspect in the context of numerous methodological difficulties noted in the extant literature; such limitations include poor inclusion of confounding variables, lack of attention to parental IQ, little control for multiple statistical comparisons, examination of extreme groups, and poor quality control in data collection. This set of arguments (which indeed can be applied to all areas of behavioral teratology) has been refuted, noting that the corpus of studies on lead exposure is commensurate in quality with those in the human development literature in general.

Meta-analysis, often useful in resolving uncertainty in the face of conflicting findings, has generated as much debate as the corpus of original empirical studies. Indeed, Kaufman's commentary in 2001 presents aggregate evidence in the domain of IQ, arriving at a relatively noncontroversial estimate of effect size of about 2–3 IQ points for the increase from 10 to 20 μg dl^{-1}. What becomes controversial, however, is the nonquantitative portion of meta-analytic procedures. High-quality meta-analyses examine not only the specific estimates of associations or group differences, but also examine variance associated with various study characteristics, including quality. It is at this point that disagreements often occur (as is true for the literature on low lead levels) as the criteria are inherently more subjective.

Polychlorinated biphenyl Exposure

PCBs are a class of compounds derived from commonly occurring hydrocarbons combined with chlorine. PCBs are very stable compounds ranging from viscous to solid, and have desirable insulating, nonflammability, and lubricating properties. Used widely in a variety of industrial applications, their use has been curtailed dramatically since environmental concerns became apparent in the 1970s. Their stability has resulted in large accumulations in various industrial sites, and PCBs have found their way into the food chain as well, mostly in adipose tissue in fish. Physical health effects have been noted, including some cancer risk, skin conditions, and liver function changes, and animal studies suggest immune system changes as well.

Early reports of health effects in workers exposed to large concentrations of PCBs in Asia, as well as effects on children born to exposed women, fueled many subsequent cohort studies focusing on prenatal exposure. Interpretation of the original Asian exposures has been difficult to interpret regarding PCBs, owing to the presence of other PCB derivatives known to be far more toxic than the PCBs themselves. Findings from early studies were contradictory, but subsequent work has converged on the presence of small (and perhaps nonspecific) subtle effects on physical and cognitive functioning. Effects include lower birth weight, smaller head circumference, poorer long-term memory, less response inhibition, longer reaction time, and changes in P300 duration (a physiological brain response to a sensory stimulus). These findings are not uncomplicated, however. Breastfeeding, for example, appears to be protective rather than additive in terms of PCB effects, perhaps because breastfeeding mothers provide more optimal contextual supports.

Mercury Exposure

As noted above, mercury enters the environment in natural ways and as part of industrial processes; it is found in the food supply and in pharmaceuticals. High-level exposures were observed in notorious industrial pollution sites in Japan. As noted in McCurry's historical description of the Minamata mercury exposure, symptoms were first noted in cats and birds, and quickly thereafter in humans. Severe neurological problems (paralysis, convulsions,

speech problems, etc.), often resulting in death, were widespread. The widespread publicity of these events (one of my own early childhood memories is seeing the compelling pictures of affected residents in *Life* magazine) resulted in substantial attention to the issue of mercury pollution, environmental controls, and subsequent interest in low-level and prenatal exposures. For example, studies of adult dental workers have identified associations among mercury levels, gene mutations affecting pro-survival proteins (brain derived neurotrophic factor), and performance deficits on simple cognitive-motor tasks.

Many studies identify associations between prenatal mercury exposure and childhood deficits in cognitive and motor performance. Associations with IQ, language, and achievement tests have been observed in a New Zealand cohort of 6–7-year-old children; analyses identify levels of about 10 mg kg^{-1} as being potential thresholds at which deficits are noted. Another cohort from the Faroe Islands exhibited associations of prenatal mercury exposure and simple motor and cognitive tasks at 14 years of age. Associations with postnatal exposure were not identified. Some investigators strike a somewhat different tone, noting that most assessments of cognitive and motor function at 9 years of age did not reveal associations with prenatal mercury exposure.

In a combined quantitative analysis of these cohorts, it is estimated that the dose–response relationships is about 0.7 IQ points μg g^{-1} of mercury detectable in hair samples. Given that the median value is 0.2 μg g^{-1} and the 90th percentile is 1.4 μg g^{-1}, the ultimate meaning of these associations is uncertain. In commenting on the Myers *et al.* findings, Lyketsos in 2003 asserts that there is no contraindication for prenatal fish consumption in most parts of the world, although in a few isolated areas where shark and whale are consumed (with higher mercury concentrations) the recommendation might be different.

Stepping outside the strict realm of behavioral teratology for the moment, perhaps the most contentious issue regarding mercury exposure concerns thiomersal use in vaccines. Many have hypothesized that the mercury exposure is related to subsequent autism and other neurodevelopmental problems. Most epidemiologic studies do not support this view. One potential reason for the lack of effect may be that the ethyl-mercury in the vaccine preservative is less toxic than the methylmercury typically found in more naturally occurring mercury. This set of studies has not, however, diminished the debate, as a brief visit to the world-wide-web reveals. Western countries have mostly eliminated thiomersal from vaccines, but less-developed countries have not in part because of expense and in part because of the need for effective preservative. Thus, discussion of the effects has become framed in terms of short- to medium-term costs and benefits of vaccine use in prevention of disease, use of public heath funds, and risks of thiomersal-containing vaccines.

Licit and Illicit Substances

Tobacco Exposure

Tobacco is a legal substance used primarily for recreational purposes. There is a large literature on the association of tobacco use during pregnancy and subsequent pregnancy and child outcomes. The vast majority of tobacco use is via cigarette smoking, particularly for women. In addition to direct use by pregnant women, there is also passive contact with environmental tobacco smoke (both to pregnant women and to young infants after birth) as a potential additional source of exposure. Still, the bulk of the literature on tobacco exposure concerns maternal smoking during pregnancy.

Approximately 20% of American women smoke during pregnancy. Rates are highest among unmarried, unemployed women from lower socioeconomic status (SES) backgrounds, likely affecting about 800 000 births per year. Although we know little about the effects on young infants, it is important to note that women who smoke during pregnancy continue to do so after pregnancy, thereby exposing children to the hazardous effects of prenatal smoking as well as to those associated with environmental tobacco smoke.

Extrapolations from existing data indicate that smoking during pregnancy is responsible for up to 4800 infant deaths as well as 26 000 infants needing neonatal intensive care annually. Smoking causes important changes in fetal neurological development and also results in increased rates of spontaneous abortion, placenta previa, placental abruption, and perhaps sudden infant death syndrome (SIDS). Furthermore, a dose–response relationship between smoking and birth weight exists, with infants born to smokers being typically 150–250 g lighter in comparison to infants of nonsmokers.

In addition to the well-documented associations of prenatal tobacco use and pregnancy outcomes, behavioral functioning of infants may be affected in the realm of poor cognitive function (especially executive processes), unregulated behavior, attention difficulties, and difficult temperament. In the first days of life, infants present as difficult and unregulated. Sucking behavior, perhaps the most basic organized function of neonates, is weaker and less efficient. Crying of tobacco-exposed infants is also affected, with high pitch and excessive crying, which is indicative of a less well-organized system. There is also indication of early difficulty on Brazelton's Neonatal Behavior Assessment Scale indexes of tremulousness, irritability, and habituation.

As children grow older, their behavior becomes more organized. With respect to regulatory behaviors, there are several indications that the early neurobehavioral differences persist into later childhood. Furthermore, these characteristics have been implicated in pathways to delinquency and substance abuse. General temperamental difficulty is increased in nicotine-exposed children, in particular activity level. From a more clinical perspective,

tobacco-exposed children exhibit more symptoms of, and are diagnosed more frequently with, attention deficit hyperactivity disorder. Regulation differences are also manifest at the physiologic level, where nicotine-exposed children exhibit lower autonomic arousal.

Cognitive functioning is also related to prenatal nicotine exposure. General effects are present in lower scores on standardized tests beginning in infancy and extending to the school years. Also, nicotine-exposed children have more difficulty with complex cognitive executive functions. Specific learning and reading problems are also evident as children enter school, and the related cognitive manifestations of attentional problems are also noted in tobacco-exposed children. As with behavioral regulation, these cognitive and attentional processes have been implicated in the development of antisocial behavior (see below).

Another notable association with prenatal tobacco exposure is conduct disorder and antisocial behavior. Beginning early in childhood, prenatally exposed children have more conduct problems. Later in adolescence and young adulthood, these conduct problems may manifest as delinquent and criminal behavior. There is, however, some concern that these associations may be more related to postnatal characteristics of families where pregnant women smoke, rather than prenatal smoking. Associations of prenatal exposure and conduct problems are particularly intriguing in the context of associations with behavior regulation, temperament, attention, and executive function. All of these characteristics have been implicated in the development of antisocial behavior in adolescents and young adults. Low physiological reactivity has also been associated with conduct problems, although there is less evidence for the association with prenatal nicotine exposure. Taken together, these findings highlight that identifying early in life the roots of behavioral dysregulation, poor attention and cognitive functioning, and difficult temperament would provide some developmental insights into the long-term effects of prenatal nicotine exposure.

Alcohol Exposure

Like tobacco, alcohol is a legal substance used primarily for recreational purposes. Although alcohol is present in some medications and foods, almost all exposure relevant to behavioral teratology is via voluntary recreational use. Alcoholic beverages are significant in almost all cultures; they have been available since ancient times when beer and wine were widely produced and were integral to economic development. Patterns of use vary widely both among cultures and individually within cultures. The association of alcohol use with adverse pregnancy/child development outcomes has been widely acknowledged over the past 30 years.

Virtually all interest with regard to alcohol exposure and young children's development concerns prenatal alcohol exposure; there is little reason to suspect that direct exposure occurs in the postnatal period. Heavy use during pregnancy is associated with fetal alcohol syndrome (FAS), which was initially identified by Jones and Smith in 1973. FAS is characterized by facial deformities, microcephaly, muscular/skeletal abnormalities, memory problems, and perhaps other cognitive deficits. Drinking thresholds for occurrence of FAS are unclear, but it is likely substantial – on the order of an average (or multiple instances of) five or more standard drinks per day for extended periods during pregnancy. Furthermore, timing of exposure may be important, with much attention on first trimester effects.

The consequence of lower levels of exposure is far less clear. Public health guidelines in the US recommend no drinking at all during pregnancy, for example, as recommended in 2004 by the National Center for Birth Defects and Developmental Disabilities. But research findings are far less clear regarding negative effects of drinking at low levels during pregnancy. Many studies have identified associations with small effect size when examining cognitive functioning in children whose mothers drank during pregnancy. These studies, however, often have conflicting findings. In many cases, specific tests are associated in some studies but not in others, or associations are found for some subgroups but not for others. When examining young children, one meta-analysis identified associations at one age (12 months) but not at two other ages. Such patterns of findings bring into question the degree to which effects of low levels of prenatal alcohol use are indeed associated with specific or nonspecific developmental problems, independent of other confounding factors.

Some have gone further and questioned whether the cultural context in which the science of alcohol effects developed has influenced interpretation of findings. Most notable among these critiques is the work of Abel and Armstrong during the past decade. Abel notes that for FAS, incidence rates among heavy drinkers are far higher in the US than in Western Europe, despite the fact that many of the European countries have higher drinking rates than the US. He likens this phenomenon to the well-known 'French paradox' where high alcohol and fat consumption are not associated with high rates of heart disease. Explanations for the 'American paradox' for FAS incidence may range from patterns of alcohol consumption to reporting biases to SES and race differences. In a more pointed analysis, Armstrong and Abel note that the response to (and public recommendations regarding) the use of alcohol during pregnancy is far different in the US than in other countries. Whereas the US Surgeon General recommends no alcohol consumption during pregnancy, European countries such as the UK recommend that drinking at low levels (less than seven standard drinks per week) during pregnancy is not dangerous to the developing fetus, while noting potential harm at higher levels

(embodied in the 1996 statement by the Royal College of Obstetricians and Gynecologists). Armstrong and Abel contend that the US response is a moral panic (i.e., an exaggerated response to a perceived social problem) that is embedded in a moral, political, and media context peculiar to this country.

Illicit Drugs

Tobacco and alcohol are the two legal psychoactive substances most often used for recreational purposes. There are, of course, many illicit psychoactive substances, many of which are used by pregnant women. Those that have received the most attention with respect to behavioral effects in young children are cocaine, marijuana, opiates, and (more recently) methamphetamine. As with tobacco and alcohol, almost all studies have focused on prenatal exposure; cocaine and methamphetamine both have the potential for passive postnatal exposure because smoking is one common route of administration, and for methamphetamine, there is also potential for passive exposure because it is often manufactured in home-based laboratories.

Much of what is known about prenatal marijuana exposure emanates from the work of two large cohort studies conducted by Fried and colleagues and Goldschmidt and colleagues. Marijuana (especially the active ingredient Δ-9-tetrahydrocannabinol (THC)) likely acts on cerebral blood flow, cerebral glucose metabolism, and binds to cannabis-specific receptor sites (which may be overrepresented in frontal cortex). Behavioral effects have been reported in infancy and early childhood (e.g., increased tremulousness), but have not been very consistent across time and study, and most comparisons have revealed no effects. Later in childhood, however, evidence converges to some extent on effects in the realm of executive function. Although a loosely defined term, executive function typically is used to convey higher-order volitional cognitive processes (e.g., sustained attention, inhibition, working memory). Beginning around age 4 years, a pattern of findings implicates a series of executive function measures, including memory, attention, visual–spatial skills, impulsivity, and problem solving. Even so, the effect sizes of the marijuana associations are small, and the pattern of findings inconsistent. These samples have been followed through early adolescence.

Cohort studies of prenatal cocaine exposure began 10–15 years later than those focused on marijuana exposure. Whereas the marijuana cohort studies were conducted largely motivated by scientific interest, the cocaine cohort studies were accompanied by a far greater degree of public concern about the fate of so-called 'crack babies'. Cocaine has a multitude of physiologic effects, most notably blocking synaptic reuptake of catecholamines (norepinephrine, dopamine) and serotonin by specific, presynaptic plasma membrane transporters. Cocaine also blocks the reuptake of catecholamines in adrenal cells, all leading to elevated circulating catecholamine levels. Sympathetic nervous system responses including hypertension, tachycardia, vasoconstriction, agitation, euphoria, and excitation are likely downstream effects, which in turn suggest many behavioral processes that may be modified.

Early in life, prenatal cocaine exposure appears to affect arousal, excitability, acoustic cry characteristics, and the auditory brainstem response. These are specifically manifest in greater excitability, many state transitions, more state transitions associated with stimulation, more rapid arousal from sleep, and increased physiological lability. More organized attention- and information-processing system deficits have been reported in cocaine-exposed infants, as have differences in mother–child dyadic interaction and attachment security. Prenatal cocaine exposure has also been shown to influence the hypothalamic–pituitary–adrenal (HPA) axis. Salivary cortisol in nonchallenging situations, as well as in the context of noninvasive and invasive challenges is low.

As cocaine-exposed children grow older, there is evidence that they may have cognitive and/or executive function deficits as well as other behavioral and physical problems. Cognition and attention functions are poorer at 4 years of age. Event-related potentials in high-density EEG assessments are longer in duration (indicating less efficient processing) in response to word stimuli in 8-year-olds. Dysmorphic physical features have been noted in some samples of prenatally exposed children. Aggression at age 5 years has also been related to prenatal cocaine exposure. Overall, the effect sizes in most studies are small, and interpretation of the degree of effect must always keep this point in mind.

Fewer follow-up studies exist for examination of opiates and methamphetamine. Neonatal abstinence syndrome has been clinically recognized for some time in response to 'withdrawal' of opiates in newborns of mothers who were chronic users. Most of what we know about later development, however, comes from follow-up of children whose mothers used methadone during pregnancy. A related issue historically was the effect of opiate medications used during labor, which is less relevant given current labor and delivery practice. Methamphetamine, on the other hand, has only recently been a focus of those interested in the effects of prenatal exposure.

With regard to opiate exposure, effects on behavior are observed in newborns and in the first years of life. As noted above, neonatal abstinence syndrome, affecting autonomic, gastrointestinal, and respiratory functions, is widely observed, although dose–response relationships are difficult to establish. Difficulties in the social–emotional realm may be present (e.g., disorganized attachment), but it may be the case that this is only true for those families with multiple contextual adversities. There is little evidence of generalized cognitive or motor deficits in opiate-exposed children. Methamphetamine exposure currently has a very small empirical knowledge base, as the first studies have been reported only in the past few years. There does, however, appear to be some indication of fetal growth restriction.

Some general issues in the substance-exposure literature are worth noting here. Most available work is focused on identifying effects of specific substances, in line with specific main-effects-type developmental models. This is the case despite the well-known phenomenon that pregnant women who use one of the licit or illicit substances reviewed here tend to use more than one. Thus, in the absence of the ability to conduct more rigidly controlled experiments, analyses of effects of single substances are almost always in the context of many other potential teratogens to which the developing fetus is exposed. Furthermore, as noted by Lester and Hans in separate commentaries in the past decade, there are also clear associations of broad contextual factors (poverty, racial/ethnic minority status) as well as more subtle lifestyle and parenting characteristics of the families in which the children are reared. Finally, it is also likely that the subtle exposure effects on children will themselves alter the developmental trajectories of the emergent parent–child relationship system.

Concluding Remarks

Several consistent themes emerge from a very diverse literature on teratogenic effects of prenatal (or early in life) exposure to a variety of substances:

- Exposures at high levels are associated with substantial developmental consequences for children, in some cases with distinct physical/behavioral syndromes.
- Exposures at low levels are far less clear cut – effects may not be present; when present, the effect sizes are small; the pattern of effects is inconsistent (across studies, or at different ages in longitudinal follow-ups of the same cohort); the functional significance of the effects may be small or nonexistent.
- Much of the focus has been on cognitive and motor performance, with less emphasis on social–emotional development.
- Investigation of multiple exposures is rare; when multiple exposures are identified, analysis tends to focus on untangling effects of individual substances.
- Exposures occur in larger social context that affects the developmental outcomes of interest – some studies address these issues well, but many do not.
- Complex developmental analyses are virtually nonexistent in this literature.

Given these general characteristics of the human behavioral teratology literature, we should remain cognizant that each set of scientific studies reviewed exist in a highly charged social and political context. On a general level, there are strong advocacy groups on both sides of the environmental pollutant debate, each of which would like to minimize or maximize the adverse developmental effects found in exposed children. The balance of economic development vs. small (and sometimes controversial) developmental effects is viewed differently on each side of this debate. In similar fashion, the literature on licit and illicit substance use (particularly in the US) exists in the framework of a declared war on drugs. Again, those concerned with eliminating drugs from the culture would have very different perspectives on research findings than those with a more *laissez faire* attitude. In other instances, the advocacy is very direct, with the issue of thiomersal exposure and neurodevelopmental problems being perhaps the best example. When science is conducted in these conditions, the end user of the science must be constantly vigilant for potential biases associated with promoting one's political or social views, need for funding, publication patterns, and degree of data mining to find results that satisfy either the publications biases or one's own scientific/social/political views.

To be more useful in the future, the field would benefit from several new or re-emphasized directions. These include examination of exposure in larger family and social context, application of more complex developmental models, examination of multiple exposures (particularly across boundaries where lines of investigation currently do not overlap), better reporting of nonsignificant findings (especially when samples are large enough to have low type II error), good meta-analyses to aggregate findings across studies, and interpretation of findings in the context of quality of life and cost-effectiveness models.

See also: Birth Defects; Endocrine System; Fetal Alcohol Spectrum Disorders; Lead Poisoning.

Suggested Readings

Abel EL (1998) Fetal alcohol syndrome: The 'American paradox'. *Alcohol and & Alcoholism* 33: 195–201.
Armstrong EM and Abel EL (2000) Fetal alcohol syndrome: The origins of moral panic. *Alcohol and Alcoholism* 35: 276–282.
Brown RT (2001) Behavioral teratology/toxicology: How do we know what we know? *Archives of Clinical Neuropsychology* 16: 389–402.
Dilworth-Bart JE and Moore CF (2006) Mercy mercy me: Social injustice and prevention of environmental pollutant exposures among ethnic minority and poor children. *Child Development* 77: 247–265.
Fraser S, Muckle G, and Despres C (2006) The relationship between lead exposure, motor function, and behavior in Inuit preschool children. *Neurotoxicology and Teratology* 28: 18–27.
Fried PA and Smith AM (2001) A literature review of the consequences of prenatal marihuana exposure: An emerging theme of a deficiency in aspects of executive function. *Neurotoxicology and Teratology* 23: 1–11.
Hans SL (2002) Studies of prenatal exposure to drugs focusing on parental care of children. *Neurotoxicology and Teratology* 24: 329–337.
Kaufman AS (2001) How dangerous are low (not moderate or high) doses of lead for children's intellectual development? *Archives of Clinical Neuropsychology* 16: 403–431.
Lester B, Lagasse L, and Seifer R (1998) Prenatal cocaine exposure: The meaning of subtle effects. *Science* 282: 633–634.
McCurry J (2006) Japan remembers Minamata. *Lancet* 367: 99–100.
Olds D (1997) Tobacco exposure and impaired development: A review of the evidence. *Mental Retardation and Developmental Disabilities Research Reviews* 3: 257–269.
Riley EP and Vorhees CV (1986) *Handbook of Behavioral Teratology.* New York: Plenum.
Sameroff AJ, Lewis M, and Miller SM (eds.) (2000) *Handbook of Developmental Psychopathology,* 2nd edn. New York: Plenum.
Testa M, Quigley BM, and Eiden RD (2003) The effects of prenatal alcohol exposure on infant mental development: A meta-analytical review. *Alcohol and Alcoholism* 38: 295–304.
Wachs TD (2000) *Necessary but not Sufficient: The Respective Roles of Single and Multiple Influences on Individual Development.* Washington, DC: American Psychological Association.
Wakschlag LS and Hans SL (2002) Maternal smoking during pregnancy and conduct problems in high-risk youth: A developmental framework. *Development and Psychopathology* 14: 351–369.

Vision Disorders and Visual Impairment

J Atkinson, University College London, London, UK
O Braddick, University of Oxford, Oxford, UK

Glossary

ABCDEFV – Atkinson Battery of Child Development for Examining Functional Vision.

Accommodation – Adjustment of the lens of the eye to bring objects at different distances into sharp focus on the retina.

Acuity – A measure of the ability to detect fine detail.

Amblyopia – A loss of visual acuity that cannot be explained by the optical effects of refractive error or by pathology of the eye. Amblyopia is believed to result from functional changes in neural connections, primarily in the visual cortex, that results from degraded visual input.

Anisometropia – A difference of refraction between the two eyes.

Aphakia – Absence of the lens of the eye.

Astigmatism – A difference in refraction of the eye between different meridians, usually caused by the cornea having different degrees of curvature in different directions.

Binocular – Using the two eyes together.

Binocular disparity – Difference between position of images of an object as viewed by the two eyes.

Cataract – An opacity in the lens of the eye.

Contrast sensitivity – The ability to detect the difference between light and dark parts of the image.

Cornea – The curved transparent surface at the front of the eye, through which light passes into the pupil.

Crowding – The effect that acuity for recognizing a letter is reduced if it is surrounded by other letters.

Cycloplegia – The relaxation of the muscles that control accommodation of the lens.

Dorsal stream – A series of cortical areas, transmitting visual information from V1 to the parietal lobe of the brain, that extracts information and provides a sense of spatial relationships and the basis for visually guided actions.

Electroretinogram (ERG) – An electrical signal recorded from the surface of the cornea, that originates in the retina and can help to diagnose disease conditions of the photoreceptors and other retinal elements.

Extrastriate cortex – The collection of visually responsive areas of cortex that surround *area V1* and receive input from it directly or indirectly. It includes areas V2, V3, V3a, V4, V5, and lateral occipital (LO).

Fixation – The act of moving the eye, or maintaining its direction, so that the object of interest is focused on the fovea. Sometimes called 'fixing' in newborns.

Form coherence – A measure of the global visual processing that integrates information about static shape and pattern in the ventral cortical stream.

Fovea – The region in the center of the retina where the cone photoreceptors are most densely packed, and which therefore provides the highest acuity.

Frontal eye fields (FEF) – A region of the frontal cortex, that is involved in eye movements control.

Fusiform face area (FFA) – A region of the brain presumed to be a specialized center for processing the visual information used to detect and recognize faces.

Glaucoma – A disorder where the pressure of fluids within the eye is abnormally high.

Habituation/recovery – A method of investigating the ability of young infants to distinguish different visual patterns. If one pattern is presented repeatedly, the time spent by the infant looking at it declines (habituation). If the looking time increases when a new pattern is presented (recovery), this is evidence that the infants can distinguish the two patterns and so respond to the novelty of the new pattern.

Hyperopia or hypermetropia – Far-sightedness.

Hypoxic-ischemic encephalopathy (HIE) – Widespread brain damage caused by a general deprivation of oxygen (hypoxia).

Lateral geniculate nucleus (LGN) – A nucleus in the thalamus where the fibers of the optic nerve terminate.

Lateral occipital (LO) – An area on the lateral and ventral aspects of the human occipital cortex, which responds strongly to intact images of objects and scenes as opposed to scrambled versions of the same images.

Mirror neuron – A neuron which responds either when an animal is executing a certain action, or when it sees that action being performed by another.

Monocular – Relating to one eye only (contrast with binocular).

Motion coherence – A measure of visual processing that detects elements moving in a consistent direction, although the remaining elements are moving in random directions.

Myopia – Near-sightedness.

Nystagmus – Repetitive oscillatory movements of the eyes.

Optokinetic nystagmus (OKN) – Nystagmus induced by motion of all, or a large part of, the field of view. The eyes repetitively follow the movement of the field and then flick rapidly back in the opposite direction.

Orthoptic – The clinical practice of exercises designed to improve eye movements, develop accurate and reliable control of vergence and encourage the establishment and maintenance of binocular function.

Parahippocampal place area (PPA) – A region of the brain, active when viewing scenes such as the interior and exterior of buildings, especially for familiar locations.

Photoreceptors – Cells within the retina that convert light energy into electrical signals that can be processed by other nerve cells in the retina and brain. Rod photoreceptors are sensitive to dim light but do not provide good acuity or color vision. Cone receptors, provide high acuity and can signal the difference between colors.

Photorefraction – A method of estimating the refractive state of the eye, by recording photographically the pattern of light returning through the pupil of the eye from a flash.

Posterior parietal cortex (PPC) – A complex of brain areas that receive information from extrastriate visual areas and form part of the dorsal stream.

Preferential looking – A method of testing infant vision by measuring the infant's preference for looking at a patterned screen compared with a blank one.

Refraction – The process of measuring the distance at which an eye is focused when relaxed.

Retina – The neural network, with supporting tissues and blood vessels, that covers the inside of the back of the eyeball.

Spatial frequency – A measure of the scale of detail present in a pattern.

Stereopsis or stereoscopic vision – The ability to perceive the relative distance and three-dimensional modeling of objects in the scene. It depends on nerve cells in visual cortex receiving and processing signals from the two eyes together, and can be impaired or abolished when strabismus prevents this from occurring.

Strabismus – A condition where the axes of the two eyes are misaligned and so look in different directions.

Striate cortex – An alternative name for area V1, named from the 'Stripe of Gennari' where the fibers of the optic radiation terminate.

Superior colliculus – A structure in the midbrain, also known as the optic tectum, which receives input from the retina by a branch of the optic nerve. It sends output to oculomotor nuclei for the control of eye movements, and so is believed to be responsible for orienting behavior, including in newborn infants whose cortex is immature.

Visual evoked potentials or visual event-related potentials (VEP/VERP) – Electrical signals recorded noninvasively from the surface of the head, that arise from visual processing events in the underlying brain structures.

Ventral stream – A series of cortical areas, transmitting visual information from V1 to the temporal lobe of the brain, which extracts information that enables the visual recognition of faces, objects, and scenes.

Vergence – An eye movement which alters the relative direction of the two eyes.

Vernier Acuity – The ability to make fine visual comparisons of position, for example, whether two vertical lines are aligned or misaligned.

V1 – (striate cortex) The primary receiving area in the ocipital lobe of the brain for visual information.

V2, V3, V3a, V4, V5 – Extrastriate visual areas of the brain.

Visual cortex – The region in the occipital lobe of the brain that carries out the early stages of processing of the visual image.

Introduction

To understand visual development and its disorders, it is necessary to understand in outline the structure and function of the visual system. This is a technical subject with a specialized vocabulary.

An optical image of the visual world is formed in the eyes and is encoded into neural signals in the retina. These signals are transformed, first by the neural network of the retina, and then by transmission through a series of interconnected brain areas. Complex brain processing is required to use incoming visual information for recognizing objects, people, and events; for location in the environment; and for guiding visuomotor actions. Developmental disorders of vision can arise from problems at all levels of this process. Furthermore, the development of the later, brain-based stages depends on the signals that are received from the eye, so disorders of the eyes can lead to more pervasive problems of visual perception and cognition.

A sharp optical image depends on the cornea (front surface of the eye) and lens focusing light rays on the retina, and on the media within the eye being clear and transparent. The retinal photoreceptor cells (rods and cones) signal the light intensity falling upon them, and a neural network in the retina lead to the optic nerve fibers that carry information to the brain. These fibers are routed so that signals from the each eye are transmitted to each side of the brain via a relay in the thalamus (the lateral geniculate nucleus LGN).

The signals arrive in the striate cortex (or area V1) in the occipital lobe of the brain, where the neurons are specialized to extract various kinds of information, notably the orientation of lines and edges, directions of motion, and to bring together information from the two eyes for depth perception based on binocular disparity (stereopsis – the 3-dimensional 3D vision). V1 is surrounded by a series of extrastriate visual areas, such as V2, V3, V4, and V5, which have distinct specializations of function; for example, area V5 (also known as MT) combines the directional information coming from V1 to detect more global patterns of motion over larger spatial areas. Pathways through these extrastriate visual areas send information to the temporal and parietal lobes of the brain. The ventral stream, involving the temporal lobe, is specialized for recognizing shapes and objects, including human faces, while the dorsal stream, involving the parietal lobe, encodes the spatial and motion information needed for visually guided actions. This whole complex of neural circuitry is called the cortical visual system. Some specialized areas for processing information about faces (fusiform face area), objects (lateral-occipital – LO), places or scenes (parahippocampal place area – PPA) have been identified in adults from Functional magnetic rescrarce imaging (FMRI) brain imaging studies. Other pools of cortical neurons are involved in specific visuomotor actions (e.g., mirror neurons in the frontal lobes) together with specific networks for discriminating emotional states from visual expressions and gestures.

The brain based processing of visual information can be called perception, cognition, spatial cognition, sensorimotor cognition, or spatial attention. In development these all involve overlapping neural circuitry. Notably, the deployment of selective attention determines how we act on visual information coming in. Visual information is integrated with other senses and with planning and on-line control of action, and gives us our ability to orient ourselves in space and to manipulate spatial information.

A minority of fibers in the optic nerve do not connect to the cerebral cortex, but to midbrain structures, in particular the superior colliculus. This pathway primarily serves to control eye movements, in particular saccades, the abrupt jerk eye movements which shift gaze from one object to another. Midbrain nuclei also control the smooth eye movements enable us to follow moving objects, and the reflex optokinetic nystagmus (OKN) that stabilizes vision when the whole field of view moves. In adults, all these eye movement functions interact strongly with the more complex analysis taking place in the cortex, via connections that run both ways between subcortical visual centers and visual cortical areas, in particular involving the frontal eye fields (FEF) and posterior parietal complex (PPC).

Techniques Used to Measure Normal and Abnormal Vision

One of the most basic measures of visual development is that of visual acuity. One measure, detection acuity, is the thinnest line or dot that can be distinguished from a uniform background. If the line to be detected has sharp high-contrast edges it may still be detected with blurred vision. An edge can be blurred either because of optical blurring in the formation of the optical image within the eye itself and/or due to processes that degrade the retinal image within the neural system. Single dots or white balls are often used in standard pediatric clinical tests of acuity (such as the STYCAR balls test) and give an approximate measure of the child's real-life visual limitations of vision under these particular viewing conditions. For measuring resolution acuity a bar or grating pattern is commonly used in the method of preferential looking. At some level of blur the grating becomes indistinguishable from a uniform gray. Grating acuity is often expressed in terms of spatial frequency.

A second basic measure is contrast sensitivity, where the bars of a grating are varied in contrast against the background as well as in width. For measurements of acuity and contrast sensitivity for children between

2 and 6 years of age various behavioral matching or searching tasks have been devised such as the Cambridge crowding cards. This test, for children aged between 4 and 7 years, conducted at a 3 m (10 ft) viewing distance (rather than 6 m (20 ft) – the standard viewing distance for letter charts for adults), gives a line equivalence of a Snellen letter chart for preschool children. Another effective standardized test for preschool children is the Lea Symbols test. These preschool tests can be used with older children with physical and mental disabilities, such as children with minimal responses with cerebral palsy. Besides these behavioral methods, acuity and contrast sensitivity have been estimated using electrophysiological techniques, visual-evoked potential (VEP) or visual event related potentials (VERP), including the sweep VEP method.

For measuring cortical responses in infants and children, marker tasks have been devised to identify responses in particular neural pathways specific for certain visual attributes (such as orientation or shape, motion, color, binocular disparity), combining results from electrophysiological and behavioral methods such as forced-choice preferential looking (FPL) and habituation. This has provided a neurobiological account of early eye–brain development, underpinning normal development of spatial vision. This model gives the sequence of developmental visual milestones, together with the broad neural processes corresponding to them, against which abnormalities can be identified.

For assessing functional vision in both normal and clinical populations, a portable battery has been standardized for testing from birth to 6 years, the ABCDEFV. This includes standard procedures for core vision tests (such as measures of acuity and control of eye movements) and additional tests for higher-level functions in the visuocognitive domain (shape matching, spatial tasks such as block construction copying). From such a standardized battery an approximate age equivalence can be given for children who are lagging behind their peers and areas of concern can be identified for further testing. Some findings using this battery are described briefly later.

Model of Normal Visual Development

Studies of human infants show that the newborn, starting with very limited visual behavior, develops over the first months of life many of the complex visual processes of pattern and depth perception. Neurophysiological and anatomical evidence, and clinical observations, show that this is achieved by a programmed sequence of maturation interacting closely with activation by the environment

Visual development goes through a number of stages, presented diagrammatically in **Figure 1**.

At birth, the infant can make saccadic eye movements and imprecise, slow head movements to orient toward high-contrast targets, a function mediated by a subcortical system involving the superior colliculus, with functioning of the visual cortex being, at best, rudimentary. This newborn 'where?' orienting system only operates well when there is no competition between targets for the newborn's attention. It is likely to operate across sensory modalities as a nonspecific alerting system, shown by the ability to orient the head and eyes to a lateral auditory stimulus in the first few hours after birth.

Over the first 6 months of life a set of specific neural networks (sometimes called channels or modules) become functional for processing different visual attributes in the cortex. Onset after birth of cortical visual processes for orientation selectivity is around 3–6 weeks of post-term age; directional motion selectivity around 2–3 months of post-term age of; and binocular interaction for stereopsis is functional around 4 months of post-term age. The infant can use perspective information for depth perception from 6 months onwards. Pools of neurons, sensitive to these different visual attributes, form the first stage of the two main cortical streams of processing, the dorsal and ventral streams. It has been suggested that because sensitivity to orientation and color develops a little earlier than channels for motion and binocular disparity that the ventral stream starts to function at these lower levels slightly earlier than the dorsal stream.

At the next stage of processing in dorsal and ventral streams, in extrastriate cortex, global cortical processing takes place. The development of global motion processing – a function of extrastriate dorsal stream processing – can be compared with global processing of form in the ventral stream, where analogous thresholds can be measured in young children. In infants, form coherence discrimination is apparent from 4 to 6 months of age from preferential looking and VEP/VERP studies. Global organization based on pattern orientation is found to be less effective in determining infant behavior than global organization based on motion coherence (sensitivity to the latter is apparent from around 9 weeks of age onwards). At this stage of dorsal and ventral stream processing, the dorsal stream areas appear to be processing stimuli for global motion coherence earlier than those in the ventral stream for global static form coherence.

Sensitivity in these channels is followed by development of integrative processes across channels within a single stream so that the infant can build up internal representations of objects, including discrimination of individuals in face recognition. However, faces are a special case, for which there may be an earlier, possibly subcortical, mechanism operating from birth, which biases visual attention to configurations that are face-like in the newborn. This may be replaced by a cortical system operating from a few months after birth for discrimination of faces using more detailed information from features. At present there is a discrepancy between the behavioral and

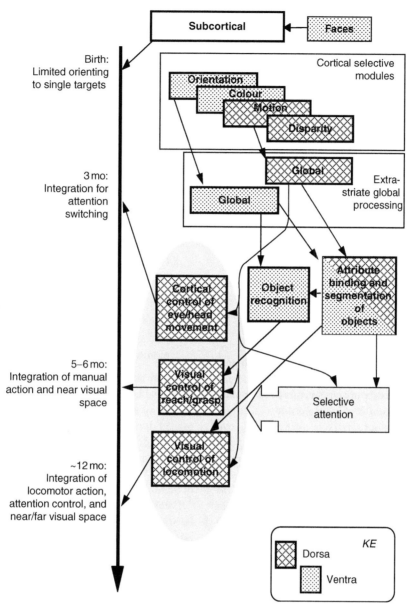

Figure 1 Schematic neurobiological model of visual development over the first year of life.

VERP data; behavioral studies indicate that infants can discriminate faces from 3 months onwards but evidence from VERP studies suggests that the maturation of the FFA, is later, toward the end of the first year.

These cortical channels for visual attributes are linked into the first functional cortical networks for selective attention. Orienting or switching attention to a peripheral novel stimulus or target, when the infant is already fixating a centrally presented stimulus, requires modulation and disengagement of the subcortical orienting system by cortical processes. In normally developing infants, the cortical system for active switches of attention between competing targets starts to function around 3–4 months of age. Evidence for the role of the cortex comes from

studies of infants who have undergone hemispherectomy, surgical removal of one complete hemisphere to relieve intractable epilepsy. Postoperatively these infants can shift gaze toward a target appearing in the peripheral field contralateral to the removed hemisphere when a initial central fixation target disappears, but fail to disengage to fixate the peripheral target when the central target remains visible, although they can do so toward a target in the intact visual field. This 'sticky fixation' when two targets are competing has also been observed in infants with focal lesions in parietal areas and infants with diffuse hypoxic ischemic encephalopathy (HIE). It resembles the problems seen in adult patients as part of the visual neglect syndrome.

Attribute binding and figure-ground segregation: Throughout development there must be interactions and integration between information in the dorsal and ventral streams. For objects to be represented, information about color, shape, and texture must be integrated with motion information at a relatively early stage, so that objects can be segregated from each other in space and separated from their background. This basic 'figure-ground' segmentation has been shown to start functioning at around 3 months of age. These processes provide object representations that must be integrated with dorsal-stream spatial information to allow the infant to act and respond, first with selective eye and head orienting action systems, then later with the emergence of action systems associated with reaching and grasping, and later still with exploratory action systems involving locomotion. These action systems require maturation and integration in both visual attentional systems and visuomotor systems and are integral parts of the dorsal stream.

Alongside emergence of these qualitative functional changes, there are steady quantitative improvements in vision in terms of visual acuity, the range of velocities for motion perception, the control of pursuit eye movements (smooth pursuit), and the range of retinal disparity for stereo vision. In tracking eye movements there is a gradual change over the first 6 months of life from slow inaccurate saccadic tracking to smooth pursuit. Anticipatory eye movements are observed from around 2 months post-term age for reappearance of an object which has disappeared from view while the infant was tracking it. There is massive improvement in visual acuity in the first 6 months of life. Using FPL, the estimated acuity for an infant at birth and over the first few weeks of life is equivalent to around 20/600 in Snellen terms. By 3 months of age acuity is 20/200, at 6 months 20/100, and at 12 months about 20/50. VEP measures give comparable results, although some studies claim higher values at the youngest ages. Although an acuity of 20/600 would be legal blindness in an adult, newborn acuity and contrast sensitivity in near space is certainly good enough for everyday recognition tasks of people and large objects (such as the mother's face or a baby bottle) and for discriminating between different adult facial expressions. The rapid improvement in acuity over the first few months of life means that older infants' behavioral limitations are unlikely to be due to lack of acuity and are more likely to be due to the visuo-cognitive or visuomotor demands of the task. After 1 year of age there is a slow rise to adult levels by 6–7 years, with adult levels of grating acuity from FPL estimates earlier at around 3 years of age. Certainly single letter matching acuity values for 3-year-olds can often be the equivalent of 20/30 Snellen letters, and by 4–5 years acuity is equivalent to adult 20/30 from crowded letter matching tests (e.g., Cambridge crowding cards), provided the child is sufficiently motivated.

Several changes in the visual system underlie the very rapid improvements in acuity and 'contrast sensitivity' in infancy.

1. While the optical media are clear at birth, and infants' refractions (on average moderately hyperopic or far sighted) should not impose a limit, infants at 0–1 month of age generally accommodate (adjust the lens focus) at a near distance (e.g., 50 cm). They are capable of some adjustment of focus, but this becomes accurate over a much wider range of distances over the first 6 months. The range of refractive errors in infants and their development is discussed later.
2. At birth, the cone photoreceptors of the fovea are small and sparsely spaced. Although this imposes a serious limit on acuity and contrast sensitivity, overall visual development probably depends more critically on neural changes, especially in the cortex.
3. Progressive myelination of the visual pathway over the first years of life.
4. The number of synaptic connections throughout the visual system increases rapidly, particularly in the first 9 months, with later pruning.

Other aspects of the child's visual capabilities change a great deal between 2 and 7 years of age. The more complex aspects of perceptual or cognitive processes are underpinned by maturation of the massive interconnectivity between different cortical areas and networks. Standardized pediatric assessment batteries (e.g., Griffiths and Bailey), and the ABCDEFV battery contain tests that measure some of these visual components, such as shape matching tests.

Ventral and dorsal stream development in childhood have been measured from comparisons of form and motion coherence thresholds (using stimuli which have been matched to give equal thresholds in adults). Motion coherence thresholds have been found to mature later than form coherence, with children reaching adult levels for form coherence at around 8 years of age and for motion coherence around 10 years of age. A consistent deficit (or delay) in motion coherence processing has been found in certain developmental disorders (discussed below). Specific areas associated with form and motion coherence tasks have been identified in fMRI studies of normal adults. Distinct circuits are activated in global processing of form and motion, although each circuit involves parts of occipital, parietal and temporal lobes.

A caveat is necessary: It is over-simple to show visual development in infancy and childhood as a linear sequence; there are likely to be important feedback loops, by which the consequences of a new development can affect the way that earlier established processes work. Furthermore, a description of the sequence is only the start. There is still much debate as to why there are timing differences in functional onset and plasticity in one system as opposed to another.

Division of Childhood Visual Disorders

A major division is normally made between childhood visual disorders related to the functioning in the eye itself and disorders related to eye–brain neural connections and functioning in the visual brain. This tends to be emphasized by the division between two branches of clinicians who study childhood visual disorders – those trained in ophthalmology, optometry, orthopics and related professions (health/education professions related to the visually impaired and their treatment), and those trained in neurology (pediatricians, pediatric neurologists, health/education related professionals in neurological disorders). There are also those trained in neuropsychology and developmental cognitive neuroscience, who tend to emphasize brain rather than eye abnormalities. In infancy and childhood the distinction between visual disorders arising from eye or brain function are sometimes hard to make, as the two interact strongly in development and different aspects may be manifest at different stages.

A second categorization of visual disorders is made in terms of severity, ranging from severe, but usually rare, abnormalities including varying degrees of 'blindness', to milder deficits, particularly common in the developed world, such as strabismus and amblyopia, dyslexia related to vision and visual attentional disorders (attention deficit hyperactive disorders ADHD).

Epidemiology of Childhood Visual Deficits

Childhood is defined by UNICEF as an individual under 16 years, and blindness as a refractively corrected visual acuity of 3/60 (20/400) or below in the better eye or a central visual field of less than 10 degrees around the point of central fixation. This definition raises problems of appropriateness and reliability when applied to infants, children, and individuals with difficulties of communication and/or additional physical and mental disabilities. In such case blindness is often difficult to separate from unawareness and lack of responses, for example, abnormal eye and head movements. In young infants, the diagnosis of congenital blindness may also be confused with what has been termed delayed visual maturation.

From registration (which is likely to be an underestimate because many children with multiple impairments are not registered as blind), the prevalence of blindness in Europe is around 0.1–0.3 per 1000 and in developing countries three to four times greater, giving at least 1.5 million children worldwide. Although these children may be registered as blind, this does not necessarily mean that they have no useful vision. Many will have good enough vision for some crude navigation, provided that light levels are adequate. Additionally, from Scandinavian registers there are around 0.08 per 1000 registered visually

impaired children (with acuity less than 6/18 = 20/60) per year. A difficulty with registers of visual impairment and blindness in children is that these cannot be static measures made for all time. Because of cascading processes of visual development throughout infancy and childhood, a measured visual loss which would not constitute a serious handicap in infancy can be a source of disability in late childhood and adulthood. For example, a moderate near acuity loss would not prevent a 9-month-old infant playing and manipulating most toys appropriate for age, but might prevent reading text in school. At present there are very few measures of quality of life appropriate for the entire age range from birth to adulthood, and although adult scales can be used with some modification for older children, there are very few measures for infants and especially for children with multiple disabilities, which may include severe cerebral visual impairment. The interactions between visual loss and other physical limitations in causing disability are still poorly characterized or standardized.

In industrialized countries genetic conditions (15–50% of blindness), and conditions occurring as a result of perinatal events, are the major causes of child blindness. In Eastern Mediterranean regions, two-thirds of blindness has been attributed to genetic causes, 50% of which is autosomal-recessive disease. Genetically related parents are known to increase the risk of recessive diseases and multifactorial disorders.

Intrauterine causes of blindness include rubella, toxoplasmosis, cytomegalovirus, drugs, alcohol, or maternal metabolic disturbance (e.g., diabetes). Perinatal causes of blindness (between 25 weeks, gestation to 28 days after term birth) are retinopathy of prematurity, the results of sexually transmitted diseases, (e.g., HIV infection, and gonorrhea), and lesions of the optic nerve and higher visual pathways in the brain. In developed countries many of these are related to birth asphyxia, with approximately 50% of those with brain lesions having additional problems such as cerebral palsy. In many cases such perinatal brain damage is associated with extreme prematurity.

Acquired diseases (measles, vitamin A deficiency) are unusual causes of blindness in children in industrialized countries, but are very important in poorer developing countries. Studies in Africa suggest that 1–3% of children develop ulcerations of the cornea following measles.

The most common of the rarer childhood visual disorders is congenital cataract, with prevalence around 2.5 per 10 000, around 40% being in one eye only. A significant proportion of blinding eye diseases does not have a determined cause (from Nordic studies, 32% of blind children, with a higher proportion in developing countries).

Less severe childhood visual loss, but the most common in developed countries, is congenital or early onset strabismus and related refractive error and amblyopia.

Childhood Visual Disorders Related to Functioning in the Eye

Retinal dystrophies. A small but significant source of visual defects in childhood is the degeneration of the photoreceptors of the retina, generally as a result of an inherited photoreceptor degeneration (IPD). These are not common diseases (6–9 per 100 000 births) but are a major fraction of childhood blindness. As many as 25 000 different genes may be expressed in the retina, and an unusually high number (30–50%) are specific to the retina. Many different genes have been identified as associated with IPDs, both in human pedigrees and in mouse models, but they are believed to act by affecting a relatively small number of molecular pathways.

Among the most severe, and a relatively large proportion, of these disorders is Leber's amaurosis, which affects both rods and cones. Although it is progressive, children are already seriously affected at birth, with nystagmus and very low acuity, and can be diagnosed by the lack of the electrical response from the retina (electroretinogram, ERG).

Some receptor disorders affect only one type of receptor. Congenital achromatopsia is a complete loss of cone function, with no color vision, very poor acuity, nystagmu, and often photophobia (aversion to bright light). Conversely, congenital stationary night blindness is a failure of rod vision from birth: children have normal acuity and color vision at high light levels, but poor vision at low levels.

Retinitis pigmentosa is a wide, and genetically diverse class of IPDs, generally progressive and affecting rods and cones, although the rod system is usually affected earlier and more severely. As a result, night-blindness is the usual symptom in childhood, with the loss is most evident in peripheral vision.

Recent advances in gene therapy and stem-cell transplantation provide an optimistic future for eradicating or lessening the impact on quality of life from these visually devastating diseases.

Retinopathy of prematurity (ROP) is a result of excessive oxygen delivered to aid survival of the premature neonate in intensive care, which adversely affects the immature vascular system of the premature retina. It emerged as a cause of blindness in the late 1940s. A lowering of the incidence of ROP in the 1970s was related to better monitoring of oxygen, but with later improved neonatal care and survival of infants under 32 weeks, gestation, there has been another increase in developed countries and in countries (e.g., in Latin America) where an increase in Cesarean delivery has led to more premature births.

In the initial phase of ROP, the growth of the retinal blood vessels is delayed after premature birth; excess oxygen in this phase causes a growth factor molecule called vascular endothelial growth factor (VEGF) to be released, which in a second phase stimulates the proliferation of vessels that distort and damage the retina. Treatments that counteract VEGF are currently being developed, but current therapy is to stop retinal damage by laser treatment or cryotherapy (local freezing). These treatments reduce the incidence of blindness by approximately 25%, although the visual outcomes are often poor. It must be recognized, however, that very premature infants requiring oxygen in intensive care are also those most likely to suffer perinatal brain damage, with visual consequences that are discussed below.

Cataract is an opacity in the lens of the eye that, if large and dense, allows only diffuse light to reach the retina. The child is deprived of pattern vision until the defective lens is removed surgically and the eye is fitted with a compensatory optical correction, either an intraocular lens implant or a contact lens. The optimal age for surgery remains controversial, although the best results seem to be achieved if surgery is very early, in the first few months of life. Early correction is desirable because the complete deprivation of pattern vision, in either one or both eyes, has strong effects on the development of visual brain mechanisms at a stage when the developing connections among visual neurons are extremely plastic. The consequences of this plasticity are amblyopia, a form of vision loss discussed in later.

Optic Nerve Problems

Optic nerve hypoplasia or atrophy is a developmental defect of the optic nerve fibers of one or both eyes (bilateral). If bilateral and severe, it leads to complete blindness. Neurological defects such as quadriplegia and hemiplegia are often associated. It can be related to maternal diabetes and to fetal alcohol syndrome. Optic atrophy is rarely isolated and is often associated with rubella virus, brain malformations, or hypoxic-ischemic encephalopathy (HIE) (brain damage caused by lack of oxygen).

Glaucoma is an increase of pressure within the eye which ultimately damages the optic nerve. It is rare in infants (1 in 10 000), with very heterogeneous causes and prognosis. It is usually treated with surgery, but the majority of children remain myopic when the pressure has successfully been reduced.

Refractive errors. Vision may be degraded if the eye does not optically bring images to a sharp focus on the retina. Such refractive errors may be myopic (short- or nearsighted; the eye cannot focus distant objects), hyperopic (long- or far-sighted; excessive effort is required to focus on close objects), or astigmatic (lines at different angles cannot be sharply focused together). As well as the immediate reduction in image quality, these conditions may have longer-term effects on development that are discussed in the section on Amblyopia and Plasticity.

In a well-focused (emmetropic) eye, the curvature of the cornea and lens bring light to a focus at the distance of the retina, so refractive error is a consequence of the shape and size of the eyeball as it matures. However, these structural aspects cannot be considered independently of visual processing. In general, as the eye grows there is a trend toward emmetropia, and there is much evidence, both from experimental animal models and from clinical conditions, that this change is actively controlled. Image blur or visual deprivation can affect the course of refractive change, and so does habitual accommodation. Furthermore, childhood refractive error is correlated with aspects of cognitive and visuomotor development.

Myopia is rare in the first year of life in Caucasian populations, but commonly has an onset between early school age and adolescence, and tends to increase progressively. There are undoubtedly familial genetic factors, but these appear to interact with environmental conditions. The latter are suggested by the increase in childhood myopia, especially in Far Eastern populations. The progression of myopia is correlated with near work (e.g., reading, extended viewing of computer screens), but there are also large individual variations in this effect. There are suggestions that reading in low light levels has a particularly strong effect; this has been related to the light-dependent release of dopamine that is known to affect eye growth in animal models.

Hyperopia. The average infant eye has a modest level of hyperopia. This is revealed when the child's accommodation is relaxed with cycloplegic drops. About 5% of infants (in Caucasian populations that have been studied) have significant hyperopic refractive errors (over $+3.5D$ at age 9 months), with many of these showing marked degrees of astigmatism. This has a number of consequences. Some hyperopic infants put in very little accommodative effort and therefore have permanently blurred visual input. Hyperopia is also associated with early onset strabismus (cross-eyed squint). It is suggested that this is a result of the link between accommodation and convergence; the hyperopic child has to make a great accommodative effort to achieve a sharp image and this induces an abnormal degree of convergence of the eyes, overcoming the control processes which keep the two eyes' images in register. However, the detailed dynamics though which hyperopia leads to disruption of the sensory–motor binocular loop is still only poorly understood. Spectacles that reduce the need for accommodation (focusing in) are frequently an effective treatment for strabismus. It has also been shown, in randomized, controlled trials that prescribing a spectacle correction for infant with significant hyperopia reduced the risk of them developing strabismus and poor acuity, without adverse effects on their emmetropization.

In addition, the association with strabismus and amblyopia, significant infant hyperopia is associated with subtle small delays in development of visual attention and in visuocognitive, visuomotor, and spatial abilities (but not language abilities), first identifiable in the second year of life and persisting into the early school years. The deficit may be particularly associated with frontoparietal systems for spatial cognition and attention. Its basis is not yet known; it is as likely to have a common neurodevelopmental origin with hyperopia, as to be a consequence of any effects of hyperopia on the visual input. It offers the possibility of early identification a group of children at risk of preschool visuocognitive problems, in particular attention deficits, which may be a significant factor for educational achievement. Anisometropia is a difference in refraction between the eyes. Such differences, particularly if one eye is markedly hyperopic, are associated with the development of strabismus and, even if the eyes remain straight, can lead to amblyopia (see below).

Childhood Disorders Related to the Control of Eye Movements

The muscular systems that move the eyes are a key aspect of functional vision since they are necessary to maintain the stability of the image on the retina, to direct the high-acuity fovea to the object of interest, and to maintain coordination of the two eyes. Disorders of these systems generally reflect disorders of central neural control systems. However, since they are manifest in external examination of the eyes, they sit between the domains of ophthalmological and neurological professionals.

A number of conditions can cause oculomotor disorders in childhood.

Disorders of the cranial nerves linked to the eye muscles can lead to paralysis of one or more of these muscles (ophthalmoplegia). Congenital ophthalmoplegia is relatively common, especially Duane syndrome or retraction syndrome, in which poor development of the sixth cranial nerve which limits the ability of the eye to turn in (abduction) and causes the eyes to narrow when an outward (adduction) movement is attempted.

Congenital ptosis (drooping eyelid) is a relatively common condition. The resulting obstruction of vision may be a cause of deprivation amblyopia (see below).

Gaze palsies may arise from lesions at many different, higher brain levels and unlike peripheral palsies affect the movements of both eyes together are due to involvement of the supranuclear pathways that control the orientation of the head and eyes. They are often associated with hemiplegia as a result of cortical damage.

Ocular motor apraxia is a condition where the child's attempts to change fixation lead to very abnormal head and eye movements. The head may turn without any change of eye position, or with eye movements in the opposite direction to the head. The origin is often unknown, but it has been reported from brain scans that 30% of the cases showed delayed myelination, agenesis of the corpus callosum and cerebellar abnormalities.

Nystagmus is involuntary, rhythmical, oscillatory eye movements. It should be distinguished from the roving eye movements of totally blind children. Congenital nystagmus (which may be delayed for several months after birth) is often associated with low visual acuity, and is believed often to be a consequence of various retinal (especially macular) disorders degrade the sensory information controlling fixation. One common link is with albinism. Albinos have wide ranging disruption of the visual system, besides the problems caused by lack of pigmentation in the eye. In particular VEP and MRI studies confirm what has been found in animal models, that the uncrossed optic nerve fibers are reduced, causing the brain mapping of the two eyes' fields to be highly anomalous representation.

Strabismus. In strabismus (often called squint in the UK) the movements of the two eyes are not properly co-ordinated, so that they look in different directions rather than fixating at the same time on a single point. Paralytic strabismus comes under the oculomotor palsies described above. In the much more common disorders of concomitant strabismus, the eyes move together but with one eye either deviating inwards (convergent strabismus or esotropia, cross eyes) or outwards (divergent strabismus or exotropia). The amount of deviation may vary with vertical gaze; for instance in a V-pattern esotropia increases as the child looks down. Such patterns are attributed to a relative imbalance in the inferior and superior oblique muscles of the eyes – a motor explanation of strabismus. In contrast, maintaining binocular fixation requires cortical binocularity – the integration of information from the two eyes in the visual cortex. Weakness or absence of this mechanism may lead to strabismus, for example, in albino children where the misrouting of optic nerve fibers described above means that fibers from the two eyes do not reach the same cerebral hemisphere. However, in many cases of strabismus, stereo vision develops before the onset of strabismus, so a deficit of sensory binocularity does not appear to be the primary cause. Rather, the sensory–motor interaction is two-way; misalignment of the eyes means that signals from corresponding points of the two images do not come together in the cortex, so that the correlated signals needed to maintain connections from the two eyes to the same cortical cell are absent, and these binocular connections break down. The readiness with which this developmental feedback loop can be broken may explain why binocularity is vulnerable in infancy, and strabismus very frequent, in all kinds of neurodevelopmental disorders (Down syndrome, prematurity, perinatal brain insult, etc.).

The role of accommodation in disrupting normal convergence of the eyes, in children with hyperopic refractive errors, has been discussed above. However, convergent squint can occur without hyperopia. The strength of the link between accommodation and convergence varies greatly between individuals and it may be that in some cases even normal levels of accommodation are enough to break the maintenance of binocular fixation. As indicated above, some cases of strabismus can be controlled by refractive correction. However, frequently, surgical adjustment of the eye muscles is required. To restore secure alignment of the eyes, these treatments have to be accompanied by orthoptic exercises to encourage the active control of vergence. In addition, following surgery, the associated amblyopia (see below) will also require treatment.

Amblyopia. Amblyopia is a reduction of visual acuity, usually in one eye, that cannot be improved with refractive correction and for which there is not a detected organic cause in the eye. It is a very common condition affecting 2–4% of the population in developed countries. It is believed to be a developmental disorder of neural connectivity in the visual cortex; an eye whose image is degraded in some way has diminished input to cortical processing, as a result of plasticity of synaptic mechanisms in competition with the other eye.

There are three major causes of amblyopia. In deprivation amblyopia, one eye has pattern vision reduced or abolished, for example, by a dense cataract or a ptosis. Poor acuity remains even after the obstruction of vision is removed. Animal models of this condition, in which cortical responses are measured following occlusion of one eye, have led to the explanation of amblyopia in terms of activity-dependent competitive interactions between cortical synapses. Such experiments have also established the existence of a critical period following birth, in which these connections are much more readily modified than later in life. This concept leads to the importance, which has been clinically supported, of correcting the amblyogenic condition at the earliest practical age.

Anisometropic amblyopia results from one eye having a defocused image due to a difference in refraction from the other eye. It can be regarded as a partial form of deprivation amblyopia, where the relative deprivation is for fine detail rather than all pattern vision. In clinical practice care is needed not to confuse genuine amblyopia with uncorrected refractive error.

Strabismic amblyopia is a reduction of acuity in the deviating eye in strabismus. It is usually seen when one eye is predominantly used for fixation, most typically in convergent strabismus. The nature of the deprivation is less well understood than in deprivation or anisometropic amblyopia, and the cortical mechanism may be different. However, in many cases both strabismus and anisometropia are present, and the contributions of the two cannot be easily separated.

Although amblyopia is usually assessed in terms of visual acuity, the actual visual deficit is more complex. First, there is a reduction of contrast sensitivity for low- and medium-spatial frequencies. Second, there is often a severe effect on visual information about the position of image features, reflected in a greatly increased crowding effect (interference between acuity targets), a loss of vernier acuity, and sometimes reports that images appear scrambled. Statistical factor analysis shows that these different effects are to some degree independent. Amblyopes who also have a loss of binocularity – typically strabismic amblyopes – have a disproportionate crowding effect and vernier acuity loss relative to their contrast sensitivity loss. These results suggest that multiple mechanisms are at work.

The usual treatment for amblyopia is partial or continuous patching of the 'good' eye, once the refractive error, strabismus, or source of deprivation has been corrected. However, this needs careful monitoring: (1) To avoid the risk that an artificial deprivation amblyopia is induced in the patched eye and (2) because following strabismus surgery cortical binocularity is fragile, and to establish and maintain it requires correlated binocular input, that is, both eyes open. The optimal compromise between these therapeutic aims depends on (1) practical considerations of compliance with patching treatment in children; (2) the benefits of treatment and how long they last when patching is stopped; and (3) the relative disability and reduction in quality of life resulting from loss of binocularity or loss of acuity and contrast sensitivity. There are few systematic data on these, and the balance will of course depend on age and the presence of any accompanying developmental conditions. However, from data from treatment trials, it appears that 2 h per day of patching can achieve significant improvements of acuity.

The importance of treating amblyopia rests in part on the long-term risk of losing vision in the 'good' eye, leading to severe visual disability. This lifetime risk has been estimated at 1.2%. The risk of injuring the good eye of an amblyope is three times that in a nonamblyopic individual.

Analysis of visual abilities in children who were treated for congenital cataract suggests that there are important aspects of plasticity in central visual processing that are not captured by measures of binocularity and acuity. Children with a few months of visual deprivation before a cataract removal in the first year, when tested at age 6–14 years, show persisting impairment in face recognition, and in tasks requiring integration of local elements in global form and motion perception. These deficits are much greater than would be expected from any remaining acuity loss. They occur even though at the age vision was restored, these aspects of high-level visual processing were quite immature. These data indicate that early visual experience is required to set up the infrastructure for later development involving both the dorsal ('where') and ventral ('what') streams.

Vision Screening

Screening refers to testing people who are asymptomatic in order to classify their likelihood of having a particular disease. It aims to identify as many as possible of those affected by the target condition as possible, while minimizing the number who are incorrectly suspected of having the disease. The criteria for worthwhile screening are that: (1) a large part of the at-risk population can be screened, (2) the condition screened for has a high prevalence, (3) it is significantly disabling, and (4) it has an effective treatment which is acceptable.

It is common to screen newborns in the neonatal ward by examination with an ophthalmoscope, to detect structural disorders in the eye and serious conditions (e.g., cataract, ROP, and retinal tumours). General surveillance methods in primary healthcare can often detect abnormalities with sufficient signs and symptoms, for example, strabismus and nystagmus. Given the importance of early correction of conditions leading to amblyopia, there have been a number of programs at later ages aiming to detect the conditions, in particular the refractive errors, which lead to amblyopia, but it is difficult to meet the screening criteria stated above. In screening children for poor acuity (the method in many preschool programs), it is often hard to achieve high attendance, and by the time acuity can be measured rapidly and reliably, it is relatively late for successful amblyopia treatment.

The Cambridge Infant Screening programs used photorefraction or videorefraction to detect potentially amblyogenic levels of hyperopia and anisometropia (as well as congenital strabismus) at 8–9 months of age, and achieved high rates of attendance (75–80% of the total targeted population). Photo- and videorefractive techniques offer the possibility of rapid, safe, reliable, inexpensive screening that is acceptable to parents and infants and children of all ages. As initial results with these measures have shown relatively successful visual outcomes, extensions of such programs across different populations (including clinical populations with multiple disorders) should lead to the prevention, reduction in number, and early effective treatment of the common visual problems of strabismus, refractive error, and amblyopia in the future. However, such programs depend on then successfully and accurately prescribing spectacle corrections, and regular frequent follow-up and counseling, which may be hard to achieve for infants and very young children in regular practice.

Childhood Disorders Related to Functioning in the Brain

Cerebral visual impairment (CVI). CVI usually refers to a severe deficit of visual behavior as a result of brain damage, usually perinatal, typically identified in infancy by poor fixation and following, and by the absence of reaching for objects in children with the motor capability to do so. It is the most common cause of permanent visual impairment in children in developed countries. Strabismus is common; nystagmus less so. There may be abnormal responses to light (either gazing at lights or photophobia). Eye examination may show anomaly of the optic nerves, but this is not severe enough to be the cause of the visual impairment exhibited.

The term cortical blindness has sometimes been used. However, cerebral visual impairment is preferred, since the damage is not necessarily cortical but may involve various parts of the central visual pathways, including white matter, and may not be anatomically well localized, e.g., when associated with epilepsy or metabolic disorders. Common causes include HIE in the term-born infant; periventricular leukomalacia (PVL) in the preterm infant; accidental or nonaccidental traumatic brain injury; neonatal hypoglycemia; infections (e.g., viral meningitis); and hydrocephalus shunt failure.

CVI is unlikely to be an isolated impairment; the underlying neurological damage will commonly lead to cerebral palsy, developmental delay, and/or other sensory impairments. It is important to discover the child's visual capabilities but these should be considered as part of an overall pattern of capability and disability for the individual child.

The term delayed visual maturation can be a source of confusion. Visual inattention in the first months of life is the presenting symptom of CVI, a condition which may show some long-term improvement but generally leaves an enduring deficit. There is, however, a distinct group of children who present with isolated visual inattentiveness in the first months and without known neurological damage. In such cases, it is common to see recovery with normal visual attentiveness by 6 months or soon after. This pattern suggests a delay in the onset of development of cortical visual mechanisms, but the reasons for such a delay are not understood.

Cerebral visual impairment should not be considered an all-or-none phenomenon. The brain basis of visual processing is complex, and perinatal brain injury can lead to a range of deficits from profound loss to more subtle impairments of specific function.

One pervasive deficit found across many clinical populations with suspected cerebral damage is an inability to change focus (accommodate) on targets at different distances, in the absence of a marked myopic or hyperopic refractive error. It seems likely that networks involving accommodative mechanisms in conjunction with cortical systems have never developed normally in infancy. Whether this is due to damage to accommodative systems *per se* or whether it is due to more central damage to cortical attentional systems, cannot be determined from these measurements alone.

Specific Cerebral Impairments of Spatial Vision: Deficits Related to Ventral Stream Function

Visual agnosia refers to a multitude of different disorders, in which recognition of objects and people is impaired. Some patients cannot recognize faces but can still recognize other objects, while others retain only face recognition. Some see only one object at a time; others can see multiple objects but recognize only one at a time. Some do not consciously perceive the orientation of an object but nevertheless reach for it with a well-oriented grasp; others do not consciously recognize a face as familiar but nevertheless respond to it. All of these conditions, known to occur in adults, have also been described for individual pediatric cases. In general lesions to occipital–temporal lobe areas have been suggested as underpinning these disorders. However, with new knowledge concerning the ventral and dorsal streams, some agnosias can be related to specific areas in these networks (see below). In a number of cases an association between agnosia and certain characteristics of autism spectrum disorder have been noted. This association (comorbidity) may relate to underlying, more pervasive attentional deficits.

Developmental prosopagnosia (DP) is an impairment in identifying faces which is present from early in life, accompanied by apparently intact visual function. DP, as strictly defined, refers to the impairment in the absence of any known lesion or neurological condition (such as autism spectrum disorder). Cases of DP are relatively rare in the literature and findings have been contradictory and inconsistent, with variability across individuals on various face processing tasks. Configural processing of faces can been divided into (1) first order – detecting that the configuration is a face because of the basic arrangements of features; (2) holistic processing – integrating features into a whole and thus rendering individual features less accessible; and (3) encoding the spacing among features. Cases of DP appear to vary in the level of deficit in these different aspects of configural processing.

Deficits Related to Dorsal Stream(s) Function

One particular clinical group, where all individuals show a common phenotype of massive visual spatial deficits across many different areas and types of task combined with relatively good (but not normal development of speech and language) is that of Williams syndrome (WS), a rare genetic disorder characterized by a deletion of around 30 genes on one arm of chromosome 7. WS infants and children generally reach all visuomotor milestones later than typically developing children, they are often delayed in learning to walk and in the development of fine motor skills, and show marked deficits on all standardized test of visuomotor and visuocognitive function. Problems that persist into later life include block construction copying and all related spatial tasks and games, uncertainty when negotiating stairs or uneven surfaces, and difficulty with the use of everyday tools and implements. This neuropsychological profile is consistent with the possibility that ventral stream processes at all levels is relatively unimpaired (but not necessarily normal) but dorsal stream function for visual control of all actions and the planning of these actions is abnormal. In tasks involving motor planning, WS individuals show great difficulties. The post-box (mailbox) task is based on a test which showed a striking dissociation in the Goodale *et al.* study of a ventral-stream impaired adult patient, who could accurately post a card (letter) through an oriented slot in the mailbox (dorsal control of action) but failed on perceptual matching of the slot orientation (ventral processing for perception and recognition). Children with WS showed the opposite deficit, with much greater inaccuracy in posting the card than in matching its orientation to that of the slot, compared with normally developing children. WS children are also poorer than normal children in matching the size of objects, in matching hand opening aperture in reaching and grasping objects of different sizes, and in 'end-state planning' when grasping an object so that it can be easily manipulated with the hand ending the action in a comfortable position. End-state planning is likely to involve the integration of ventral stream information in recognizing the object and dorsal stream information, with prefrontal areas involved in inhibiting inappropriate actions and coordinating the elements of action sequences. WS individuals also show many problems with executive function tests related to frontal lobe processing, and problems of spatial memory for location which is likely to involve additional frontal, hippocampal, and parahippocampal processing.

Studies comparing dorsal stream versus ventral stream development using motion versus form coherence thresholds (see above) have also found relative deficits in global motion processing in many individuals (even high-functioning adults) with WS. This apparent dorsal stream deficit has also been found in a subset of dyslexics, autistic children, children with hemiplegia and fragile X syndrome. This widespread pattern has been called dorsal stream vulnerability. It is important to make such a claim only when direct comparisons of dorsal and ventral stream function have been made using comparable tasks

with the same children. The basic cause of this difference in plasticity between dorsal stream and ventral stream modules for global coherence is not yet well understood. It may have its origin in very low-level timing mechanisms in subcortical or early cortical areas, it may depend on a misbalance between the number of functional magnocellular and parvocellular cells and their integration, or it may reflect faulty integration of information from processing in many different occipital, parietal and frontal areas across both dorsal and ventral streams. Support for this relative deficit in dorsal stream networks in WS comes from recent studies using structural and fMRI. It seems that the transmission of spatial information to frontal systems within the dorsal stream is specifically disrupted in WS.

Children born very prematurely, who show a range of cognitive problems, have especially marked deficits in the visuospatial and visuomotor domains. On visual location memory tasks there are subgroups with differential patterns of impairment. For example, impairments to spatial updating for changes of viewpoint, produced when a child sees a toy hidden in one location and then walks to a point with a different viewpoint, may be related to poor detection of coherent motion, related to visual processing of optic flow, while performance on the perspective problem (changes of viewpoint produced by movement of the stimulus array) has been found to be correlated with frontal tests of inhibition and response selection, suggesting that frontal control processes are also involved in this task. Adults with WS showed only marginal ability to use local landmarks to solve the perspective problem, solved by typical children at 5 years. Young WS children tended to use an egocentric frame of reference in these tests. Success on all these spatial tasks must involve integration between visual processing in occipital, parahippocampal, parietal, and prefrontal areas and a failure at one stage of development may be different in its underpinnings from a failure at a different stage of development.

In cases of early focal cortical injury in the right hemisphere there are deficits in organizing spatial elements coherently into whole forms, while left hemisphere injury is associated with poor encoding of detail in complex forms. WS individuals have great difficulty copying the overall shape of relatively simple block constructed forms which is similar to deficits in children with right focal lesions. However, the deficit may be more marked and persistent in the case of WS. This suggests that in some developmental anomalies there may be a failure or difference in the level of hemisphere specialization and consequent visual processing.

Deficits in spatial attention in childhood: In conditions where two targets are competing for attention, infants with early focal lesions, HIE, and a subset of infants born very prematurely with white matter changes identified on structural MRI, have problems disengaging attention from the fixated target to a newly appearing target in the periphery (this is similar to the disengagement problem to one side of space for children who have undergone hemispherectomy). Early damage involving parietal and frontal areas is likely to underpin these deficits, although the exact location of the damage may vary considerably across individuals. These deficits of attention, identified early in the first few months of life with this fixation-shift paradigm, have been shown to correlate with later deficits on many visuocognitive and attentional tasks.

In school-age children there are many studies of spatial attention and spatial deficits related to visual attention. Three different components of attention have been identified from adult studies and patient populations, each with rather different neural underpinnings. The first component is linked to selective visual attention in visual search tasks. The second component is sustained attention which can be measured in vigilance tasks, and the third component involves inhibiting a prepotent response to switch task and make a new association, an aspect of executive control. Many studies have documented age-related improvements in these various components of attention, with some indication that developmental trajectories differ for different attention components. A small number of tasks have been developed to examine executive function in visuomotor tasks in preschool children demonstrating improvement between the age of 3 and 6 years. These tasks involve inhibition of a prepotent visuomotor response, an example being the test of counterpointing. The child first has to point as rapidly as possible to a visual target which appears to either the left or right of a fixation spot and reaction time is measured. The rule is then changed and the child is asked to point as rapidly as possible to the opposite side to where the target appears. This inhibitory control is achieved on average by 4 years of age in typically developing children, but is considerably delayed in children with WS and in a large subgroup of children born very prematurely who have suffered early brain damage. These tasks are likely to have some frontal lobe neural circuitry in common with that required for overcoming the 'A not B error' in Piagetian tasks of object permanence, where infants under 1 year of age fail to search for a toy if it is hidden in front of them in a new spatial location from where it has previously been hidden on a number of occasions. This perseverative failure persists in older infants and children with generalized brain damage (HIE), WS individuals, and in some autistic children.

Conclusions

The current level of understanding in both diagnosis and treatment for pediatric visual problems varies considerably both in identification of anatomical differences and differences of processing and function. Progress in terms of underlying genetics is rapid, but this alone is only one side of the starting point for understanding the much more difficult problem: how does the expression and interaction of genes become altered by subtle but pervasive environmental factors, from conception to adult maturity? In some cases we may serendipitously find the cure before we understand the underlying processes. Progress will only be made in improving quality of life for children with visual problems if we pool our knowledge and understanding across areas in interdisciplinary research and clinical practice.

Acknowledgments

The authors would like to thank the Medical Research Council for research funding and University College London, the University of Cambridge, and the University of Oxford for their support.

See also: Developmental Disabilities: Cognitive; Neurological Development.

Suggested Readings

Aicardi J (ed.) (1998) Disorders of the ocular motor and visual systems, In: *Disorders of the Nervous System in Childhood,* ch. 18. London: MacKeith Press.
Atkinson J (2007) *The Developing Visual Brain.* Oxford: Oxford University Press.
Atkinson J and Nardini M (2007) Visual spatial development. In: Reed J and Rogers JW (eds.) *Child Neuropsychology.* Oxford: Blackwell.
Braddick O, Atkinson J, and Wattam-Bell J (2003) Normal and anomalous development of visual motion processing: Motion coherence and 'dorsal stream vulnerability'. *Neuropsychologia* 41(13): 1769–1784.
Daw NW (1995) *Visual Development.* New York: Plenum Press.
Maurer D, Lewis TL, and Mondloch CJ (2005) Missing sights: Consequences for visual cognitive development. *Trends in Cognitive Science* 9: 144–151.
McKee SP, Levi DM, and Movshon JA (2003) The pattern of visual deficits in amblyopia. *Journal of Vision* 3: 380–405.
Moore AT (2000) *Paediatric Ophthalmology (Fundamentals in Clinical Ophthalmology).* London: BMJ Books.
Simons K (ed.) *Early Visual Development: Normal and Abnormal.* New York: Oxford University Press.
Stiles J (2001) Spatial cognitive development. In: Nelson CA and Luciana M (eds.) *Handbook of Developmental Cognitive Neuroscience* Ch. 27. Cambridge, MA: MIT Press.

SUBJECT INDEX

This index is in letter-by-letter order, whereby hyphens and spaces within index headings are ignored in the alphabetization, and it is arranged in set-out style with a maximum of three levels of heading. Major discussion of a subject is indicated by a bold page range.

A

ABCDEFV 379, 382
Abdominal reflex 318, 318*f*
  assessment 325
Academic achievement/performance
  leukemia survivors 124
  premature infants 126
  See also Education; Schools/schooling
Accommodation
  definition 379
Achilles (ankle jerk) reflex 318–319
  clinical significance 324
Achondroplasia 83, 84*f*
Acid reflux, definition 34
Acoustic blink reflex 319
Acoustics
  crying *See* Crying
  observer based psychoacoustics (OBP) 45
Acquired immunodeficiency syndrome *See* AIDS
Action potential(s) 280
  auditory system 42
Active case ascertainment, definition 181
Activities, ICF model of health and
    well-being 120–121
Acuity *See* Visual acuity
Acuity scales, definition 379
Acupuncture, nocturnal enuresis 67
Acute lymphoblastic leukemia (ALL)
  definition 118
  incidence 123
  treatment approaches 123
Acute stress disorder (parental) 296
Adaptation/adaptive behavior
  accommodation 379
  assessment 228
  congenital heart disease and 126
  definition 226, 228
  intellectual disability 228
Adaptive immune system
  cellular immunity 222, 222*f*
  components 218*t*, 219
    B lymphocytes 219
    immunoglobulins 220, 220*f*
    T lymphocytes 222, 222*f*
  disorders
    autoimmunity *See* Autoimmunity/autoimmune
      disorders
    immunodeficiency
      cell-mediated immunity and 225
      humoral immunity and 224
  humoral immunity 219, 224
  memory 220
  passive immunity 220
Adaptive response
  sensory processing 330
    definition 329
  See also Sensory processing
Addison's disease 155
ADHD *See* Attention deficit hyperactivity disorder
    (ADHD)
Adherence
  definition 14
  HIV treatment 21
Adipocyte, definition 285
Adiponectin, obesity 288
Adiposity rebound
  definition 285
  obesity in later life 287
Adjustment
  child
    risk of maladjustment, maternal depression 307
  See also Adaptation/adaptive behavior

Adolescence
  cancer survivors/patients 125
  maternal postnatal depression effects 310
Adrenal glands 148
  hormones 149–150
Adrenal insufficiency 155
  Addison's disease 155
Adrenergic receptors
  alpha adrenergic 2A receptor gene,
    ADHD and 9
  beta-adrenergic receptors
    beta agonists, asthma 40
    beta-blocker, definition 34
Adrenocorticotropic hormone (ACTH)
  infant rumination syndrome 164–165
Adverse food reactions 29
Affect
  definition 103
  negative 104
  See also Mood
Affective disorders *See* Mood disorders
Afferent(s)
  reflex arc 315
Aggression
  genetic studies 204
    monoamine oxidase A (MAO-A) 204
Agonist muscle, definition 315
Aicardi syndrome, as X-linked dominant
    condition 211
AIDS **14–23**, 225
  caregivers 21
  changing context 15
  comorbid physical conditions 17
  epidemiology 15
  family functioning 21
  future directions 22
  medical aspects 17
  orphans due to 15, 15*f*
  psychological aspects 18
    coping 20
    distress 19
    quality of life 20
  psychosocial intervention 22, 22*f*
  transmission to infant 16
    during birth 16
    breastfeeding 16
    prevention 16
    in utero 16
  treatment 18
  treatment, percentage of children 18*f*
  See also HIV infection
Air pollution
  asthma 38
Airway
  definition 33
  hyperresponsiveness
    asthma 27, 35–36
    definition 33
Albinos, visual disruptions 388
Albright's hereditary osteodystrophy,
    obesity 287–288
Albuterol, definition 34
Alcohol
  prenatal exposure
    disorders caused by *See* Fetal alcohol spectrum
      disorders (FASDs)
    risk recognition 183
  teratogenic effects 184, 374
Alcohol-related birth defects (ARBD) 181–183
Alcohol-related neurodevelopmental disorder
    (ARND) 181–183
  diagnostic criteria 182*t*
Alimentary reflexes 321

Allele(s)
  definition 1, 209
  variations *See* Polymorphism
Allergens
  definition 23, 34
  environmental control 32
Allergic response 24, 24*t*
Allergic rhinitis 25, 26*f*
  classification 26
  examination 26
  risk factors 26
  symptoms 25
  treatment 26, 32
Allergy/allergic disease **23–33**
  allergy definition 34
  diagnostic tests 31
  immunoglobulin E and *See* Immunoglobulin E (IgE)
  management 32
    education 33
    immunotherapy 32
    pharmacological therapy 32
  natural history 37
Alogia, definition 293
Alström syndrome, obesity 287–288
Amblyopia 388
  definition 379
American Association of Mental Retardation (AAMR)
    227, 251
American Heart Association (AHA), weight
    guidelines 291*t*
American Lung Association (ALA), asthma 35
'American paradox,' 375
Amniocentesis
  Down syndrome 85
Amygdala
  shyness, role in 349
  size, autism spectrum disorder 55
Anaclitic depression 103, 104–105
Anal reflex 318
Analysis of variance (ANOVA) interaction model,
    teratology 368
Anaphylaxis 30
  risk factors 30
  symptoms 30
  treatment 30
Androgen insensitivity syndromes 204
Androgens 150
  autism 206
  insensitivity 204
  normal growth and 152
Anemia
  sickle-cell, genetic screening 214–215
Anencephaly 275
Aneuploidy
  Down syndrome *See* Down syndrome
  screening 85
Angelman syndrome
  behavioral phenotypes 256
Angioedema 31
Anhedonia
  childhood depression 103, 106–107, 109
  definition 293
Animal dander
  allergic response 25
  control of 32
Anisometropic amblyopia 388
Anistometropia 387
  definition 379
Ankle jerk (Achilles) reflex 318–319
  clinical significance 324
Anorexia, infantile *See* Infant anorexia syndrome
Anterior, definition 77
Anterior pituitary 148

Printed and bound by CPI Group (UK) Ltd, Croydon, CR0 4YY

08/06/2025

01896878-0001